Introduction to Nutrition, Exercise, and Health

FRANK I. KATCH

Professor
Department of Exercise Science
University of Massachusetts
Amherst, Massachusetts

WILLIAM D. McARDLE

Professor
Queens College
Department of Health and Physical Education
City University of New York
Flushing, New York

Introduction to Nutrition, Exercise, and Health

FOURTH EDITION

LEA & FEBIGER, Philadelphia/London

1993

Executive Editor: J. Matthew Harris
Project Editor: Frances M. Klass
Production Manager: Thomas Colaiezzi

Lea & Febiger
Box 3024
200 Chester Field Parkway
Malvern, PA 19355–9725
(215) 251-2230

Drs. Katch and McArdle are actively engaged in experimental research in the exercise sciences. Having published over 220 articles in national and international scientific journals, and presented their research at over 300 scientific meetings and conferences, they are also the authors or co-authors of 7 books. The recipients of numerous research grants from government and private industry, both doctors serve as reviewers and associate editors of various professional journals. Professors Katch and McArdle are elected Fellows of the Research Council of the American Association of Health, Physical Education, Recreation, and Dance, and the American College of Sports Medicine. They serve on the Scientific Advisory Boards for numerous companies in the health and fitness field. They also contribute articles to and are consultants for popular magazines such as Vogue, Harper's Bazaar, Mademoiselle, Self, Shape, Muscle and Fitness, Weight Watchers, Woman's Day, and Time-Life Books.

Library of Congress Cataloging-in-Publication Data
Katch, Frank I.
Introduction to nutrition, exercise, and health / Frank I. Katch, William D. McArdle. — 4th ed.
p. cm.
Rev. ed. of: Nutrition, weight control, and exercise. 1988.
Includes bibliographical references and index.
ISBN 0–8121–1555–4
1. Nutrition. 2. Reducing. 3. Exercise—Physiological aspects.
4. Food—Caloric content. I. McArdle, William D. II. Katch, Frank I.
Nutrition, weight control, and exercise. III. Title.
[DNLM: 1. Exercise. 2. Nutrition. 3. Obesity—prevention & control. QT 255 K186n]
RA784.K32 1992
613.7—dc20
DNLM/DLC
for Library of Congress 92–10386
CIP

Print No. 4 3 2 1

With Love and Affection
To Our Families

PREFACE

The three previous editions of *Nutrition, Weight Control, and Exercise* covered a 15-year period between 1977 and 1992. Our primary objective in these editions was to bridge the gap between many introductory topics usually covered in nutrition courses and those courses that emphasized topics related to exercise and physical fitness. Our target audience was undergraduate majors enrolled in physical education and exercise science elective courses such as sports nutrition, human performance, and nutrition, as well as in diverse courses integrating introductory material on physical activity, diet, and weight control. While this approach seemed appropriate to these relatively focused areas, we always believed that basic information about nutrition and exercise should be part of many different curricula, not just a few.

The explosion of new information in the last five years about such topics as the interrelated and protective role of both nutrition and physical activity in many disease processes, including coronary heart disease, cancer, osteoporosis, and obesity, has refocused our attention on course content. To this end, we have broadened our original textbook, starting with a new title, *Introduction to Nutrition, Exercise, and Health.* The term "health" in the title is added because our coverage in the area is more robust, and the relationship between exercise and nutrition and health is more direct. Examples include sections on exercise, nutrition, and osteoporosis, basic nutrition and cancer, physical activity and coronary heart disease prevention, primary and secondary risk factors and their relation to both diet and exercise, physical activity and pregnancy outcome, and the clear interrelationships among nutrition, weight control, and exercise.

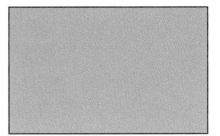

For the fourth edition, the pages are designed in a two-column format; this was done to present current and relevant text and graphics close to the chapter's main text. There are also two new introductory chapters to make it easier for non-science majors to integrate the basics of biology and chemistry, as well as the physiology of digestion and absorption, with the nutrition, exercise, and health content of the remaining 18 chapters. We believe these two chapters are essential to the expanded scope of the fourth edition. While they can serve as the starting point for most courses, this is not a requirement. The text content is of sufficient breadth to allow the instructor to select specific chapter groupings to meet a course's goals and requirements. There are also new chapters on food advertising, food packaging, and food labeling, and separate chapters devoted to carbohydrates, lipids, proteins, vitamins, minerals, and water. The 12 remaining chapters have been revised significantly to include the most recent scientific literature.

Other changes in the fourth edition include:

- Color graphics. There are a total of 245 new illustrations.

- New Appendices with updated information.
  Appendix A is an expanded version of our previous caloric expenditure tables for various physical activities. It now includes the most popular recreational and household activities for both men and women.
  Appendix B presents the nutritive value of common foods, including the grouping of foods into nine major categories (breads, cakes, cookies, candy bars, and desserts; cereals; cheese; fish; fruits; meats and eggs; milk and dairy products; vegetables) expressed in one-ounce portions. Thus, all foods are now comparable for the important nutrients on a per ounce basis, including a new food category that consists of soups, sandwiches, and dressings, oils, and condiments. We present new caloric information on alcoholic and nonalcoholic beverages, including the latest nutrition facts for many popular fast-food restaurants such as McDonald's, Burger King, and Taco Bell, from our last edition.
  Appendix E lists dependable scientific journals and popular newsletters in the nutrition and exercise science areas. This information should be helpful to the student who desires to obtain primary source materials, as well as to augment his or her professional library.
  Appendix F lists reliable sources of information about nutrition, exercise, and health. After compiling a list of possible sources, we wrote to each and asked for consumer information materials. Our list is not inclusive, but those federal agencies and companies that responded to our request and provided enough information so we could evaluate the content of their offerings are mentioned.
  Appendix G includes relevant conversions to metric and SI units.

- Up-to-date references for each chapter.

- *Student Study Guide and Workbook.* This is a resource companion to the textbook. Its purpose is to facilitate student understanding of text content by focusing on key terms and concepts, and on specific questions within each chapter. Also included are sample test questions (Fill-In, True-False, and Multiple Choice), and as far as we know, the first crossword puzzles dealing with nutrition, exercise, and health. Section II includes six self-assessment tests. These tests are designed to provide a realistic appraisal of your status on important measures of nutrition, health, and fitness. Along with the answers to the questions and crossword puzzles, Section III also contains helpful hints for studying and preparing for exams. In two years of testing with the *Student Study Guide and Workbook,* there was an overall 87% student approval rating. Students improved their course grade significantly by using the workbook, often by a full letter grade or more. It is our firm conviction that integrating textbook material with assignments in the *Student Study Guide and Workbook* will augment the learning process.

- In the textbook, key words and concepts are designated with **bold type**. These same key words and concepts are included in the *Student Study Guide and Workbook* in the order in which they appear in the textbook.

As in the three previous editions, no attempt is made to be all inclusive or to cover the numerous related topics often attempted in some introductory texts. We believe the content is appropriate for introductory level courses in nutrition, especially those that emphasize exercise and health, obesity, weight control, and the evaluation of body composition. These areas are not covered in sufficient depth in introductory nutrition textbooks. The content is also appropriate for some classroom courses dealing with physical fitness and wellness at the university level, and for the formal professional preparation of individuals who specialize in exercise science, nutrition, health education, and some medically related disciplines in the health science fields such as nursing, physical therapy, and chiropractic.

The book is divided into three main parts with chapter subdivisions. Part I is organized into 13 chapters. The introductory chapter is a review of biology and chemistry basics related to nutrition and exercise. The focus is on definitions of common terms and major concepts that are important in studying the interactions among nutrition, exercise, and health. The subsequent chapters take a closer look at the five nutrients and attempt to answer the following questions: What are they? Where do they come from? What are their functions? In what foods are they found? How are they digested and absorbed? Chapter 9 discusses per capita food consumption patterns, food advertising, food packaging, and food labeling. The concept of optimal nutrition is explored in Chapter 10, and practical recommendations and guidelines are provided for the active man and woman. Chapter 11 emphasizes the importance of the food nutrients in sustaining physiologic function during moderate and more strenuous physical activity, while Chapter 12 focuses on the role of the ventilatory and circulatory systems in exercise. In Chapter 13, we discuss the energy value of foods, and how energy is extracted from food to power various forms of physical activity.

Part II deals with topics relevant to body composition, obesity, and weight control. Chapter 14 discusses the underlying rationale for the evaluation of body composition and estimation of body fat and lean body weight. In Chapter 15, we define the term "overweight" in terms of the acceptable limits of body fat for a particular age range for men and women. We discuss the interrelated factors often associated with obesity, as well as the efficacy of diet and exercise as a treatment for the overfat condition. Chapter 16 deals with weight control. We discuss the questions of weight loss and weight gain within the framework of the "energy balance equation." In addition, a strategy is presented for quantifying food intake, and incorporating exercise and caloric restriction to achieve a desired rate of weight loss. Chapter 17 is concerned with the application of the principles of behavior modification, with emphasis on weight reduction by means of dietary modification and increased energy expenditure through moderate physical activity.

Part III considers training for muscular strength and conditioning for anaerobic and aerobic power, as well as aging, exercise, and cardiovascular health.

The graphics in the textbook were rendered by Bobby Starnes of Electragraphics, Inc., Blountville, Tennessee, simply the best electronic artist we know. To those who have ever tried to master the intricacies of modern computer drawing tools, or are thinking of trying, we hope you are as fortunate in your search for artistic help as we were when we hooked up with Bobby Starnes. His creative energy, when merged with Apple's high-speed Macintosh computer and Aldus Freehand 3.01, was pure magic. We hope that the quality of the artwork has enhanced the educational relevance of the textbook. Finally, we are grateful to the technical staff at Lea & Febiger for providing expert assistance in all phases of production. We are particularly thankful to Tom Colaiezzi and his professional and dedicated staff for their technical excellence; to John Spahr, Jr. and Richard Perry for believing in us and giving us the freedom and resources to pursue our ideas; and to our new editor, Matt Harris, for his encouragement and assistance. We also would like to thank our many former and current students who were helpful in so many ways in providing constructive ideas that have been incorporated into the fourth edition. We are grateful to our friend Bill Pearl for allowing us to use original photographs.

To the new generation of students, we hope you enjoy the textbook. If you have suggestions or comments, we would love to hear from you.

Amherst, Massachusetts — *Frank I. Katch*
Sound Beach, New York — *William D. McArdle*

CONTENTS

NUTRITION AND ENERGY FOR BIOLOGIC WORK

I

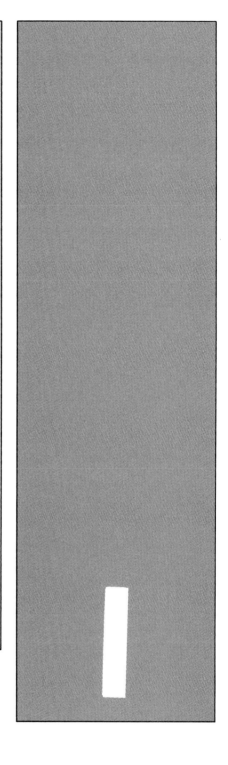

The nutrients consumed in the daily diet provide the energy necessary to maintain bodily functions both at rest and during various forms of physical activity. Although the raw fuel for biologic work takes the form of carbohydrates, lipids, and proteins, the efficient extraction and utilization of energy from these foods requires a delicate blending of other nutrients in the finely regulated watery medium of the cell. The different vitamins and minerals play important and highly specific roles in activating and facilitating energy transfer and tissue synthesis throughout the body. Fortunately, the minute, yet crucial quantities of these substances are readily obtained in the foods consumed in well-balanced meals. With proper food selection and preparation, the need to consume vitamin or mineral supplements is both physiologically and economically wasteful.

Six categories of nutrients compose the foods we eat; these are the three main groups of macronutrients—carbohydrates, lipids, and proteins—and the small quantity of micronutrients, the vitamins and minerals. Water is also included with this group because of its importance in the regulation of diverse bodily functions. The nutrients consumed in the diet are the basic substances used for many vital processes that can be broadly classified as follows:

- Maintenance and repair of body tissues
- Regulation of the thousands of complex chemical reactions that occur in cells
- Provision of energy for biologic work
- Conduction of nerve impulses
- Secretion by glands
- Synthesis of the various compounds that become part of the body's structures
- Growth
- Reproduction

The sum of these processes in which the energy and nutrients from foods are made available to and utilized by the body is referred to as *metabolism.* An understanding of the nutrition-metabolism interaction is important because proper nutrition not only affects the normal functioning of the body at rest, but also contributes to its efficient operation during different intensities of physical activity.

In the transition from rest to more vigorous physical activity, for example, the energy for muscle contraction is provided in several ways. Certain biochemical reactions can generate considerable energy quite rapidly for short periods of time without consuming oxygen. In sprint activities or all-out bursts of exercise, the body's capacity for this form of rapid energy release is critical in maintaining a high standard of performance. From a nutritional perspective, such performance depends upon adequate carbohydrate intake and subsequent storage in the liver and specific muscles. For exercise that lasts longer than a minute or two, however, energy must be extracted from a blend of carbohydrates, lipids, and some proteins through reactions that do require oxygen. To be effective, the physiologic conditioning process must be based on an understanding of how energy is supplied as well as the energy requirements of a particular activity. This knowledge is also fundamental in formulating an effective, yet prudent program of weight control through diet and exercise.

Part I of this text is organized into 13 chapters. The introductory chapter reviews biology and chemistry basics as they relate to nutrition and exercise. The focus is on definitions of common terms and major concepts that are important in studying the interactions between nutrition, exercise, and health. Chapter 2 deals with the digestion and absorption of food nutrients in the mouth, stomach, and small and large intestines. Chapters 3 through 8 take a closer look at the macronutrients and micronutrients, and attempt to answer the following questions: What are they? Where do they come from? What are their functions? In what foods are they found? How are they digested and absorbed?

Chapter 9 discusses per capita food consumption patterns, food advertising, food packaging, and food labeling. The concept of optimal nutrition is explored in

Chapter 10, and practical recommendations and guidelines are provided for the active man and woman. Emphasis in Chapters 11 and 12 is on the importance of the food nutrients in sustaining physiologic function during moderate and more strenuous physical activity. In Chapter 13, we discuss the energy value of foods, and how energy is extracted from food to power various forms of physical activity.

1

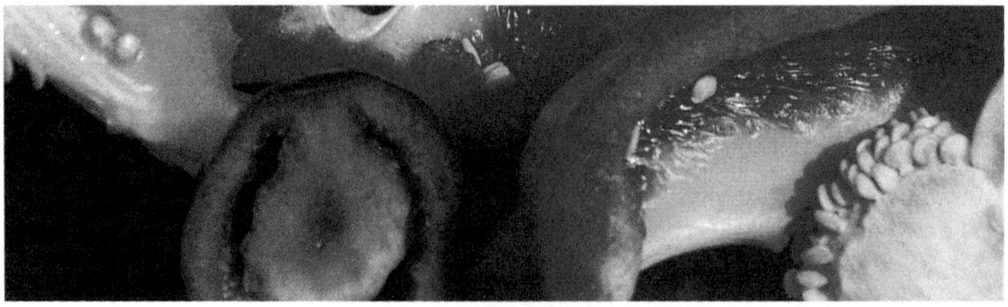

BIOLOGY AND CHEMISTRY BASICS: THE LINK TO A BETTER UNDERSTANDING OF NUTRITION, EXERCISE, AND HEALTH

Biology and chemistry serve as the foundation for understanding almost every aspect of nutrition, exercise, and health. Sometimes the picture is fairly clear: the energy imbalance in obesity is associated with excessive television viewing and snacking, and a reduced level of physical activity. Often, however, interactions are more complex, as during the digestion and absorption of carbohydrates, lipids, and proteins or in the processes of energy transfer from these nutrients during diverse forms of physical activity.

In this introductory chapter, we review some basic definitions and concepts in biology and chemistry as they relate to nutrient intake and assimilation and to energy expenditure. Knowledge of these fundamentals will help you to appreciate what goes on "behind the scenes" as the various nutrients undergo chemical transformations during tissue synthesis or their conversion to useful energy while at rest or during physical activity.

MATTER

Chemistry is the science that studies the structure and composition of matter: the solids, liquids, and gases that are the basic building blocks of our universe. ***Matter** is defined as a material substance (composed of atoms or molecules, or a mixture of the two) that occupies space and has mass.* All the biologic substances in the body are matter, and thus all of these substances have mass. A fundamental property of all matter is **inertia,** the resistance to change in speed or position when a force is applied. We clearly observe this resistance to movement when we try to move something heavy.

Mass. *The **mass** of an object is the quantitative measure of the inertia, or resistance to acceleration, of that object.* Under ordinary circumstances, the mass of any object remains constant whether it is submerged under water or is nearly weightless beyond the earth's atmosphere. The greater the mass, the larger its inertia and the smaller the change produced when a force is applied.

The metric system. Scientific measurement is generally presented in terms of the metric system. This system uses units that are related to each other by some power of ten. The prefix centi- means one hundredth, milli- means one thousandth, and the prefix kilo- is also derived from a word that means one thousand. Consequently, 1 kilogram (kg) is 1000 grams (g) or 2.2 pounds (lb). In general, we will use metric units throughout this text, although the English system will also appear where applicable.

Weight. The term **weight** is often used interchangeably (but imprecisely) to mean the same as mass; weight is related to mass but is not identical to it. *The weight of an object is the measure of its gravitational attraction by the earth or other celestial body.* Weight varies depending on the location of the object. When describing a person's weight, we could say that the force of attraction the earth exerts on a particular individual is 70 kg. On the surface of the moon, with its smaller gravitational force, this person would weigh only one-sixth as much, or 11.7 kg, yet the mass would remain unchanged. Even on earth, the weight of an object is slightly more at the South Pole (greater gravitational pull) than at the Equator (less gravitational pull). Although the weight of an object changes according to where it is located, its mass remains the same independent of location. So, if you want to be precise, the next time you weigh yourself, remember that what you have measured is the attractive or gravitational force the earth exerts on you. If you weigh 93 kg (205 pounds), then the gravitational force is 93 kg. At the Equator, the North Pole, or Mt. Shasta, California, you may weigh slightly more or less.*

Density. Matter takes up space and occupies a volume. *The mass of a unit volume of a material substance is referred to as its **density**.* This is computed by the equation: density = mass ÷ volume, and is usually expressed as grams per cubic centimeter (g/cc^3). Knowing the density of a substance is important in nutrition and for the evaluation of body composition. In nutrition, the physical density of a food is determined by its mass in relation to the volume it occupies. For example, the density of a fatty food is lower than that of a food composed mostly of protein or carbohydrate (yet as we will see in Chapter 13, the caloric content or "energy density" of the fat-laden food is nearly twice as high!).

The concept of density is also relevant when comparing the body composition of two people of the same stature and mass. Although both have the same mass, their proportion of fat to muscle could differ radically. One person's fat content, for example, could be 38% of total mass, whereas the

*A physicist would remind us that Newton's second law of physics states that force equals mass times acceleration ($F = ma$) and that weight equals mass times the acceleration of gravity ($W = mg$), the latter expressed as 32.2 feet per second squared. A unit of mass that is widely used by engineers is the slug, a term that comes from the word *sluggish,* implying resistance to change. The unit of force is the pound, and is defined as the force that will produce an acceleration of 1 foot-pound per second squared (1 fps^2) in a body of 1 slug mass, or 32.2 pounds. By rearranging terms, $m = W/g$, the mass of a 205-pound person would be calculated as $205 \div 32.2 = 6.3665$ slugs. Although the slug may have meaning to some people, most of us prefer to compute a person's weight from the relationship $W = mg$. In this case, the person's weight would be 205 pounds (6.3665×32.2), or 92.97 kg.

TABLE 1–1. THE 105 KNOWN ELEMENTS IN NATURE*

ELEMENT	ATOMIC NUMBER	OUTER SHELL ELECTRONS	ELEMENT	ATOMIC NUMBER	OUTER SHELL ELECTRONS
Hydrogen (H)	1	1	Cesium (Cs)	55	1
Helium (He)	2	2	Barium (Ba)	56	2
Lithium (Li)	3	1	Lanthanum (La)	57	2
Beryllium (Be)	4	2	Cerium (Ce)	58	2
Boron (B)	5	3	Praseodymium (Pr)	59	2
Carbon (C)	6	4	Neodymium (Nd)	60	2
Nitrogen (N)	7	5	Promethium (Pm)	61	2
Oxygen (O)	8	6	Samarium (Sm)	62	2
Fluorine (F)	9	7	Europium (Eu)	63	2
Neon (Ne)	10	8	Gadolinium (Gd)	64	2
Sodium (Na)	11	1	Terbium (Tb)	65	2
Magnesium (Mg)	12	2	Dysprosium (Dy)	66	2
Aluminum (Al)	13	3	Holmium (Ho)	67	2
Silicon (Si)	14	4	Erbium (Er)	68	2
Phosphorus (P)	15	5	Thulium (Tm)	69	2
Sulfur (S)	16	6	Ytterbium (Yb)	70	2
Chlorine (Cl)	17	7	Lutetium (Lu)	71	2
Argon (Ar)	18	8	Hafnium (Hf)	72	2
Potassium (K)	19	1	Tantalum (Ta)	73	2
Calcium (Ca)	20	2	Tungsten (W)	74	2
Scandium (Sc)	21	2	Rhenium (Re)	75	2
Titanium (Ti)	22	2	Osmium (Os)	76	2
Vanadium (V)	23	2	Iridium (Ir)	77	2
Chromium (Cr)	24	1	Platinum (Pt)	78	1
Manganese (Mn)	25	2	Gold (Au)	79	1
Iron (Fe)	26	2	Mercury (Hg)	80	2
Cobalt (Co)	27	2	Thallium (Tl)	81	3
Nickel (Ni)	28	2	Lead (Pb)	82	4
Copper (Cu)	29	1	Bismuth (Bi)	83	5
Zinc (Zn)	30	2	Polonium (Po)	84	6
Gallium (Ga)	31	3	Astatine (At)	85	7
Germanium (Ge)	32	4	Radon (Rn)	86	8
Arsenic (As)	33	5	Francium (Fr)	87	1
Selenium (Se)	34	6	Radium (Ra)	88	2
Bromine (Br)	35	7	Actinium (Ac)	89	2
Krypton (Kr)	36	8	Thorium (Th)	90	2
Rubidium (Rb)	37	1	Protactinium (Pa)	91	2
Strontium (Sr)	38	2	Uranium (U)	92	2
Yttrium (Y)	39	2	Neptunium (Np)	93	2
Zirconium (Zr)	40	2	Plutonium (Pu)	94	2
Niobium (Nb)	41	1	Americium (Am)	95	2
Molybdenum (Mo)	42	1	Curium (Cm)	96	2
Technetium (Tc)	43	1	Berkelium (Bk)	97	2
Ruthenium (Ru)	44	1	Californium (Cf)	98	2
Rhodium (Rh)	45	1	Einsteinium (Es)	99	2
Palladium (Pd)	46	—	Fermium (Fm)	100	2
Silver (Ag)	47	1	Mendelevium (Md)	101	2
Cadmium (Cd)	48	2	Nobelium (No)	102	2
Indium (In)	49	3	Lawrencium	103	2
Tin (Sn)	50	4	Rutherfordium	104	2
Antimony (Sb)	51	5	Hahnium	105	2
Tellurium (Te)	52	6			
Iodine (I)	53	7			
Xenon (Xe)	54	8			

* The list includes the atomic number and the number of electrons in the outer valence shell. The element's atomic symbol is shown in parentheses. A chemistry textbook should be consulted for further details about the Periodic Table of the Elements.

second person could possess one-tenth the fat, or only 3.8% of body mass. Because fat and muscle occupy different volumes per unit mass (i.e., they possess different densities), the volume occupied by each person varies considerably, depending on individual differences in body composition, even though body mass may be identical. Chapter 14 focuses on the concept of body density in relation to body fat content.

ELEMENTS

Matter in the universe is composed of fundamental materials or **elements.** Table 1–1 lists the 105 elements that have been identified. Of these, 90 occur in nature, either free or in combination with other elements; the remaining 15 are produced artificially. *An important characteristic of an element is that it cannot be decomposed into a simpler substance by ordinary chemical processes.* Water, for example, is not an element because it can be chemically separated into the elements hydrogen and oxygen.

Each of the elements is abbreviated by a one- or two-letter atomic symbol, a practice first used by the Swedish chemist Jöns Berzelius in the early 1800s. Twelve elements are identified by the first letter of their name; most of the others are identified by the first two letters. In several cases the atomic symbol is derived from the Latin name for the element: Fe stands for iron (Latin ferrum), Pb for lead (Latin plumbum), Ag for silver (Latin argentum), and Na is from the Latin natrium, the shorthand term for sodium.

DISTRIBUTION OF ELEMENTS IN THE BODY

In humans, the most abundant elements are oxygen (O; 65%), carbon (C; 18%), hydrogen (H; 10%), and nitrogen (N; 3%). Combined, their composition by weight, shown in Figure 1–1, constitutes approximately 96% of body mass. These elements serve as the chief constituents for five of the six basic nutrients—carbohydrates, lipids, proteins, vitamins, and water—and comprise the structural units for most biologically active substances in the body. The remaining group of nutrients includes major minerals such as the elements calcium (1.5%), phosphorus (1.0%), potassium (0.4%), sulfur (0.3%), sodium and chlorine (0.2%), and magnesium as well as such exotic elements as vanadium, gold, silver, silicon, molybdenum, manganese, copper, cobalt, selenium, chromium, tin, and even arsenic. They are present in the body only in trace amounts, usually as integral parts of protein catalysts or enzymes (see "Enzymes" later in this chapter) and their reactions. For example, copper (Cu) forms part of the enzymes associated with absorption and metabolism of the mineral iron. Copper is also intimately involved in the release of cholesterol from the liver; it helps to clot blood and, when bound to certain enzymes, aids in the synthesis of important neurotransmitters.

Major minerals. There are seven major minerals; calcium, phosphorus, potassium, sulfur, sodium, chlorine, and magnesium. They are considered major because they are present in the body in amounts greater than 0.1% of body mass, or are required in the diet in amounts over 100 milligrams (mg) a day. The remaining essential elements are called trace minerals.

CELLULAR ORGANIZATION

Many types of cells make up biologic systems. The basic processes that sustain life among all cells are fairly similar, even though different cells carry out unique functions that necessitate special structures. Cells with

High turnover rate of some elements. The mineral content of the body does not remain fixed. Some elements are continually replaced. During the growth cycle, for example, the mineral calcium is in a continual state of flux; more calcium is used than is broken down. Thus, there is a large turnover in bone during the first year of life. During adolescence, up to 32% of the skeleton mass per year can be rebuilt.

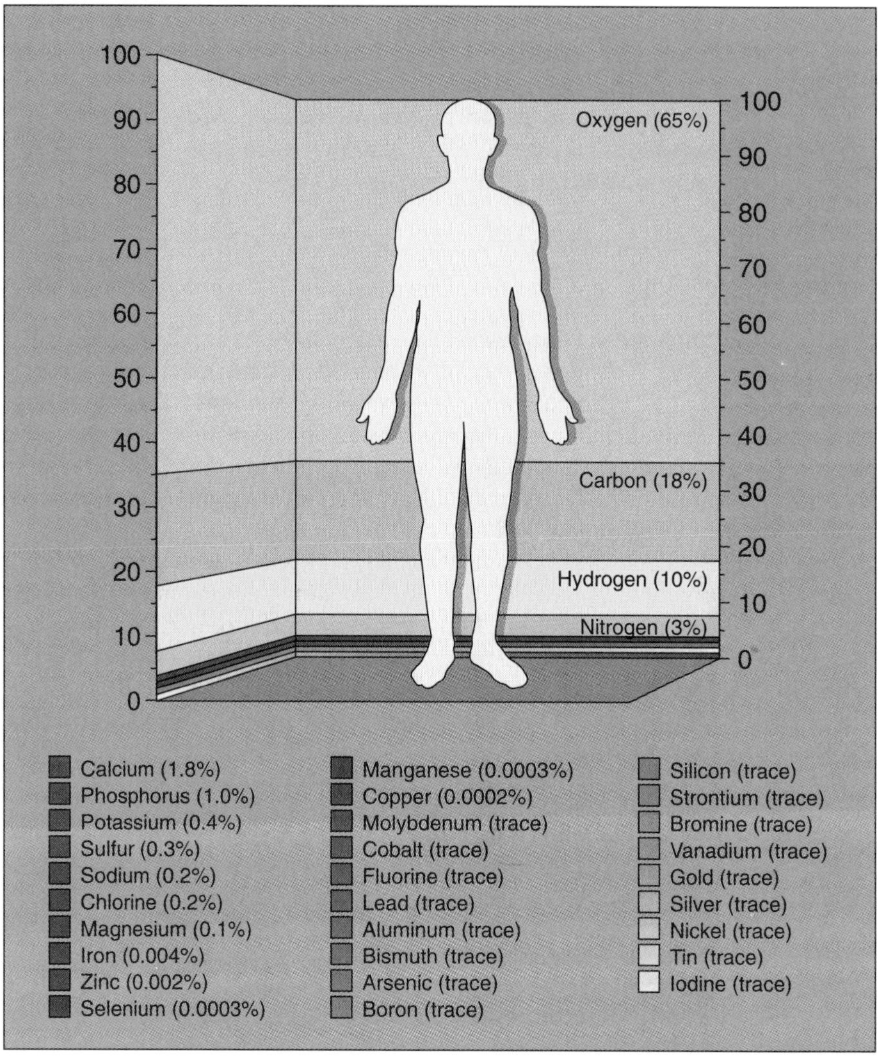

FIG. 1–1. Elemental composition of the human body. The percent values represent the approximate percentage of a 60 kg person's body mass.

different functions also contain essentially the same chemicals; they differ only in the proportion and arrangement of these chemicals. Figure 1–2 shows the complexity of the body's biologic organization. Humans are a collection of diverse systems, each comprising highly specialized organs and tissues. The tissues are composed of numerous cells, and the cells are made up of molecules. Molecules, in turn, are constructed from individual atoms.

ORGAN SYSTEMS

The body is a collection of various **organ systems** including the digestive, urinary, nervous, integumentary, skeletal, muscular, endocrine, pulmonary, lymphatic, reproductive, and cardiovascular. In turn, each organ system is made up of combinations of specialized tissues. For example, highly specific cells make up the three main components of the integu-

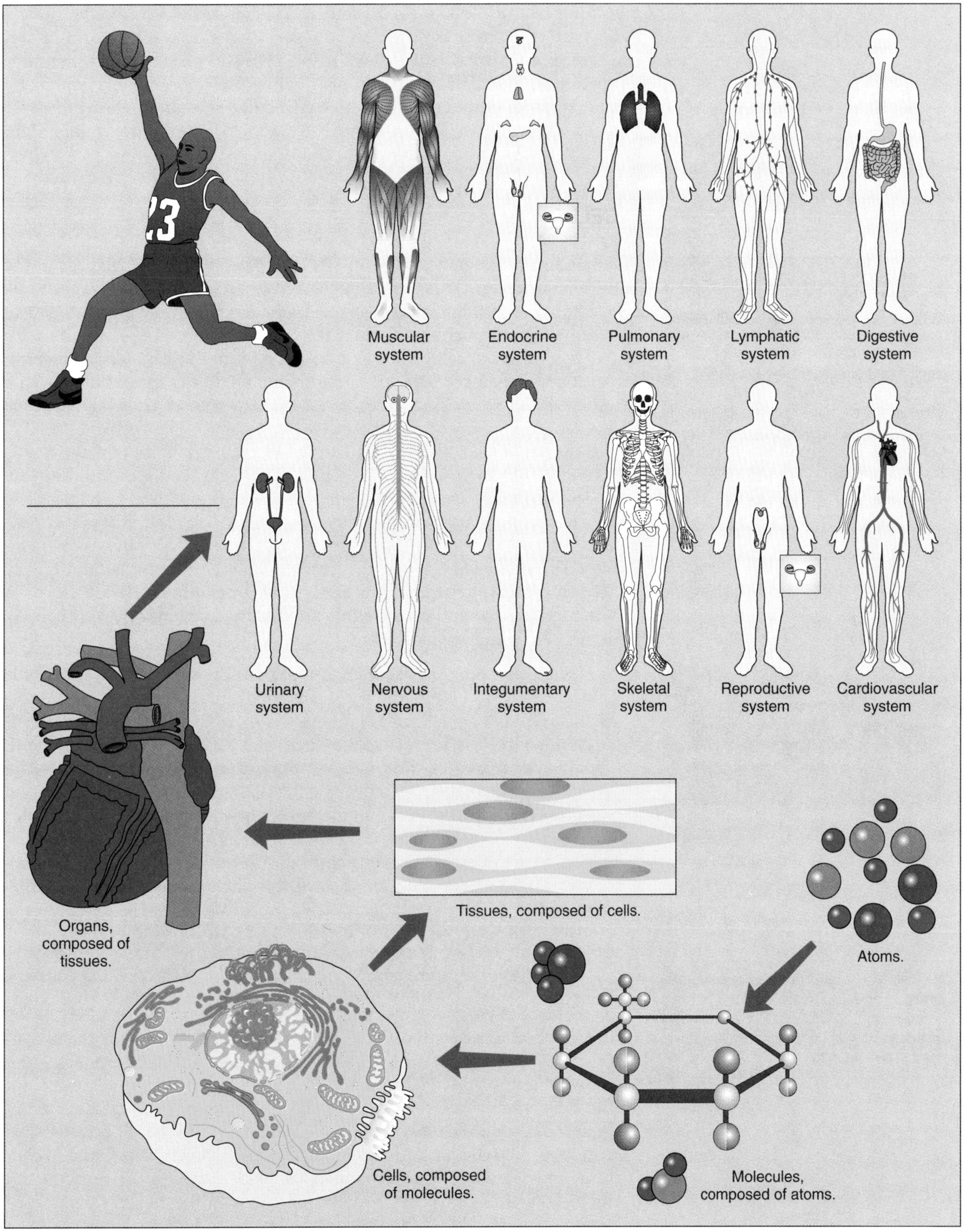

FIG. 1–2. Complexity of the body's biologic organization.

mentary system: the skin, hair, and nails. This system forms the body's outer protective layer to shield the deeper tissues from injury or invasion by outside organisms, as well as to respond to stimuli evoked by pressure, temperature, and pain. The skin also is the formation site of vitamin D. All the organ systems have their own particular and unique functions, yet each usually works in harmony with the others to maintain an optimal state of bodily function.

CELLS

Organ systems. An organ is a collection of tissues joined together to perform a common function. For example, muscle, nervous, connective, and epithelial tissue make up the heart, whose function is to pump blood throughout the body. An organ system comprises a collection of organs that serve together in a common function, such as the cardiovascular system, the endocrine system, and the digestive system.

The next level of organization consists of the nearly 100 trillion cells in the adult human body. **Cells,** which represent *the basic units of life,* vary in size and shape depending on their specific function. Most have a diameter of approximately 10 micrometers (a micrometer, or μm, is $^1/_{1000}$ of an inch), but an egg or ovum cell can be as large as 140 μm in diameter. Cell length can also vary tremendously, from approximately 8 μm for red blood cells, to a muscle cell 30 cm long, or a nerve cell that stretches up to 1 meter (100 cm) in length!

The shapes of cells also differ. The red blood cell is both oval (and thus adapted for carrying oxygen and carbon dioxide) and flat (for rapid uptake or release of these gases in appropriate tissues). Some digestive cells have many convolutions and depressions, which increase their surface-area-to-volume ratio and permit greater absorption of nutrients through their membranes. The epithelial cells on the inside of the mouth are flat and tightly packed to protect the underlying tissues from penetration by bacteria.

Although unique and often highly specific in function, cells share many structures in common (Figure 1–3):

DNA. DNA is a highly specialized series of proteins called nucleic acids that exist in all cell nuclei. Nucleic acids code, store, and transmit the character of inherited traits of the organism through generations.

- A **plasma membrane,** a "sandwich-type" double structure made of lipids and proteins, separates the cell's contents from the surrounding extracellular fluid. The cell membrane is semipermeable, so only materials of certain sizes can be exchanged between the cell and its environment. The bilayer serves as the basic constituent of the membrane; the core of the bilayer contains the fatty acid "tails" of the phospholipid, and the inner portion of the membrane prevents water-containing molecules from simply passing through the membrane. This part of the membrane is said to be *hydrophobic* (water-fearing). The outside of the bilayer membrane contains the polar "heads" of the phospholipid molecule. This part of the membrane is *hydrophilic* (water-loving); it is in continual contact with water on both the inside and outside of the cell.

RNA. RNA is formed in the cell under the direction of DNA. This compound is the messenger by which the coded information in DNA is transmitted for the process of protein synthesis.

- A central command center, the **nucleus,** is the largest structure in the cell and regulates its many functions. The nucleus contains chromatin, a precursor of chromosomes that carry the hereditary material. The **DNA** (deoxyribonucleic acid) of the chromosomes directs cellular protein synthesis; **RNA** (ribonucleic acid) is the messenger protein responsible for translating the genetic instructions of DNA into proteins that carry out the cell's vital functions. The nucleus is surrounded by a plasma membrane that separates its cytoplasmic fluid from the rest of the cell. The endoplasmic reticulum joins the double nuclear membrane and is continuous with it. Communication takes place between the nucleus and the cellular fluid through pores or channels in the nuclear membrane and by way of microtubular channels in the endoplasmic reticulum.

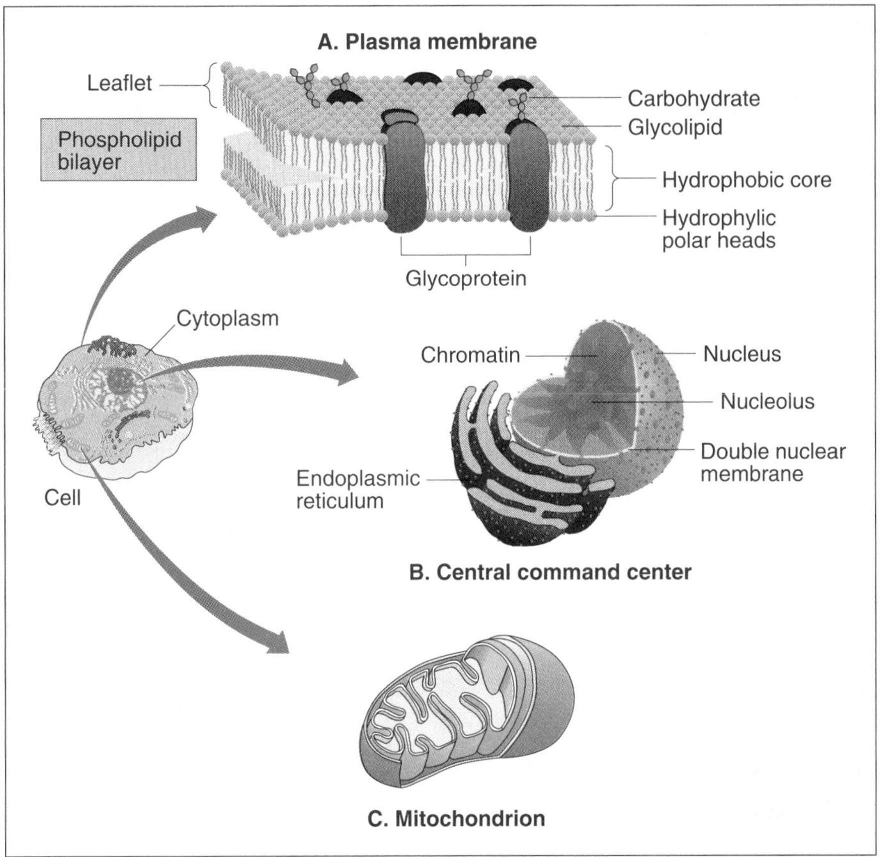

FIG. 1–3. Three common structures characteristic of living cells. **A.** The plasma membrane, a double "sandwich-type" structure composed of lipids (mostly phospholipids) and interspersed with proteins. Note that the bilayer can be cleaved into two halves, or leaflets. Each leaflet is responsible for binding specific protein structures. An elaborate network of tubules and microchannels serves as "inner scaffolding" to provide structure to the gel-like contents of the cell. **B.** The central command center, the nucleus, is the largest structure in the cell and regulates its many functions. Note that the endoplasmic reticulum joins the double nuclear membrane and is continuous with it. **C.** Mitochondria, the power plants of the cell, convert food nutrients into energy.

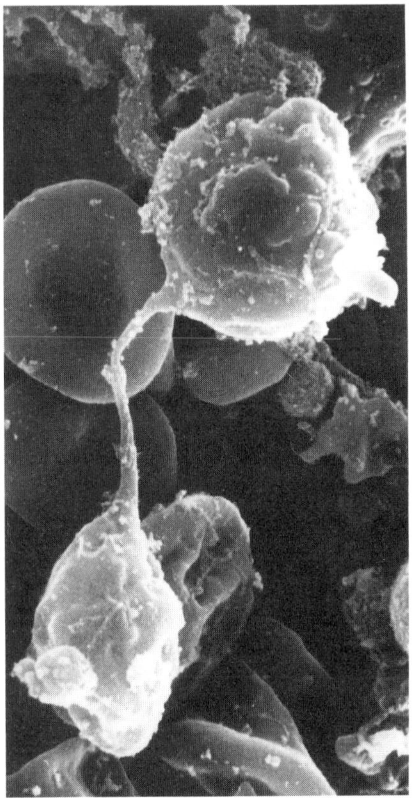

An "up-close" view. The scanning electron microscope has penetrated the submicroscopic structure of cells. This technology provides an intimate look at the organizational details that comprise the cells and how they function. (From Lee, G.R.: Normochromic anemias. In Wintrobe's Clinical Hematology. 9th Ed. Edited by G.R. Lee, et al. Philadelphia, Lea & Febiger, 1993.)

- **Mitochondria,** the cell's "power plants," convert food nutrients into energy. In these structures, the potential energy in food is extracted and harvested within the energy-rich bonds of ATP (adenosine triphosphate), the unique energy currency of each cell. The mitochondria and other cellular organelles are bathed in cytoplasm, the intracellular watery medium containing minerals, enzymes, and other specialized solutions, compounds, and mixtures. The cytoplasm permits volleys of neural impulses to travel within the cell and also between cells and their surroundings.

MOLECULES

A **molecule** is defined as a minimum of two atoms bonded together strongly enough to create a stable identity. *The molecule represents the smallest unit of a substance that still retains the compositional and chemical identity of that substance.* Further fragmentation of the molecule involves breaking of the chemical

Chemistry is linked to physics. Marie Curie, a chemist who discovered the radioactive elements radium and polonium, was awarded the Nobel Prize in 1911 for her discoveries. Physicists then went on to explore the subatomic properties of the atom.

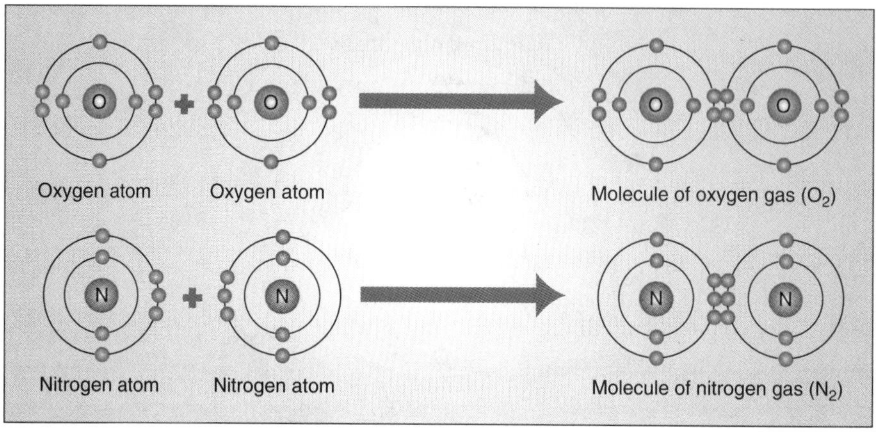

FIG. 1–4. Molecules of specific elements are composed of identical atoms.

bonds that hold it together. The chemical properties of a molecule are changed by altering the configuration of its chemical bonds.

Figure 1–4 shows that a molecule made up of a specific element always has identical atoms. Examples are the gases nitrogen ($N + N = N_2$) and oxygen ($O + O = O_2$), shown in the figure, as well as hydrogen ($H + H = H_2$) and chlorine gas ($Cl + Cl = Cl_2$).

ATOMS

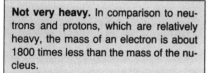

Not very heavy. In comparison to neutrons and protons, which are relatively heavy, the mass of an electron is about 1800 times less than the mass of the nucleus.

Molecules are composed of atoms, particles up to 4 billionths of an inch in diameter that serve as the basic building blocks of matter. *The **atom** is the unit into which elements (matter) can be divided without the release of charged particles.* An atom consists of four main subatomic particles: nucleus, neutrons, protons, and electrons. The composition of atoms differs according to the number of subatomic particles they contain.

The dense core, or **atomic nucleus,** is the central portion of the atom. It can contain positively charged particles, called **protons,** and particles with a neutral electric charge, called **neutrons.** The protons and neutrons within the nucleus are bound tightly together and account for nearly 100% of the mass of the atom. Surrounding the nucleus is a cloud of **electrons,** negatively charged particles with almost no mass. Because opposite electric charges attract, the electrons are bound to the positively charged nucleus. An atom is usually electrically neutral; consequently, every atom has an equal number of positively charged protons and negatively charged electrons. For example, an atom of hydrogen has 1 proton and 1 electron; oxygen has 8 protons and 8 electrons; calcium has 20 protons and 20 electrons; and zinc has 30 protons and 30 electrons.

Discovery of the neutron. The neutron was discovered in 1932 by the English scientist, James C. Chadwick.

Figure 1–5A shows a **planetary model** of the atomic structure and subatomic particles for atoms of hydrogen and helium. For each atom, the number of "orbits" is determined by the number of electrons. A maximum of 2 electrons can fill the first orbit, or shell. Depending on the particular atom, up to seven remaining shells, or energy levels, can exist.

An alternative presentation, shown in Figure 1–5B for helium, is called the **orbital model.** Here, the atom's 2 electrons move randomly about the nucleus, which holds 2 protons and 2 neutrons. The electrons are repre-

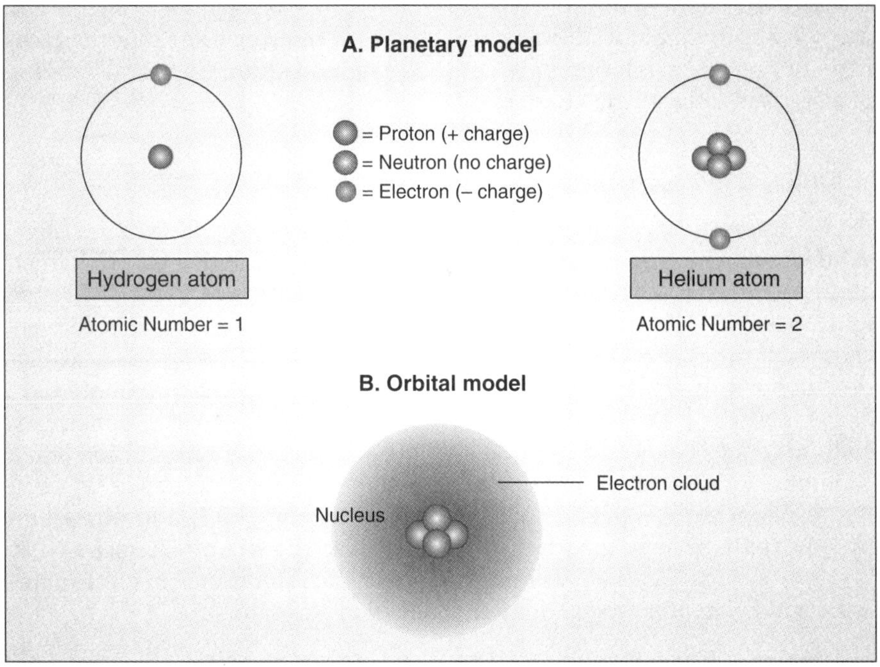

FIG. 1–5. Atomic structure and subatomic particles for atoms of hydrogen and helium. **A.** Planetary model for hydrogen and helium. **B.** Orbital model for helium.

Compared to the size of the atom, the nucleus is small. The nucleus of an atom is about one hundred thousandth of the diameter of the atom.

sented as a cloud of electric charges. Hydrogen has 1 proton and 1 electron. The lone electron squirts unpredictably about the nucleus, somewhat as a bee buzzes about its hive. Sometimes the electron is near the nucleus and sometimes it is farther away. Thus, the electron at one time or another occupies the relatively vast empty space around the nucleus. The electrons form an electric field about the nucleus that gives the atom its volume and simultaneously excludes other atoms from occupying its space. Each atom is electrically neutral because the total positive charge of the nucleus equals the total negative charge of the swarming electrons that move haphazardly about the nucleus.

The number of protons in the nucleus determines the **atomic number** of an element. Thus hydrogen, with 1 proton, has an atomic number of 1 and helium, with 2 protons, has an atomic number of 2. For the remaining 103 elements, the atomic numbers range consecutively from 3 for lithium to 105 for hahnium. Additionally, numbers 106 to 109 have been reserved for four other possible elements that have yet to be named or whose existence has not yet been confirmed.

In addition to its atomic number, an atom has a **mass number** that is equal to the sum of its neutrons and protons. For example, helium has a mass number of 4 (2 neutrons plus 2 protons) and is symbolized in chemical terms as $^{4}_{2}He$. The number 4 to the left of the atomic symbol is the mass number; we can deduce how many electrons there are since there are an equal number of protons and electrons in an atom. Thus, He has 2 electrons, and the number 2 to the left of the atomic symbol is the atomic number. For nitrogen ($^{14}_{7}N$), the number 14 is the atomic mass and the number 7 is the atomic number. By deduction, there are 7 electrons (equal to the number of protons). For oxygen, the atomic mass is 16 and the atomic number is 8 ($^{16}_{8}O$), while for carbon, the symbol is $^{12}_{6}C$. Since the atomic mass for the element hydrogen is 1, we can state that the mass of the carbon atom is approximately 12 times more than for hydrogen, or that the mass of an oxygen atom is 4 times greater than a helium atom. Chemical bonding is discussed later in the chapter.

IONS

An ***ion*** *is any atom or group of atoms with a positive or negative electric charge.* When an atom holds fewer electrons than protons, it is positively charged and is referred to as a positive ion or **cation;** an example is the hydrogen ion, labeled H^+. An atom that has more electrons than protons is negatively charged (**anion**), for example, the chloride ion (Cl^-). The strong acid, hydrochloric acid, (HCl) can separate or *dissociate* into the simple ionic form of H^+ and Cl^-. The reaction is written $HCL \rightarrow H^+ + Cl^-$. Similarly, a sodium cation (Na^+) and chloride anion (Cl^-) are present in solution when sodium chloride (NaCl), or table salt, dissolves and dissociates in water in the reaction $NaCl \rightarrow Na^+ + Cl^-$. Ions such as Na^+, Cl^-, and potassium (K^+) in solution are called **electrolytes** because the solutes dissociate into positive or negative ions. More is said about the importance of electrolytes later in this chapter (see Oxidation-Reduction Reactions).

ISOTOPES

If the nucleus of an atom contains more neutrons than protons, the atom takes on different chemical properties and is known as an ***isotope.*** For example, Figure 1–6 shows that the nucleus of a hydrogen atom can contain more than a single proton. The nucleus of the most abundant of hydrogen atoms has only a single proton and no neutron. The most common isotope of hydrogen is called *deuterium* (^2H), and contains 1 neutron in addition to its single proton. *Tritium* (^3H) is a third isotope of hydrogen, and its nucleus contains 2 neutrons and 1 proton.

The isotopes of atoms emit energy from their nuclei during decomposition. This property of isotopes is called radioactivity, and the isotopes are referred to as radioactive. Isotopes are important in nutritional research because they allow the scientist to monitor and "trace" metabolic pathways and physiologic functions both at rest and during exercise. For example, radioisotopes can be injected into different nutrients as a "chemical cocktail" to trace the pathways of a particular nutrient in the body. This technique

Isotopic tracers are used in diagnostic medicine. The iodine-131 isotope, for example, is used to detect disorders of the thyroid gland, and the isotopes radium-226 and cobalt-60 are used to detect the metabolic activity, and therefore the size, of various tumors.

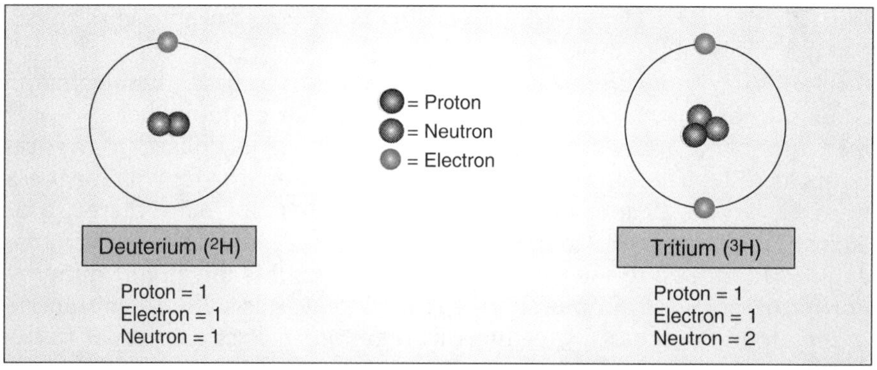

FIG. 1–6. Deuterium and tritium are two isotopes of hydrogen.

has been used to keep track of the body's pool of amino acids as they undergo various chemical transformations. The labeling of carbon atoms in the glucose molecule has provided insight into the eventual fate of glucose during varying intensities of physical activity as well as its resynthesis in the recovery process. The topic of exercise metabolism is discussed further in Chapter 11. Potassium-40, a naturally occurring isotope present in lean tissue, is essentially absent in fat. By "counting" the emissions of this isotope, an observer can estimate the lean and fat content of the body. Chapter 14 presents several simpler methods for estimating body composition.

CHEMICAL BONDING: FORCES OF ATTRACTION THAT HOLD ATOMS TOGETHER

The interaction of one atom's electrons with those of another creates forces of attraction or ***chemical bonds*** *between atoms.* The union of these atoms occurs in such a way that the total energy of the product is less than the total energy of the sum of its component atoms. This energy lowering is the bonding energy.

Recall that electrons literally hover in a space about the nucleus in electronic energy shells. The maximum number of shells is eight, and each energy shell can contain a specified number of electrons. The shell closest to the nucleus contains up to 2 electrons; the second shell can accommodate up to 8 electrons, while the third shell can hold up to 18 electrons. The additional shells can hold even greater numbers of electrons. One of the unique properties of an atom is that its electrons will fill the innermost energy shell before they occupy the next successive outer shell. If there are more than 8 electrons in the outermost shell, only those electrons in excess of 8 (or multiples of 8) are chemically reactive.

Figure 1–7 shows the electronic configuration of four common atoms: hydrogen, carbon, oxygen, and sodium. Hydrogen has only 1 electron and it occupies shell 1, leaving space for an additional electron in this shell. For carbon, with a total of 6 electrons, 2 fill shell 1 and the remaining 4 occupy shell 2, leaving space for up to 4 additional electrons. Oxygen, with 8 electrons, has 2 in shell 1 and 6 in shell 2 with room for 2 additional electrons. The sodium atom is slightly different: it has 11 electrons so its first two energy levels are filled (2 electrons in shell 1 and 8 in shell 2), leaving only 1 electron to occupy the third shell. A key concept is that the number of electrons in the outermost energy shell, or **valence shell,** of an atom determines the number of bonds that atom can form. For example, hydrogen has a valence of 1 and oxygen's valence is 2; thus, oxygen can combine with two atoms of hydrogen to form a molecule of water.

When the outer shell carries its maximum number of electrons, the atom is said to be stable and its electrons are unavailable to react chemically with other atoms. In such cases, the atom is said to be inert. This is true for the helium atom, which has only 2 electrons that both occupy the first shell. Atoms of other inert gases such as neon, argon, krypton, xenon, and radon are similarly saturated with electrons in the outer shell. Even though these atoms have different atomic numbers, and therefore different numbers of protons in the nucleus, they all have 8 electrons in their outer shell with no "extra" space for additional electrons.

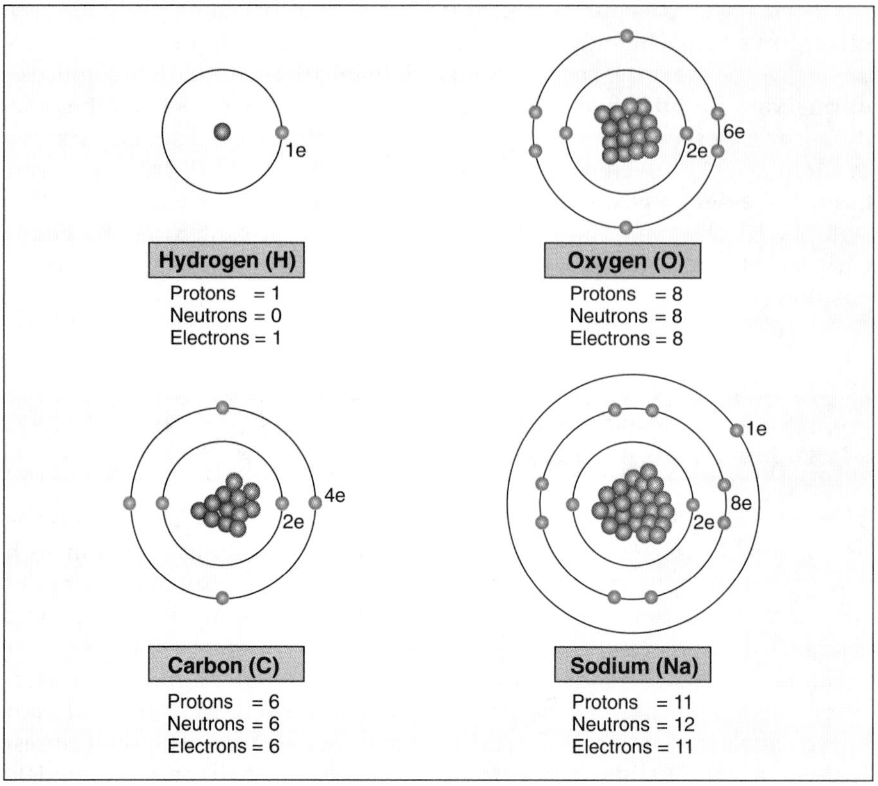

FIG. 1–7. Electronic configuration for hydrogen, carbon, oxygen, and sodium.

When a shell is filled with electrons, any excess electrons in the outer shell are chemically reactive and take part in bonding. These participatory electrons are referred to as bonding or valence electrons. Fluorine, for example, with 7 electrons in its outer shell, is highly reactive because it can readily join with another atom that has an available electron to "share." For carbon, with 4 electrons in its outer shell, there is room for 4 additional electrons to fill the valence shell. Thus, it can combine with a variety of other atoms to saturate this shell.

In essence, chemical bonding involves the sharing of an atom's valence electrons with those of another atom. Different atoms become bonded when their interaction produces stability in the energy level of a particular valence shell. Except for helium, which fills its lone energy shell with 2 electrons, bonding in other atoms occurs when 8 electrons are accommodated in the valence shell. Electron sharing among atoms provides the necessary force of attraction or "electrostatic cement" so the resulting molecule achieves maximum stability.

There are three main types of chemical bonding: ionic bonds, covalent bonds, and hydrogen bonds.

IONIC BONDS

An **ionic bond,** the simplest of chemical bonds, involves the transfer of electrons between two neutral atoms. The resulting electrostatic force holds the atoms together. The atom that gains 1 or more electrons during this process is called an **anion** and it bears a negative charge; the atom that

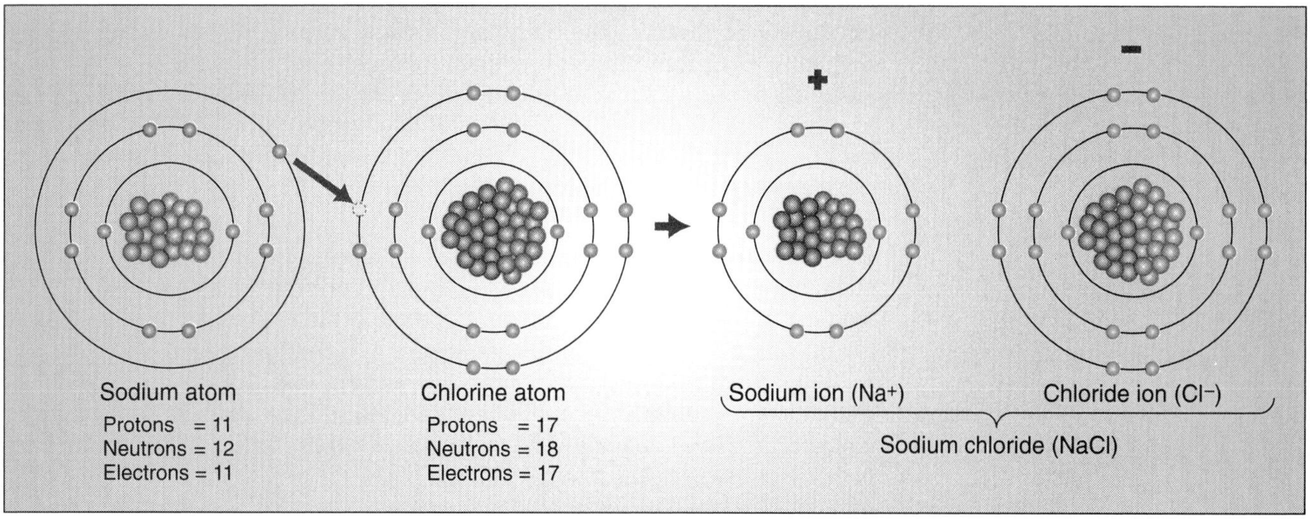

FIG. 1–8. Atomic configuration for atoms of sodium and chlorine, and how they join chemically to form sodium chloride.

gives up an electron is called a **cation** and it has a positive charge. Common table salt, formed from the union of sodium and chlorine atoms, is an excellent example of ionic bonding.

Figure 1–8 displays the configuration for atoms of sodium and chlorine and how they join chemically to form sodium chloride. Notice that the outer valence shells for the two atoms are not completely filled: sodium (atomic number 11) has a single electron in its valence shell, while chlorine (atomic number 17) has 7 electrons in its outer shell. The sodium atom can more easily donate its outer shell electron to chlorine than accept 7 new electrons from chlorine. Similarly, it is easier for the chlorine atom to accept sodium's lone electron than to transfer its 7 electrons to sodium.

When sodium transfers its single outer-shell electron to chlorine, the sodium atom becomes a cation and achieves stability because its outermost shell is filled. Before the transfer, the sodium atom had a net electric charge of zero (11 positive charges in the nucleus and 11 minus charges represented by 11 electrons). With the donation of 1 electron, sodium now achieves a net electric charge of plus 1 (11 positive charges and 10 negative charges due to the loss of 1 electron). Similarly, the chlorine atom, by accepting sodium's electron, now fills its valence shell with 8 electrons and becomes an anion with a net negative charge. This is achieved because with the acceptance of sodium's negatively charged electron, chlorine attains a net electric charge of minus 1 and a completely filled valence shell. The oppositely charged sodium (Na^+) and chloride (Cl^-) ions are attracted to each other by electrostatic force, and the resulting ionic compound is known chemically as sodium chloride.

In their individual states, sodium and chlorine exhibit quite dissimilar chemical properties: sodium is a silvery white metal that burns on exposure to air, while chlorine is a toxic, yellow-green gas. When sodium and chlorine ions chemically unite, however, they form the ubiquitous white crystalline substance we often consume in excess by sprinkling it liberally on the foods we eat. When this salt is dissolved in water, it immediately dissociates into its separate ions (Na^+ and Cl^-) to form an electrolyte solution. Some athletes consume electrolyte drinks to replace the salt lost during sweating. Research indicates, however, that except for extreme sweat loss, electrolytes are effectively replaced in the daily diet. One does not have to resort to commercially prepared "sport" drinks to replace electrolytes lost through sweating.

COVALENT BONDS

Covalent bonding involves the sharing of electrons in the atom's valence shell. Figure 1–9 shows examples of covalent bonding for the gases methane, oxygen, and nitrogen. The creation of a molecule of methane gas (depicted chemically as CH_4: four hydrogen atoms bonded to one carbon atom) illustrates the formation of four single covalent bonds. Each hydrogen atom, with a single electron in its valence shell, shares this electron with 1 of the 4 electrons in the valence shell of carbon. Because one carbon atom has 4 valence electrons available for sharing, four discrete covalent bonds form with the four hydrogen atoms.

When two oxygen atoms combine to form one molecule of oxygen gas (O_2), 2 of the valence electrons from each atom are shared by both atoms. This provides the 8 electrons to fill the valence shell and creates a stable energy state for the oxygen molecule. Because the two oxygen atoms share

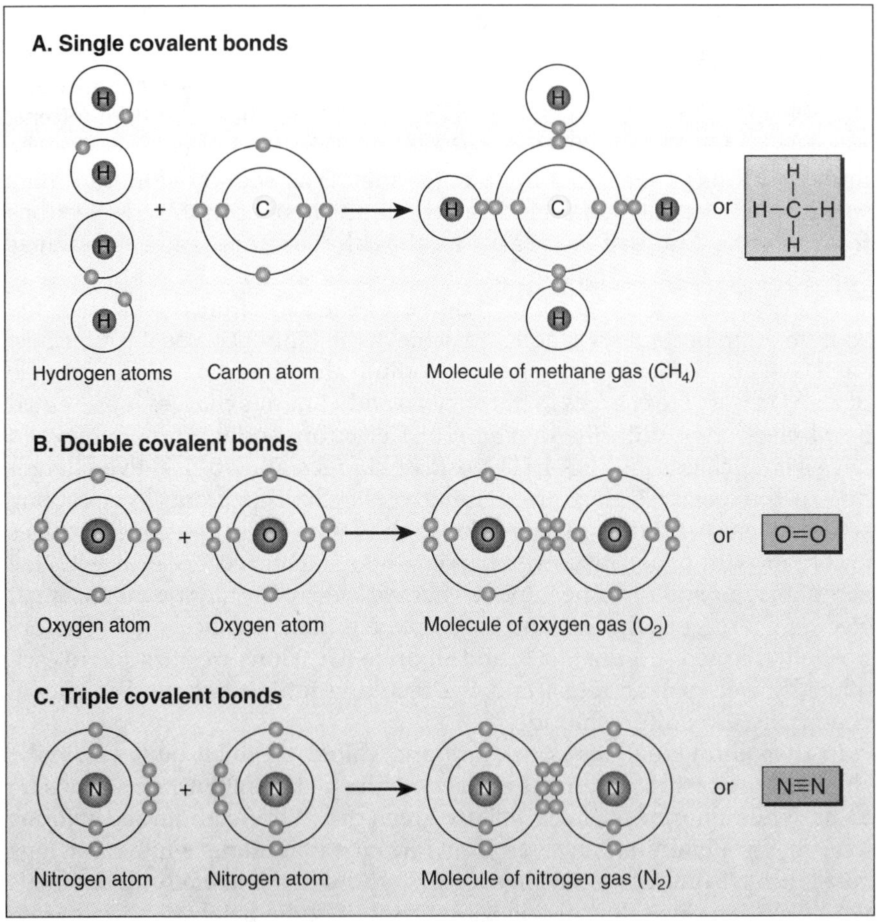

FIG. 1–9. Covalent bonding. **A.** Single covalent bonding for methane. **B.** Double covalent bonding for oxygen. **C.** Triple covalent bonding for nitrogen.

two pairs of electrons, the bond is known as a double covalent bond. When two atoms of nitrogen join chemically, the two nitrogen atoms share three pairs of electrons so they can fill the outer shell with a total of 8 electrons. This type of bonding is called a triple covalent bond.

The shape of a particular molecule determines how that molecule interacts with other atoms or molecules. When the electron pairs in covalent bonding are not shared equally among atoms, the shared electron pair spends more of its time in the vicinity of one of the atoms. This inequality is referred to as polarity, and it can affect the chemical characteristics of a molecule.

A water molecule is a dipolar molecule; Figure 1–10 shows that the two hydrogen atoms, with a positive electric charge, are located toward one end of the larger oxygen atom, which has a slightly negative charge. The two poles of electric charge on the H_2O molecule cause it to orient its negatively charged oxygen side to the positive side of other molecules, such as large, positively charged proteins, which prevents them from settling out of solution. This dipole nature allows water to surround other molecules and shield them from chemically reactive substances. In this way, water serves as a universal solvent to help transport substances throughout the body. These include the five nutrients—carbohydrates, lipids, proteins, vitamins, and minerals—as well as the respiratory gases carbon dioxide and oxygen, and the metabolic wastes that are filtered through the kidneys and eliminated as urine.

In contrast to a polar covalent bond, a nonpolar covalent bond is one in which the electron pairs are shared equally with the electric charge balanced among the atoms. Carbon dioxide gas (two oxygens connected to a carbon, symbolized as CO_2 or O═C═O) exhibits nonpolar covalent bonding. *Compounds that contain carbon atoms, such as CO_2, CH_4, or $C_6H_{12}O_6$, are referred to as* ***organic compounds;*** all organic compounds are joined together chemically by either polar or nonpolar covalent bonding.

HYDROGEN BONDS

Hydrogen bonds form when the positively charged hydrogen atom that is covalently bonded to a slightly negative atom is attracted by another slightly negative atom. In essence, the hydrogen bond serves as a relatively weak bridge between two electronegative atoms such as oxygen or nitrogen.

Figure 1–10 illustrates how single water molecules readily join together because their positive ends become attracted to the negative ends of other nearby water molecules. Hydrogen bonds are weaker compared to ionic and covalent bonds, which have relatively strong forces of attraction. Large molecules such as DNA and many other proteins have hydrogen bonding. The bonds are located in discrete parts of these complex molecules, and serve to stabilize them to help maintain their spatial configuration.

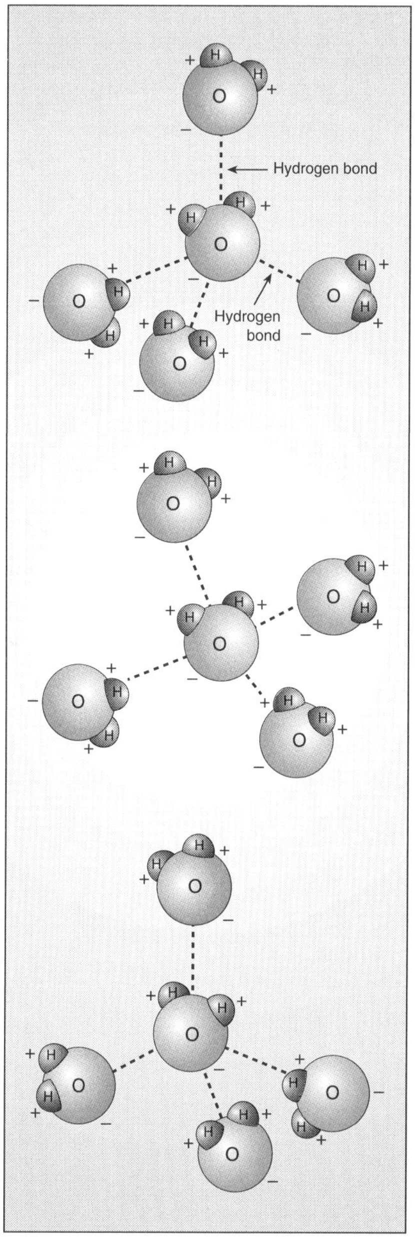

FIG. 1–10. Water is a dipole molecule: the positive ends of a molecule orient with the negative ends of other water molecules.

Smooth operation. The dipole nature of water enables it to serve as an essential component of the body's many lubricants. Examples include saliva and mucus, which become part of ingested food particles so they can move more easily through the digestive tract, tears to bathe the eyeballs so they rotate smoothly in their sockets, and the lubricating synovial fluids of joints that prevent the grinding of bony surfaces.

COMPOUNDS AND MIXTURES

COMPOUNDS

A ***compound*** *is a substance formed from two or more different elements.* The simple water molecule (H_2O), for example, is a compound formed from the union of one atom of oxygen (O) and two hydrogen atoms (H + H).

Similarly, glucose is a compound because it is formed by the chemical joining of six carbons (6 C), twelve hydrogens (12 H), and six oxygens (6 O) to form one molecule of $C_6H_{12}O_6$. At an extreme of complexity, the nucleic acid compounds contain thousands of atoms linked together. When a compound is formed, it becomes a different substance than its constituent parts with discrete color, state, and chemical properties.

MIXTURES

Most common materials are mixtures of various chemical compounds. *A **mixture** is created when two or more different substances are physically combined.* Mixtures differ from compounds in the following ways: (1) mixtures are not linked by chemical bonds; (2) mixtures can be separated into their individual components by physical processes such as filtering, straining, centrifugation, or distillation (evaporation); compounds can only be separated into their constituent elements by chemical reactions in which bonds between atoms are broken; and (3) unlike a compound, a mixture is not a chemically pure substance. A mixture can be a heterogeneous substance such as a particular enzyme, hormone, or vitamin; it can also be a combination of food nutrients such as strawberries and whipped cream or chocolate chip cookies.

There are three types of mixtures:

- Solutions. *A **solution** is a homogeneous mixture of either a gas, liquid, or solid that is composed of at least two substances.* Oxygen and carbon dioxide are in solution in the fluids of the body, as are the products of digestion as they are transported to and from different tissues. The air we breathe is a solution because it is a mixture of gases (approximately 79.04% nitrogen, 20.93% oxygen, and 0.03% carbon dioxide with trace amounts of several inert gases). The largest quantity of a substance in a solution is customarily called the *solvent,* while the smaller amount—usually a solid or gas—is the *solute.* In the body, water is the chief solvent. (Chapter 8 is all about this important substance.)
- Suspensions. *A **suspension** is a mixture of substances that may have visible solutes, but with little chemical attraction for the solvent.* If a snapshot is taken of blood flowing through the vascular system, it looks like a well-mixed, heterogeneous solution. But if a sample is collected in a small tube and spun at high speed, there would be three distinct parts. The top part, the plasma, would be a relatively clear liquid representing about 55% of the sample. There would be a minute middle layer of white blood cells (leukocytes) and platelets; and the third layer, consisting of red blood cells, would settle to the bottom and occupy about 45% of the sample. The different layers of substances are the *suspensions.*
- Colloids. *A **colloid*** is somewhat similar to a suspension, but the substances in the mixture are often translucent and do not precipitate like the solutes in blood. The cell cytoplasm and its lattice-like microstructures, for example, have a gel-like consistency that keeps the various molecules dispersed throughout this mixture. Many important metabolic reactions take place within the gel-like colloidal fluids of the cytoplasmic structures.

ISOMERS

The glucose molecule is an example of an **isomer** because it can exist in two different geometric configurations with the same chemical formula but with its atoms joined together in different ways. Isomers play a vital role in metabolism because of their specific interaction with enzymes. Often enzymes will interact only with the specific isomer of a compound. Figure 1–11 shows the difference between the D and L mirror images of glucose. In D-glucose, three of the four hydroxyl groups (OH) are located on the right side of the carbon chain; in L-glucose, three of the four OH groups are positioned on the left side of the carbon chain. In actuality, glucose exists as a ring structure shown in Figure 1–12.

The D and L nomenclature relates to the direction that polarized light bends when it passes through a solution of the substance (the D stands for dextrorotary, or turning toward the right, and L is levulorotary, or turning toward the left). The D configuration of the glucose isomer is the form metabolized in the body; it is in this form that glucose occurs in the diet. The body's enzymes cannot act on L-glucose. There are also D and L forms of amino acids and fatty acids. Figure 1–13 shows the two isomers of the amino acid alanine. Mainly the L form of the amino acids is present in proteins, and only limited metabolism is possible for the D-form amino acids.

Cis and Trans Isomers. Another aspect of isomers is the configuration of their hydrogen atoms in relation to their bonding with carbon. Figure 1–14 shows the two common forms of such isomers. In a cis isomer present in fatty acids, the H atoms are positioned on the same side of the carbon's double bond; this isomeric form takes on a U shape. The presence of ad-

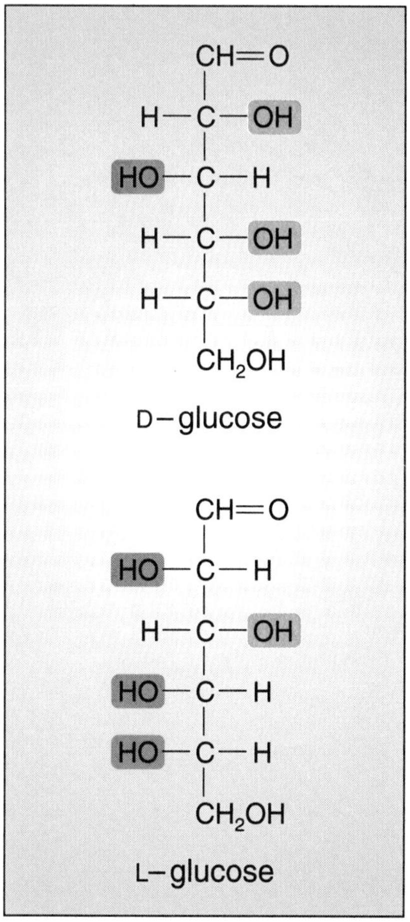

FIG. 1–11. Glucose is an example of an isomer because it can exist in two different geometric configurations with the same chemical formula but with its atoms joined differently.

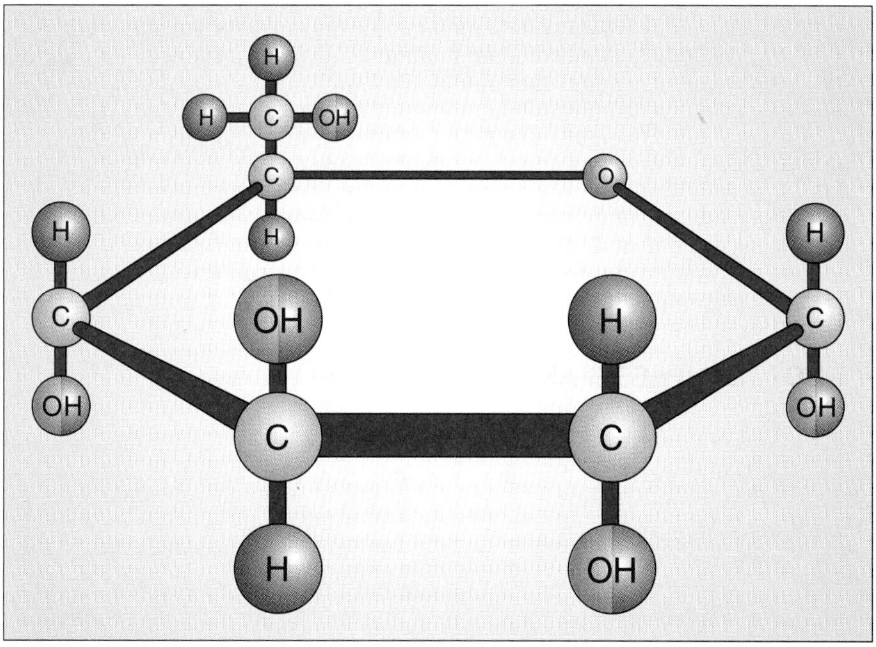

FIG. 1–12. Three-dimensional ring structure of the simple sugar molecule glucose. The molecule resembles a hexagonal plate to which H and O atoms are attached.

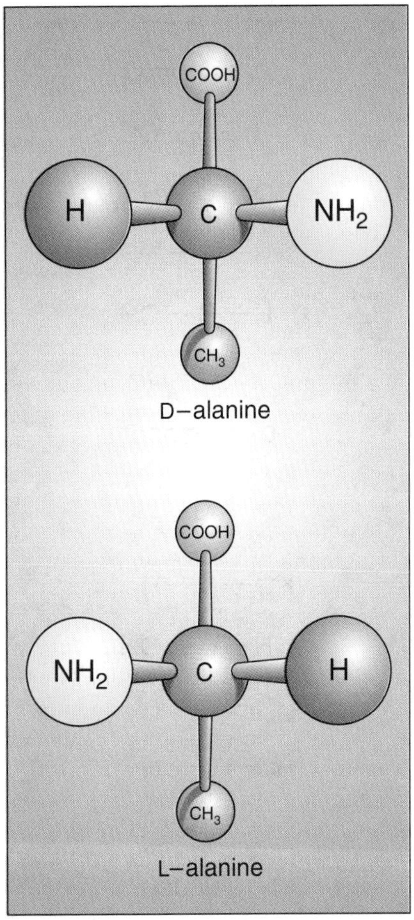

FIG. 1–13. Two isomers of the amino acid alanine.

Interconversions of energy. The underlying principle is that energy is not produced, consumed, or used up: it is merely transformed from one form into another.

ditional double bonds means that the molecule becomes even more convoluted. In **trans fatty acids,** the H atoms lie across from each other in relation to the double bond between carbons. Trans fatty acids are more linear in structure and are similar in shape to long-chain fatty acids.

In the manufacture of margarine, trans fatty acids are formed as shown in Figure 1–14 for trans elaidic acid. Note that the two H atoms lie on opposite sides of the double bond between the two C atoms. The cis form of this fatty acid differs from the trans form only in the position of the two H atoms. From a health standpoint, however, the trans form of fatty acids may elevate a potentially harmful form of cholesterol and depress a beneficial form. The structural differences between margarine and butter and the possible medical consequences of the various forms of cholesterol are discussed more fully in Chapter 4.

ENERGY

All forms of biologic work are powered by the direct transfer of chemical energy. Performance in swimming, jogging, aerobic dancing, or competitive tennis is greatly influenced by our capacity to extract energy from food nutrients and ultimately transfer it to the contractile proteins of skeletal muscle. But unlike the physical properties of matter, it is difficult to define energy in concrete terms of size, shape, or mass. Rather, all forms of energy are associated with motion; this suggests a dynamic state related to a condition of *change,* because the presence of energy is revealed only when a change has taken place. *Within this context,* ***energy*** *is related to the performance of work.* As work increases, the transfer of energy increases so that a change occurs.

THE FIRST LAW OF THERMODYNAMICS

The ***first law of thermodynamics*** *states that energy is neither created nor destroyed, but is transformed from one form to another.* In essence, this is the immutable principle of the conservation of energy that applies to both living and nonliving systems. The large amount of chemical energy in fuel oil, for example, is readily converted to heat energy in the home oil burner. In the body, however, not all of the chemical energy trapped within food nutrients is immediately lost as heat; rather, a large portion is conserved as chemical energy and then changed into mechanical energy (and ultimately heat energy) by the action of the musculoskeletal system. Figure 1–15 illustrates the interconversions for six different forms of energy.

PHOTOSYNTHESIS AND RESPIRATION

The most fundamental examples of energy conversion in living cells are the processes of photosynthesis and respiration.

PHOTOSYNTHESIS

In the sun, with a temperature of several million degrees Fahrenheit, part of the potential energy stored in the nucleus of the hydrogen atom is released by the process of nuclear fusion. This energy, in the form of gamma radiation, is then converted to radiant energy.

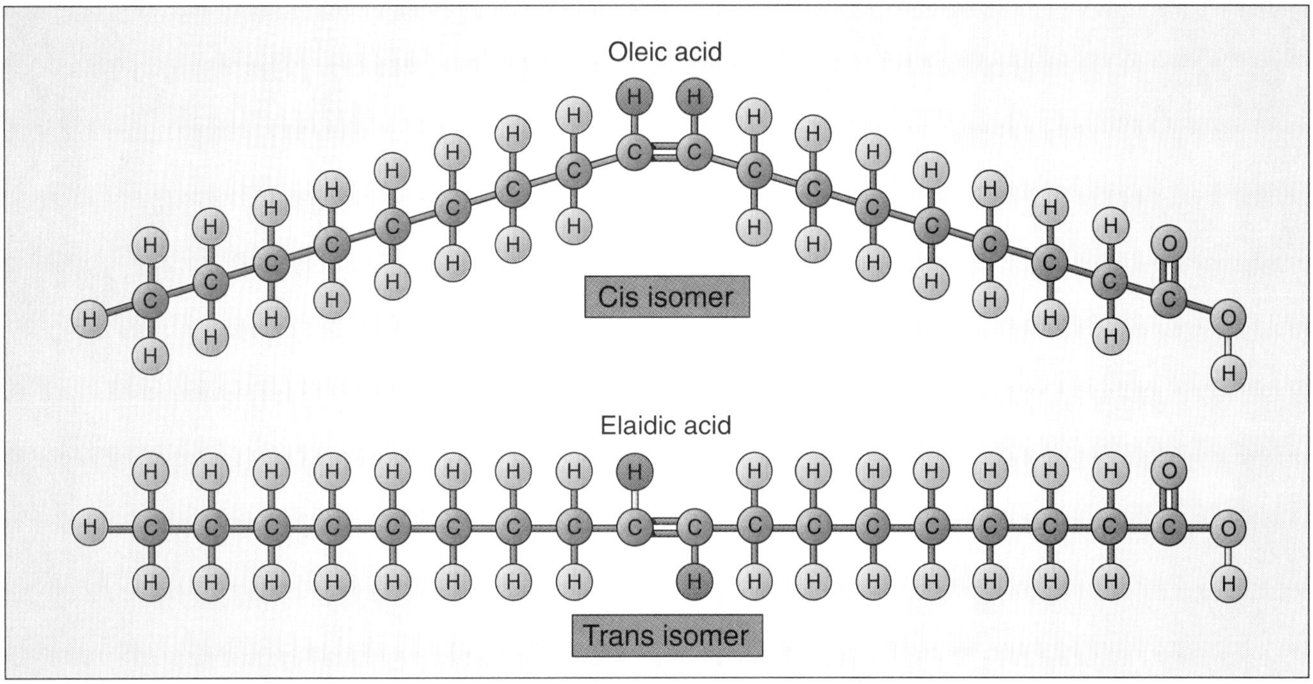

FIG. 1–14. Cis and trans isomers of two fatty acids.

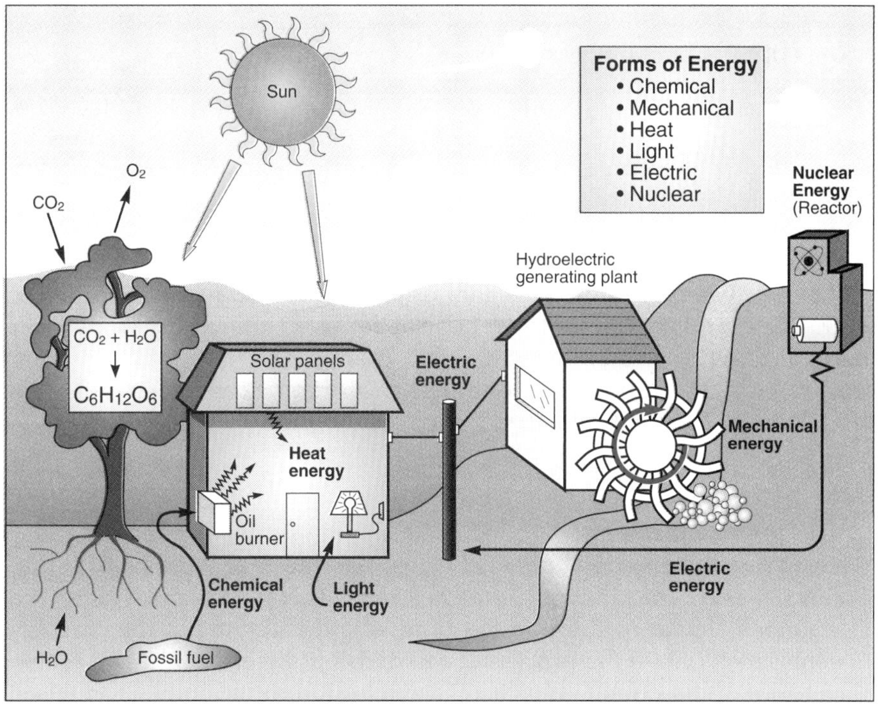

FIG. 1–15. Interconversions of the six different forms of energy.

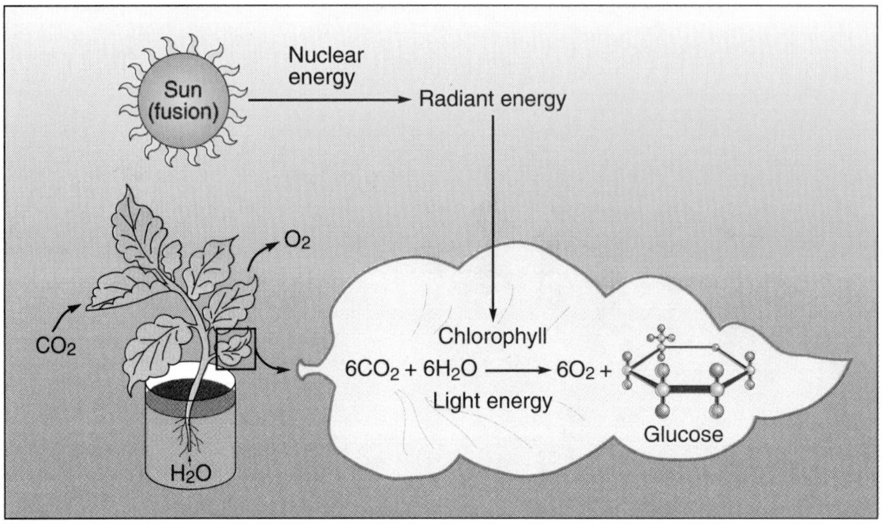

FIG. 1–16. The process of photosynthesis.

Figure 1–16 illustrates that during **photosynthesis,** the plant pigment chlorophyll is contained in *chloroplasts,* the large organelles located in leaf cells, and absorbs radiant (solar) energy to facilitate the synthesis of energy-rich chemical compounds. The end result of photosynthesis creates glucose from carbon dioxide and water, and releases oxygen. Glucose and oxygen are subsequently used by animals in the process of respiration. In plants, carbohydrates can be converted to fats and proteins for storage as a reserve of potential energy for future use. Animals then ingest the plant nutrients to serve their own energy needs. *In essence, solar energy coupled with photosynthesis powers the animal world with food and oxygen.*

CELLULAR RESPIRATION

The process of **respiration** is the reverse of photosynthesis. During these reactions, the chemical energy stored in glucose, fat, and protein molecules is extracted in the presence of oxygen. A portion of the energy released can be conserved in other chemical compounds and then used by the body for its energy-requiring processes; the remaining energy flows to the environment as heat.

Biologic work. Biologic work encompasses all of the energy-requiring, life-sustaining processes of the cell.

The energy released during cellular respiration is used to sustain **biologic work.** This can take one of three familiar forms as shown in Figure 1–17: mechanical work of muscle contraction, chemical work that involves the synthesis of cellular molecules, or transport work that concentrates various substances in the intracellular and extracellular fluids.

- Mechanical work. The most obvious example of energy transformation in the body is the **mechanical work** generated by muscle contraction. The protein filaments of the muscle fibers directly convert chemical energy into mechanical energy. However, this is not the body's only form of mechanical work. In the cell nucleus, for example, contractile elements similar to those found in muscle literally tug at the chromosomes to facilitate the process of cell division. Mechanical work is also performed by specialized structures such as cilia that are part of many cells.

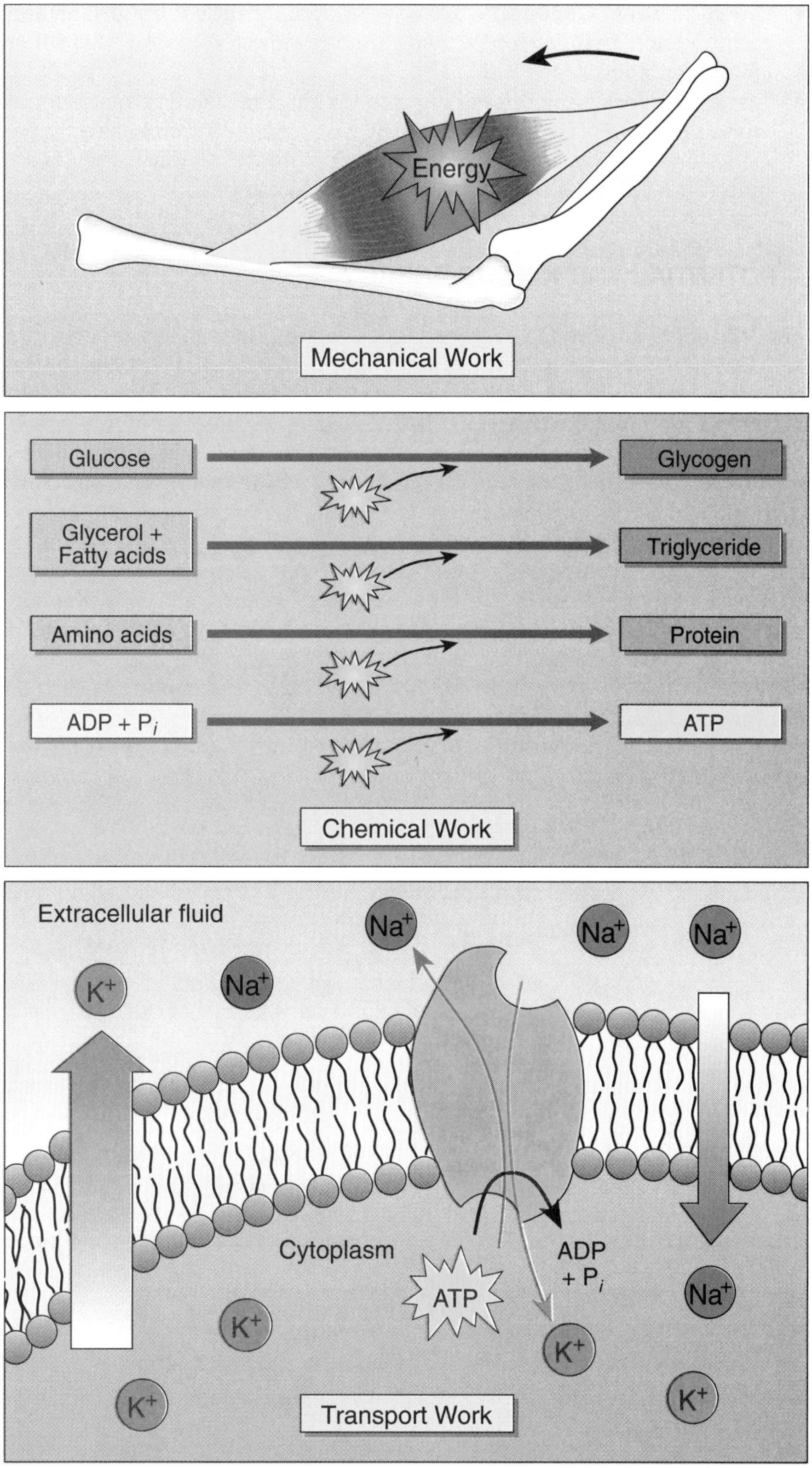

FIG. 1–17. The process of respiration generates energy for mechanical work, chemical work, and transport work.

- Chemical work. **Chemical work** is performed by all cells for growth and maintenance. Cellular components are continually synthesized as other components are destroyed.
- Transport work. Much less conspicuous than mechanical or chemical work is **transport work,** or the biologic work of concentrating substances in the body. A continual expenditure of stored chemical energy is required to accomplish this "quiet" form of biologic work.

POTENTIAL AND KINETIC ENERGY

The total energy of any system consists of two components: potential energy and kinetic energy. Figure 1–18 illustrates that **potential energy** can be energy of position, such as the energy possessed by water at the top of a hill before it flows downstream. In this example, the energy change is proportional to the vertical drop of the water. Potential energy can also be light energy, electric energy, or bound energy within the internal structure of a nutrient. *When potential energy is released, it is transformed into **kinetic energy,** or energy of motion.* In some cases, the bound energy in one substance can be directly transferred to other substances to increase their potential energy. Energy transfers of this type are necessary for the body's chemical work of **biosynthesis.** In this process, specific building-block atoms such as carbon, hydrogen, oxygen, and nitrogen are activated and join other atoms and molecules to synthesize important biologic compounds such as cholesterol, enzymes, and hormones. Some of the newly created compounds serve structural needs, such as the protein-rich contractile elements of muscle or the fat-containing membranous covering of cells. Other energy-

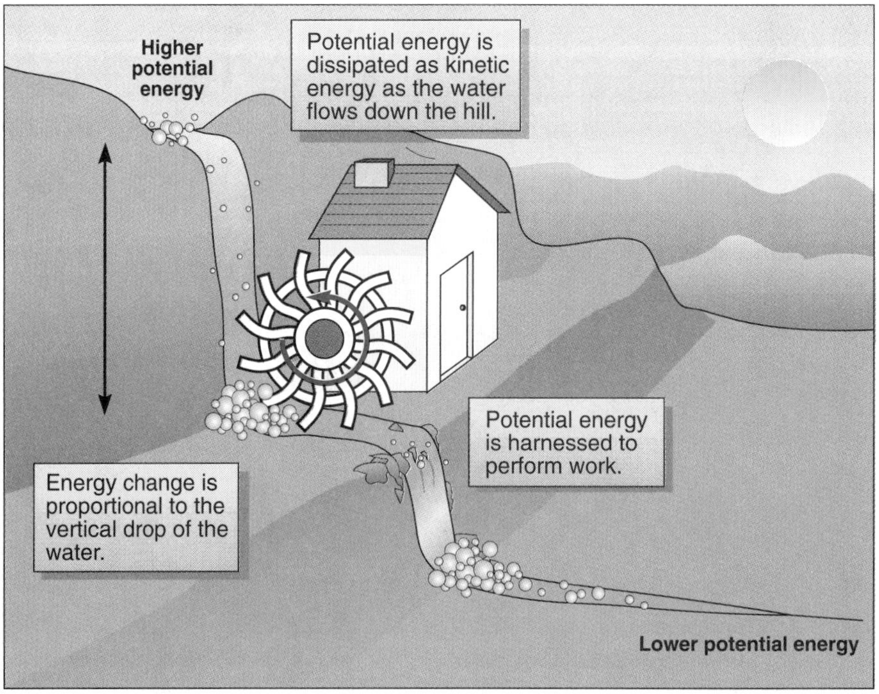

FIG. 1–18. Potential energy that performs work is transformed into kinetic energy.

rich compounds can serve the cell's energy needs; this occurs, for example, when ATP is "split" apart during its own chemical breakdown.

Enzymes work extremely fast. In a typical mitochondrion, there may be as many as 10 billion enzyme molecules, each carrying out millions of operations within a short time period. During exercise, the rate of increase in enzyme activity within the cell speeds up tremendously.

ENZYMES

*An **enzyme** is a catalyst that tremendously accelerates the forward and reverse rates of chemical reactions within cells without being consumed or changed in the reaction.* Within the fluids of a single cell there can be as many as four thousand different enzymes, each performing a specific function. Almost every chemical reaction within a cell is catalyzed by its specific enzyme. Enzymes make contact at precise locations on the surfaces of cell structures, and they often work within the structure itself. Many enzymes also are operative outside the cell, such as in the bloodstream, in the digestive mixture, and in the fluids of the small intestine.

Enzymes are usually named for the function they perform. For example, the suffix *-ase* is often appended to the specific molecule on which the enzyme operates. Hydrol*ase* adds water during hydrolysis reactions, prote*ase* interacts with protein, oxid*ase* adds oxygen to a substance, and ribonucle*ase* splits apart RNA. What is truly remarkable is that enzymes do not all operate at the same rate: some operate slowly, while others act quite rapidly. Enzymes often work cooperatively among their binding sites. While one enzyme is "turned on" at a particular site, its neighbor is "turned off" until the job is completed; the operation can then be reversed, with one enzyme becoming inactive and the other active. When a substance is acted on by an enzyme, the term **substrate** is used to denote that the enzyme functioned as a catalyst on that substance. Enzymes also can act along small regions of the substrate and begin their task over again, each time working at a different rate than previously! Some enzymes delay when they begin to work. A good example is the precursor enzyme trypsinogen that is manufactured by the pancreas. Following a delay, trypsinogen is secreted into the small intestine where it functions as the active enzyme trypsin to digest complex proteins to simple amino acids (referred to as *proteolytic action*). Without a delay in its activity, trypsinogen would literally digest the pancreatic tissue that produced it. Other enzymes are inactivated once they perform their specific function. For example, once the blood-clotting enzymes have carried out their coagulation functions, they cease activity; if they did not, the blood vessels would become clogged with continually clotting blood.

Catalysts: chemical facilitators. The increased rate of a catalyzed reaction can be 10^6 to 10^{12} times faster than an uncatalyzed reaction under similar conditions.

Digestive enzymes. The maltase enzyme (facilitates the conversion of maltose to 2 glucose molecules) is synthesized in the intestinal wall, as are the enzymes sucrase (that interacts with sucrose to form glucose and fructose), lactase (that binds with lactose to form glucose and galactose), aminopeptidase (that catalyzes peptides to create amino acids and smaller peptides), and enterokinase (that forms trypsin after it acts on its substrate trypsinogen).

A unique characteristic of an enzyme, as illustrated in Figure 1–19, is its interaction with one specific substrate to perform a specific function. The enzyme becomes turned on when its active site is joined in a "perfect fit" with the active site on the substrate. The example shows the sequence of steps for interaction of the enzyme maltase with its substrate maltose in the intestinal wall. *Step 1* is to achieve a fit between the active sites of the enzyme and substrate to form an **enzyme-substrate complex.** In *Step 2*, the enzyme catalyzes (speeds up) the chemical reaction with the substrate. Note that a water molecule is liberated during this hydrolysis process. *Step 3* produces an end product. In the example, the major end product is glucose.

The enzyme-substrate interaction resembles a key fitting into a lock, and is known as the **lock and key mechanism.** This interactive process assures that the correct enzyme "mates" with its specific substrate to carry out a particular function. Once the enzyme and substrate are joined, a confor-

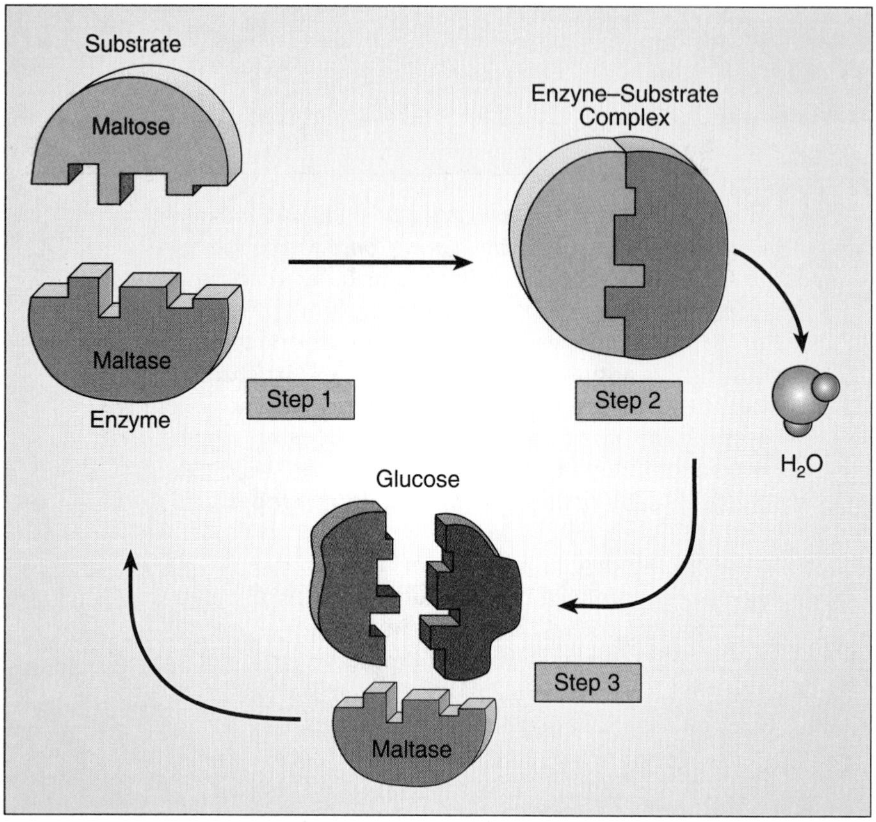

FIG. 1–19. Sequence of steps in the "lock and key" mechanism of an enzyme with its substrate. The example shows the formation of glucose following interaction of the enzyme maltase with its substrate maltose.

mational change in shape of the enzyme takes place as it molds to its substrate.

Conformational change. Even if an enzyme happens to link with a substrate, unless the specific conformational change in shape of the enzyme takes place, the enzyme will not interact chemically with the substrate.

The lock and key mechanism is essentially protective in that only the correct substrate becomes activated by the correct enzyme. A typical example involves the enzyme hexokinase, which accelerates a chemical reaction when it links with a glucose molecule. When this occurs, a phosphate molecule is transferred from ATP to a specific binding site on one of glucose's carbon atoms. Once the two binding sites join to form a glucose-hexokinase complex, the substrate is degraded in stepwise fashion to less complex molecules in the process of energy metabolism. This process by which energy is extracted from carbohydrate, lipid, and protein molecules for use by the body is discussed in Chapter 11.

HYDROLYSIS AND CONDENSATION: THE BASIS FOR DIGESTION AND SYNTHESIS

HYDROLYSIS REACTIONS

Hydrolysis *is a basic digestive process in which complex organic molecules such as carbohydrates, lipids, and proteins are degraded, or catabolized, into simpler forms that the body can more easily assimilate.* During the chemical decomposition process of hydrolysis, energy is released when covalent bonds are broken by addition of the constituents of water (H and OH) to the by-products of the reaction. Examples of hydrolysis are the digestion of the food nutrients: starches and disaccharides to monosaccharides, proteins to amino acids, and lipids to fatty acids. The hydrolysis of each nutrient is catalyzed by its specific enzyme. For the disaccharides lactose, sucrose, and maltose, for example, the specific enzymes are lactase, sucrase, and maltase, respectively. The lipid enzymes are called lipases; they degrade the lipid molecule when water is added, causing the fatty acids to be cleaved from their glycerol backbone. During the digestion of proteins, the protease splitting enzymes require water to degrade the peptide linkages to their simple amino acids. More detailed information about the digestive process is presented in Chapter 3 for carbohydrates, Chapter 4 for lipids, and Chapter 5 for proteins.

The general form for all hydrolysis reactions is as follows:

$$AB + HOH \rightarrow A\text{-}H + B\text{-}OH$$

When water is added to the substance AB, the covalent bond that joins AB is decomposed to produce the breakdown products A-H (H is a hydrogen atom from water) and B-OH (OH is the remaining hydroxyl group from water). Figure 1–20A shows the hydrolysis reaction for the disaccharide sucrose to its end-product molecules glucose and fructose; also illustrated is the hydrolysis of a dipeptide (protein) into its two constituent amino acid units. Intestinal absorption occurs quickly following hydrolysis of the carbohydrate, lipid, and protein nutrients.

CONDENSATION REACTIONS

Because the reactions illustrated for hydrolysis can also occur in the opposite direction, that is, they are reversible, the compound AB can be synthesized from A-H and B-OH in the process of **condensation.** In this building, or anabolic, process a molecule of water is formed. The structural components of the nutrients are bound together in condensation reactions to form more complex molecules. Figure 1–20B shows the condensation reaction for the synthesis of maltose from two glucose units and the creation of a more complex protein from two amino acid units. In the synthesis of proteins, note that a hydroxyl is removed from one amino acid, and a hydrogen from the other, to create a water molecule. For the protein, the new bond is called a **peptide bond.** A similar production of water occurs in the synthesis of complex carbohydrates from simple sugars, and for fats from the union of their glycerol and fatty acid components.

OXIDATION AND REDUCTION REACTIONS

Literally thousands of simultaneous chemical reactions occur in the body that involve the transfer of electrons from one substance to another. ***Oxidation*** *reactions are those that involve the transfer of either oxygen atoms, hydrogen atoms, or electrons.* When hydrogen is removed from a substance, for example, there is a net *gain* of valence electrons. In **reduction** reactions, electrons are gained from a substance and there is a net *loss* of valence electrons.

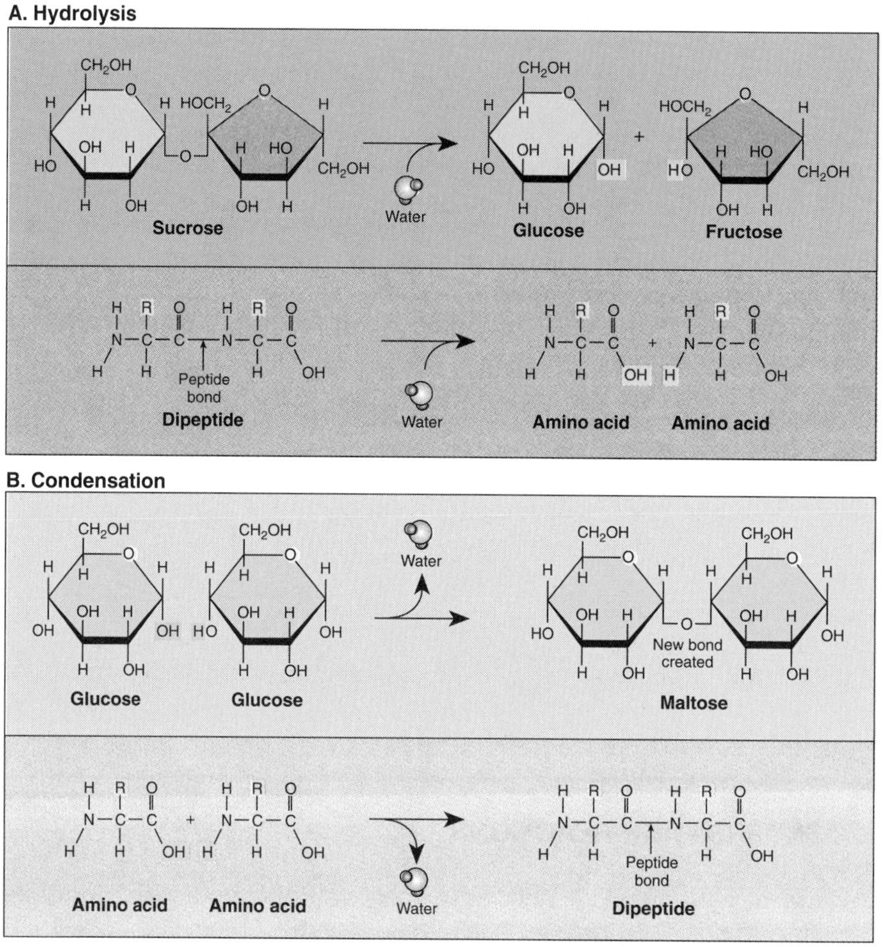

FIG. 1–20. **A.** Hydrolysis reaction for the disaccharide sucrose to the end-product molecules glucose and fructose, and a hydrolysis chemical reaction for a dipeptide (protein) into two amino acid end-product units. **B.** Condensation reaction for the synthesis of maltose from two glucose units, and the creation of a protein polymer from two amino acid units. The latter reaction is the reverse of the hydrolysis reaction for the dipeptide. The symbol *R* represents the remainder of the amino acid molecule.

Oxidation and reduction reactions are characteristically coupled: whenever oxidation occurs, the reverse reaction of reduction also takes place and the electrons lost from one substance are gained by the other. An oxidation-reduction reaction is also called a **redox reaction.** Reduction *involves any process in which the atoms in an element gain electrons with a corresponding decrease in valence.*

An excellent example of an oxidation reaction is the transfer of electrons in the mitochondria. Here, hydrogen atoms are oxidized and the removed electrons are passed by special carriers to be delivered ultimately to oxygen, which becomes reduced. The source of hydrogen is the carbohydrate, lipid, and protein nutrient substrates. The enzymes that speed up the redox reactions are called dehydrogenases or oxidases. Two of the hydrogen-accepting coenzymes are the vitamin-B–containing nicotinamide-adenine dinucleotide **(NAD)** and flavin adenine dinucleotide **(FAD).** Energy in the form of ATP is harnessed during the transfer of electrons from NAD to FAD.

The transport of electrons by specific carrier molecules constitutes the **respiratory chain.** This is the final common pathway in aerobic (oxidative) metabolism and is referred to as **electron transport.** For each pair of hydrogen atoms, two electrons flow down the chain and reduce one atom of oxygen. To complete the process, oxygen also accepts hydrogen to form water. This coupled redox process constitutes the oxidation of hydrogen and subsequent reduction of oxygen. Much of the energy generated in cellular oxidation-reduction reactions is trapped or conserved as chemical energy to power the cell's various forms of biologic work.

Figure 1–21 illustrates a redox reaction during vigorous physical activity. As exercise becomes intense, more hydrogen atoms are stripped from the carbohydrate substrate than can be oxidized in reactions in the respiratory chain that utilize oxygen. For energy metabolism to continue, these non-oxidized excess hydrogens must be "accepted" by a chemical other than oxygen. This is exactly the case, as a molecule of pyruvic acid, an intermediate compound formed in the initial phase of carbohydrate metabolism, temporarily accepts a pair of hydrogens (electrons). This reduction of pyruvic acid by accepting hydrogens forms a new compound called lactic acid. The more intense the exercise, the greater the flow of excess hydrogens to pyruvic acid, and lactic acid increases rapidly. During recovery, the excess hydrogens used to form lactic acid can now be oxidized (electrons removed and passed to NAD) and the oxidized pyruvic acid molecule is reformed.

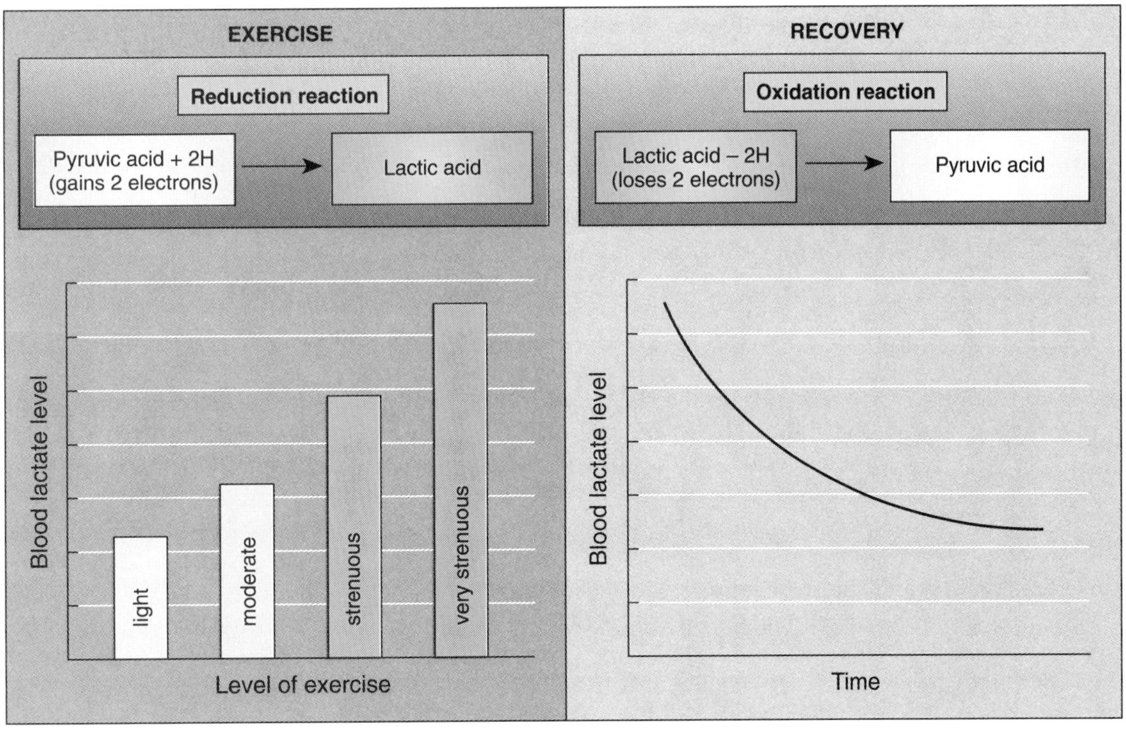

FIG. 1–21. Example of a redox (oxidation-reduction) reaction: pyruvic acid ↔ lactic acid.

ACID-BASE CONCENTRATION AND pH

Acid. *An **acid** is any substance that ionizes in solution to give off positive hydrogen ions (H^+).* Acids taste sour, turn litmus indicators red, react with bases to form salts, and cause some metals to liberate hydrogen. Examples of acids in the body include hydrochloric, phosphoric, carbonic, citric, and carboxylic acids.

Base. *A **base** is any substance that forms hydroxide ions (OH^-) in water solutions.* Alkaline solutions taste bitter, are slippery to the touch, turn litmus indicators blue, and react with acids to form salts. Examples of bases in the body include sodium and calcium hydroxide, and water solutions of ammonia that form ammonium hydroxide.

pH and H^+. There is an inverse relation between pH and the concentration of H^+. Because the pH scale is logarithmic, a one-unit change in pH is associated with a tenfold change in H^+ concentration. For example, lemon juice and gastric juice (pH = 2.0) have 1000 times greater H^+ concentration than black coffee (pH = 5), while hydrochloric acid is about one million times greater in H^+ concentration compared to blood!

pH. *The **pH** is a quantitative measure of the acidity or alkalinity (basicity) of a liquid solution.* Specifically, pH refers to the concentration of protons, or H^+. Solutions with relatively more OH^- than H^+ have a pH above 7.0 and are called **basic** or alkaline. Conversely, solutions with more H^+ than OH^- have a pH below 7.0 and are termed **acidic.** Chemically pure or distilled water is considered neutral with an equal amount of H^+ and OH^- and thus a pH of 7.0. The pH scale shown in Figure 1–22 was devised in 1909 by the Danish chemist Sören Sörensen. It ranges from +1.0 to +14.0. The pH of body fluids ranges from a very low pH of 1.0 for the digestive acid hydrochloric acid to a slightly basic pH of between 7.35 and 7.45 for arterial and venous blood and most other body fluids.

Foods are referred to as "acid forming" or "alkaline forming" depending on how they ultimately affect the pH of urine. An acidic residue is formed when the elements phosphorus, sulfur, and chlorine are completely oxidized; a basic residue remains when the elements sodium, potassium, calcium, and magnesium are oxidized. **Acid-forming foods** include meat, eggs, cereal products, bread, corn, and many foods with high protein content. In contrast, the **alkaline-forming foods** include most fruits (except plums, prunes, and cranberries, which contain benzoic and quinic acids), vegetables, and milk products (despite their high protein content). When the acid content of the stomach is high, the body does its best to neutralize or buffer excess H^+ with alkaline secretions from the pancreas. Buffers are discussed in the following section.

pH drops during maximal exercise. During maximal exercise, the arterial blood pH drops from a resting value of about 7.4 to a pH of about 7.0 or slightly lower. The pH is then restored to the resting value during recovery.

Enzymes and pH. Many chemical processes in the body occur only at a specific pH. An enzyme that works at one pH becomes inactivated when the pH of its surroundings change. The fat-digesting enzyme gastric lipase, for example, is effective in the highly acidic stomach environment but ceases to function within the slightly alkaline small intestine. The same is true for salivary amylase, the enzyme that begins starch breakdown in the mouth. The pH of the salivary fluids ranges between 6.4 and 7.0. When passed to the stomach (pH 1.0 to 2.0), this enzyme ceases its digestive function and is itself digested like any other protein by the stomach acids. As a general rule, extreme changes in pH produce irreversible damage to enzymes. For this reason, the body's pH (acid-base) balance is maintained within narrow limits.

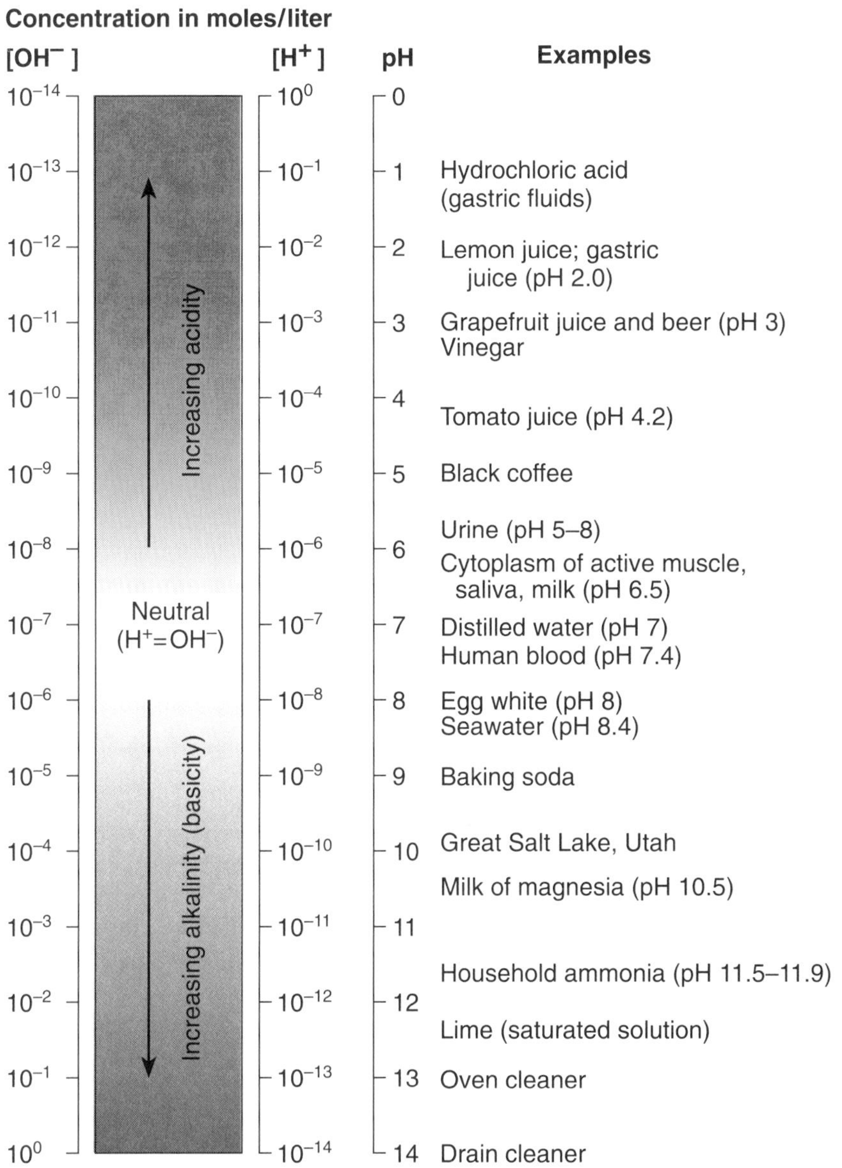

FIG. 1–22. The pH scale is a quantitative measure of the acidity or alkalinity (basicity) of a liquid solution.

BUFFERS

The term buffering is used to designate reactions that minimize changes in H^+ concentration; the chemical or physiologic mechanisms that prevent this change are termed **buffers.** In the body, any decrease in pH above the normal, slightly alkaline average of 7.4 is the result of an increase in H^+ concentration and is referred to as **acidosis.** Conversely, a decrease in H^+ concentration (increase in pH) is termed **alkalosis.** If the buffer system is unable to neutralize deviations in H^+, effective bodily function becomes disrupted with the end result of coma or eventual death. Three mechanisms control the acid-base quality of our internal environment: chemical buffers, pulmonary ventilation, and kidney function.

CHEMICAL BUFFERS

The **chemical buffering** system consists of a weak acid and a base or salt of that acid. The body's bicarbonate buffer, for example, consists of the weak carbonic acid and its salt, sodium bicarbonate. Carbonic acid is formed when the bicarbonate binds H^+. As long as H^+ concentration remains elevated, the reaction continually converts stronger acids to the weaker carbonic acid because the excess H^+ are bound in accordance with the general reaction:

$$H^+ + \text{Buffer} \rightarrow \text{H-Buffer}$$

The strong stomach acid, hydrochloric acid, is changed into the much weaker carbonic acid by combining with sodium bicarbonate. As a result, only a slight reduction is noted in pH. If the body's buffer response is inadequate and stomach acidity remains elevated, many individuals seek "outside help" in the form of ingested neutralizing agents (Rolaids, Maalox, and Mylanta) to provide buffering relief.

If, however, the concentration of H^+ decreases and the body fluids become more alkaline, the buffering reaction moves in the opposite direction. In the process, H^+ are released and acidity increases:

$$H^+ + \text{Buffer} \leftarrow \text{H-Buffer}$$

In addition to digestive juices, other acids are continually being produced in the body. Much of the carbon dioxide generated in energy metabolism reacts with water to form carbonic acid ($CO_2 + H_2O \rightarrow H_2CO_3$). This then dissociates into H^+ and HCO_3^-. Likewise, lactic acid, a strong metabolic acid, is buffered by sodium bicarbonate to form sodium lactate and the relatively weak carbonic acid; in turn, carbonic acid separates and increases the H^+ concentration of bodily fluids. Other organic acids such as fatty acids dissociate and liberate H^+, as do the sulfuric and phosphoric acids produced during protein breakdown.

Other chemical buffers available to the body include the phosphate buffers, consisting of phosphoric acid and sodium phosphate. These chemicals act in a manner similar to the bicarbonate system. The phosphate buffers regulate the acid-base quality of the kidney tubules and intracellular fluids, in which there is a relatively high concentration of phosphates. Carbonic acid is buffered by the protein-containing hemoglobin compound as well as by other plasma proteins.

VENTILATORY BUFFER

Any increase in H^+ concentration in body fluids stimulates the respiratory center to increase breathing. This adjustment causes a greater than normal amount of carbon dioxide to leave the blood. Recall that a large amount of this gas is transported dissolved in the blood and combined with water as carbonic acid. Thus, reducing the carbon dioxide content of the body acts directly as a **ventilatory buffer** to reduce the quantity of carbonic acid, and the body fluids become more alkaline. Conversely, reducing normal ventilation causes carbon dioxide to build up, and the fluids become more acidic.

RENAL BUFFER

The excretion of H^+ by the kidneys, although more time-consuming than the action of the chemical and ventilatory buffers, is required if the long-term acid-base quality of body fluids is to be maintained. To this end, the kidneys stand as final sentinels. Acidity is controlled by the **renal buffer** through alterations in the amount of bicarbonate ions, ammonia, and H^+ ions secreted into the urine and the alkali, chloride, and bicarbonate that is reabsorbed.

FACTORS AFFECTING pH BALANCE

Severe diarrhea and vomiting, diabetes, and intense physical activity are all factors that can dramatically alter the acid-base balance of the body.

Diarrhea. With diarrhea, sodium bicarbonate is depleted to produce an imbalance in the important bicarbonate buffering system. Loss of sodium bicarbonate leads to increased acidity that, in extreme cases, causes severe metabolic acidosis and even death. Sorbitol, one of the common ingredients in dietetic foods, can precipitate diarrhea if consumed in excess of 50 g daily because it is not easily digested and absorbed. Sorbitol is found in fruit drinks, chocolate, marmalade, canned fruits, sugarless gums, and "diabetic-type" foods.

Vomiting. Severe vomiting depletes the stomach's acidic gastric juices. This loss of hydrochloric acid produces a net decrease of total acid in the extracellular fluids and resulting metabolic alkalosis.

Diabetes. When insulin production is normal, energy is provided primarily from a mixture of carbohydrate and fat. In **diabetes,** however, the lack of insulin limits carbohydrate utilization, and fat becomes the major energy source. Such reliance on fat for energy produces acid by-products that can lead to an acidotic condition. Additional water and sodium are lost as these acids are excreted by the kidneys. This limits the availability of sodium to form the strong chemical buffer sodium bicarbonate. If the imbalance continues, the person will eventually lapse into a coma from the resulting metabolic acidosis. Immediate countermeasures include ingestion of carbohydrate and injection of synthetic insulin to facilitate glucose transport into the cell.

Effects of Strenuous Exercise. In strenuous exercise, large amounts of the metabolic by-product lactic acid leave active muscle and enter the bloodstream. This acid production can dramatically alter local muscle and blood pH, as shown in Figure 1–23. At the point of physical exhaustion, the blood pH is often as low as 6.8. The individual becomes disoriented and nauseated, and suffers severe headaches. Even though the body's buffering systems are attempting to maintain an acid-base balance throughout exercise, it is only when exercise ceases that the blood pH quickly stabilizes and returns to normal. In addition to the bicarbonate buffer, the protein-containing compound hemoglobin along with phosphate buffers serve as important neutralizing agents in the blood during vigorous physical activity.

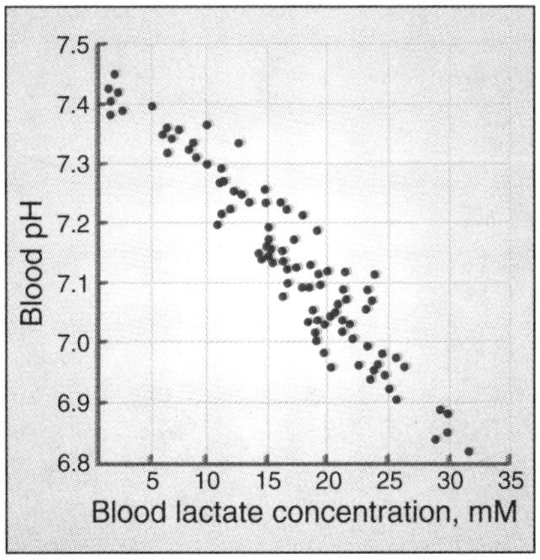

FIG. 1–23. The relationship between blood pH and blood lactic acid concentration at rest and during increasing intensities of short-duration exercise up to the maximum.

TRANSPORT OF NUTRIENTS ACROSS CELL MEMBRANES

At any moment, literally thousands of chemicals such as ions, vitamins, minerals, acids, salts, water, gases, hormones, and carbohydrate, protein, and lipid components traverse the bilayer plasma membrane as exchange takes place between the cell and its surroundings. The plasma membrane, however, is highly permeable to some substances but not to others. Such selective permeability allows the cell to maintain reasonable consistency in its chemical composition. When this equilibrium, or homeostasis, is disrupted, immediate adjustments occur to restore constancy in the cell's internal "milieu." **Homeostasis** *is a concept in biology that reflects the dynamic action of the body's various physiologic systems to regulate and maintain a relatively stable physical state and chemical composition.* This is accomplished by two processes: **passive transport** of substances through the cellular membrane, where no energy is required; and **active transport** through the membrane, where metabolic energy in the form of ATP is used to "power" the exchange of materials.

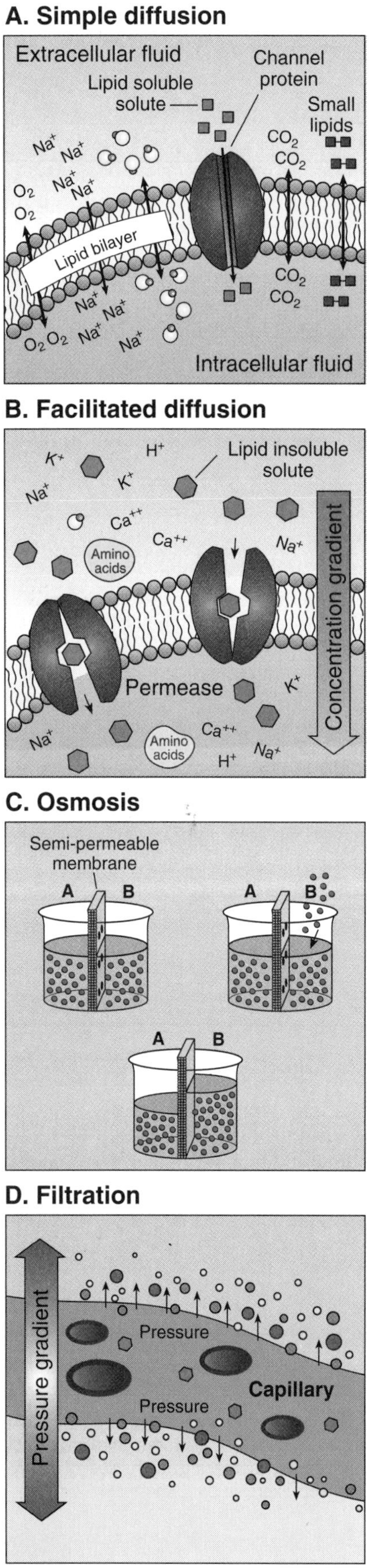

FIG. 1–24. A. Simple diffusion. **B.** Facilitated diffusion. **C.** Osmosis. **D.** Filtration.

PASSIVE TRANSPORT PROCESSES

There are four types of passive transport: simple diffusion, facilitated diffusion, osmosis, and filtration. Figure 1–24 shows an example of each.

SIMPLE DIFFUSION

In the cellular environment, **simple diffusion** involves the free and continuous net movement of molecules in aqueous solution across the plasma membrane. In the example, note that water molecules, small lipids, and gases move unimpeded from outside the cell through the lipid bilayer to the intracellular fluid. In simple diffusion, a substance will move from an area of initial higher concentration to one of lower concentration until it becomes evenly dispersed. This is an entirely passive process, powered only by the kinetic energy of the molecules themselves, with no expenditure of cellular energy. When sugar is added to water, for example, the sugar molecules dissolve and become evenly dispersed through their continuous, random movement. If the water is hot, diffusion speeds up because a higher temperature increases molecular movement and thus the rate of diffusion. If the particles stay within a closed system, they will eventually become evenly distributed throughout the solution and the net movement of particles will cease.

Simple diffusion across the plasma membrane occurs for water molecules, the dissolved gases such as oxygen, carbon dioxide, and nitrogen, small uncharged polar molecules such as urea and alcohol, and various lipid-soluble molecules. The reason these substances diffuse so quickly is because the plasma membrane consists of sheet-like, watery structures composed mainly of lipids. This allows relatively small, uncomplicated molecules to traverse the membrane with ease. When a molecule of oxygen, for example, diffuses from a higher concentration outside the cell toward a lower concentration on the inside, it is said to move down or along its **concentration gradient.** It is this concentration gradient that determines the direction and magnitude of molecular movement. This is why oxygen molecules continuously diffuse into cells. In contrast, the concentration of carbon dioxide, an end product of energy metabolism, is high within the cell; thus, carbon dioxide moves down its concentration gradient and continually diffuses from the cell into the blood.

FACILITATED DIFFUSION

Unlike simple diffusion, in which molecules pass unaided through the semipermeable cell membrane, **facilitated diffusion** involves the passive, yet highly selective binding of lipid-insoluble molecules and other large molecules to a lipid-soluble carrier molecule. The carrier molecule is a protein called a transporter or permease that spans the plasma membrane; its function is to help transfer membrane-insoluble chemicals such as hydrogen, sodium, calcium, and potassium ions, as well as glucose and amino acids, down their concentration gradients across the plasma membrane.

The transport of glucose into the cell is an excellent example of facilitated diffusion. Glucose is a rather large, lipid-insoluble, uncharged molecule. Without its specific permease (technically D-hexose permease), it would have difficulty passing into the cell. With facilitated diffusion, however, the glucose molecule first attaches to a binding site on its specific permease in the plasma membrane. A structural change then occurs in the permease that creates a "passageway" enabling the glucose molecule to cross through the permease into the cytoplasm.

Facilitated diffusion moves chemicals rapidly. If simple diffusion were the only means for glucose to enter a cell, its maximum rate of uptake would be nearly 500 times slower compared to glucose transport by facilitated diffusion.

It is indeed fortunate that facilitated diffusion occurs, because glucose is an important energy fuel that should always be in ready supply. It is also fortunate that energy from ATP is not required to "power" glucose transport; if it were, this would only increase the demands on limited reserves of this high-energy compound. Consequently, facilitated diffusion should be considered an energy-conserving mechanism that spares cellular energy for other vital functions.

OSMOSIS

Osmosis is a special case of diffusion. It involves the movement of water through a selectively permeable membrane because of a difference in the concentration of water molecules on both sides of the membrane. Through this passive process, water is distributed throughout the fluid-containing compartments (intracellular, extracellular, plasma) of the body.

In the example in Figure 1–24C, a semipermeable membrane separates compartments A and B. When there are an equal number of solute particles on sides A and B, the same water volume is present in both compartments. If a solute is added to an aqueous solution, the concentration of the solution increases by the amount of solute added; as more solute is added, its concentration of particles increases and the concentration of water molecules correspondingly decreases. In the example, adding the solute to side B forces water from side A to move through the semipermeable membrane to side B. When this happens, the volume of water now becomes greater on side B than side A. More water flows into an area where there are more particles, leaving less water on the side with fewer solute particles. Even-

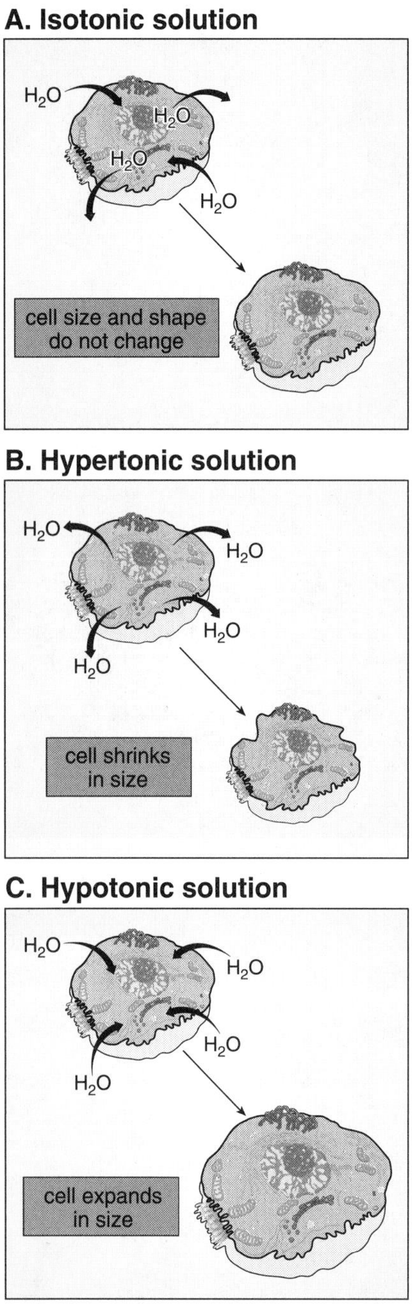

FIG. 1–25. A. Isotonic solutions. The cell retains its shape because the concentration of the solute is equal inside and outside the cell. **B.** Hypertonic solutions. The cell shrinks (crenates) because there is a higher concentration of nonpenetrating solutes outside the cell membrane than inside. **C.** Hypotonic solution. The concentration of nondiffusible solutes in the solution is diluted compared to the concentration within the cell. The cell will take on water by osmosis, and can actually burst (lyse).

tually, the concentration of solute particles on sides A and B becomes equal.

The total concentration of particles from all solutes in a solution is known as its **osmolarity.** In living tissues, there is always a difference in the osmolarity of the body's various fluid compartments. This is because the semipermeable membrane that separates different solutions retards the passage of many solute substances, particularly certain ions and intracellular proteins. This maintains a difference in solute concentration on both sides of the membrane. Because water diffuses freely through the plasma membrane, a net movement of water occurs as the system attempts to equalize osmolarity on both sides of the membrane. This often results in dramatic volume changes in the two fluid compartments. At some point, water is unable to gain further entry to the cell because the hydrostatic pressure of water on one side of the cell balances the pressure tending to draw water through the membrane. *The pressure on one side of a membrane required to prevent the osmotic movement of water from the other side is known as the **osmotic pressure** of the solution.*

Altering the internal water volume of a cell changes its shape or "tone," a characteristic referred to as tonicity. When a cell neither loses nor gains water when placed in a solution, the solution is said to be **isotonic** (Figure 1–25A). In isotonic solutions, the concentration of a nonpenetrating solute such as sodium chloride is equal on the inside and outside of the cell, and there is no net movement of water. An example of an isotonic solution is the body's extracellular fluid under normal conditions.

A solution is **hypertonic** if it contains a higher concentration of nonpenetrating solutes outside the cell membrane than inside. When this occurs, water migrates out of the cell by the process of osmosis and the cell shrinks in size. Hypertonic solutions are infused into the bloodstream when the objective is to decrease excessive accumulation of water in the tissues, a condition referred to as **edema.**

When the concentration of nondiffusible solutes outside the cell becomes diluted compared to that within the cell, the extracellular solution is considered **hypotonic.** In such cases, the cell takes on water by osmosis and appears bloated. If the condition goes uncorrected, cells can actually burst apart. Hypotonic solutions are administered during dehydration to return the tissues to isotonic conditions.

If the membrane is permeable to both the solute and water (sugar in water is a good example), then both solute and solvent molecules will diffuse until the sugar molecules are equally distributed. On the other hand, if the membrane is impermeable to the solute, then osmotic pressure will draw water in the direction that equalizes the solute concentration on both sides of the membrane. This movement of water will occur until solute concentration is equalized or until the hydrostatic pressure on one side of the membrane counteracts the force exerted by osmotic pressure.

FILTRATION

Filtration is a passive process whereby water and its solutes flow from a region of higher pressure to one of lower pressure. Filtration is the mechanism that allows plasma fluid and its solutes to move across the capillary membrane to literally bathe the tissues. The movement of plasma filtrate (the fluid portion of the blood with no significant amount of proteins) through the kidney tubules also occurs by filtration.

ACTIVE TRANSPORT PROCESSES

If a substance is unable to move across the cell membrane by one of the four passive transport processes, then energy-requiring active transport processes come into play.

Fluids that reduce swelling. Intravenous feeding of hypertonic solutions to edematous patients causes their tissues to become less swollen, as water is literally drawn from the tissue spaces into the blood and eliminated by the kidneys.

SODIUM-POTASSIUM PUMP

Figure 1–26 illustrates the operation of the **sodium-potassium pump,** one of the active transport mechanisms for moving substances through semipermeable membranes. In this process, energy from ATP serves to "pump" ions "uphill" against their electrochemical gradients through the membrane. This is accomplished by a specialized carrier protein enzyme, sodium-potassium ATPase, that serves as the basic pumping mechanism. Recall that substances usually diffuse along their concentration gradients, from an area of higher to lower concentration. In the living cell, however, diffusion alone cannot provide for the optimal distribution of cellular chemicals. Charged particles such as sodium and potassium ions, and large amino acid molecules that are insoluble in the lipid bilayer, must often move against their concentration gradients to carry out their normal functions. Sodium ions, for example, exist in relatively low concentration inside the cell, so there is a tendency for Na^+ to remain there and not pass through the membrane barrier to the outside. In contrast, potassium ions normally exist in higher concentration inside the cell and the tendency is for extracellular K^+ to remain there. However, during normal nerve and muscle function, both of these ions are continually moved against their concentration gradients so that Na^+ becomes concentrated extracellularly, whereas K^+ builds up within the cell. This ability of the sodium-potassium pump to counter the normal tendency of solutes to diffuse is indeed fortunate, for it is this mechanism that establishes the normal electrochemical gradients so that nerve and muscle can be stimulated.

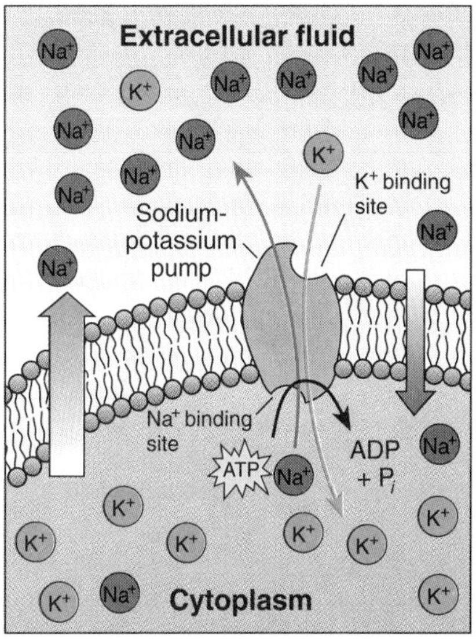

FIG. 1–26. Operation of the sodium-potassium pump.

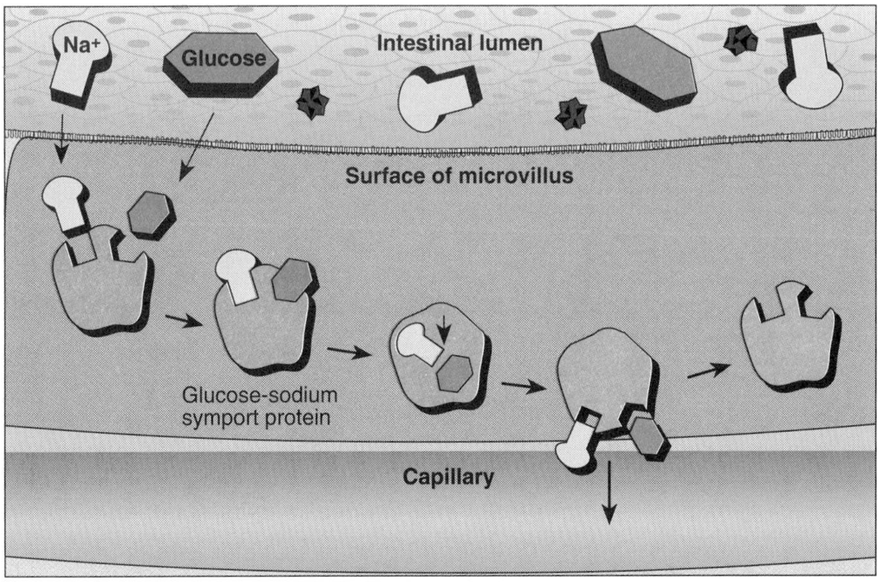

FIG. 1–27. Example of coupled transport. A molecule of glucose and a sodium ion move together in the same direction through the plasma membrane in a symport protein.

COUPLED TRANSPORT

In addition to its role in transporting sodium, potassium, and protein across cellular membranes, active transport is crucial in absorbing nutrients from the digestive tract and for reabsorbing important chemicals filtered by the kidneys. Absorption of glucose, for example, takes place by a form of active transport called **coupled transport.** In this process illustrated in Figure 1–27, a molecule of glucose and a Na^+ ion join together before they enter an intestinal villus; they then move in the same direction as they are "pumped" through the plasma membrane to the inside of the cell and finally into the bloodstream. Amino acids also join with Na^+ and pass

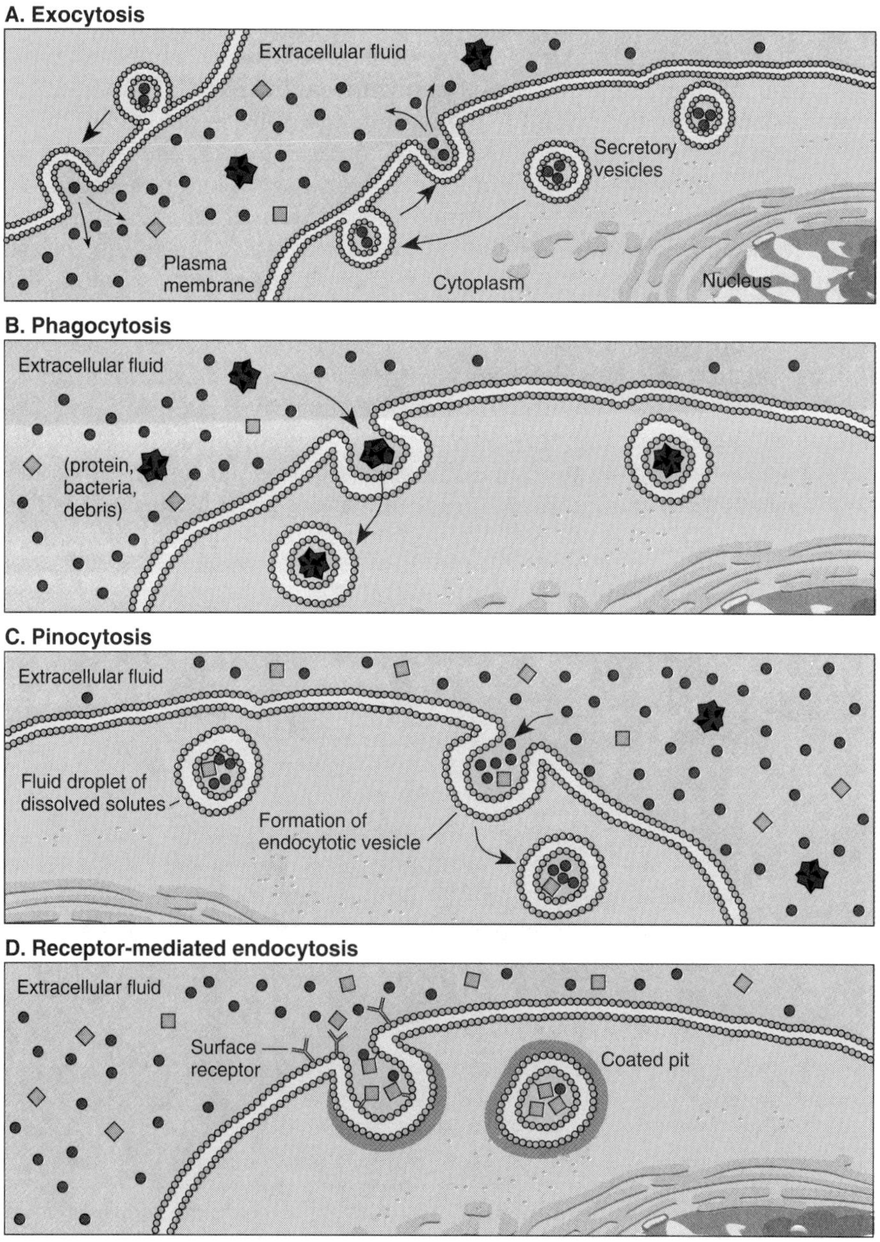

FIG. 1–28. **A.** Exocytosis. **B.** Phagocytosis. **C.** Pinocytosis. **D.** Receptor-mediated endocytosis.

through the intestinal villi. The simultaneous transport of two chemicals in the same direction is called **symport,** and each symport has its own specialized permease with a specific binding site for each substance. Coupled transport is unidirectional, so when the glucose-sodium and amino acid–sodium symports leave the intestines to enter the blood, they cannot move backward and re-enter the intestines.

Liposomes—new disease fighters. The liposome, a microscopic sphere constructed from the same lipid-like structures as the cell bilayer, may ultimately play a crucial role in fighting a variety of diseases. The ultimate shape of the liposome is physically altered by manipulating the chemistry of its internal structures. The core of the liposome is filled with a specific disease-fighting substance that travels throughout the circulation to "attack" a specific target site. By encapsulating a drug inside the liposome, the liposome and its medication become "magic bullets," efficiently delivering their healing cargo to a specific diseased site. The usefulness of this kind of cellular drug-delivery system is that there is minimal infiltration of the beneficial medication to nontarget sites. This minimizes deleterious side effects that often occur when powerful chemotherapeutic agents are administered in conventional drug therapy.

BULK TRANSPORT

Bulk transport is an energy-requiring process for moving large particles and macromolecules through cell membranes. There are two ways in which this is accomplished: exocytosis and endocytosis. Examples of both processes are illustrated in Figure 1–28.

Exocytosis. This transfer process moves substances such as hormones, neurotransmitters, and mucous secretions from the intracellular to extracellular fluids. As shown in Figure 1–28A, there are three distinct phases to **exocytosis.** First, the substance to be transferred is enclosed within a membranous, sac-like pouch. The pouch then migrates to the plasma membrane; once it fuses to the membrane, its contents are ejected into the extracellular fluids.

Endocytosis. In this transfer process of **endocytosis** substances are surrounded by the cell's plasma membrane which then pinches away and moves into the cytoplasm. Figure 1–28B–D shows three examples of endocytotic processes. In **phagocytosis,** large substances are literally engulfed by the plasma membrane. In **pinocytosis,** fluid and dissolved solutes are engulfed by the plasma membrane to form a vesicle called a coated pit that has a protein coating. In **receptor-mediated endocytosis,** receptor proteins bind specific molecules such as insulin, iron, and low-density lipoproteins. When the coated pit combines with a lysosome (a small spherical organelle containing numerous acidic hydrolytic enzymes), the engulfed substances are digested and released into the cytoplasm. The attached receptors and protein membrane are then recycled back to the plasma membrane.

2

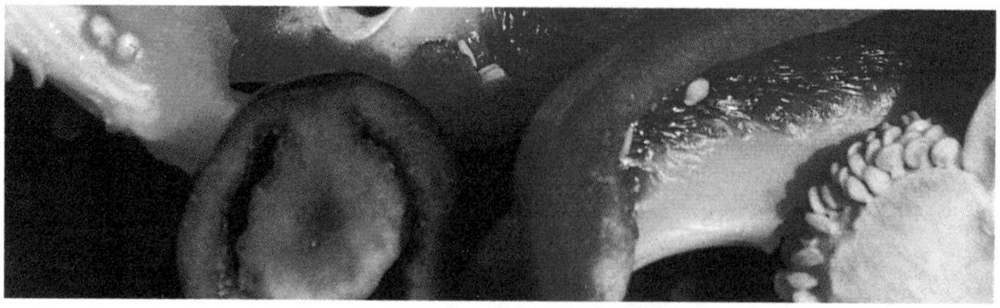

DIGESTION AND ABSORPTION OF FOOD NUTRIENTS

Hormone. A **hormone** is an organic protein-like (e.g., insulin) or fat-like (e.g., estrogen) substance produced by a gland in one part of the body and carried in the blood to exert its effect on another, often distant part. These "chemical messengers" regulate a variety of physiologic activities and contribute to the maintenance of stability, or *homeostasis*, in the internal environment.

The ultimate purpose of eating is to provide an uninterrupted supply of energy and tissue-building nutrients to sustain life. This involves complex physiologic and metabolic processes that usually progress unnoticed for a lifetime. Hormones and enzymes work nonstop in concert throughout the digestive tract to facilitate the breakdown, or hydrolysis, of more complex nutrients into simpler ones. During digestion, food is processed into simpler substances for absorption through the lining of the intestines into the blood and lymph. Self-regulating processes within the digestive tract usually move food along at a rate slow enough to allow its complete absorption, yet just rapidly enough to assure timely delivery of its nutrient contents.

THE GASTROINTESTINAL TRACT

Figure 2–1 illustrates the various structures of the **gastrointestinal tract,** which includes the esophagus, gallbladder, liver, stomach, pancreas, small intestine, large intestine, rectum, and anus. In essence, the gastrointestinal (GI) tract—also referred to as the **alimentary canal**—can be thought of as a long tube that runs from the mouth to the anus. This tube's main function is to supply the body with water and nutrients. Figure 2–1A shows the highly specialized connective tissue **mesentery** that weaves around and gives support to the approximately 2 kg mass of intestinal organs. This membrane contains a diffuse network of capillaries that transport absorbed nutrients. Figure 2–1B shows that these vessels eventually converge to become the large **hepatic-portal vein** that delivers nutrient-rich blood to the liver. Here, the nutrients are processed and then returned to the general circulation to be delivered throughout the body.

MOUTH AND ESOPHAGUS

The journey of a bite of food begins in the mouth, where food is subjected to crushing forces of up to 90 kg as it is cut, ground, softened, and mashed. This increases the surface area of the food particles, making them easier

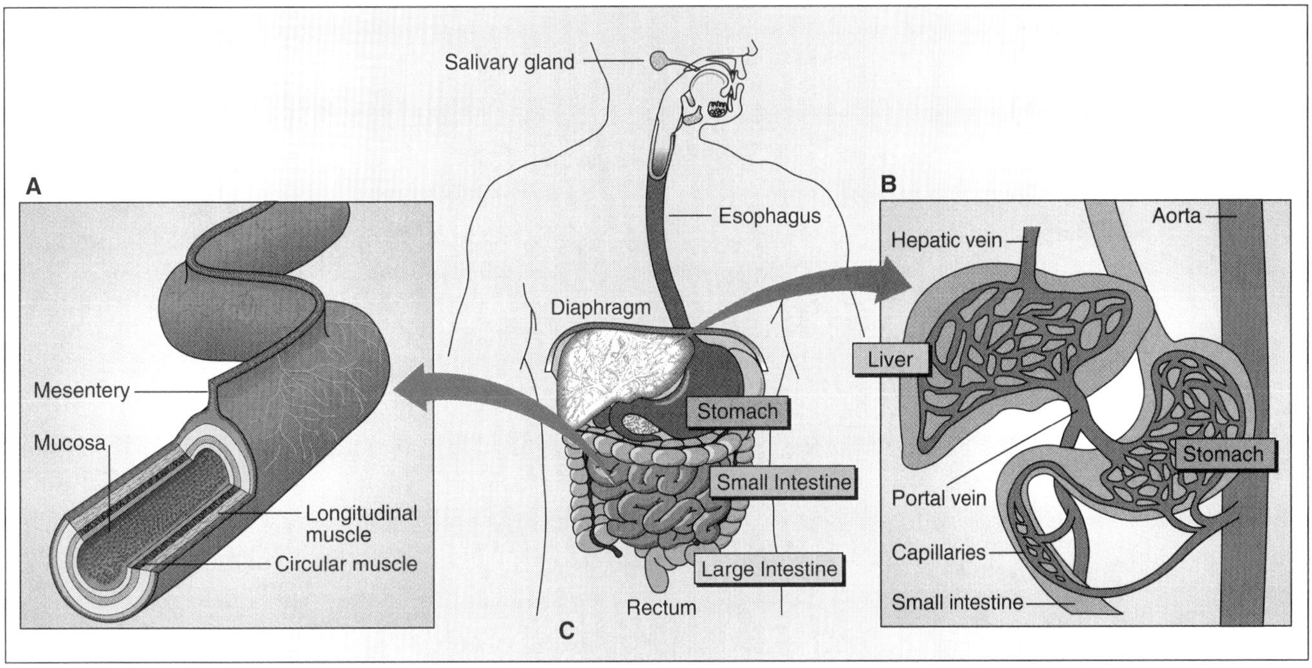

FIG. 2–1. Structures of the gastrointestinal (GI) tract. **A.** Mesentery, which weaves around and gives support to the intestinal organs. **B.** The large portal vein collects blood from the mesenteric area and transports it to the liver for processing before it is returned to the general circulation.

to swallow and more accessible to enzymes and other digestive substances that begin the breakdown process. As a result of swallowing, the bolus of food passes through the pharynx at the back of the mouth and enters the **esophagus.** The length of the esophagus is ringed by two layers of muscle tissue: the inner layer consists of circular bands of muscle, while in the outer layer the muscle tissue runs longitudinally. When the circular muscles contract and the longitudinal muscles relax, the esophagus constricts; when the reverse occurs, the esophagus bulges. The food bolus is propelled down the esophagus by these powerful waves of rhythmic contractions and relaxations, called **peristalsis.** At the end of the esophagus a one-way valve, the esophageal **sphincter,** relaxes to allow the food mass entry into the next part of the GI tract, the **stomach.** The stomach serves as the temporary reservoir for the partially digested food.

Peristalsis. Peristalsis involves progressive and recurring waves of smooth muscle contractions that compress the alimentary tube in a squeezing action, causing its contents to be mixed and moved along. This intrinsic means of food propulsion can take place in zero gravity; peristalsis will occur even if you are upside down!

Sphincter. A sphincter is a ring or valve of smooth muscle that regulates the movement of food through the digestive tract.

STOMACH

Figure 2–2 shows structural details of the approximately 25 cm long stomach; the inset details the stomach wall, containing the gastric glands. The parietal cells of the gastric glands secrete **hydrochloric acid** and powerful enzyme-containing digestive juices that continue to degrade the nutrients once they leave the esophagus and enter the stomach. Mucus is secreted from the mucous neck cells to protect the mucosal lining of the gastric tissue; the chief cells produce pepsinogen, the inactive form of the protein-digesting enzyme *pepsin.* Simple sugars are the easiest nutrients to digest, followed by proteins and lipids. *Little absorption takes place in the stomach except for some water; it is only alcohol that is readily absorbed.*

The stomach truly is a temporary holding tank for food. On average, the

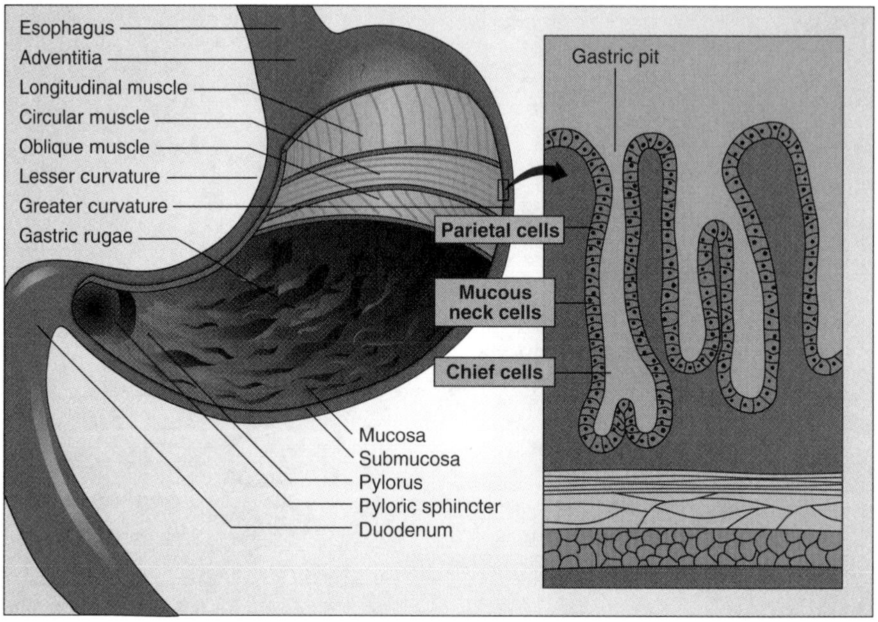

FIG. 2–2. Structure of the stomach and gastric glands. The parietal cells secrete hydrochloric acid, the neck cells secrete mucus, and the chief cells produce pepsinogen.

stomach's volume is about 1.5 liters, but it can hold a volume ranging from about 50 ml when "empty" to nearly 6.0 liters when fully distended after an excessively large meal. The contents of the stomach are mixed with chemical substances to produce **chyme,** a slushy, acidic mixture of food and digestive juices. The chyme moves along the 6 to 8 m of GI tract on its journey to the large intestine where it is finally eliminated through the **rectum.**

Stomach's capacity reduced. Research indicates that the capacity of the stomach decreases dramatically when a person reduces food intake. In the first such experimental demonstration in humans, the stomach's capacity shrank by about 30% in a group of obese subjects who consumed a formula diet of 600 calories a day, compared to a nondieting control group.

After eating, the stomach takes 2 to 3 hours to empty depending on the relative concentration of each nutrient and the volume of the meal—a large meal takes longer to clear the stomach than a smaller one. The nervous system, through hormonal regulation, largely controls the time and rate of stomach emptying through the action of peristaltic waves that travel from the stomach toward the opening of the **small intestine.** There is also a self-regulating feedback control between the stomach and small intestine: if the stomach becomes too distended because of volume overload, signals are sent to the sphincter at the intestinal entrance causing it to relax so more chyme can enter; conversely, distention of the first portion of the intestines or the presence of excessive protein, lipid, or highly concentrated or acidic solutions reflexly slows gastric emptying.

SMALL INTESTINE

Approximately 90% of digestion takes place in the first two sections of the 3 m long small intestine. This coiled structure consists of three sections: the duodenum (first 0.3 m), jejunum (next 1–2 m, where most of digestion occurs), and ileum (last 1.5 m). The smaller digested units of carbohydrates, proteins, and lipids, in addition to water, alcohol, vitamins, and minerals, are absorbed through millions of specialized protruding structures of the intestinal mucosa. These finger-like protrusions that move in wave-like fashion are called **villi.** As shown in Figure 2–3, the highly vascularized surfaces of the villi contain small projections known as **microvilli.** The membrane that surrounds these structures allows amino acids, glucose, fatty acids, and other substances to be absorbed by the body. The villi increase the absorptive surface of the intestine by up to 600-fold compared to a flat-surfaced tube of the same dimensions. This large surface greatly enhances the speed and capacity for nutrient absorption. Within each villus are small lymphatic vessels called **lacteals.** The lacteals mainly transport fatty materials from the liver into the lymphatic vessels that drain into the large veins near the heart.

Intestinal absorptive surface. If spread out, the 300 square meter surface area of the small intestine would cover an area the size of an entire tennis court, or about 150 times the external surface of the body!

If all goes well, the transit through the GI tract from the time the food

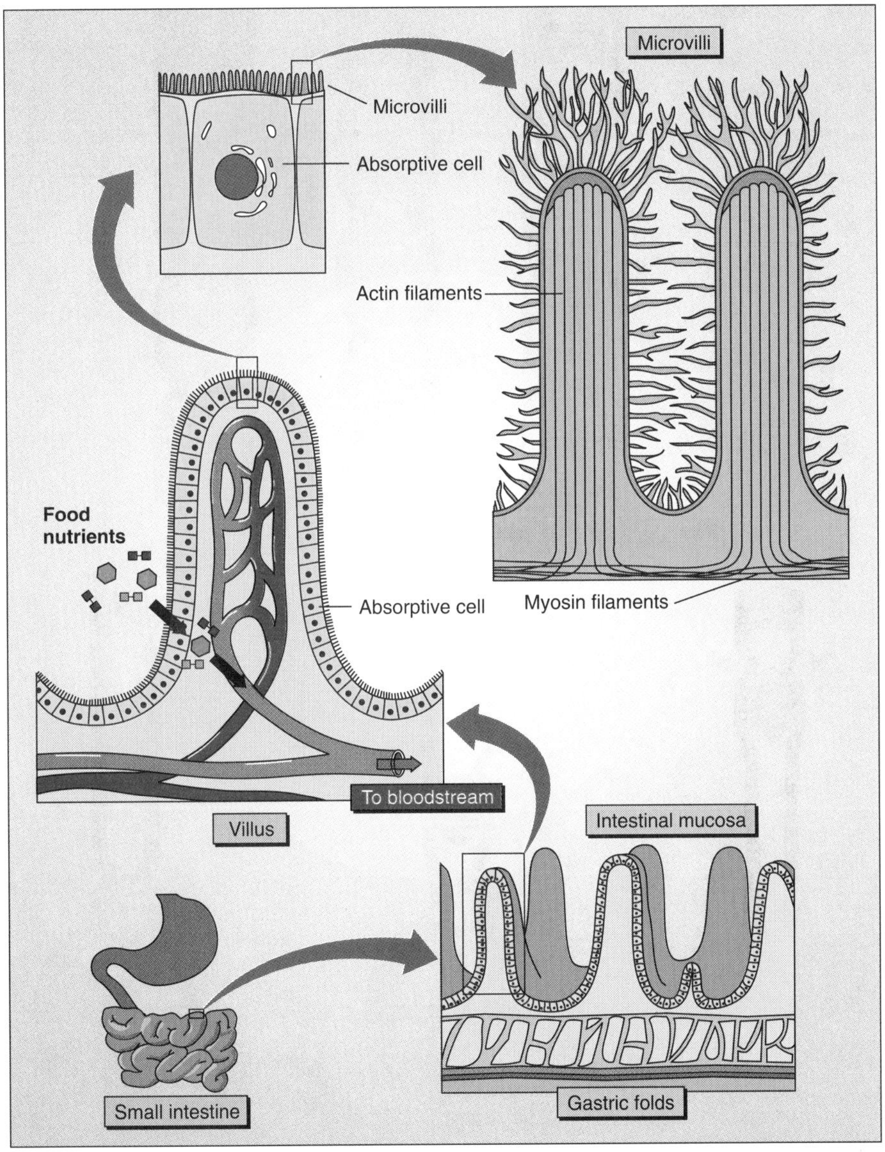

FIG. 2–3. The microscopic structure of the small intestine. The villi and microvilli are referred to as the *brush border.* These tiny projections tremendously increase the surface area of the mucosal cell's plasma membrane for the purpose of nutrient absorption.

is first eaten until its elimination usually takes 1 to 3 days. The movement of chyme through the small intestine takes from 3 to 10 hours and is assisted by intermittent oscillating contraction and relaxation, called **segmentation contractions,** of the intestinal wall's circular smooth muscle. Figure 2–4A shows that segmentation contractions give this section of the GI tract a "sausage-link" look. This occurs because the alternating contractions and relaxations occur in nonadjacent segments of the intestine. Thus, instead of propelling food directly forward as occurs in peristalsis (Figure 2–4B), the food actually moves slightly backward before advancing. This gives digestive juices additional time to mix with the food mass before it moves on its way. During segmentation contractions, the propulsive movements

pH of the small intestine is normally regulated. The intestinal lining cannot withstand the highly acidic nature of the gastric juices from the stomach. Consequently, neutralizing the acid is crucial in protecting against duodenal damage, which in extreme form causes tissue ulceration or what is commonly referred to as "ulcers."

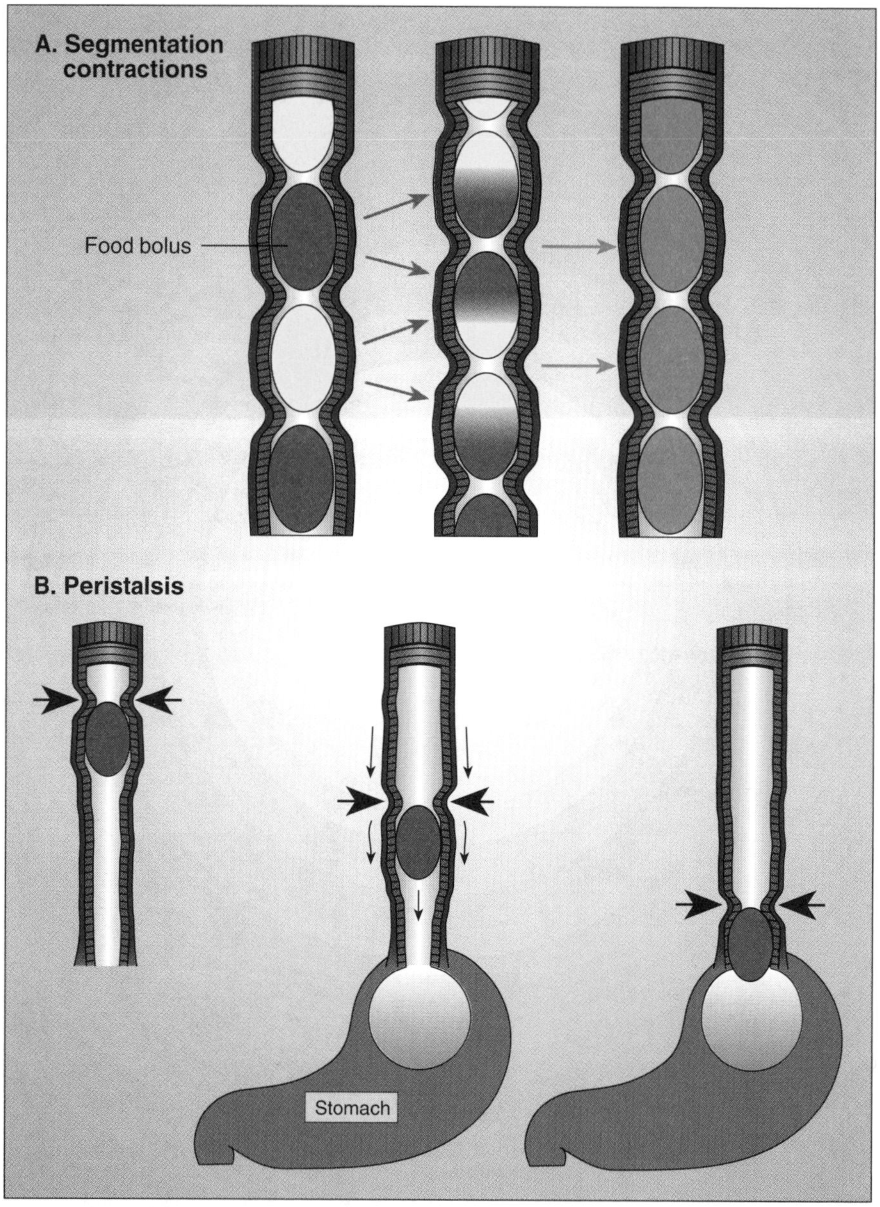

FIG. 2–4. Propulsion of nutrients through the GI tract. **A.** Segmentation contractions. **B.** Peristalsis.

continue to churn and mix the chyme before it passes the pyloric sphincter into the **large intestine.**

During digestion, **bile** produced in the **liver** and stored and secreted by the **gallbladder** helps to increase the solubility and digestibility of lipid droplets by emulsifying them. The **pancreas** secretes alkali-containing substances (bicarbonates) to help buffer the hydrochloric acid from the stomach that remains in the intestinal chyme. At a higher pH, pancreatic enzymes, released by nervous and hormonal mechanisms, come into play to degrade the larger protein, carbohydrate, and lipid nutrients into smaller subunits for further digestion and ultimate absorption.

Emulsification. The lipid content of intestinal chyme stimulates the gallbladder's pulsatile release of bile into the duodenum. In a manner similar to the action of many household detergents, bile salts break up fat into numerous smaller droplets that do not coalesce. This renders the fatty acid end products of fat digestion insoluble in water so they can be absorbed by the intestines.

LARGE INTESTINE

Figure 2–5 depicts the structures of the large intestine, which serves as the final pathway for digestion, especially the absorption of water and electrolytes and storage of digestive residues as fecal matter. This terminal 1.2 m (4 ft) portion of the GI tract contains no villi and is known as the **colon** or bowel. Its major anatomic sections include the ascending and descending colon, transverse colon, sigmoid colon, rectum, and anal canal. Within the large intestine, the digested food remnants, almost thoroughly mixed and devoid of all

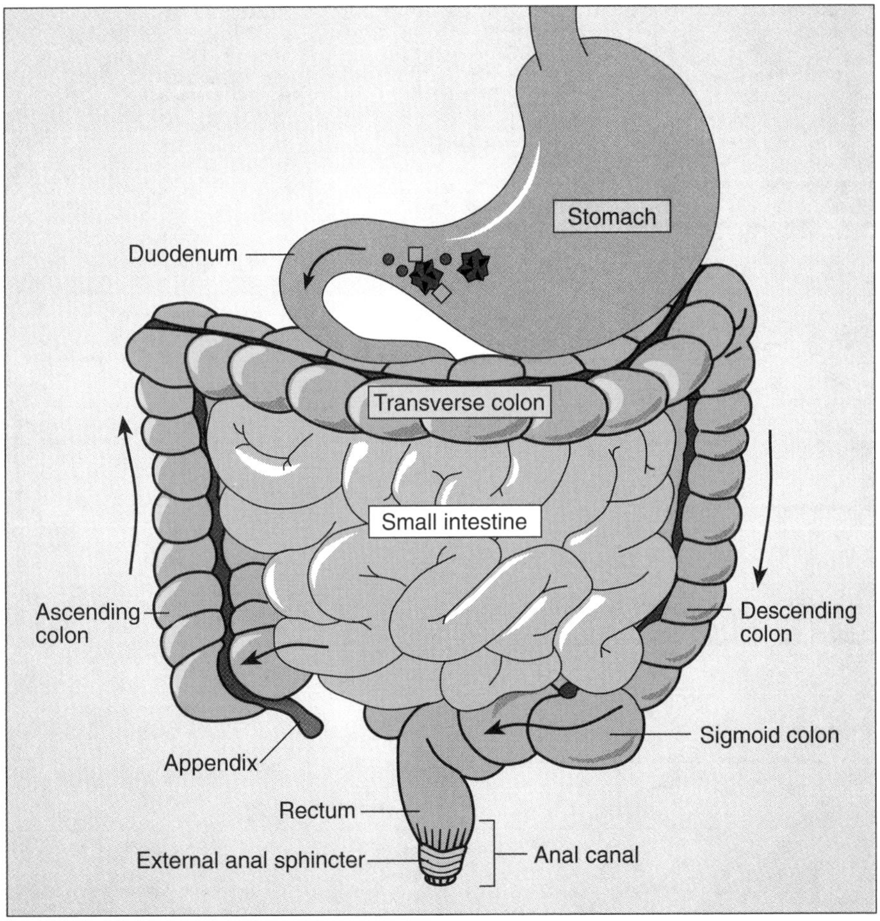

FIG. 2–5. Gross anatomical structures of the large intestine.

but about 5% of their useful nutrients, are further acted upon by bacteria that ferment the remaining undigested food residues. The bacteria, through their own process of metabolism, synthesize small amounts of the vitamin K and B-vitamin *biotin* that become absorbed. Bacterial fermentation also produces about 500 ml of gas (flatus) each day. This gas is a mixture of hydrogen, nitrogen, methane, hydrogen sulfide, and carbon dioxide. A small amount produces no outward effects, but excessive flatus can cause severe abdominal pain. This occurs when we consume large quantities of

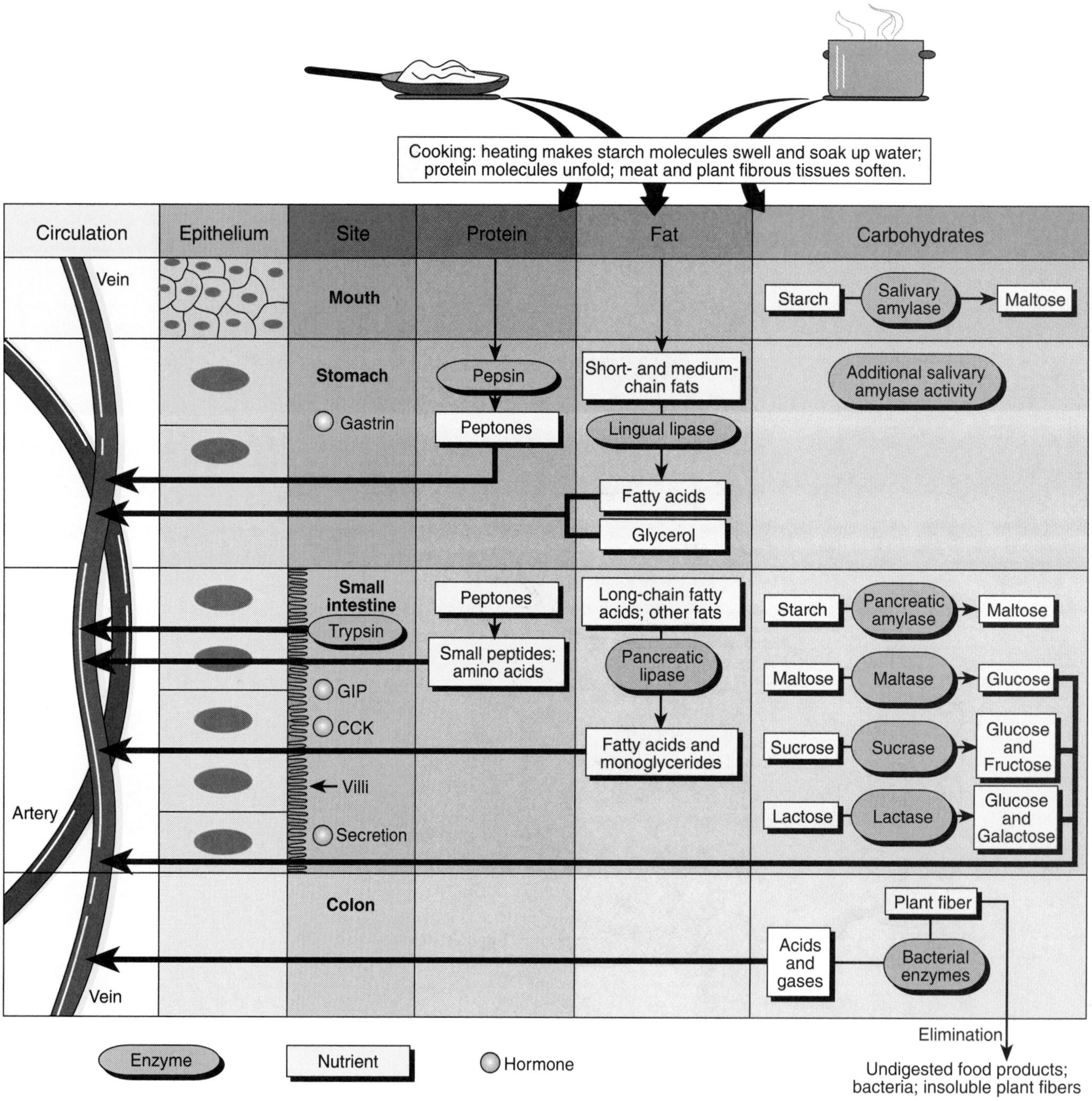

FIG. 2–6. Overview of human digestion. (GIP, gastric inhibitory peptide. CCK, cholecystokinin.)

foods such as beans or dairy products, which leave partially digested sugars that produce a larger than normal amount of gas. Mucus is the only significant secretion of the large intestine. It serves to protect the intestinal wall and contributes to holding fecal matter together.

THE DIGESTIVE PROCESS

The sequence of events during digestion occurs almost entirely under involuntary control. When something goes awry, however, we often voluntarily attempt to alter the process. For example, we consume **antacids** to tame an excessively acidic or "upset" stomach, we battle various intestinal ailments such as diarrhea and constipation with specially formulated "over-the-counter" compounds, and we seek medical treatment to combat the debilitating effects of more painful conditions such as heartburn, ulcers, diverticulitis, and hemorrhoids. As we look more closely at the process of digestion and absorption in the following chapters, keep in mind that these specialized functions usually work in harmony under exquisite neural and hormonal control. This helps to maintain the relative constancy of the body's internal environment.

Involuntary control. The entire GI tract is controlled by the autonomic nervous system: the parasympathetic aspect generally increases gut activity, while the sympathetic aspect generally inhibits it. Even if nervous control is lost, this intrinsic autoregulatory control can eventually return gut function to a near-normal level.

Figure 2–6 presents an overview of human digestion in terms of the pathways that nutrients follow through the GI tract. Indicated are the major enzymes and hormones that act on protein, lipid, and carbohydrate as they pass from the mouth to the stomach, small intestine, and colon. In the chapters on carbohydrates, lipids and proteins that follow, the last section contains a discussion of the digestion and absorption of each of these nutrients.

SUMMARY

1. In the process of digestion, complex molecules are broken down into simpler substances for absorption by the body. Self-regulating processes within the digestive tract largely control the liquidity, mixing, and speed of movement of the digestive mixture.
2. In the mouth, food is physically altered in a manner that makes it easier to swallow, while at the same time increasing its accessibility to enzymes and other digestive substances. As a result of swallowing, the food mixture is passed into the esophagus where peristalsis propels it into the stomach.
3. In the stomach, the food contents are further mixed as hydrochloric acid and enzymes continue the breakdown process. Little absorption takes place in the stomach except for some water and alcohol. Actually, it is only the alcohol that is readily absorbed.
4. About 90% of the digestion of all food nutrients takes place along the first half of the 3 m long small intestine. Highly specific intestinal enzymes act on more complex carbohydrate, lipid, and protein structures, splitting them into simpler subunits. Bile, produced in the liver and secreted by the gallbladder, emulsifies lipid droplets, thus facilitating the action of digestive enzymes.

5. The villi of the small intestine provide a tremendous surface through which digested nutrients are absorbed into the body.
6. The large intestine serves as the final path for digestion. It is here that water and electrolytes are absorbed and the undigested food residue or feces is stored.

RELATED LITERATURE

Guthrie, H.A.: Introductory Nutrition, 7th ed. St. Louis, C.V. Mosby, 1988.

Guyton, A.C.: Textbook of Medical Physiology, 7th ed. Philadelphia, W.B. Saunders, 1986.

Hunt, S.M., and Groff, J.L.: Advanced Nutrition and Human Metabolism. St. Paul, West Publishing Company, 1990.

Kanarek, R.B., and Marks-Kaufman, R.: Nutrition and Behavior. New Perspectives. New York, Van Nostrand Reinhold, 1991.

Marieb, E.N.: Human Anatomy and Physiology. Redwood City, CA, Benjamin Cummings, 1989.

Shils, M.E. and Young, V.R. (Eds.): Modern Nutrition in Health and Disease, 6th ed. Philadelphia, Lea & Febiger, 1988.

Vander, A.J., et al.: Human Physiology, 2nd ed. New York, McGraw-Hill, 1985.

Wardlaw, G.M., and Insel, P.M.: Perspectives in Nutrition. St. Louis, Times Mirror/Mosby, 1990.

Weiss, L. (Ed.): Cell and Tissue Biology, 6th ed. Baltimore, Urban & Schwarzenberg, 1988.

Whitney, E.N., et al.: Understanding Nutrition. 5th ed. St. Paul, West Publishing Company, 1990.

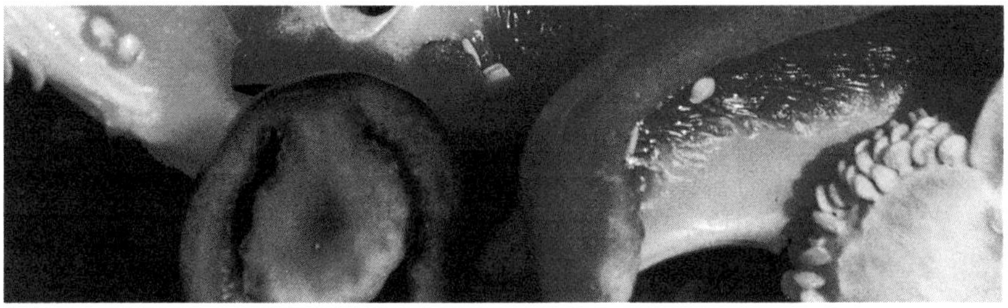

3

CARBOHYDRATES

Carbohydrates make up only 3% of the body's organic matter, but play a major role in supplying energy for bodily function. These naturally occurring, water-soluble substances are usually consumed in the diet as sugars, starches, and cellulose. In most higher animals, including humans, the simple six-carbon glucose molecule is the quick and accessible form in which carbohydrates ultimately contribute to energizing metabolic processes.

WHAT ARE CARBOHYDRATES?

Carbohydrates *are compounds constructed in a ratio of one atom of carbon and two atoms of hydrogen for each oxygen atom.* The general formula for a simple carbohydrate is $(CH_2O)_n$, where *n* can be from three to seven carbon atoms. Many of the simple carbohydrates or sugars have five carbon atoms and are called **pentoses;** those with six carbon atoms are referred to as **hexoses.** Ribose and deoxyribose, the essential ingredients of nucleic acids, are examples of pentoses. The simple sugar glucose is a hexose. A change in the spatial orientation of individual atoms within the sugar molecule can dramatically alter its properties. For example, fructose and galactose, both hexose sugars, are identical in chemical formula to glucose except for a reversal of the atoms attached on one of the carbons along the chain. These slight distinctions in atomic configuration give the compounds their unique biologic function. While glucose exists freely in cells throughout the body, the other hexoses are more commonly associated with specialized protein and lipid structures.

MONOSACCHARIDES

Monosaccharides. The basic chemical structure of a simple sugar molecule consists of a chain of from three to seven carbon atoms with hydrogen and oxygen atoms attached by single bonds. The most typical sugar is glucose.

Among more than 200 **monosaccharides** found in nature, the most common are the six-carbon sugar units **glucose, fructose,** and **galactose.** Glucose, also called dextrose or blood sugar, is composed of a chain of six carbon atoms to which are attached six oxygen and 12 hydrogen atoms. The chemical formula that describes this molecule in terms of its atomic structure is $C_6H_{12}O_6$. Figure 3–1 shows that the glucose molecule can be linear, or can exist in one of two ring structures. The hexagonal ring shape is generated from the linear structure when the carbon (labeled in the figure as 1) attaches to the hydroxyl OH at carbon position 4 or 5. Glucose can be used in any of three ways: (1) directly by the cell for energy, (2) stored as glycogen in the muscles and liver, or (3) converted to fat for energy storage.

Fructose or fruit sugar, the sweetest of the sugars, is present in large amounts in fruits and honey; the sugar galactose is produced in the mammary glands of lactating animals. The body easily converts both fructose and galactose to glucose. Because glucose is an important form of usable food energy, it is desirable to maintain a plentiful supply of this nutrient. Among both plants and animals, a ready reservoir of glucose is kept available, stored in alternative forms such as disaccharides or polysaccharides.

DISACCHARIDES

The joining of two simple sugar molecules forms a double sugar or **disaccharide,** of which **sucrose, maltose,** and **lactose** are examples. Sucrose (common table sugar) is formed from glucose and fructose. It is found in most plants, notably in sugar cane and sugar beets. Maltose, composed of two glucose molecules, is formed during the digestive breakdown of large carbohydrate molecules. The disaccharide lactose, the chief sugar present in milk, is dismantled to glucose and galactose during digestion.

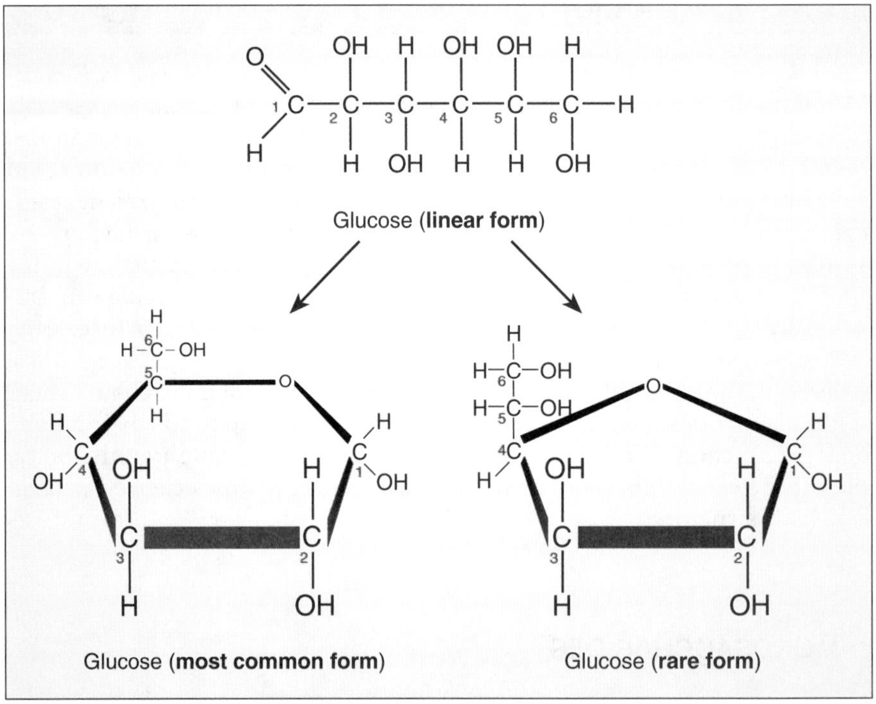

FIG. 3–1. Three alternative formations of the glucose molecule. The linear configuration can be changed to one of the ring structures by rearrangements along parts of the carbon chain. The most common glucose molecule resembles a hexagonal plate with attachments of H and O atoms.

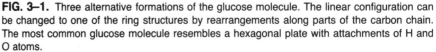

SIMPLE SUGARS AND SUGAR SUBSTITUTES

The monosaccharides and disaccharides collectively make up what are commonly referred to as the **simple sugars.** These sugars are packaged under a variety of guises: brown sugar, corn syrup, invert sugar, corn sugar, sorbitol, levulose, fructose, dextrose, honey, and "natural sweeteners." Interestingly, honey contains the same two monosaccharides that make up table sugar. While sweeter because of its high fructose content, honey is no more "natural" than sucrose, nor is it superior nutritionally or as an energy source.

Products are also commercially available that are not true sugars, but provide the same sweet taste as sucrose with little or no caloric content.* These include saccharin (first produced in 1979 and due for further review by the Food and Drug Administration in 1992 because of possible links to cancer), aspartame (trade name *NutraSweet* when added to foods and *Equal* when sold as a powder), and acesulfame (trade name *Sunette*). Aspartame yields 4 calories per gram (g), the same as sucrose, but requires only minute amounts for equivalent sweetness. Acesulfame contributes no calories to the diet. Paradoxically, excessive use of artificial sweeteners may increase subsequent voluntary caloric intake compared to food sweetened with natural sweeteners.

Excessive intake of simple sugar will draw fluid from the body into the intestinal tract; this reduces fluid uptake and can cause gastrointestinal distress. Simple sugars also are rapidly absorbed, and a large sugar influx can trigger a hormonal response that actually causes blood sugar to drop.

More of our carbohydrate from simple sugars. The average American consumes about 50% of dietary carbohydrate as simple sugars, mostly in the form of sucrose and high-fructose corn syrup. This amount includes more than 16 teaspoons a day, or 60 pounds of table sugar and about 50 pounds of corn syrup each year, as contrasted to an average person's annual intake of only four pounds of table sugar 100 years ago!

POLYSACCHARIDES

The term **polysaccharide** *is used when three or more sugar molecules combine.* This is the form in which most natural carbohydrates occur. The most common polysaccharides are starch, fiber, and glycogen.

STARCH

Three hundred to thousands of individual sugar molecules may join together in a **starch** molecule. Starch, a plant polysaccharide, is found in corn and in various grains used to make bread, cereal, spaghetti, and pastries. Large amounts of starch are also present in beans, peas, and potatoes.

FIBER

Cellulose and most other fibrous materials constitute another form of plant polysaccharide. They make up the structural part of plant cell walls, and are present in the leaves, stems, roots, seeds, and edible skins and peels of vegetables and fruits. They are also present as mucilage and gums within the plant cell. Cellulose is found in the protective outer layer of whole grains referred to as the **bran layer.** Fibers are resistant to human digestive enzymes.

Dietary Fiber. Although technically not a nutrient, **dietary fiber** has received considerable attention from researchers and the lay press. The Western diet is high in fiber-free animal foods and loses much of its natural

Diverse forms of fiber. There are two categories of dietary fiber: water-insoluble and water-soluble. The five kinds of dietary fiber are cellulose, hemicellulose, lignins, pectins, and gums. Eating a variety of plant foods will insure that all types of fibers are consumed.

* A **calorie** is a unit of heat used to express the energy value of food.

plant fiber through processing. Low dietary fiber intake has been linked to the prevalence of intestinal disorders in the United States compared with countries that consume a more "primitive-type" diet high in unrefined, complex carbohydrates. For example, diets from Africa and India range between 40 and 150 g whereas the typical American diet contains a daily fiber intake of only about 12 g.

Unrefined, complex carbohydrates. This term generally refers to plant polysaccharides as they occur in their natural state. **Unrefined complex carbohydrates** include the plant's coarse, fibrous coverings as well as materials contained within the structure of the plant itself.

Fibers hold considerable water and thus give "bulk" or "roughage" to food residues in the small intestine, often increasing stool weight and volume by 40 to 100%. This bulking action may aid gastrointestinal function by exerting a scraping action on the gut wall. Fibers may also bind or dilute harmful chemicals or inhibit their activity, or they may shorten the transit time for food residues (and possibly cancer-producing materials) to pass through the digestive tract. Through these actions, fiber may reduce the chances of contracting colon cancer and various other gastrointestinal diseases later in life.

Fiber intake, especially of **water-soluble fibers** such as pectin and the guar gum present in oats, beans, peas, carrots, and fruits, may also lower blood cholesterol. These fibers may depress the synthesis and absorption of cholesterol in the gut, while at the same time bind existing cholesterol to facilitate its excretion in the feces. Alternatively, the addition of fiber may simply replace other cholesterol-laden items in the diet. In contrast, the **water-insoluble fibers** such as some hemicelluloses, lignin, and cellulose, found in brown rice, corn, and wheat bran (the coarse, outer layer of the whole-grain kernel), show no cholesterol-lowering effect.

Upgrade your fiber intake. When shopping for high-fiber foods, look for whole-grain cereals and breads, and for fruits and vegetables with edible stalks, skins, and seeds such as broccoli, apples, prunes, figs, pears, and strawberries.

*The **recommended fiber intake** is about 20 to 35 g a day as an important part of a well-structured diet for the average American adult.* The ratio of insoluble to soluble fiber should be about 3 to 1 and should be derived in natural form from foods, not from synthetic fiber supplements. If fiber intake is pegged to caloric intake, daily fiber intake would be approximately 12 g for each 1000 calories of food consumed.

Figure 3–2 displays the fiber content in 1-ounce portions of high-fiber foods. The inset table shows the dietary fiber in edible portions of common vegetables. As with most nutrients, excessive intake may be counterproductive. An excess of dietary fiber carries the risks of intestinal distress, and decreases absorption of the minerals calcium, iron, magnesium, zinc, and phosphorus. A diet too high in fiber could thus lead to a mineral imbalance, especially in individuals whose nutrition level is marginal.

GLYCOGEN

Glycogen, or animal starch, is a large molecule. It is formed by glucose molecules, ranging from a few hundred to ten thousand or more, linked together in long chains. Glycogen is not present to any large extent in the foods we eat. Instead, when the glucose derived from food enters the muscles and liver, it is trapped, synthesized, and stored for later use as glycogen. Liver glycogen can constitute up to 10% of the weight of the liver, or approximately 100 g. The process of transforming glucose to glycogen in the liver is known as **glycogenesis.** When glucose is needed as an energy source, liver glycogen is reconverted to glucose and transported in the blood for use by the active muscles. The term **glycogenolysis** is used to describe this reconversion process. The muscles are a larger storage site for glycogen than the liver, and hold approximately 325 g as muscle gly-

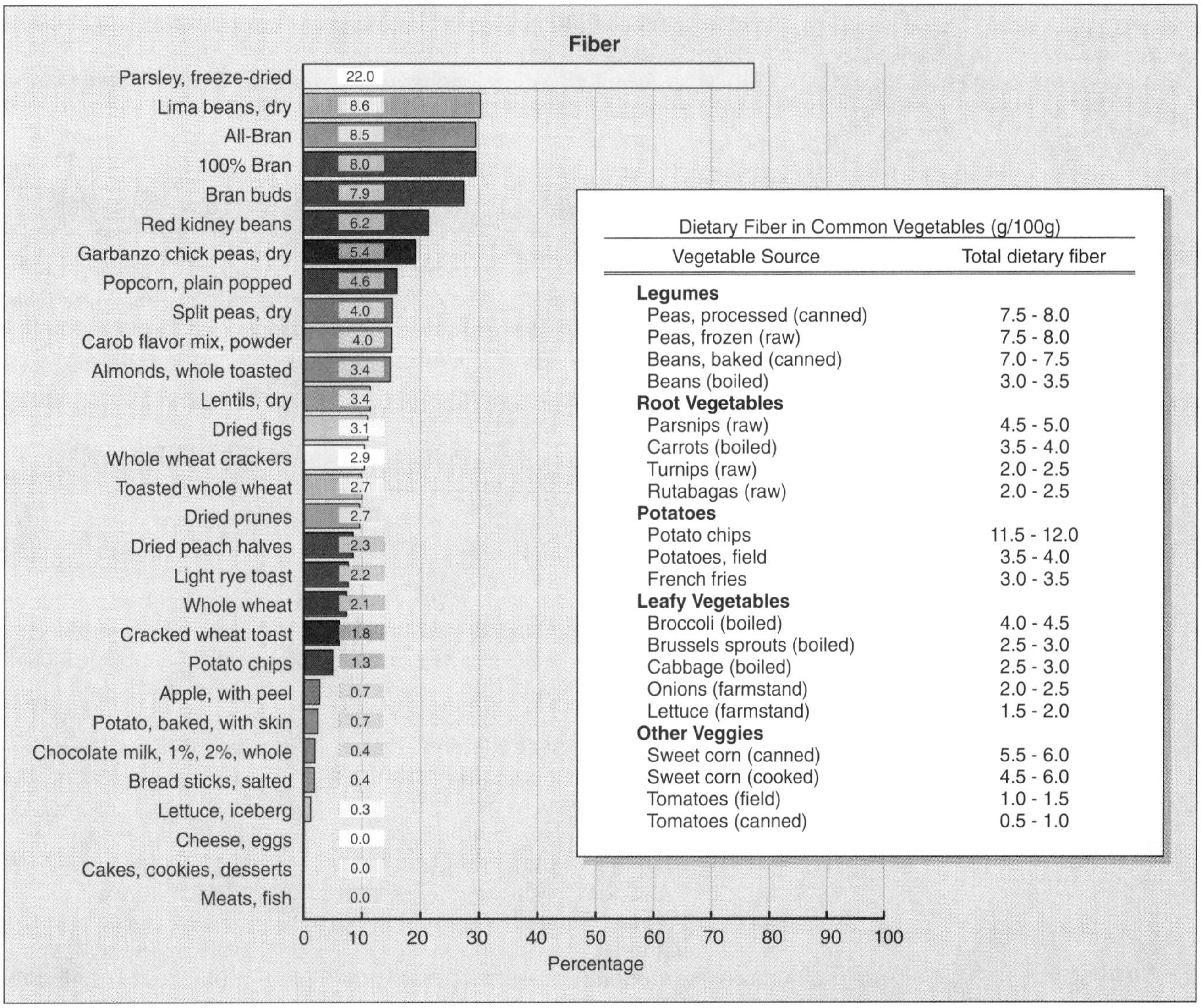

Dietary Fiber in Common Vegetables (g/100g)

Vegetable Source	Total dietary fiber
Legumes	
Peas, processed (canned)	7.5 - 8.0
Peas, frozen (raw)	7.5 - 8.0
Beans, baked (canned)	7.0 - 7.5
Beans (boiled)	3.0 - 3.5
Root Vegetables	
Parsnips (raw)	4.5 - 5.0
Carrots (boiled)	3.5 - 4.0
Turnips (raw)	2.0 - 2.5
Rutabagas (raw)	2.0 - 2.5
Potatoes	
Potato chips	11.5 - 12.0
Potatoes, field	3.5 - 4.0
French fries	3.0 - 3.5
Leafy Vegetables	
Broccoli (boiled)	4.0 - 4.5
Brussels sprouts (boiled)	2.5 - 3.0
Cabbage (boiled)	2.5 - 3.0
Onions (farmstand)	2.0 - 2.5
Lettuce (farmstand)	1.5 - 2.0
Other Veggies	
Sweet corn (canned)	5.5 - 6.0
Sweet corn (cooked)	4.5 - 6.0
Tomatoes (field)	1.0 - 1.5
Tomatoes (canned)	0.5 - 1.0

FIG. 3–2. Percentage of fiber in commonly served foods. The actual grams of fiber per ounce (28.4 g) of the food is shown within the bar. In the inset table, the number of grams of dietary fiber per 100 g of the vegetable is shown for edible portions of common vegetables.

cogen. Only about 15 to 20 g of carbohydrate remains unstored and circulates as blood glucose.

When glycogen is depleted by dietary restriction or exercise, some "new glucose" can be produced in the liver and kidneys. With the aid of the hormone **cortisol,** this glucose is derived from structural components of the other nutrients, especially proteins, in a process termed **gluconeogenesis.** Because of our limited capacity to generate glucose, carbohydrate intake is essential. *Starvation diets and diets with reduced-calorie or lowered carbohydrate content, as well as strenuous exercise programs, will deplete glycogen reserves. This places demands on body protein, and lean (muscle) tissue will be lost.*

The hormone **insulin,** secreted by the pancreas, plays an important part in liver and muscle glycogen storage by controlling the level of circulating blood sugar. If the blood sugar level is high, the pancreas secretes additional insulin and excess circulating glucose is taken up by the cells. This type of

Cortisol. Cortisol, also called hydrocortisone, is the major steroid hormone secreted from the cortex of the adrenal glands. It regulates various aspects of metabolism including the synthesis of glucose from amino acids.

Insulin. Insulin is a peptide hormone, secreted by beta cells of the pancreas that aids the movement of nutrients—primarily glucose but also amino acids—into most cells by facilitated diffusion. Insulin also stimulates the synthesis of glycogen, protein, and fat.

Glucagon. Glucagon, termed the "insulin antagonist" hormone, is secreted by alpha cells of the pancreas. Glucagon's major function is to raise the blood glucose level by stimulating both glycogenolysis and gluconeogenesis in the liver.

"feedback" regulation maintains blood glucose at an appropriate and safe physiologic concentration. In contrast, if blood sugar falls below normal, insulin's opposing hormone, **glucagon,** is immediately secreted to normalize the blood sugar level.

WHERE DO CARBOHYDRATES COME FROM?

As discussed in Chapter 1, carbohydrates are synthesized in plants by the process of photosynthesis. When a carbohydrate molecule is formed, oxygen is released to the atmosphere for use by most organisms in the life-sustaining process of energy metabolism.

FUNCTIONS OF CARBOHYDRATES

ENERGY SOURCE

The immediate and most important function of carbohydrates is to provide a continuous energy supply to the body. To be useful, complex carbohydrate molecules are broken down during digestion into simple six-carbon sugar molecules that are absorbed and transported in the bloodstream to individual cells throughout the body. Inside the cell, glucose can be synthesized to glycogen or used directly for energy. During energy metabolism, the bonds of the glucose molecule are broken through specific chemical reactions; the liberated energy is used to power the cell's many functions.

Carbohydrate must be regularly ingested to maintain the body's glycogen stores. If the amount of incoming glucose is inadequate, glycogen reserves are tapped and the "backup" glucose stored as glycogen is recruited for energy. The blood normally contains about 70 to 110 milligrams of glucose per 100 milliliters of blood (the measurement is usually expressed as milligrams per deciliter, or mg/dl). This usual range of blood glucose is said to be **normoglycemic.** The level of sugar in the blood is elevated immediately after a meal; concurrently, insulin is released to facilitate glucose transport into the cell. Under normal conditions, any excess incoming sugar is converted to its storage form, glycogen, and held in reserve for later use. Once the cell's capacity for glycogen storage is reached, sugars are readily converted to fat and stored as triglyceride in the adipose (fat) tissues beneath the skin. This action helps to explain how body fat increases even when we consume excess calories in the form of carbohydrate!

PROTEIN SPARER

Adequate carbohydrate intake helps to maintain tissue protein. Under normal conditions, protein serves its vital role in the growth and repair of body tissues. When carbohydrate reserves are reduced, however, metabolic pathways exist for the synthesis of glucose from protein (gluconeogenesis). This provides a metabolic option for maintaining some carbohydrate in the face of depleted glycogen. The price the body pays is a temporary reduction in protein "stores," especially of muscle protein. In extreme conditions, lean tissue can be significantly reduced and the kidneys burdened as they excrete the nitrogen-containing by-products of protein breakdown.

METABOLIC PRIMER

Carbohydrate serves as a "primer" for fat metabolism. If an insufficient level of carbohydrate breakdown exists, either through a limitation in glucose transport into the cells as occurs in diabetes, or when glycogen is depleted through improper diet or prolonged exercise, the body will mobilize fat to a greater extent than it can use. The result is incomplete fat breakdown and the accumulation of acid by-products called **ketones** (see p. 280). Ketones can cause a harmful increase in the acidity of body fluids.

FUEL FOR THE CENTRAL NERVOUS SYSTEM

Carbohydrate is essential for proper functioning of the central nervous system. Under normal conditions, the brain uses blood glucose almost exclusively as its fuel and has essentially no stored supply of this nutrient. Because of the specific role blood glucose plays in generating energy for use by nervous tissue, blood sugar is regulated within narrow limits.

Hypoglycemia. When blood sugar falls below normoglycemic levels, hormones stimulate the liver to release its glucose into the bloodstream. If blood sugar continues to fall, the symptoms of **hypoglycemia** occur: hunger, dizziness, anxiety, tachycardia (rapid heart beat), weakness, and excessive sweating. This condition also impairs exercise performance and may partially explain the fatigue associated with prolonged exercise, which puts tremendous demands on glycogen reserves. (Anxiety and emotional stress can trigger a "pseudohypoglycemic" effect that resembles the symptoms of hypoglycemia.)

Hyperglycemia. When the blood sugar level becomes excessive, the condition is known as **hyperglycemia.** This state is often associated with diabetes mellitus, a disease that currently afflicts about 12 million Americans and ranks sixth among primary causes of death. Maintaining a normal blood insulin level is important because of the hormone's role in regulating glucose uptake by cells.

Diabetes mellitus. In diabetes mellitus, hormonal control of plasma glucose is defective. The cause may be due to inadequate insulin production or decreased sensitivity to insulin by peripheral tissue. As a result, glucose fails to enter the cells in normal amounts, and abnormally high levels remain in the bloodstream. A simple test for hyperglycemia is the presence of sugar in the urine.

RECOMMENDED INTAKE OF CARBOHYDRATES

The typical American diet includes between 40 to 50% of its total calories in the form of carbohydrate. For a sedentary 70-kg person, this amounts to a daily intake of about 300 g of carbohydrate. For this person, the stability of the relatively limited quantity of muscle and liver glycogen is probably maintained. For more active people and those involved in exercise training, about 60% of daily calories (400 to 600 g) should be in the form of carbohydrate, predominantly of the complex variety. This amount will be sufficient to replenish the carbohydrate used to power the increased level of physical activity.

Excellent sources of complex carbohydrates, and the percentage of calories derived from them.	
FOOD	% CALORIES
Rice cakes	90
Wasa crackers	88
Pita bread, whole wheat	86
Spaghetti, tomato sauce with cheese	81
Popcorn, no oil used	80
Pretzels	78
Soup, vegetable and tomato	77
Chili, all veggies and no meat	74
Bagel, plain	73
Soup, split pea	71

Our national "sweet tooth.". This year, the average American will consume more sugar-flavored soft drinks than milk!

Potato chips, a popular snack food. In 1990, the average person consumed 6.1 pounds of potato chips. Tortilla chips were second at 3.9 pounds, followed by snack nuts (1.6 pounds), pretzels (1.4 pounds), and microwave popcorn (1.3 pounds).

Ranked #1. Bananas are America's most popular fruit; the average person consumes about 25 pounds each year.

Diet can significantly alter the storage of glycogen. Changes in diet can rapidly affect carbohydrate reserves. Even temporary fasting for as little as one day can be considered a form of semistarvation that disrupts the body's normal carbohydrate stores. For example, a 24-hour fast nearly depletes liver and muscle glycogen. If semistarvation persists, the "fuel" to power biologic work is derived largely from fat (with undesirable ketone buildup) and increasing amounts of protein extracted from lean tissue by gluconeogenetic processes. On the other hand, consuming a carbohydrate-rich diet (80% of total calories) for several days can raise the body's carbohydrate stores to almost twice the levels obtained with a normal, well-balanced diet. This increased carbohydrate storage can enhance performance during prolonged exercise. Chapter 10 provides details about the technique of "carbohydrate loading."

CARBOHYDRATES IN FOODS

The percentage of starch consumed in the American diet has decreased by about 30% since the turn of the century, while the consumption of simple sugars has increased to represent the other 50% of our current carbohydrate intake. This amounts to a yearly intake of approximately 55 kg of simple sugar for the average person. Of this total, high-fructose corn syrup represents 21 kg, and cane and beet sugar 27 kg, while the remainder comes from various other sweeteners. Intake of the noncarbohydrate chemical sweeteners saccharin and aspartame amounts to about 7 kg per year.

While simple sugars occur naturally in fruits, vegetables, and dairy products, sugars are also present in soups, sauces, spaghetti, cereals, yogurt, fruit drinks, cereals, frozen dinners, condiments such as ketchup (one teaspoon of sugar per tablespoon), most canned goods, and various types of soft drinks. According to some clinical nutritionists, an increase in sugar consumption is linked in a causal way with an increase in dental caries; it has yet to be proven that excessive sugar intake contributes to the development of adult onset diabetes, obesity, or coronary heart disease.

Cookies, candies, cakes, and white bread consist predominantly of carbohydrates. Figure 3–3 graphically displays the percentage of carbohydrates in some common foods. The values are based on the carbohydrate percentage in relation to total food weight, including water content. This makes fruits and vegetables appear to be less valuable carbohydrate sources. The dried portion of these foods, however, is almost pure carbohydrate! Table 3–1 lists the percentage of carbohydrate in popular breakfast cereals. Of the 83 brands listed, 53 contain at least 75% carbohydrate.

DIGESTION AND ABSORPTION

Carbohydrate digestion and absorption, illustrated in Figure 2–6, begins in the mouth. The **salivary glands,** located along the underside of the jaw, continually secrete lubricating mucous substances that combine with food particles during the chewing process. The enzyme salivary amylase attacks starch and begins to reduce it to the simpler dissacharide form, maltose. When the food-salivary mixture enters the acidic environment of the stom-

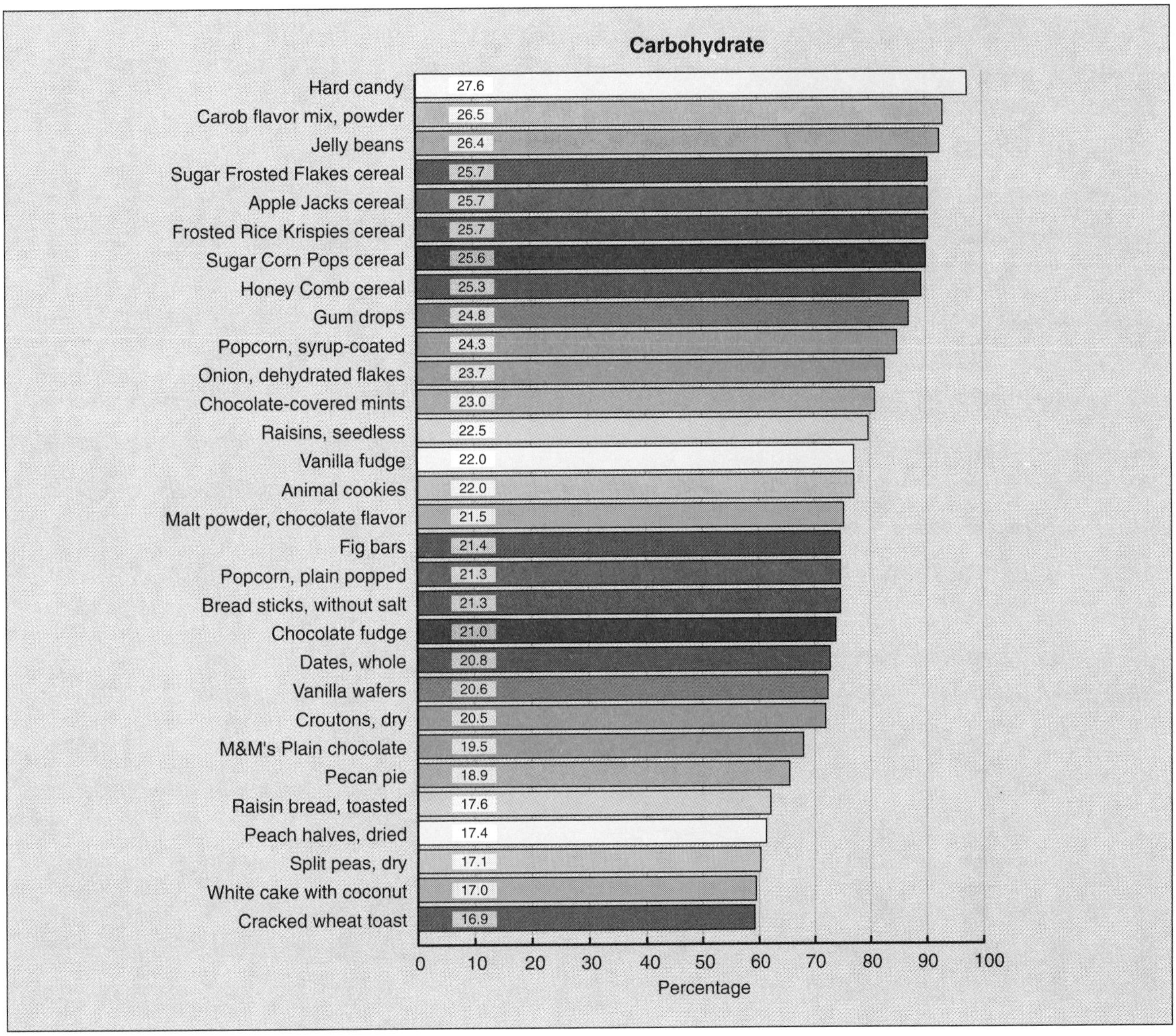

FIG. 3–3. Percentage of carbohydrates in commonly served foods. The insert bars display the number of grams per ounce.

ach, some additional starch breakdown occurs but is quickly halted as salivary amylase becomes inactive under acidic conditions.

When food leaves the stomach for the small intestine, a more powerful enzyme released from the pancreas, **pancreatic amylase,** in conjunction with other enzymes, completes the breakdown of starch into simple monosaccharides. For example, **maltase** breaks down maltose to its glucose components, **sucrase** reduces sucrose to the simple sugars glucose and fructose, and **lactase** degrades lactose to glucose and galactose. The simple sugars are then taken up by the process of active transport in the microvilli and villi (see Fig. 2–3). If intestinal enzymes or the villi themselves are affected by disease, the gastrointestinal (GI) tract can indeed become "upset" and may take several weeks to resume normal functioning. For example, carbohydrates cannot be completely broken down if the digestive

TABLE 3–1. PERCENTAGE OF CARBOHYDRATE IN POPULAR BREAKFAST CEREALS*					
RANK	CEREAL	% CHO	RANK	CEREAL	% CHO
1	Apple Jacks	90.5	43	Bran Chex	79.6
2	Frosted Rice Krispies	90.5	44	Wheat & Raisin Chex	79.6
3	Sugar Frosted Flakes	90.5	45	Wheaties	79.6
4	Sugar Corn Pops	90.1	46	Fruitful Bran	79.2
5	Super Golden Crisp	90.1	47	Shredded Wheat	79.2
6	Puffed Rice	89.8	48	Puffed Wheat	78.9
7	Honey Comb	89.1	49	40% Bran Flakes, Kellogg's	78.2
8	Cocoa Krispies	88.7	50	Fruit & Fiber, with apples	77.5
9	Rice Chex	88.7	51	Bran Buds	76.1
10	Froot Loops	88.0	52	Raisin Bran, Kellogg's	75.4
11	Corn Chex	87.7	53	Special K	75.0
12	Trix	87.7	54	All-Bran	73.9
13	Cocoa Pebbles	87.0	55	100% Bran	72.9
14	Sugar Smacks	87.0	56	Fortified Oat Flakes	72.2
15	Alpha Bits	86.6	57	Roman Meal, dry	71.8
16	Corn Flakes, Kellogg's	85.9	58	C.W. Post, plain	71.5
17	Corn Flakes, Post Toasties	85.9	59	Life	71.5
18	Fruity Pebbles	85.9	60	Cheerios	68.3
19	Team	85.6	61	Cracklin Oat Bran	68.3
20	Raisin Bran, Post	85.2	62	Rolled Oats	66.9
21	Rice Krispies	85.2	63	100% Natural, with apples	66.9
22	Golden Grahams	84.9	64	Granola-Nature Valley	66.5
23	Buc Wheats	84.5	65	100% Natural	63.4
24	King Vitamin	84.5	66	Granola, homemade	54.9
25	Nutri-Grain, corn	84.5	67	Wheat Germ, toasted	49.3
26	Nutri-Grain, rye	84.5	68	Instant Oatmeal, with cinnamon spice	21.8
27	Nutra-Grain, wheat	84.5	69	Instant Oatmeal, with maple	20.4
28	Corn Bran	84.2	70	Instant Oatmeal, with raisins/spice	20.1
29	Quisp	83.1	71	Instant Oatmeal, with apples	17.6
30	Product 19	82.7	72	Instant Oatmeal, with bran/raisins	15.5
31	Frosted Mini-Wheats	82.4	73	Roman Meal, cooked	13.7
32	Nutri-Grain, barley	82.4	74	Whole wheat cereal, cooked	13.7
33	Honey & Nut Corn Flakes	82.0	75	Cream of Wheat	12.0
34	Kix	82.0	76	Wheatena, cooked	12.0
35	Wheat Chex	82.0	77	Cream of Rice	11.6
36	Grape Nuts	81.7	78	Ralson, cooked	11.3
37	Grape Nuts Flakes	81.7	79	Whole Wheat Berries	11.3
38	Honey Bran	81.7	80	Malt-O-Meal	10.9
39	Crispy Wheat 'n Raisins	81.3	81	Oatmeal, prepared	10.9
40	Lucky Charms	81.3	82	Farina, cooked	10.6
41	Cap'n Crunch	80.6	83	Maypo, cooked	0.4
42	Honey Nut Cheerios	80.3			

* Cereals are ranked for the most carbohydrate per ounce (Apple Jacks, Frosted Rice Krispies, and Sugar Frosted Flakes, 90.5%) to least carbohydrate (Maypo, 0.4%).

enzymes become altered. When partially digested food is passed to the colon, sugar fermentation can cause excessive gas formation and abdominal discomfort. A person recovering from diarrhea or a bacterial infection of the abdomen has a transient **lactose intolerance** and should avoid food products containing lactase. When appropriate lactose concentration is re-established, this sugar can once again be ingested without undesirable consequences. In about 70% of the world's population, intestinal levels of the enzyme lactase decrease to a degree that affects the digestion of this sugar.

Monosaccharides are absorbed from the small intestine into the bloodstream and are transported via capillaries to the hepatic-portal vein, which feeds directly to the liver. The pathway of circulatory transport from the GI tract is called the **hepatic-portal circulation.** Blood drainage from the intestines does not pass directly back to the heart but travels first to the liver, where its nutrients are processed before the blood finally enters the general circulation. The hepatic-portal circulation transports blood from the intestinal capillaries to the liver; this unique shunt also drains blood from portions of the stomach and the pancreas. The colon is the final stop for undigested carbohydrates, including fibrous substances. Some further digestion and water reabsorption occurs here; then the remaining semisolid contents—the **feces,** or stool—are pushed into the rectum by peristaltic and segmentation action and expelled through the anus.

Fecal matter. The stool consists of undigested fragments of plant fiber and connective tissue from animal foods, plus bacteria and water.

Consuming too much dietary fiber can produce an overly mushy stool, but inadequate dietary fiber can cause the stool to become hard. Considerable pressure during a bowel movement must then be exerted to expel the stool. This can damage supporting tissues and expose blood vessels in the rectum, an often painful condition called **hemorrhoids.** Hemorrhoidal bleeding during defecation may require surgery to correct. Gradually increasing fiber content in the diet often relieves hemorrhoidal symptoms.

SUMMARY

1. Simple sugars consist of a chain of three to seven carbon atoms with hydrogen and oxygen attached in a ratio of 2 to 1. Glucose, the most common simple sugar, contains a six-carbon chain and is expressed as $C_6H_{12}O_6$.
2. There are three kinds of carbohydrates: monosaccharides (sugars such as glucose, fructose, and galactose); disaccharides (sucrose, lactose, and maltose); and polysaccharides, which contain three or more simple sugars to form starch, fiber, and glycogen.
3. Dietary fiber may aid gastrointestinal function, with the water-soluble fibers perhaps helping to lower blood cholesterol. Current recommendations advise increasing fiber intake to about 20 to 35 g a day with the ratio of insoluble to soluble fiber at about 3 to 1.
4. The transformation of glucose to glycogen in the body is called glycogenesis; glycogenolysis is the process of reconverting glycogen to glucose, and gluconeogenesis refers to synthesis of glucose by the body, especially from protein sources.
5. Carbohydrates, which are stored in limited quantity in liver and muscle, serve (1) as a major source of energy, (2) to spare the breakdown of proteins, (3) as a metabolic primer for fat metabolism, and (4) as fuel for the central nervous system.
6. Americans typically consume about 40 to 50% of their total calories as carbohydrates. Only half this amount is in the form of fruits, grains, and vegetables; the remainder is simple sugars, predominantly in the form of sucrose and high-fructose corn syrup.
7. Muscle glycogen and blood glucose are important fuels during intense exercise. Individuals involved in heavy exercise and training should consume about 60% of their daily calories (400 to 600 g) as carbohydrates, predominantly in unrefined, complex form.

8. The major portion of the digestion of carbohydrate takes place in the small intestine through the action of pancreatic amylase. The simple sugars are then absorbed by the intestinal villi and delivered throughout the body.

RELATED LITERATURE

Bell, L.P., et al.: Cholesterol-lowering effects of soluble-fiber cereals as part of a prudent diet for patients with mild to moderate hypercholesterolemia. Am. J. Clin. Nutr., 52:1020, 1990.

Bergstrom, J., et al.: Diet, muscle glycogen and physical performance. Acta Physiol. Scand., 71:140, 1967.

Block, G. et al.: Nutrient sources in the American diet: quantitative data from the NHANES II survey. Am. J. Epidemiol., 122:13, 1985.

Cara, L., et al.: Effects of oat bran, rice bran, wheat fiber, and wheat germ on postprandial lipemia in healthy adults. Am. J. Clin. Nutr., 55:81, 1992.

Coyle, E.F.: Carbohydrates and athletic performance. Sports Science Exchange (Gatorade Sports Institute), 1(7), 1988.

Crapo, P.A.: Sugar and sugar alcohols. Contemp. Nutr., 7(12), 1981.

Felig, P., et al.: Hypoglycemia during prolonged exercise in normal men. N. Engl. J. Med., 306:895, 1982.

Felig, P., and Wahren, J.: Fuel homeostasis in exercise. N. Engl. J. Med., 293:1078, 1975.

Guthrie, H.A.: Introductory Nutrition, 7th ed. St. Louis, C.V. Mosby, 1988.

Guyton, A.C. Textbook of Medical Physiology, 7th ed. Philadelphia, W.B. Saunders, 1986.

Hultman, E. Liver as a glucose supplying source during rest and exercise, with special reference to diet. In: Nutrition, Physical Fitness and Health. Edited by J. Parizkova and V.A. Rogozkin, Baltimore, University Park Press, 1978.

Jansson, E., and Kaijser, L.: Effect of diet on the utilization of blood-borne and intramuscular substrates during exercise in man. Acta Physiol. Scand., 115:19, 1982.

Kashtan, H., et al.: Wheat bran and oat bran supplements' effects on blood lipids and lipoproteins. Am. J. Clin. Nutr., 55:976, 1992.

Kay, R.M.: Dietary fiber. J. Lipid Res., 23:221, 1982.

Koelslag, J.H.: Post-exercise ketosis and the hormone response to exercise: a review. Med. Sci. Sports Exerc., 14:327, 1982.

Kromhout, D., et al.: Dietary fiber and 10 year mortality from coronary heart disease, cancer, and all causes. Lancet, 2:518, 1982.

Levine, A.S., et al.: Effect of breakfast cereals on short-term food intake. Am. J. Clin. Nutr., 46:790, 1987.

McArdle, W.D., et al: Exercise Physiology: Energy, Nutrition, and Human Performance, 3rd ed. Philadelphia, Lea & Febiger, 1991.

Miller, V.C. et al.: Adaptations to high-fat diet that increases exercise endurance in male rats. J. Appl. Physiol., 56:78, 1984.

Saltin, B., and Gollnick, P.D.: Fuel for muscular exercise: role of carbohydrate. In: Exercise, Nutrition, and Energy Metabolism. Edited by E.S. Horton and R.L. Terjung. New York, Macmillan, 1988.

Sharon, N.: Carbohydrates. Sci. Am., 243:90, 1980.

Sherman, W.A., and Wimer, G.S.: Insufficient dietary carbohydrate during training: does it impair athletic performance? Int. J. Sports Nutr., 1:28, 1991.

Shils, M.E., and Young, V.R. (Eds.): Modern Nutrition in Health and Disease, 6th ed. Philadelphia, Lea & Febiger, 1988.

Superko, H.F., et al.: The effect of solid and liquid gum on the reduction of plasma cholesterol in patients with moderate hypercholesterolemia. Am. J. Cardiol., 62:51, 1988.

Swanson, J.E., et al.: Metabolic effects of dietary fructose in healthy subjects. Am. J. Clin. Nutr., 55:851, 1992.

Williams, P.T., et al.: Relationship of dietary fat, protein, cholesterol, and fiber intake to athrogenic lipoproteins in men. Am. J. Clin Nutr., 44:788, 1986.

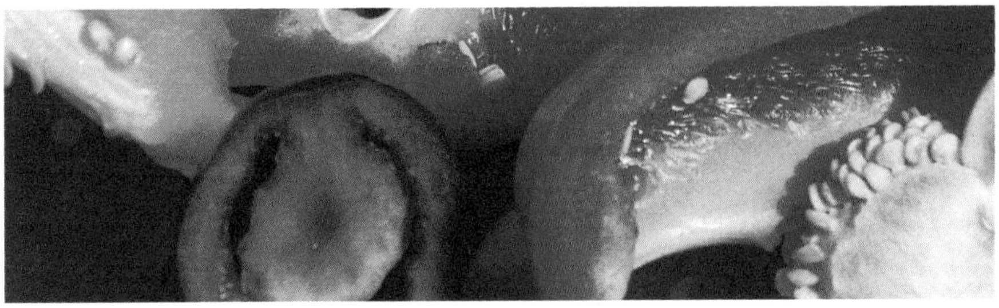

4

LIPIDS

Fats, or lipids, consist of any organic substance of plant or animal origin that is oily or greasy to the touch, insoluble in water, and nonvolatile. In humans, a major function of lipids is to provide cellular fuel through enzyme-regulated oxidative reactions. This is because, on a weight basis, fat contains more than twice as much energy as protein or carbohydrate. In addition to serving as a food reserve to supply energy, lipids fulfill numerous other functions related to optimal physiologic regulation.

WHAT ARE LIPIDS?

Lipid is the name given to a family of compounds that includes **fats, oils,** and other lipid-like substances. The distinction is that fats are solid at room temperature; oils, by contrast, are lipids that liquefy at room temperature. For ease in reading and comprehension, we will use the terms lipids and fat interchangeably where applicable.

Like carbohydrate, a lipid molecule is composed of carbon, oxygen, and hydrogen atoms linked together in a specific and unique way. Figure 4–1 shows that the chemical structure of the major lipids consists of two different clusters of atoms. One cluster, **glycerol,** is the basic building block that forms the backbone of the triglyceride molecule, and is composed of three atoms of carbon combined with three hydroxyl (OH) groups. *When glycerol and three fatty acid molecules are joined chemically, they produce a molecule of "neutral fat" or* ***triglyceride.*** Besides the neutral or simple fats, two additional groups are recognized: **compound fats,** composed of simple fats in combination with other chemicals (phospholipids, glucolipids, and lipoproteins), and **derived fats** (notably cholesterol) made up from simple and compound fats.

Triglyceride, the most common fat. By far, triglycerides represent the most plentiful fat in the body. More than 95% of body fat is in this form.

FATTY ACIDS

The **fatty acids** give each fat its unique qualities of flavor and texture, making corn oil very different from chicken fat. Fatty acids have two unique char-

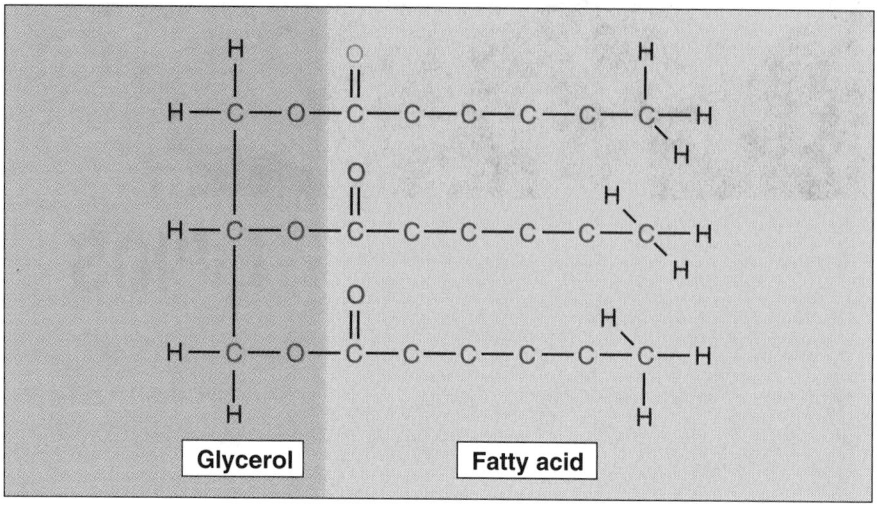

FIG. 4–1. A combined glycerol and a fatty acid molecule forms a triglyceride.

acteristics: they differ in (1) the length of their carbon chain, and (2) the bonding of carbon atoms and arrangement of hydrogens along the carbon chain.

Short-chain fatty acids have four to eight carbons (dairy fats), **medium-chain fatty acids** have eight to 12 carbons (coconut and palm oil), and **long-chain fatty acids** have more than 12 carbon atoms (many animal fats). The most common fatty acids in the diet come from animal sources; they contain between 16 and 18 atoms of carbon in each molecule. Oils are usually of the short-chain variety, while the long-chain fatty acids from animal sources are the solid fats.

Fatty acids are of two types, depending on their carbon bonding. *Fatty acids with only single bonds linking carbons together are known as **saturated fatty acids.** Fatty acids with at least one double bond in the carbon chain are referred to as **unsaturated fatty acids.***

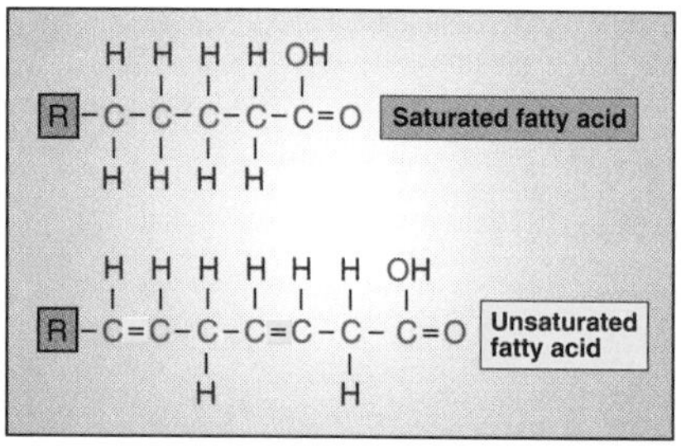

FIG. 4–2. The major structural difference between saturated and unsaturated fatty acids is the presence or absence of double bonds between the carbon atoms. R represents the glycerol portion of the triglyceride molecule.

Figure 4–2 illustrates the general differences in bonding and arrangement of hydrogens in saturated and unsaturated fatty acids. For simplification, the symbol R represents the glycerol portion of the molecule. Only single bonds link the carbon atoms in saturated fatty acids, so at least two hydrogen atoms can attach to each carbon along the main chain. Because the interconnected chain of carbon atoms holds as many hydrogens as is chemically possible, the molecule is said to be saturated with respect to hydrogen atoms; hence its name. Saturated fats are found primarily in animal products including beef, lamb, pork, and chicken. They are also present in egg yolk and in the dairy fats of cream, milk, cheese, and butter. Coconut and palm oil, vegetable shortening, and margarine (discussed later in this chapter) are sources of saturated fat from the plant kingdom and are present to a relatively high degree in commercially prepared cakes, pies, and cookies. Chocolate—a plant product—is rich in saturated fat, and nondairy creamers, because they contain coconut oil, have more saturated fat than does real cream.

In contrast, an unsaturated fatty acid contains one or more double bonds along the main carbon chain. Each double bond takes the place of two hydrogen atoms; the fatty acid can have either the cis or the trans configuration (see Chapter 1) with cis the more common type. If the carbon chain of the fatty acid has only one double bond, it is called **monounsaturated;** examples are olive, peanut, or canola oil. If there are two or more double bonds along the main carbon chain, the fatty acid is said to be **polyunsaturated;** sunflower, soybean, corn, and safflower oil are all polyunsaturated. Fats from the plant kingdom are generally unsaturated. Regardless of the degree of saturation, all lipids have essentially the same number of calories per unit weight. One gram of fat contains approximately 9 calories of energy.

WHERE DO LIPIDS COME FROM?

Both plants and animals provide ready sources of fat. Plants manufacture lipids by photosynthesis, the same process they use to make carbohydrates. Animals use or store the fat they ingest, or can synthesize fat from the carbon, hydrogen, and oxygen atoms present in excess quantities of ingested carbohydrates and proteins.

Fish Oils May Be Healthful. Considerable research has focused on the potential health benefits of ingesting an **omega-3 family of fatty acids** found primarily in the oils of cold-water fish such as Atlantic halibut, mackerel, herring and salmon, Pacific herring, sardines, lake trout, bluefish, albacore tuna, and coho, pink, and king salmon. This group of polyunsaturated fatty acids includes eicosapentaenoic acid (abbreviated EPA), a 20-carbon fatty acid with five double bonds; arachidonic acid, also a 20-carbon fatty acid; and docosahexaenoic acid (DHA), a 22-carbon-chain fatty acid. The body cannot synthesize these fatty acids, so they can only be obtained in the diet.

Consider fish. When 27 hyperlipidemic men were fed a daily fish-oil supplement (15 g/day) for eight weeks, there was a 40% decrease in serum triglycerides, a 12% increase in HDL cholesterol, and a significant decrease in blood viscosity, whereas a vegetable-oil placebo had no effect.

The Inuit Eskimos of Greenland have a low heart attack rate but, paradoxically, consume more total calories and calories from fat than their typical American counterparts. Analysis of their diet showed that their food intake is particularly high in omega-3 fatty acids from fish oil sources. In relation to heart disease risk, the molecular structure of the omega-3 fatty acids may help to prevent blood clots from forming on artery walls, lower blood pressure, and increase plasma HDL, and decrease LDL cholesterol. Of course substances in fish besides the omega-3 fatty acids may contribute to the positive effect on cardiovascular disease risk. While research continues, it seems reasonable to include fish (or perhaps fish oil) at least two or three times a week as part of our regular diet. This would amount to about 10 ounces, or 280 g, weekly. Plant sources of omega-3 fatty acids include tofu (soybean curd), walnuts, dried beans, lecithin, and wheat germ, soybean, and canola oil.

PHOSPHOLIPIDS AND RELATED FATS

Phospholipids are a type of compound fat present in the body. They are mainly synthesized in the liver from a combination of fatty acids, phosphorus, and nitrogen compounds. In chemical terms, a phospholipid is a lipid that has a phosphorus-containing unit in place of a fatty acid chain. Phospholipids are a component of all cells. As discussed in Chapter 1, they serve as the structural framework for both the bilayer that constitutes each cell's unique plasma membrane as well as the membranes that enclose the organelles within a cell, such as the nucleus, endoplasmic reticulum, lysosomes, and mitochondria. In addition to helping maintain a cell's structural integrity, phospholipids are important in blood clotting and in the structure of the insulating sheaths around nerve fibers (see Chapter 1).

The best known of the phospholipids is **lecithin,** a compound that consists of two fatty acids and the vitamin-like compound choline. Lecithin functions as an emulsifier in the small intestine and helps to regulate the passage of lipids through a cell's phospholipid membrane. In the body, the highest concentration of lecithin is found in nerve cells. Examples of lecithin-rich foods include soybeans, peanuts, calf's liver, ham, lamb, beef, egg yolk, oatmeal, and wheat germ. In prepared foods, lecithin acts as an emulsifying agent so oils and water can mix, as in salad dressings, ice cream, chocolate, and cookie and cake mixes.

Because lecithin is so readily available in the diet, it is not considered an essential ingredient and has no recommended requirement. People who take lecithin supplements, usually in excess of 30 g daily, may suffer minor but unpleasant side effects including diarrhea, nausea, sweating, and vomiting. The concentration of lecithin, as sold commercially in capsule, liquid, and granular form, may be only 10 to 40%; taking several capsules, therefore, may provide no more lecithin than is contained in daily food intake. Even if taken in amounts up to 60 g or more daily, lecithin has no magic properties to help lower blood cholesterol, reduce excess body fat, improve memory, or alleviate symptoms of Alzheimer's disease.

Other compound fats include the **glucolipids** (fatty acids bound with carbohydrate and nitrogen) and lipoproteins (discussed in detail later in this chapter). These lipids are formed primarily in the liver from the union of either triglycerides, phospholipids, or cholesterol with protein.

Foods high in cholesterol based on a 100-g (3.5 oz) serving.

FOOD	CHOLESTEROL (MG)
Beef brains, pan fried	1995
Beef liver, fried	482
Egg, raw	410
Egg salad	344
Chicken gizzards, simmered	194
Cheesecake	185
Quiche Lorraine	162
Waffles, home-made	136
Crab, cooked	100
Lemon meringue pie	98

The leaner the better. Recent research indicates that beef fat, and not the lean portion, is related to elevated blood cholesterol. If beef is trimmed of all visible fat and the diet is low in saturated fat, lean beef can be included in a cholesterol-lowering diet.

CHOLESTEROL

Cholesterol *is a fatty-like substance belonging to a class of compounds known as sterols that are present in all animal cells.* Sterols are not fats per se, as they contain no fatty acids. They do, however, exhibit some of the physical and chemical characteristics of fat.

Cholesterol is either consumed in foods of animal origin **(exogenous cholesterol)** or synthesized within the body, usually when dietary cholesterol is inadequate **(endogenous cholesterol).** Even more endogenous cholesterol is produced when the diet is high in saturated fat! Cholesterol is *not* contained in vegetable food sources and is negligible in egg whites and skimmed milk. The richest source of cholesterol in foods is egg yolk. Because plants contain no cholesterol, advertising that a particular product of vegetable origin is "cholesterol free" is simply intended to hype the product. Cholesterol is also plentiful in red meats, in organ meats such as liver, kidney, and brains, as well as in dairy products such as ice cream, butter, cream cheese, and whole milk.

THE LIPOPROTEINS

Fat carriers in the bloodstream. The **lipoproteins are important because they allow lipids to be transported in the watery medium of the blood.**

If blood lipids were not bound to protein, they would literally float to the top like cream in milk that was not homogenized. Figure 4–3 illustrates the structural details of a lipoprotein.

Lipids are carried by lipoproteins whether they originate from dietary sources in food or from synthesis by the liver. In either case, the triglyceride is coated with a shell composed of protein, phospholipid, and cholesterol so it is easily transported in the plasma. In essence, the lipoprotein structure is a lipid droplet surrounded by a shell. The protein component of the lipoprotein shell controls its specific function and is known as an **apoprotein.**

Once a triglyceride is formed from dietary fat during digestion in the small intestine, it combines with phospholipids and a small amount of cholesterol to form a **chylomicron.** A chylomicron is a small lipid droplet that consists mainly of triglyceride and fatty acids with some cholesterol, phospholipids, and proteins. Chylomicrons are formed during fat absorption in the small intestine and are transported by the lymphatics. The chylomicron enters the bloodstream via the lymphatic system that empties into the thoracic duct and eventually drains into a large vein in the neck. Once chylomicrons are in the bloodstream, their lipoproteins are de-

Apoprotein. The apoproteins are a class of specific proteins embedded in the outer shell of the lipoprotein particle that (1) increase the solubility of the lipoprotein's cholesterol and triglyceride components, (2) act as ligands for specific lipoprotein receptors in cell membranes, and (3) act as important cofactors to activate enzymes important in lipoprotein metabolism. Researchers now believe that the specific apoproteins may be a more reliable indicator of our proneness to heart disease than the total cholesterol level. This may explain why many individuals with "normal" cholesterol levels nevertheless develop heart disease.

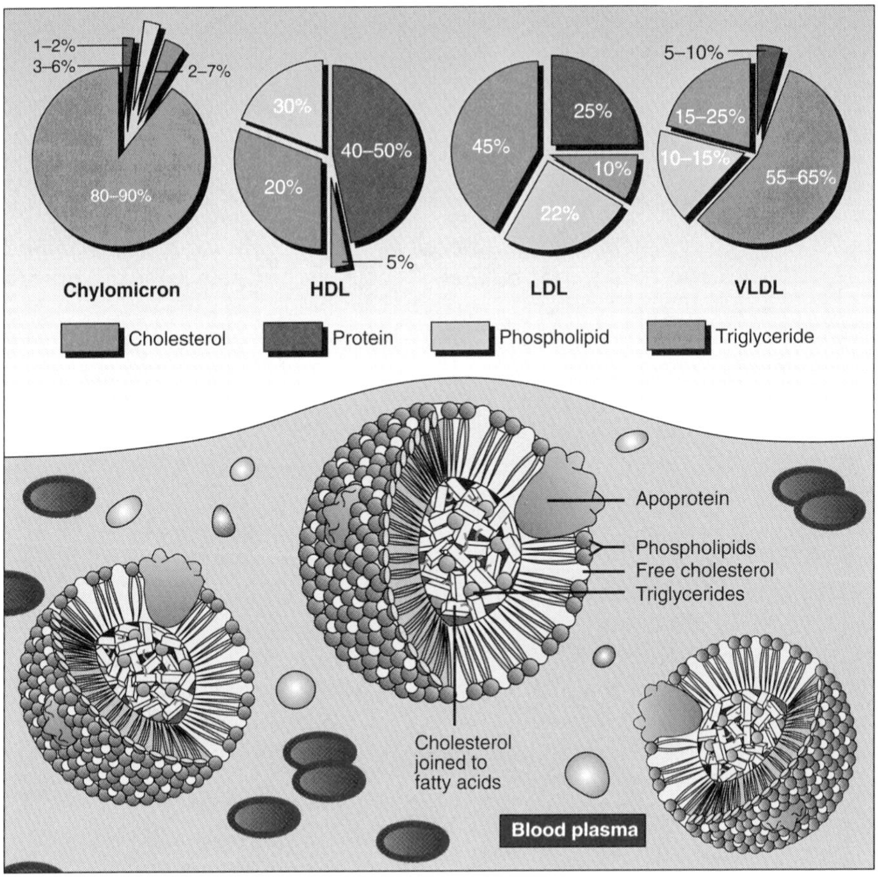

FIG. 4–3. Structural details and composition of lipoproteins. Free cholesterol and triglyceride are carried in the chylomicron. The chylomicrons transport the absorbed lipids from the intestines to the cells of the body. The VLDL and LDL subfractions carry fats made in the liver to the cells. The LDL delivers cholesterol to cells, while the HDL transports cholesterol away from cells to the liver.

esterified (broken down) by the enzyme **lipoprotein lipase** into free fatty acids and glycerol. Thereafter, the fate of the "freed" fatty acids is to be taken up for use as fuel by muscle cells or to become re-esterified (reformed) once again as triglyceride and stored in adipose tissue. In addition to triglyceride obtained in the diet, the liver synthesizes triglycerides and cholesterol from nondietary (endogenous) sources provided by body protein, fat, and carbohydrate. The compound in the liver that functions most like the small intestine's chylomicron is the triglyceride-rich very low density lipoprotein **(VLDL).** Of all of the lipoproteins, the VLDL contains the greatest percentage of lipid (95%) of which about 60% is in the form of triglycerides.

Lipoprotein lipase. This fat-degrading enzyme is attached to capillary walls and facilitates the hydrolysis of triglyceride into its glycerol and fatty acid components.

A person being tested for blood triglyceride content must go a minimum of 14 hours without food prior to testing to ensure that all chylomicrons have been cleared from the bloodstream. In this way, a fatty meal will have no residual effect on the test results. When testing is done only for total blood cholesterol, fasting is unnecessary. Abnormal blood cholesterol readings should be confirmed within an eight-week period. This will allow for a person's normal fluctuation in cholesterol level as well as variation in test results, even from the same laboratory. Desirable levels of cholesterol are discussed more fully in Chapter 20.

HIGH- AND LOW-DENSITY LIPOPROTEINS

There are basically two main types of lipoproteins. High-density lipoproteins **(HDL)** are produced in the liver and small intestine and contain the largest amount of protein and correspondingly, the smallest amount of cholesterol. A low-density lipoprotein **(LDL)** is a remnant of a VLDL. Once the VLDL is acted on by the enzyme lipoprotein lipase to de-esterify triglycerides in the chylomicron, it becomes denser because it now contains less lipid; this forms an intermediate-density lipoprotein **(IDL).** Approximately 50% of IDLs return to the liver; the remainder are converted to LDLs. The LDL and VLDL fractions contain the greatest fat and least protein components.

"Bad" cholesterol. Among the lipoproteins, the LDLs, which normally carry almost 50% of the total cholesterol, have the greatest affinity for the arterial wall. They help to carry cholesterol into arterial tissue where it is chemically modified and ultimately participates in the proliferation of smooth muscle cells and further changes that damage and narrow the artery in the process of coronary heart disease. When LDLs enter a cell, they are separated into their cholesterol and protein fractions, which are then used to build compounds such as the hormone estrogen or parts of the cell membrane. In this sense, the LDL should not really be considered "bad." A high level of LDL cholesterol, however, is considered undesirable because it is implicated in **plaque** formation on the inner walls of blood vessels. In this sense, an excessively high level of LDL cholesterol is properly thought of as "bad" cholesterol.

Consider the monounsaturates. Increasing monounsaturated fatty acids in the diet helps to lower LDL cholesterol without also reducing the "good" HDL cholesterol.

Arterial plaque. Plaque is made up of disk-shaped, cholesterol-rich deposits that form on the inner surface of a blood vessel and eventually become calcified. Plaque formation is intimately involved in atherosclerosis, the narrowing process of coronary arteries, that progressively reduces the blood vessel's capacity for blood flow and oxygen delivery to the heart.

"Good" Cholesterol. Unlike LDL, HDL may operate as so-called good cholesterol to protect against heart disease in one of two ways: (1) to act as a scavenger of cholesterol, removing it from the arterial wall and transporting it to the liver where it is incorporated into bile and subsequently excreted via the intestines, and (2) to compete with the LDL fragment for receptor sites on the arterial wall, thus blocking the entrance of LDL cholesterol into the cell.

The quantity of LDL and HDL, as well as the specific ratio of these lipoproteins and subfractions, may provide a more meaningful signal of our risk for coronary heart disease than total cholesterol per se. The LDL/HDL ratio is improved with a diet low in calories and saturated fat. Regular aerobic exercise and abstinence from cigarette smoking also increase the HDL level and can favorably affect the LDL/HDL ratio. This will be discussed more fully in Chapter 20.

High-density lipoproteins. HDL is composed of the greatest percentage of protein (about 50%), the least total lipid (about 20%), and the least cholesterol (about 20%) of all the lipoproteins. High levels of HDL relate to a low risk for heart disease.

FUNCTIONS OF LIPIDS

Lipids serve diverse, yet essential functions in the body. Their roles include energy metabolism, cushioning and protection, insulation, cell membrane formation, hormone synthesis, vitamin transport and storage, and control of hunger pangs and feelings of satiety.

ENERGY SOURCE

Energy is derived in approximately equal amounts from the body's stores of carbohydrates and lipids during rest and moderate muscular exercise. In prolonged exercise of one hour or longer, the amount of lipid utilized for energy significantly increases so that as exercise continues lipids may supply nearly 90% of the energy requirement. On the other hand, in intense but short-term exercise such as all-out running or swimming, essentially all of the energy comes from glycogen stored in the specific muscles used in the activity.

An Energy-Rich Fuel. In terms of its capability for energy storage, fat is remarkably efficient because more than twice the energy is stored in a gram of fat as in the same amount of carbohydrate or protein. Humans and many animals would be considerably larger in body size if their energy reserves depended predominantly on carbohydrate storage. This high energy density comes mainly from the large amount of hydrogen in a fat molecule: the union of glycerol and three fatty acids to form a triglyceride produces three molecules of water. In contrast, when glucose is stored as glycogen, 2.7 g of water are retained for each gram of glycogen. Thus, fat exists in a relatively water-free, concentrated form, whereas the addition of water to the glycogen molecule makes this a heavy fuel. Excess calories from nutrients other than fat are readily converted to fat for storage. In this way, fat serves as the major storehouse of excess nutrient energy. As with carbohydrate, the use of fat as an energy fuel "spares" protein for its important functions of tissue synthesis and repair.

The potential energy stored in the triglyceride molecules of an average-size young adult male is about 81,000 calories. Excluding the essential body fat required for vital functions, this would leave approximately 65,000 calories available for energy. Theoretically, if this 74-kilogram (kg) man jogged at a pace of nine minutes per mile (which would burn about 117 calories a mile), the available fuel energy from stored fat could power a 555-mile run from Hollywood in Southern California north to the wine country of Napa, California. Contrast this to the 2000-calorie energy reserve of stored carbohydrate, which could provide only enough energy for about a 20-mile run!

Essential body fat. Essential body fat is that required for normal physiologic functioning. It is incorporated into cell membranes, bone marrow, and various organs, especially the lipid-rich tissues throughout the nervous system. Females possess additional gender-specific essential fat that is biologically important for childbearing and other hormone-related functions.

Migrating animals would be unable to complete their often long and uninterrupted journey if carbohydrate were their main source of energy. Experiments have shown that during continuous flights of up to three days' duration, birds rely almost exclusively on fat for energy. Several days before migration, the fat stored in the adipose tissue increases considerably. Warblers captured immediately after a transoceanic flight have a 25 to 40% decrease in body mass, mainly from loss of body fat. Lipid stores enable some birds to fly nonstop for over 60 hours! In fact, the balance between fuel storage and energy expenditure is so delicate that if a bird encounters an unexpected headwind, it may be unable to continue and will fall exhausted into the water, sometimes only a few miles from land.

The preceding discussion does not intend to minimize the role of carbohydrate in energy metabolism for prolonged work. Although significantly less carbohydrate than fat is used in long-term exercise, a minimum amount of carbohydrate must be available for energy so exercise can continue. The functions of the macronutrients in both short- and long-term exercise are discussed more fully in Chapters 10 and 11.

PROTECTION OF VITAL ORGANS

Approximately 4% of the total body fat serves as a shock absorber and protective shield against trauma to vital organs such as the heart, liver, kidneys, spleen, brain, and spinal cord. Even during protracted periods of food deprivation, the protective fat layer surrounding these organs is reduced only slightly compared to the quantity of fat depleted from the fat storage tissues beneath the skin.

INSULATION

Fat stored in the subcutaneous tissues acts as an insulator against the stress of a cold environment. Although this benefit may provide a comfortable rationalization for many of us who are exquisite insulators, it probably is of real value to relatively few people such as ocean swimmers or occupational deep sea divers, who must work while submerged in cold water for prolonged periods. In fact, the insulation provided by excess body fat is a liability to temperature regulation in hot environments. The obese in particular are disadvantaged in dissipating body heat. Fat people sweat readily on warm days, while those who are lean and possess less insulation maintain body temperature for some time before relying on the cooling benefits of sweating. The problem of heat regulation in the obese is magnified during physical activity, in which the body's heat production can increase 10 to 20 times above the resting level.

Anorexia nervosa. This extreme eating disorder consists of voluntary food deprivation, usually among teen-age girls and women who have a distorted body image. Body mass is reduced to such an extent that the ultimate result is medical disability and even death. The condition requires skilled medical, nutritional, and psychological treatment and is best dealt with by trained personnel in a supervised setting. Anorexia nervosa is especially prevalent among dancers, gymnasts, and other competitive athletes for whom extremes of weight control are usually prerequisites for success.

In extreme fat loss, as in the disease **anorexia nervosa,** most of the body's insulating fat layer is depleted. Anorectics not uncommonly reduce their body mass by up to 35% as they become emaciated. One of the body's defenses against this inordinate fat loss is to develop additional hair, which traps air at the body surface to aid in insulation.

OTHER FUNCTIONS

Vitamin Carrier. Fat acts as a carrier and storage medium for the fat-soluble vitamins A, D, E, and K. Ingesting about 20 g of fat daily can serve this purpose. Decreasing the amount of lipid in the diet will reduce the availability of these important vitamins, and diets consistently low in lipid content can lead to a deficiency in one or more of them. Dietary fat is also believed necessary for the absorption of vitamin A precursors from nonfat sources such as carrots.

Satiety. Many people who nibble on carbohydrate-rich foods throughout the day often comment that they feel continually hungry. Adding a small quantity of fat to the diet will help with this problem. Acidic gastric juices take longer to digest fat than carbohydrates. Also, fatty food fragments remain in the stomach longer than do carbohydrates and proteins because of the lipid's lower density. Thus, some fat in the diet helps to delay the onset of "hunger pangs" and promotes a feeling of fullness and satiety. This is one reason why reducing diets containing moderate amounts of fat are considered more effective than diets low in fat. In addition, the flavors in food are fat soluble and their smell can be "sensed" in the mouth. A food with good flavor often "feels good" when it is tasted. Such foods often have a relatively high fat content.

Biologic Membranes. As pointed out in Chapter 1, phospholipids and cholesterol are integral components of cell membranes. The fatty acids in the phospholipid bilayer of the membrane, in conjunction with a specific protein, control the passage of substances into and out of the cell and organelles within the cell.

Essential Nutrients. Several of the polyunsaturated fatty acids, notably linolenic and linoleic acid, are required for good health. Unlike other fatty acids that can be synthesized from macronutrients in the body, these cannot be made endogenously and must be consumed in the diet. For this reason, they are referred to as essential fatty acids. Fortunately, the essential fatty acids are present in abundance in many foods that are part of the typical American diet. The common vegetable oils contain approximately 50% of their fatty acids as linoleic acid.

The way it's cooked is important. The cooking method can add considerable fat to the daily diet. Consider the potato: bake it and there is hardly any fat, but slice it up and deep fry it in oil, and the fat content jumps to nearly 20 g!

RECOMMENDED INTAKE OF LIPIDS

In the United States, dietary fat represents approximately 40 to 50% of total calorie intake. The latest report from the U.S. Department of Agriculture reveals that each person in the United States consumes approximately 30 kg of fats and oils a year! The largest contributor to this lipid intake is salad and cooking oils (11.8 kg), followed by shortening (10 kg), margarine (4.5 kg), butter (2.3 kg), and lard (1.0 kg). Over the last 20 years, lard consumption has decreased and intake of vegetable oil has increased dramatically. Unfortunately, the total intake of fats over this time has increased by approximately 21%.

Quite a bit of energy! The per capita yearly fat consumption in the United States, extrapolated over a population of 250 million people, amounts to 16.5 billion total pounds of dietary fat, or the equivalent of 839 billion calories!

While standards for optimal fat intake have not been firmly established, many nutritionists and medical personnel believe that to promote optimal health, fat intake should not exceed 30% of the energy content of the diet. Of this fat intake, at least 70% should be in the form of unsaturated fatty acids. For dietary cholesterol, the American Heart Association recommends the consumption of no more than 300 mg (0.01 oz) of cholesterol each day, limiting intake to no more than 100 mg per 1000 calories of food ingested. Three hundred mg of cholesterol is almost the amount contained in the yolk of one large egg and just about one-half the cholesterol ingested by the average American male. Reducing daily cholesterol intake towards 150 to 200 mg may be even more desirable.

HIGH-FAT DIETS AND HEART DISEASE

The real dietary culprit. Saturated fatty acids in the diet may stimulate a greater rise in blood cholesterol than comes from dietary cholesterol itself.

Saturated fat intake has steadily increased in the American diet to the point that the average person now consumes about 15% of total calories, or over 23 kg, as saturated fat per year! Most of this fat is of animal origin. Our pattern is in contrast to groups such as the Tarahumara Indians of Mexico, whose diet of high-complex, unrefined carbohydrate contains only 2% of the total calories as saturated fat. Coinciding with increased consumption of saturated fats has been a rise in coronary heart disease. The explanation probably is that a diet high in saturated fat facilitates cholesterol synthesis by the liver. This relationship has led nutritionists and medical personnel to recommend replacing at least some saturated fat in our diet with monounsaturated and polyunsaturated lipids such as those derived from vegetable sources (e.g., olive oil and corn oil) or the polyunsaturated oils present mainly in cold-water fish.

Ratio of Polyunsaturated to Saturated Fats. The ratio of polyunsaturated to saturated fats, known as the **P/S ratio,** provides an index of the relative contribution of these two types of fatty acids in food. The recommended P/S ratio is at least 1 to 1 and preferably 2 to 1. Based on dietary surveys, the ratio in the United States is only 0.43 to 1.0. It should be noted that the P/S ratio has some limitations and cannot be exclusively relied upon as a guide to fat intake. For example, the ratio does not consider the potential cholesterol-lowering role of some monounsaturated fatty acids if they replace saturated fatty acids in the diet. Also, not all saturated fats increase serum cholesterol. Nevertheless, the P/S ratio provides the consumer useful information about the fatty acid content of food, provided the food source lists the types of fatty acids. Table 4–1 lists examples of foods high and low in saturated fat, foods high in monounsaturated fat, and the P/S ratio for common fats and oils.

Less is better. A prudent recommendation is that saturated fat should represent no more than 10%, and preferably only 6%, of total calories.

Ratio of Saturated to Monounsaturated to Polyunsaturated Fatty Acids. Taking a slightly different approach, the American Heart Association recommends that consumers consider the ratio of the various fatty acids in the diet. By these guidelines, total fat intake should be less than 30% of total calories with the calories from fat distributed in a ratio of 10:10:10 for saturated to monounsaturated to polyunsaturated fatty acids. If food labels included such detailed information about lipid composition, the consumer would be aware of the food's "desirability" relative to risk for coronary heart disease.

TABLE 4–1. EXAMPLES OF FOODS HIGH AND LOW IN SATURATED FAT, FOODS HIGH IN MONOUNSATURATED FAT, AND THE POLYUNSATURATED TO SATURATED FAT (P/S) RATIO OF COMMON FATS AND OILS

HIGH SATURATED, %		LOW SATURATED, %		HIGH MONOUNSATURATED, %	
Coconut oil	88	Popcorn	0	Olives, black	80
Palm kernal oil	82	Hard candy	0	Olive oil	74
Butter	61	Yogurt, nonfat	2	Almond oil	70
Cream cheese	57	Crackerjacks	3	Canola oil	60
Coconut	56	Milk, skim	4	Almonds, dry	52
Hollandaise sauce	54	Cookies, fig bars	4	Avocados	51
Palm oil	49	Graham crackers	5	Peanut oil	46
Half & half	45	Chicken breast, roasted	6	Cashews, dry roasted	42
Cheese, Velveeta	43	Pancakes	8	Peanut butter	39
Cheese, mozzarella	41	Cottage cheese, 1%	8	Bologna	39
Ice cream, vanilla	38	Milk, chocolate, 1%	9	Beef, cooked	33
Cheesecake	32	Beef, dried	9	Lamb, roasted	32
Chocolate almond bar	29	Chocolate, mints	10	Veal, roasted	26

HIGH POLY-UNSATURATED, %		P/S RATIO, FATS & OILS	
Safflower oil	81	Coconut oil	0.2/1.0
Sunflower oil	73	Palm oil	0.2/1.0
Corn oil	59	Butter	0.1/1.0
Walnuts, dry	51	Olive oil	0.6/1.0
Sunflower seeds	47	Lard	0.3/1.0
Margarine, corn oil	45	Canola oil	5.3/1.0
Canola oil	32	Peanut oil	1.9/1.0
Sesame seeds	31	Soybean oil	2.5/1.0
Pumpkin seeds	31	Sesame oil	3.0/1.0
Tofu	27	Margarine, 100% corn oil	2.5/1.0
Lard	11	Cottonseed oil	2.0/1.0
Butter	6	Mayonnaise	3.7/1.0
Coconut oil	2	Safflower oil	13.3/1.0

Data compiled from the Science and Education Administration, Home and Garden Bulletin 72, Nutritive Value of Foods, Washington, DC, US Government Printing Office, 1985, 1986; Agricultural Research Service, United States Department of Agriculture, Nutritive Value of American Foods in Common Units. Agricultural Handbook No. 456, Washington, DC, US Government Printing Office, 1975.

Fat substitute eliminates the fat! A recently introduced substance called Simplesse takes the fat out of formerly fat products. It blends egg white and milk proteins to give a creamy, rich fluid that tastes like fat but has few fat calories. *Simplesse is manufactured by the NutraSweet Company.* Source: The NutraSweet Company, USDA handbook No. 8, and product labels.

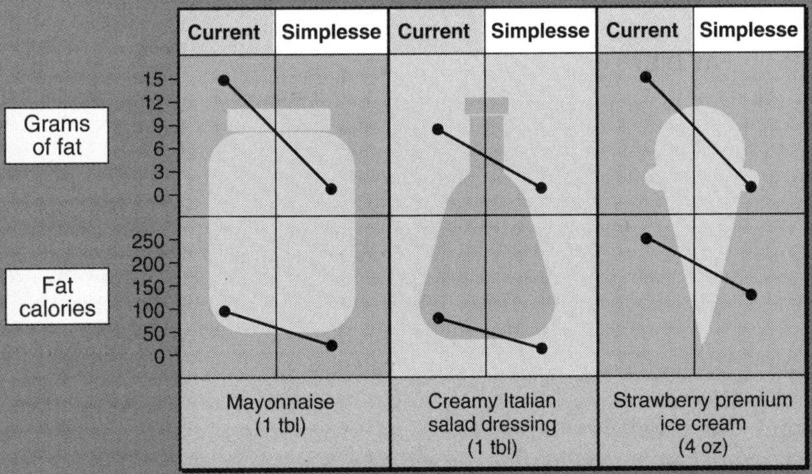

Simplesse is manufactured by the NutraSweet Company.

TABLE 4–2. THREE DIFFERENT DAILY MENUS, EACH CONSISTING OF 2000 CALORIES, BUT WITH DIFFERENT PERCENTAGES OF TOTAL FAT

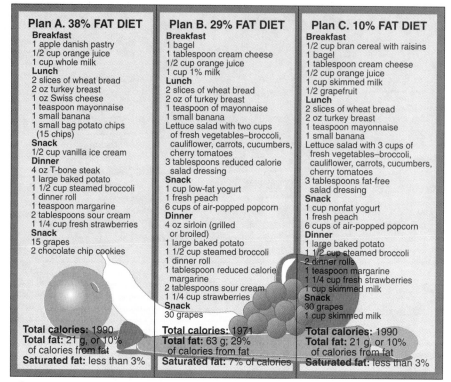

Plan A. 38% FAT DIET

Breakfast
1 apple danish pastry
1/2 cup orange juice
1 cup whole milk

Lunch
2 slices of wheat bread
2 oz turkey breast
1 oz Swiss cheese
1 teaspoon mayonnaise
1 small banana
1 small bag potato chips (15 chips)

Snack
1/2 cup vanilla ice cream

Dinner
4 oz T-bone steak
1 large baked potato
1 1/2 cup steamed broccoli
1 dinner roll
1 teaspoon margarine
2 tablespoons sour cream
1 1/4 cup fresh strawberries

Snack
15 grapes
2 chocolate chip cookies

Total calories: 1990
Total fat: 21 g, or 10% of calories from fat
Saturated fat: less than 3%

Plan B. 29% FAT DIET

Breakfast
1 bagel
1 tablespoon cream cheese
1/2 cup orange juice
1 cup 1% milk

Lunch
2 slices of wheat bread
2 oz of turkey breast
1 teaspoon of mayonnaise
1 small banana
Lettuce salad with two cups of fresh vegetables–broccoli, cauliflower, carrots, cucumbers, cherry tomatoes
3 tablespoons reduced calorie salad dressing

Snack
1 cup low-fat yogurt
1 fresh peach
6 cups of air-popped popcorn

Dinner
4 oz sirloin (grilled or broiled)
1 large baked potato
1 1/2 cup steamed broccoli
1 dinner roll
1 tablespoon reduced calorie margarine
2 tablespoons sour cream
1 1/4 cup strawberries

Snack
30 grapes

Total calories: 1971
Total fat: 63 g; 29% of calories from fat
Saturated fat: 7% of calories

Plan C. 10% FAT DIET

Breakfast
1/2 cup bran cereal with raisins
1 bagel
1 tablespoon cream cheese
1/2 cup orange juice
1 cup skimmed milk
1/2 grapefruit

Lunch
2 slices of wheat bread
2 oz turkey breast
1 teaspoon mayonnaise
1 small banana
Lettuce salad with 3 cups of fresh vegetables–broccoli, cauliflower, carrots, cucumbers, cherry tomatoes
3 tablespoons fat-free salad dressing

Snack
1 cup nonfat yogurt
1 fresh peach
6 cups of air-popped popcorn

Dinner
1 large baked potato
1 1/2 cup steamed broccoli
2 dinner rolls
1 teaspoon margarine
1 1/4 cup fresh strawberries
1 cup skimmed milk

Snack
30 grapes
1 cup skimmed milk

Total calories: 1990
Total fat: 21 g, or 10% of calories from fat
Saturated fat: less than 3%

Source: Kim Galeaz Gioe, spokeswoman for the American Dietetic Association. Adapted from Julie Stacey, USA TODAY.

The dietary guidelines work. US sailors successfully completed a 6-month experiment in which they had unlimited access to foods prepared according to American Cancer Society Guidelines, consisting of 30% or less of total calories from fat. Compared to sailors who ate traditionally prepared meals (highly buttered foods, gravies, fried foods, whole milk, rich desserts, hard candy, and fatty meats), the sailors on the experimental diet (low-fat milk and desserts, leaner cuts of meat, fat-free dressings, seasonings, and gravies, and heavy emphasis on fresh fruits and vegetables) achieved the following:

- Significantly reduced serum cholesterol
- 2 inch (5.1 cm) reduction in abdominal girth
- 12 pound (5.5 kg) decrease in body weight

Besides the obvious health benefits, there was almost universal acceptance of the stricter dietary plan.

Examples of Fat Levels in the Diet. Table 4–2 presents three daily menus, each consisting of 2000 calories but with different percentages of total fat. Meal plan A, consisting of 38% of total calories from fat, is the most typical North American diet. Meal plan B contains 29% total fat, a value recommended by most health professionals. Meal plan C, with 10% fat, is desirable but difficult to maintain for long periods in our culture.

Deli meats are high in fat. The fat content of popular deli meats often exceeds 70%!

DELI FOOD (1 oz portion)	TOTAL KCAL	TOTAL FAT, G	% KCAL AS FAT
Bologna, beef	88.7	8.0	81.6
Knockwurst	87.1	7.9	81.4
Bologna, beef & pork	88.8	8.0	81.1
Pepperoni sausage	140	12.5	80.4
Polish sausage	91.8	8.1	79.7
Kielbasa sausage	88.3	7.7	78.5
Salami, beef & pork	120	9.8	73.1
Italian sausage	91.4	7.3	71.7
Salami, beef	71.5	5.7	71.6
Corned beef	71.0	4.2	53.7
Ham, baked	51.5	3.0	52.4
Turkey pastrami	36.8	1.8	42.8

HIGH-FAT DIETS AND CANCER

Cancer is the second leading cause of death among adults in the United States. There is concern over an association between high-fat diets (both saturated and unsaturated) and colon cancer, as well as the possibility that these diets promote the growth of other cancers such as breast, prostate, and endometrial cancer.

The National Cancer Institute states that improper composition of the diet is the single largest cause of cancer. In a study of female breast cancer, those countries with a high proportion of calorie intake as lipids (The Netherlands, United States, Canada, United Kingdom) had a significantly higher age-adjusted mortality for breast cancer than countries with a low dietary lipid intake (Thailand, Japan, Portugal). In fact, recent data indicate that switching from a high-fat to a low-fat diet reduces the risk of breast cancer by as much as 30%. Clearly, numerous factors are associated with the development of cancer, and most evidence concerning the specific role of nutrition is preliminary. While saturated fat is one of the nutrients implicated in the diet-cancer connection, the key may lie in the composition of the total diet and not simply a particular component. Additional studies are required before definitive answers will be possible.

Lowering blood cholesterol. Diet and exercise are the first steps in treating elevated blood cholesterol. Drug treatment is considered if these are ineffective after six months.

HIGH-CHOLESTEROL DIETS AND HEART DISEASE

Contrary to popular belief, cholesterol is an important nutrient normally required for many of the complex functions of the body. It is a component in the synthesis of bile and of estrogen, androgen, and progesterone, the hormones responsible for development of male and female secondary sex characteristics. Cholesterol also is part of cell membranes and is required for vitamin D synthesis.

Cholesterol and triglycerides, however have been implicated in the development of heart disease, and people have attempted to reduce or eliminate these substances from their diets. Although the diet–heart disease controversy still rages, current research indicates that lowering blood cholesterol has a direct and significant effect on reducing the incidence and severity of heart attacks. Diminishing heart disease risk correlates with a decrease in blood cholesterol by a factor of 1 to 2; i.e., a 1% reduction in cholesterol is associated with an approximately 2% reduction in risk. *Consequently, reducing blood cholesterol by 25% cuts the risk of heart attack by 50%!*

Such findings are encouraging because they provide an important "missing link" in the diet–heart disease theory. They also add support to the efforts of health professionals who encourage people to reduce their serum lipids through good nutrition, increased exercise, and weight control. This relationship provides another reason why it is prudent to replace a portion of saturated fats and cholesterol in the diet with unsaturated fats. Even when we attempt to maintain a "cholesterol-free" diet, however, the body produces about 1.0 to 2.0 g of endogenous cholesterol a day. There is evidence that some people react more favorably than others to a high-cholesterol challenge. A genetic predisposition to process excessive exogenous cholesterol effectively would help to explain why some people can eat high-cholesterol foods for years without increasing their total blood cholesterol level while, for others, consuming even moderate amounts of cholesterol-rich foods results in abnormally high blood cholesterol levels.

Table 4–3 lists the cholesterol and saturated fat content of some common foods. Recall that the intake of saturated fat has a distinct serum cholesterol raising effect, regardless of the cholesterol content of the diet.

The data are not all in. While it is definitely prudent to apply the appropriate methods of nutrition, exercise, and weight control to achieve desirable levels of plasma lipids, the cholesterol–heart disease controversy is far from resolved. Recommendations to the general population concerning blood cholesterol and heart disease risk are generally based on inferences generated from studies of middle-aged men with high cholesterol levels. For example, there are no controlled studies of cholesterol lowering and heart disease risk in women. We do not know whether cholesterol lowering is necessary or effective for the elderly. Clinical trials in middle-aged men given powerful cholesterol-lowering drugs yielded disturbing results: a significant reduction in heart disease was not accompanied by an increased life span; for reasons unknown, the group receiving treatment had an increase in the incidence of violent and accidental deaths, as well as an excess of gastrointestinal disorders.

The ubiquitous egg. It is generally well known that eggs have a relatively high content of cholesterol, and that cutting down on cholesterol intake is desirable in terms of lowering heart disease risk. But cholesterol by itself may not be the real culprit! Recent evidence suggests that the key is the saturated fat content of the food. While a food may be relatively high in cholesterol content (as it is in the egg), it's the saturated fat content that should be looked at carefully. In terms of saturated fat content, 1 oz of raw egg ranks relatively low (18.9%) compared to 1 oz of pork spareribs (26.5%), bacon (27.4%), bologna (31.3%), and premium quality vanilla ice cream (37.9%).

Fat facts about cheese. Cheese is an excellent source of calcium, but the fat content is high for many popular cheeses. Fat-free and low-fat cheeses are good bets to reduce fat, because these cheeses are high in moisture content and thus lower in fat content. But for many so-called low-fat, "lite," or reduced-fat cheeses, fat content can still be relatively high.

CHEESE	TOTAL KCAL	TOTAL FAT, G	% KCAL AS FAT
Cream cheese	98.8	9.9	89.9
American, processed	106	8.8	75.1
Brie	94.8	7.8	74.4
Cheddar	114	9.4	74.1
Monterey jack	106	8.6	72.7
Camembert	84.9	6.9	72.7
Swiss, processed	94.8	7.0	66.2
Swiss, regular	107	7.8	65.5
Mozzarella, with whole milk	79.9	5.8	64.8

TABLE 4–3. CHOLESTEROL AND SATURATED FAT CONTENT FOR 100 G OF COMMON FOODS

FOOD	SATURATED FAT (mg)	CHOLESTEROL (mg)
Butter	50.7	219
Peanut butter	8.5	0
Chocolate fudge	7.3	4
French fries, McDonald's	6.8	13
Ice cream, vanilla	6.2	44
Taco, beef	6.2	57
Doritos, taco flavor	4.8	0
KFC,* breast	4.2	76
Hamburger, Big Mac	3.6	36
Pizza, cheese	3.4	47
Egg, raw	3.0	410
Beef liver, fried	2.8	482
Chicken breast, fried with skin	2.5	90
Chocolate milkshake	2.3	13
Milk, whole	2.1	14
Swordfish, broiled	1.4	50
Chicken breast, fried, without skin	1.3	91
Milk, lowfat 2%	1.2	9
Yogurt, plain low-fat	1.0	6
Shrimp, raw	0.3	152

* Kentucky Fried Chicken.

LIPIDS IN FOOD

One of the distinguishing properties of an unsaturated fat is its relatively low melting point. These lipids take liquid form at room temperature. In general, the less firm the fat, the greater the degree of unsaturation. Unsaturated fats present as liquids are called oils. The more common vegetable oils are corn oil, cottonseed oil, canola oil, and soybean oil. Oils can be changed to semisolid compounds by a chemical technology called **hydrogenation.** The most common hydrogenated fats include lard and margarine. Hydrogenation, as the name implies, adds hydrogen, thus reducing a double bond in the unsaturated fat to a single bond. This allows more hydrogen atoms to attach to the carbon atoms in the chain, and causes the lipid to behave as a saturated fat. By this process, vegetable oils are changed to more solid or semisolid form.

Calculate your daily fat limit. Here's how to compute how many grams of fat you should be eating each day. First, estimate your daily caloric requirement (see p. 225 for an average estimate). Second, multiply this estimate by the percentage of fat you would like to consume in your diet. If you require about 2500 calories a day and you desire a fat intake of 30%, you can eat 2500 calories × 30% (.30) = 750 calories from fat. Since each gram of fat contains 9 calories, your daily fat intake would be 750 ÷ 9 = 83 g of fat.

MARGARINE VERSUS BUTTER

The distinguishing characteristic between margarine and butter is not in caloric content, as they are about equal, but in the composition of their fatty acids. Approximately 62% of the fatty acids in butter are saturated compared with about 20% in margarine. During the manufacture of margarine, hydrogen atoms are pumped into unsaturated corn, soybean, or sunflower oil by hydrogenation; the manufacturer uses these oils because they are plentiful and inexpensive. Hydrogenation rearranges the original polyunsaturated vegetable oil to a fat that is more hardened (saturated), but not as hard as butter.

When one of the hydrogen atoms along the carbon chain moves to the opposite side of the double bond that separates two carbon atoms, the fatty

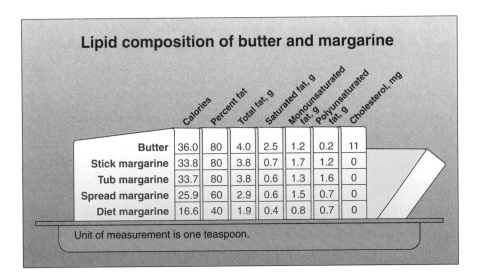

Lipid composition of butter and margarine

	Calories	Percent fat	Total fat, g	Saturated fat, g	Monounsaturated fat, g	Polyunsaturated fat, g	Cholesterol, mg
Butter	36.0	80	4.0	2.5	1.2	0.2	11
Stick margarine	33.8	80	3.8	0.7	1.7	1.2	0
Tub margarine	33.7	80	3.8	0.6	1.3	1.6	0
Spread margarine	25.9	60	2.9	0.6	1.5	0.7	0
Diet margarine	16.6	40	1.9	0.4	0.8	0.7	0

Unit of measurement is one teaspoon.

acid is referred to as a **trans fatty acid** (see p. 21). From 17 to 25% of the fatty acids in margarine are trans fatty acids, compared with only 7% in butter fat. Because margarine is made from vegetable oil, it contains no cholesterol; butter, on the other hand, is made from a dairy source and contains between 11 and 15 mg of cholesterol per teaspoon.

A Health Risk in Trans Fatty Acids? The current controversy over margarine versus butter centers on the possible detrimental health effects of trans fatty acids. A recent study from The Netherlands showed that a diet high in trans fatty acids increased LDL and decreased HDL concentration to about the same degree as a diet high in saturated fat. If it turns out that trans fatty acids do indeed place individuals at increased risk for heart disease, then manufacturers will surely change their methods of producing many foods. As it now stands, many popular foods are made with partially hydrogenated vegetable oils. These include donuts, Girl Scout and most other cookies, frozen pastries, imitation cheeses, packaged french fries, frozen fish sticks and chicken nuggets, most candies, ready-made frosting, and many popular brands of ice cream. The possible negative health effect of trans fatty acids on heart disease risk, while of concern, requires further study. Table 4–4 compares the nutrient composition, including some minerals and vitamins, of butter and three common styles of margarine.

FAT CONTENT OF COMMON FOODS

Figure 4–4 shows the approximate contribution of some common food groups to the lipid content of the typical American diet. The typical American diet contains about 37% fat, although many people consume much more. About 30 to 40% of total fat in the American diet is present as "visible fats" in butter, lard, mayonnaise, cooking oils, and the visible fat in meat, while the remainder is derived from "invisible fats" in eggs, milk, cheese, meat, nuts, vegetables, and cereals. For every 4.5 kg of lipid consumed, about 1.6 kg come from vegetables, while the remaining 2.9 kg are supplied from animal sources.

Fat in the plant kingdom. Not all fruits are low in fat. The avocado carries 8.3 g per serving (½ cup), while a serving of coconut contains a whopping 14.1 g!

In terms of total caloric content, the common vegetable oils are 100% fat, whereas margarine and mayonnaise possess about 80% fat. Most foods from animal sources range between 4 and 80% in fat content. As a frame

TABLE 4–4. COMPARISON OF THE NUTRIENT COMPOSITION OF ONE PAT OF BUTTER AND THREE STYLES OF MARGARINE (APPROMIXATELY 1 TEASPOON, OR 5 G)

Component	Butter	Margarine: Spread, hard (80% fat)	Margarine: Hard (60% fat)	Margarine: Spread, soft (60% fat)
Water, %	16	16	37	13.2
Calories	34	36	25	27
Fat, g	4	4	3	3
Saturated fat, g	2.5	0.8	0.7	0.6
Monounsaturated fat, g	1.2	1.8	1.3	1.6
Polyunsaturated fat, g	0.2	1.3	0.9	0.7
Cholesterol, mg	11	0	0	0
Protein, g	<0.1	1<0.1	<0.1	<0.1
Carbohydrate, g	<1	0.1	0	0
Dietary fiber, g	0	0	0	0
Calcium, mg	1	0	0	0
Iron, mg	<0.01	0.1	0	0
Zinc, mg	<0.01	0.01	<0.01	<0.01
Magnesium, mg	<1	<1	<1	<1
Phosphorus, mg	1	1	1	1
Potassium, mg	1	2	1	1
Sodium, mg	41	47	50	50
Vitamin A, RE	38	50	50	50
Thiamine, mg	0	0	0	0
Riboflavin, mg	<0.01	<0.01	<0.01	<0.01
Niacin, mg	<0.01	<0.01	<0.01	<0.01
Folacin, μg	<1	1<1	<1	<1
Vitamin B_6, mg	0	0	0	0
Vitamin C, mg	0	0	0	0

Granola cereals: source of hidden fat. Most regular, granola-type cereals contain a variety of whole grains, but they also are laden with fat. The accompanying table compares the percentage of calories from fat in 5 granola cereals (one low-fat) with Wheaties and Cheerios.

TYPE	TOTAL KCAL	FAT, G	KCAL FROM FAT (FAT, G × 9)	% KCAL FROM FAT
Erewhon Honey almond	130	6.0	54.0	41.5
Good Morning Pecan Splendor	130	6.0	54.0	41.5
Quaker 100% Natural	130	5.0	45.0	34.6
Homemade with nuts, raisins	138	7.7	69.0	50.0
Kelloggs Low-fat	120	2.0	18.0	15.0
Wheaties	99	0.5	4.5	4.5
Cheerios	110	1.8	14.7	15.0

of comparison, we have computed the fat content of popular fast-food items from Appendix D. Expressed as a percentage of total calories, a McDonald's Big Mac is 52.8% fat, a Burger King Whopper is 51.0% fat, and a Wendy's double burger on a white bun is 54.6% fat! Other items are as follows: Roy Rogers bacon cheeseburger (60.4%), Jack-in-the-Box Super Taco (54.6%), Burger King chicken sandwich (54.8%), McDonald's McNuggets (6 pieces

Food weight versus number of calories. While the number of grams of fat in McDonald's french fries represents only 17.7% by weight, the percentage of total calories as fat is 48.3%! You'll never see this fact displayed in advertising. Instead, McDonald's claims: "And our new cooking process also reduces the saturated fat by almost 50% in a serving of fries, while preserving 100% of the original flavor."

FOOD: McDonald's french fries, large
WEIGHT: 122.3 g (4.3 oz)

Nutrient	Weight, g	Kcal	% of Weight	% of Kcal
Protein	6	24	4.9	6.0
Carbohydrate	45.9	183.6	37.5	45.7
Fat	21.6	194.4	17.7	48.3
Ash	3.2	0	2.6	0
Water	45.6	0	37.3	0
	122.3	402	100	100

* Conversion factors: protein and carbohydrate, 4 Kcal/g; fat, 9 Kcal/g.

Source of nutrient information: McDonald's Nutrition Information Center, McDonald's Corporation, Oak Brook, ILL 60521; phone: (708) 575-FOOD. © 1990 McDonald's Corporation.

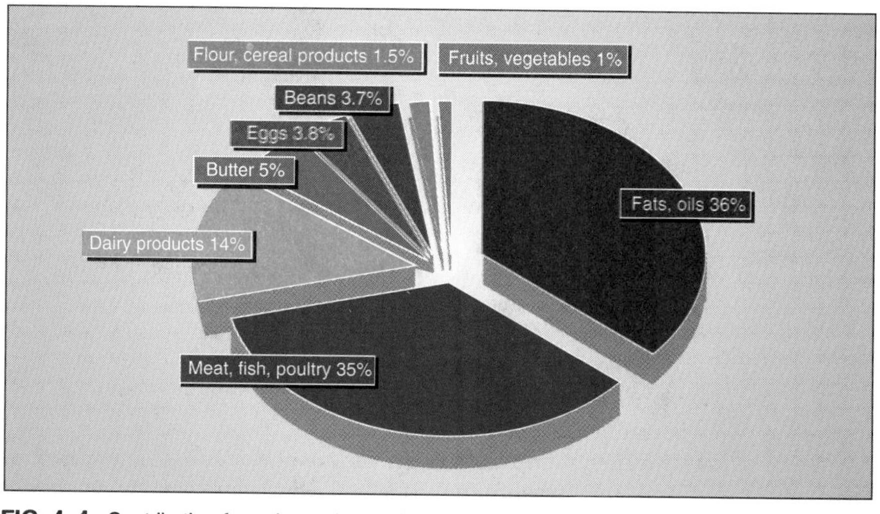

FIG. 4–4. Contribution from the major food groups to the fat content of the American diet.

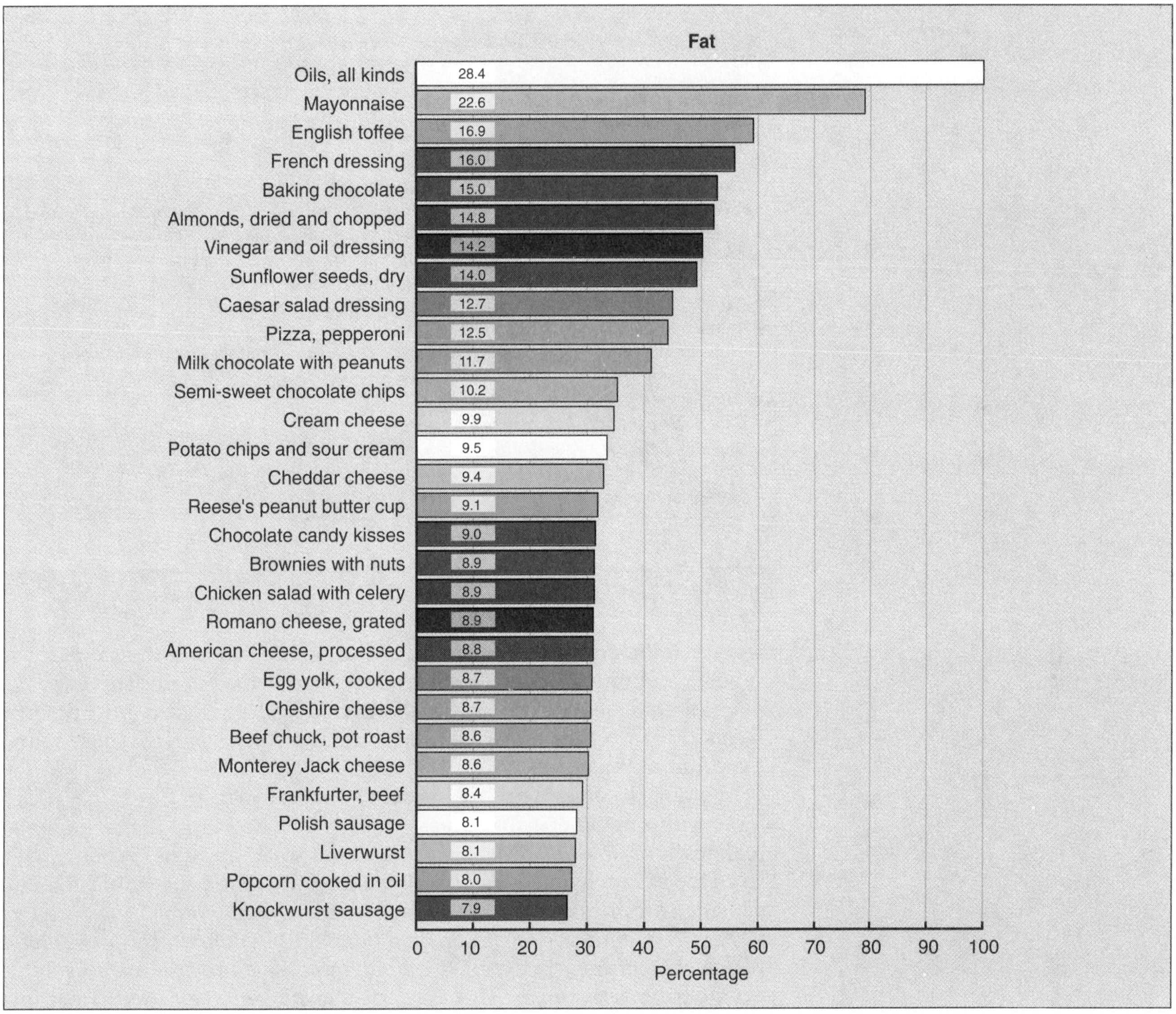

FIG. 4–5. Percentage of fat in commonly served foods. The insert bars display the number of grams per ounce.

without sauce, 54.5%), onion rings from various sources (50% and higher), while a chocolate, vanilla, or strawberry shake has "only" 20 to 30% fat.

To counter the adverse health-related publicity for such high-fat foods, many companies currently offer specialty items having a lower fat content. McDonald's, for example, has introduced a new "McLean Delux" hamburger. Compared to the McD.L.T. at 57.4% fat (37 g of fat and 580 calories), this new version has a reduced fat content of 28.1% (10 g of fat and 320 calories). Arby's offers a "New Light Menu," Burger King and Weight Watchers are testing numerous diet breakfast and dinner items, Hardee's has the "Real Lean Delux," and Kentucky Fried Chicken offers "Skinfree Crispy" chicken.

Figure 4–5 lists the percentage of fat in 1 oz of commonly served foods. The bars display the number of grams per ounce.

Table 4–5 provides a convenient checklist for cutting down on the intake of dietary fat.

Chocolate still king of candyland. Ninety percent of Americans over age 18 eat chocolate, which amounts to an expenditure of approximately $11.5 billion annually, and averages $46 per person a year. This translates to the equivalent of 9,225 fat calories, or 36 oz of lipid consumed a year!

TABLE 4–5. CHECKLIST FOR CUTTING DOWN ON DIETARY FAT

- Substitute cold cuts with 1 g of fat per 1-oz serving for regular bologna, salami, or pickled beef
- Substitute frozen yogurt or sherbet with 4 g or less of fat per 4-oz serving for high-fat ice cream
- Substitute air-popped popcorn and pretzels for party chips
- Substitute whole-grain breads and crackers for croissants and corn bread
- Substitute a variety of cereals for high-fat granola preparations
- Substitute cheese with less than 4 to 5 g of fat per ounce for high-fat cheeses
- Substitute egg whites for egg yolks, or use a dehydrated egg substitute
- Substitute light or fat-free mayonnaise for regular mayonnaise
- Substitute 2% or 1% milk for whole milk
- Substitute a variety of herbs or use low-calorie salad dressings instead of oil-rich or creamy salad dressings
- Avoid frozen vegetables in rich sauces
- Buy beef and pork with the words "round" or "lean" in the name
- Buy low-fat cake mixes
- Do not add oil or butter to water when cooking pasta, macaroni, or oatmeal
- Make hamburgers from ground round or ground sirloin

DIGESTION AND ABSORPTION

Figure 4–6 illustrates that some digestion of fats starts in the stomach by the action of **lingual lipase,** an enzyme secreted in the mouth. This enzyme, which operates effectively in the stomach's acid environment, primarily digests short- and medium-chain saturated fatty acids such as those found in coconut and palm oil.

The stomach secretes **gastric lipase,** its own fat-digesting enzyme, which works with lingual lipase to digest a very small amount of fat. The major breakdown of lipids, however, occurs in the small intestine. When chyme leaves the stomach and enters the small intestine, the fat is emulsified into very small droplets by the action of **bile.** Although bile contains no digestive enzymes, its emulsifying action facilitates fat breakdown by providing a greater contact area between the lipid molecules and the water-soluble enzyme **pancreatic lipase.** This main fat-digesting enzyme exerts its strong effect on the surface of the fat globule to degrade some of the triglyceride molecules still further to monoglycerides (one fatty acid connected to glycerol) and fatty acids. In this simpler form, monoglycerides are more easily absorbed by the intestine. The absorbed glycerol, fatty acid, and monoglyceride molecules are then free to recombine to reform triglycerides.

Pancreatic lipase is particularly effective in digesting the long-chain fatty acids commonly present in animal fats and certain plant oils. The release of enzymes into the stomach and intestine, in addition to bile from the gallbladder, is controlled by the peptide hormone **cholecystokinin** released from the wall of the duodenum, the first portion of the small intestine. This hormone regulates gastrointestinal functions including stomach motility and secretion, gallbladder contraction and bile flow, and enzyme secretion by the pancreas.

The peptide hormones **gastric inhibitory peptide** and **secretin,** released when there is a high fat content in the stomach, reduce gastric motility. This causes chyme to be retained in the stomach for a longer time. It also explains why a high-fat meal prolongs digestion and gives a feeling of fullness compared to a meal of lower fat content.

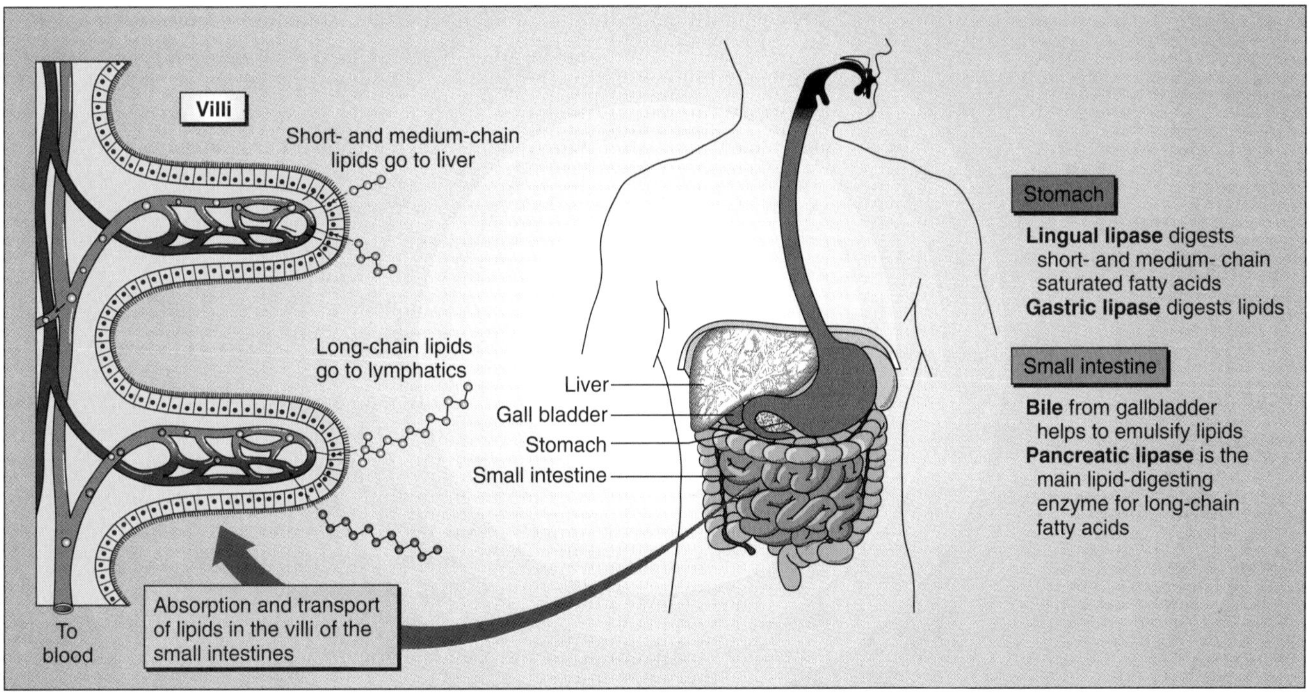

FIG. 4–6. The digestion of dietary fat.

Upon absorption through the outer brush border of the intestinal villi, the fat-bile mixture splits and bile is returned to the liver. The fatty acids take one of two routes depending on their chain length. Short- and medium-chain fatty acids proceed to the portal vein and empty into the liver. If the fatty acid is long chain, it is first reconverted to a chylomicron and then transported upward via the second route, the lymphatic system. Cholesterol can also bind to the triglyceride and be transported through the lymphatics into the systemic veins that empty into the heart.

SUMMARY

1. Like carbohydrates, lipids contain carbon, hydrogen, and oxygen atoms. Essentially, a lipid molecule consists of one glycerol molecule and three fatty acid molecules to form a triglyceride.
2. Saturated fatty acids contain as many hydrogen atoms as is chemically possible; thus, the molecule is said to be saturated with respect to hydrogen. Saturated fats are present primarily in animal meat, egg yolk, dairy products, and cheese, and in plant form as coconut and palm oil, vegetable shortening, and hydrogenated margarine.
3. Unsaturated fatty acids contain fewer hydrogen atoms attached to the carbon chain. Instead, the carbon atoms are joined by double bonds, and they are said to be either monounsaturated or polyunsaturated with respect to hydrogen.
4. Lipids are synthesized by plants and animals. They can be classified into three groups: simple fats (glycerol and three fatty acids), compound fats composed of simple fats in combination with other chemicals (phos-

pholipids, glucolipids, and lipoproteins), and derived fats such as cholesterol, an animal product made from simple and compound fats.

5. A high intake of saturated fats has been linked to the development of coronary heart disease. This is most likely because this form of dietary fat facilitates cholesterol synthesis by the liver. Increasing the proportion of unsaturated fats in the diet may help to limit heart disease risk. The polyunsaturated, omega-3 family of fatty acids found in fish oil may offer unique protection against heart disease.
6. Lowering blood cholesterol, especially that carried by LDL, provides significant protection against coronary heart disease. Elevating the cholesterol carried as HDL (through exercise and not smoking) will also reduce heart disease risk.
7. Dietary fat intake probably should not exceed 30% of total calories ingested. Of this, at least 70% should be in the form of unsaturated fatty acids. Daily cholesterol intake should not exceed 300 mg.
8. During light and moderate exercise, fat contributes about 50% of the energy requirement. As exercise continues, the role of stored fat becomes more important, and, during prolonged work, the fatty acid molecules may provide nearly 90% of the body's energy needs.
9. Fats in the form of triglycerides provide the largest nutrient store of potential energy to power biologic work, representing about 325 times more energy than stored carbohydrate. Stored body fat also protects vital organs, is involved in hormone synthesis, and provides insulation from the cold. Dietary fat also acts as the carrier of the fat-soluble vitamins. About 20 g of fat daily can serve this purpose.
10. The primary digestion of fats occurs in the stomach and small intestine through the action of gastric lipase and pancreatic lipase, respectively. In the small intestine, bile acts to emulsify fat into very small droplets, which further facilitates enzyme action.
11. Upon absorption through the intestinal villi, the fatty acids are either transported to the liver via the portal vein or reconverted to a chylomicron and transported into the lymphatics that empty into systemic veins leading to the heart.

RELATED LITERATURE

Barr, S.L., et al.: Reducing total dietary fat without reducing saturated fatty acids does not significantly lower total plasma cholesterol concentrations in normal males. Am. J. Clin. Nutr., 55:682, 1992.

Bønaa, K.H., et al.: Effect of eicosapentaenoic and docosahexaenoic acids on blood pressure in hypertension. N. Engl. J. Med., 322:795, 1990.

Burke, L.M., et al.: Dietary intakes and food use of groups of elite Australian male athletes. Int. J. Sport Nutr., 1:378, 1991.

Byers, T., and Graham, S.: The epidemiology of diet and cancer. Adv. Cancer Res., 41:1, 1984.

Caggiula, A.W. et al.: The Multiple Risk Factor Intervention Trial (Mr. Fit): IV. Intervention on blood lipids. Prev. Med., 10:443, 1981.

Childs, M.T., et al.: Effects of shellfish consumption on lipoproteins in normolipidemic men. Am. J. Clin. Nutr., 51:1020, 1990.

Clevidence, B.A.: Plasma lipid and lipoprotein concentrations of men consuming a low-fat, high-fiber diet. Am. J. Clin. Nutr., 55:689, 1992.

Conner, W.E., et al.: The plasma lipids, lipoproteins, and the diet of the Tarahumara Indians of Mexico. Am. J. Clin. Nutr., 31:1131, 1978.

Frick, M.H., et al.: Helsinki Heart Study: primary-prevention trial with gemfibrozil in middle-aged men with dyslipidemia. Safety of treatment, changes in risk factors, and incidence of coronary heart disease. N. Engl. J. Med., 317:3217, 1987.

Ginsberg, H.N.: Reduction of plasma cholesterol levels in normal men on an American Heart Association Step 1 or a Step 2 diet with added monounsaturated fat. N. Engl. J. Med., 322:574, 1990.

Gordon, D.J., et al.: High-density lipoprotein cholesterol and coronary heart disease in hypercholesterolemic men: the Lipid Research Clinics Coronary Primary Prevention Trial. Circulation, 74:12176, 1986.

Green, P., et al.: Effects of fish-oil ingestion on cardiovascular risk factors in hyperlipidemic subjects in Israel: a randomized, double-blind crossover study. Am. J. Clin. Nutr., 52:1118, 1990.

Grundy, S.: Cholesterol and coronary heart disease. JAMA, 264:3053, 1990.

Grundy, S.M., et al.: Comparison of monounsaturated fatty acids and carbohydrates for reducing raised levels of plasma cholesterol in man. Am. J. Clin. Nutr., 47:965, 1988.

Guyton, A.C.: Textbook of Medical Physiology, 7th ed. Philadelphia, W.B. Saunders, 1986.

Harris, W.S., et al.: Fish oils in hypertriglyceridemia: a dose response study. Am. J. Clin. Nutr., 51:399, 1990.

Hoeg, J.M., et al.: An approach to the management of hyperlipoproteinemia. JAMA, 255:512, 1986.

Hunter, J.E., and Applewhite, T.H.: Reassessment of trans fatty acid availability in the U.S. diet. Am. J. Clin. Nutr., 54:363, 1991.

Levy, D., et al.: Stratifying the patient at risk for coronary disease: new insights from the Framingham Heart Study. Am. Heart J., 119:712, 1990.

Lipid Research Clinics Program: The Lipid Research Clinics Coronary Primary Prevention Trial results: I. Reduction in incidence of coronary heart disease. JAMA, 251:351, 1984.

Manninen, V., et al.: Lipid alterations and decline in the incidence of coronary heart disease in Helsinki Heart Study. JAMA, 260:641, 1988.

Martin, M.J., et al.: Serum cholesterol, blood pressure, and mortality: implications from a cohort of 361,662 men. Lancet, 2:933, 1986.

McArdle, W.D., et al.: Thermal adjustment to cold-water exposure in exercising men and women. J. Appl. Physiol., 56:1572, 1984.

McArdle, W.D., et al.: Exercise Physiology: Energy, Nutrition, and Human Performance, 3rd ed. Philadelphia, Lea & Febiger, 1991.

Mensink, R.P., and Katan, M.B.: Effect of monounsaturated fatty acids versus complex carbohydrates on high-density lipoproteins in healthy men and women. Lancet, 1:122, 1987.

Nestel, P.J., et al.: Plasma cholesterol-lowering potential of edible-oil blends suitable for commercial use. Am. J. Clin. Nutr., 55:46, 1992.

Pugh, L.C.G.E., and Edholm, O.G.: The physiology of channel swimmers. Lancet, 2:761, 1955.

Satabin, P., et al.: Metabolic and hormonal response to lipid and carbohydrate diets during exercise in man. Med. Sci. Sports Exerc., 19:218, 1987.

Saudek, C.D., and Felig, P.: The metabolic events of starvation. Am. J. Clin. Nutr., 60:117, 1976.

Shils, M.E., and Young, V.R. (Eds.): Modern Nutrition in Health and Disease, 6th ed. Philadelphia, Lea & Febiger, 1988.

Simopoulos, A.P.: Omega-3 fatty acids in health and disease and in growth and development. Am. J. Clin. Nutr., 54:438, 1991.

Sims, E.A.H., and Danforth, E., Jr.: Expenditure and storage of energy in man (perspective). J. Clin. Invest., 79:1019, 1987.

Small, D.M., et al.: Chemistry in the kitchen—making ground meat more healthful. N. Engl. J. Med., 2:73, 1991.

Stamler, J., et al.: Is relationship between serum cholesterol and risk of premature death from coronary heart disease continuous or graded?: findings in 356,222 primary screenees of the Multiple Risk Factor Intervention Trial (Mr. Fit). JAMA, 256:2823, 1986.

Stampfer, M.J., et al.: A prospective study of cholesterol, apolipoproteins, and the risk of myocardial infarction. N. Engl. J. Med., 325:373, 1991.

Stephen, A.M., and Wald, N.J.: Trends in individual consumption of dietary fat in the United States, 1920–1984. Am. J. Clin. Nutr., 52:457, 1990.

Warner, J.G., Jr., et al.: Combined effect of aerobic exercise and omega-3 fatty acids in hyperlipidemic persons. Med. Sci. Sports Exerc., 21:498, 1989.

Willett, W.C.: Dietary fat and the risk of breast cancer. N. Engl. J. Med., 316:22, 1987.

Williams, M.H.: Nutritional Aspects of Human Physical and Athletic Performance. Springfield, IL, Charles C Thomas, 1985.

Williams, P.T., et al.: Relationship of dietary fat, protein, cholesterol, and fiber intake to atherogenic lipoproteins in men. Am. J. Clin. Nutr., 44:788, 1986.

5

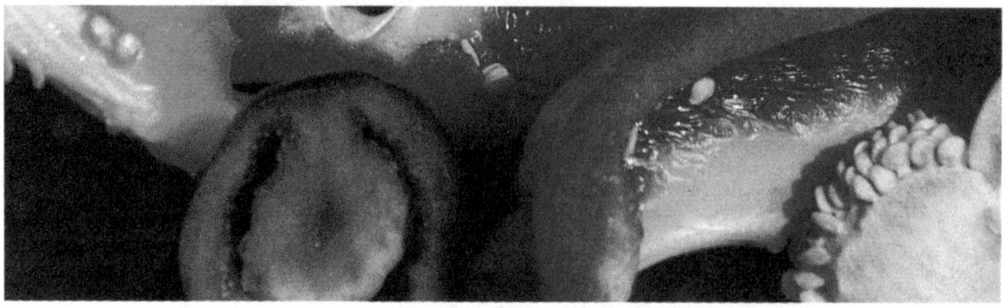

PROTEINS

Proteins represent a group of large, nitrogen-containing organic compounds for which amino acids are the basic structural units. In fact, proteins are the most abundant organic compounds in the body. They are found in all living matter and function primarily in the growth and repair of body tissue (anabolism). Although amino acids are not used to any large extent as cellular fuel, the carbon structures of some are reactive compounds in various energy-yielding reactions (catabolism). Consequently, this gives protein the potential for contributing to the body's energy needs.

WHAT ARE PROTEINS?

Proteins, from the Greek word meaning "of prime importance," are similar to carbohydrates and lipids in that each molecule contains atoms of carbon, oxygen, and hydrogen. The major difference is that proteins also contain nitrogen, which makes up approximately 16% of the molecule, along with sulfur, phosphorus, and iron.

AMINO ACIDS

The basic units or "building blocks" of protein are ***amino acids.*** These are small organic compounds that contain at least one amino radical and one radical called an organic acid (technically termed a carboxyl group). An amino radical consists of two hydrogen atoms attached to an atom of nitrogen (NH_2). The organic acid is made up of one carbon atom, two oxygen atoms, and one hydrogen atom (COOH). The difference between the various amino acids is their side chain. The chemical structure of the amino acid alanine is illustrated at the top of Figure 5–1.

Peptide bonds. Peptide bonding consists of a sequence of covalent chemical bonds between the carboxyl group of one amino acid and the amino group of the next amino acid. Amino acid bonding forms the backbone for building more complex protein compounds.

Amino acids are joined together by **peptide bonds;** the joining of two amino acids produces a **dipeptide,** and three amino acids linked together form a **tripeptide.** A linear configuration of up to as many as 1000 amino

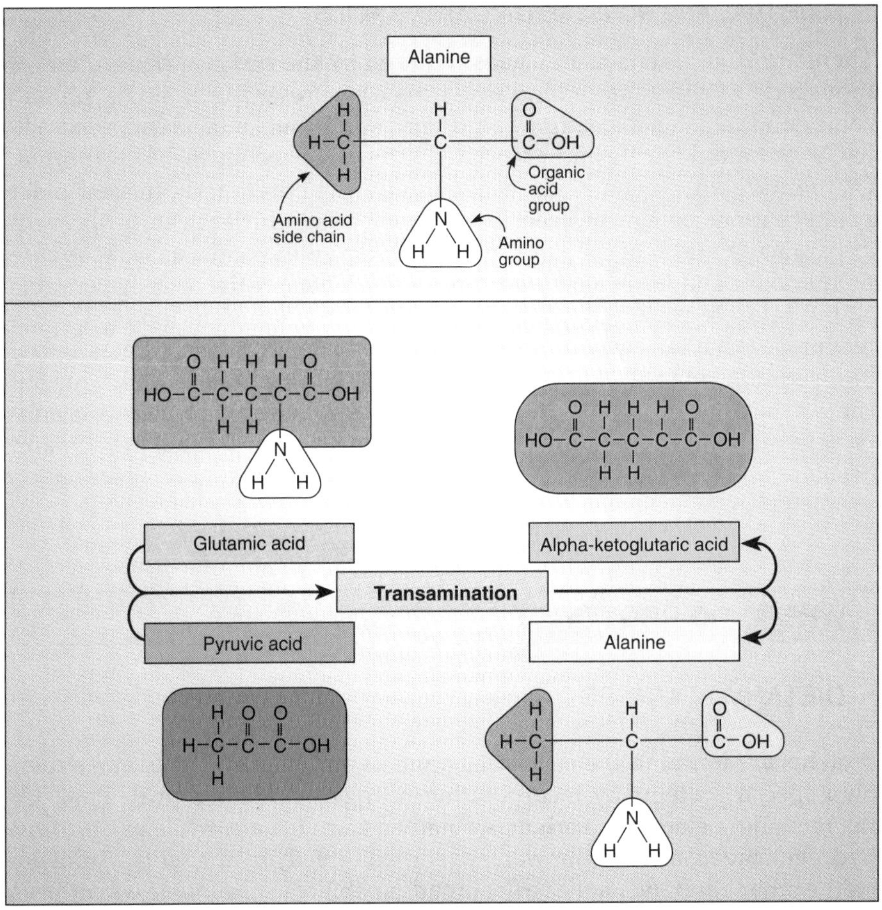

FIG. 5–1. Chemical structure of alanine and the process of transamination.

Transamination. Transamination involves the shifting of an amino group (NH_2) from a donor amino acid to an acceptor acid (keto acid), the acceptor acid thus becoming an amino acid. This allows certain amino acids to be constructed from non-nitrogen-carrying organic compounds formed in metabolism.

acids is known as a **polypeptide.** A polypeptide, however, does not exist as a simple linear string. Instead, proteins can fold into different three-dimensional shapes. They can be threadlike or fibrous, or more compact and globular. The long-chain polypeptide molecules are often referred to as **structural proteins** because their function is literally to hold the cell together. Structural proteins are present in the membranes that surround both the cell and its nucleus, as well as in the specific structures contained within the cell.

In terms of overall size, a protein molecule usually contains a minimum of 100 amino acids. The core of the protein structure has a definitive sequence of amino acids that determines its unique function. If there is an "error" in this sequencing, even a minor one, a major defect may occur in the protein molecule. Such a defect can occur, for example, in the protein **hemoglobin.** An incorrect sequence in one of the amino acids of its 287 amino-acid chain causes a deformation in the shape of the red blood cell. Instead of being a normal biconcave structure, the cell forms a crescent or "sickle" shape that affects its ability to deliver oxygen to the tissues. The resulting disease, which primarily affects blacks, is known as **sickle-cell anemia.** The imperfection in amino acid sequencing is due to an incorrect "pattern" in the DNA (itself a protein) of the chromosomes within the cell nucleus.

Hemoglobin. Hemoglobin is an iron-containing protein pigment that is a main component of the body's 25 trillion red blood cells. This compound increases the blood's oxygen-carrying capacity about 65 to 70 times above the amount normally dissolved in plasma.

ESSENTIAL AND NONESSENTIAL AMINO ACIDS

There are 20 different amino acids required by the body, although tens of thousands of the same amino acids may be present in a single protein compound. In the formation of protein, the number of possible combinations of amino acids and associated structures becomes almost infinite. Of the different amino acids, eight (nine in children and stressed older adults) cannot be synthesized in the body at a sufficient rate to prevent impairment of normal cellular function. These amino acids, as was the case with linoleic and linolenic fatty acids, are called **essential** or indispensable amino acids because they must be obtained preformed in foods. The remaining 12 that can be manufactured by the body are termed **nonessential** or disposable amino acids. This does not mean they are unimportant, but simply that the body can synthesize them from ingested protein and nonprotein nutrients at a rate that meets the demands for normal growth and tissue repair.

WHERE DO PROTEINS COME FROM?

DIETARY SOURCES

Proteins are found in the cells of all animals and plants. Plants make their own special proteins by incorporating nitrogen contained in the soil. Of the remaining elements, carbon is obtained from the air, while oxygen and hydrogen are available from water absorbed directly by the roots. Animals, on the other hand, do not have the broad capability for amino-acid synthesis possessed by plants. They must rely on ingested protein sources such as fruits and vegetables, or the animal protein in meat and in animal by-products such as eggs and milk.

SYNTHESIS IN THE BODY

Nonessential amino acids can be synthesized in the body from the carbon, oxygen, and hydrogen fragments of carbohydrates and lipids. This process, called **transamination,** is illustrated in the bottom of Figure 5–1 where a molecule of pyruvic acid combines with the amino group (NH_2) from the amino acid glutamic acid to create the amino acid alanine. As a result of transamination, the glutamic acid without its amino group becomes a different compound called alpha-ketoglutaric acid. This compound is now available to be metabolized for energy or to receive an amino group to rebuild an amino acid.

The process opposite to transamination is **deamination,** in which an amino group is removed from the amino acid molecule. The remaining carbon skeleton can then be converted into a carbohydrate or lipid, or used for energy. The split-off amino group forms urea in the liver and is then excreted by the kidneys. About 100 g of body protein is broken down and rebuilt throughout each day. The urinary nitrogen by-product of this protein turnover represents about 80 g of protein daily; the remaining nitrogen is eliminated in feces and sweat.

Deamination. Deamination involves the removal of an amino group (NH_2) from an amino acid molecule. A new amino acid can be synthesized after deamination (transamination), or the remaining deaminated carbon compound can be converted into carbohydrate or fat or metabolized for energy.

FUNCTIONS OF PROTEIN

Amino acids provide the major substance for the synthesis of cellular components in addition to the formation of new tissue. The amino acid requirement for these tissue-building or anabolic processes can vary considerably. During periods of rapid growth, as occur in infancy and childhood, over one-third of the protein intake is retained for tissue anabolism. As growth rate declines, so does the percentage of protein retained for growth-related processes. Once growth stabilizes, however, there is still a continual turnover of tissue protein.

A larger protein requirement in children. The protein demand per unit of body mass during infancy and childhood ranges between 2.5 and 5 times that required by adults.

STRUCTURAL COMPONENTS OF BODY TISSUES

The function of protein is intimately related to the varied structural components of body tissues. The protein content of the average cell is approximately 16% of its total mass. This amount, however, can vary considerably. A brain cell, for example, is only about 10% protein, whereas protein constitutes 20% of the mass of the red blood cells and the cells of skeletal muscles, heart, liver, and glands.

The protein content of cells is not always fixed. The protein in skeletal muscle, which represents about 65% of the body's total protein, can be increased dramatically with resistance training. *Simply ingesting large amounts of dietary protein, however, does not cause a muscle cell to increase in size.* If it did, then just eating an excess 100 g of protein daily, an amount consumed by many athletes, would theoretically increase the muscle mass by about 500 g a day! Fortunately, this does not occur; instead, this extra protein increases the work of the liver to deaminate the excess amino acids (so they can be used for energy) and the excretory function of the kidneys. Furthermore, if the extra protein calories consumed during the day exceed the daily energy expenditure, that protein will rapidly be converted to and stored as fat! The proper procedure for increasing the strength and size of muscles is discussed in Chapter 18.

Aside from contributing to the structure of muscle, protein is a component of many other tissues and compounds:

- Hair, fingernails, and the protective outer layer of skin are composed of the structural protein keratin.
- The specialized cells that form bone, the **osteoblasts,** secrete a protein substance that ultimately forms the major portion of new bone.
- The plasma proteins thrombin, fibrin, and fibrinogen are intimately involved in the clotting of blood.
- In muscles, the structural protein **myofilaments** actin and myosin "slide" past each other as a muscle shortens during movement.
- **Hemoglobin,** a carrier of oxygen and carbon dioxide in the red blood cells, consists of an iron-containing compound, heme, and a large protein molecule, globin. Ferritin is a protein-iron compound that acts as the storage form of iron in the tissues.
- Amino acids are essential building blocks of many **hormones.** These chemical messengers, secreted by **endocrine glands,** regulate bodily processes. For example, the front portion of the tiny pituitary gland, located beneath the base of the brain, secretes at least six specific hor-

Endocrine glands. Endocrine glands are ductless glands that secrete their hormones directly into the extracellular space that surrounds the gland. These chemicals then diffuse into the blood for transport to receptor sites throughout the body.

mones. Underproduction of pituitary hormones can retard growth, slow metabolism, and significantly affect electrolyte balance, fertility, and the metabolism of carbohydrates, lipids, and proteins. The thyroid hormones T_3 and T_4 are synthesized from amino acids; the important carbohydrate-regulating hormone insulin is a polypeptide. When these hormones are administered for medical reasons, they are injected because oral doses would be "digested" by the strong stomach acid and intestinal enzymes.

- Protein is a component of some antibodies that make up part of the body's immune system. Protein substances are present in the serum to work in coordinated fashion with the white blood cells to engulf and digest invading disease-producing micro-organisms.
- Proteins found in the nuclei of cells (nucleoproteins) transmit hereditary characteristics and are responsible for continued protein synthesis within the cell.
- Lactalbumin constitutes the major protein in breast milk. This protein is much easier for a baby to digest than the casein protein in cows' milk. There are also immunoglobulin proteins in breast milk that offer immune protection from some bacterial diseases.

OTHER FUNCTIONS OF PROTEINS

Proteins play an important role in regulating the acid-base quality of the body fluids. This buffering function is important during intense exercise, when large quantities of acid metabolites are produced. Proteins are present in blood and assist with the body's fluid balance. Globulins and albumins, two plasma proteins, exert osmotic pressure within the bloodstream. This counters the tendency of the blood's fluid (serum) component to seep out of the capillaries into surrounding tissues from the force of arterial blood pressure. The plasma proteins are far too large to leave the capillaries, and their high osmolality means that they draw fluid to them. This helps to maintain plasma volume by preserving the serum within the blood vessels.

RECOMMENDED INTAKE OF PROTEIN

THE RECOMMENDED DIETARY ALLOWANCE

The Recommended Dietary Allowance, or RDA, for protein as well as for the various vitamins and minerals required by the body are standards for nutrient intake developed by the Food and Nutrition Board of the National Research Council/National Academy of Science. These standards have been revised ten times since their initial publication in 1943. RDA levels are expressed as an average and are believed to represent a liberal, yet safe level of excess to meet the nutritional needs of practically all healthy people. The RDA was established to reflect the nutritional needs of a population over a long time period, rather than for individuals. The RDA should be viewed as a probability statement for adequate nutrition: as nutrient intake falls below the RDA, the probability for malnourishment for a particular person is increased, and this probability becomes progressively greater as the nutrient intake becomes lower. Malnutrition is the cumulative result of weeks, months, and even years of reduced nutrient intake. Of the approximately 40 nutrients known to be necessary for health, only 19 have an established RDA. The Food and Nutrition Board believes there is inadequate information about the role or requirement of the remaining nutrients to establish their RDA.

THE UNITED STATES RECOMMENDED DAILY ALLOWANCE

In 1974, the Food and Drug Administration established the **U.S. RDA** in conjunction with laws on food labeling. The U.S. RDA are based on the 1968 RDA standards and have been established for four age categories: children over 4 years old through adults, infants less than 1 year old, toddlers aged 1 to 4 years, and pregnant and lactating women. Most food labels use the adult U.S. RDA, but specialty foods display the nutrient amount provided based on the recommended values for a specific category of food. Examples include infant formula, baby foods, and vitamin supplements for pregnant women. When a label states that a particular nutrient satisfies some percentage of the U.S. RDA, this means that children aged 4 through adults, excluding pregnant and lactating women, will obtain at least the specified percentage of their RDA from one serving of that particular food. One ounce of Cheerios cereal, for example, provides 6% of the adult **U.S. RDA for protein.** The interpretation of this RDA percentage is that adults will obtain at least 6% of the total protein RDA by consuming 1 ounce of Cheerios. If one-half cup of milk is added, the percentage of the U.S. RDA for protein increases to 15%. Table 5–1 presents the U.S. RDA for protein, 12 vitamins, and seven minerals for the four categories of children and adults. The lower half of the table shows the recommended dietary intake of protein for adults expressed as grams per kilogram of body mass (g/kg).

On average, the recommended dietary intake of protein for adults is 0.8 g per kilogram of body mass. This was determined by dividing the U.S. RDA for protein (63 g) by the median body mass for a given age and gender in the U.S. For example, for a 25-year-old male, the median body mass is 79 kg; thus, the U.S. RDA for protein is 63 g ÷ 79 kg = 0.8 g/kg. For an average-sized man who weighs slightly less, at 70 kg (154 lb), the protein intake should be approximately 57 g. For a woman who weighs 56 kg (123 lb), protein intake should be 45 g. For infants, a higher intake of protein is recommended (2 to 4 g/kg of body mass). Also, protein intake should be increased by 10 g a day for pregnant women and 20 g daily for nursing mothers.

Adult protein requirement. The U.S. RDA for protein of 0.8 g per kilogram of body mass includes a reserve of approximately 25% to account for individual differences in protein requirement.

The protein requirement tends to decrease somewhat with age; conversely, stress, disease, injury, and prolonged heat exposure increase the protein requirement. The body has no protein reserve for storage; once the protein requirement is met, any excess is either used for energy or stored as fat.

The latest RDA is presented in four tables that appear on the inside covers: (1) Protein, 11 vitamins, and seven minerals; (2) Recommended energy intakes; (3) Estimated safe and adequate daily dietary intakes **(ESADDI)** for two additional vitamins not included with the RDA (biotin and pantothenic acid) and five trace mineral elements (copper, manganese, fluoride, chromium, and molybdenum); and (4) Estimated minimum requirements for the electrolytes sodium, chloride, and potassium. International agencies and other countries have developed their own versions of the RDA, including the Food and Agriculture Organization (FAO) and the World Health

TABLE 5–1. UNITED STATES RECOMMENDED DAILY ALLOWANCES (U.S. RDA) FOR PROTEIN, VITAMINS, AND MINERALS, AND THE RECOMMENDED DIETARY INTAKE OF PROTEIN FOR ADULTS EXPRESSED AS GRAMS PER KILOGRAM OF BODY MASS (G/KG)

U.S. RECOMMENDED DAILY ALLOWANCES (U.S. RDA)

Vitamins and Minerals	Unit of Measurement	Adults and Children 4 or More Years of Age	Infants	Children Under 4 Years of Age	Pregnant or Lactating Women
Vitamin A	International units	5000	1500	2500	8000
Vitamin D	International units	400	400	400	400
Vitamin E	International units	30	5.0	10	30
Vitamin C	Milligrams	60	35	40	60
Folic acid	Milligrams	0.4	0.1	0.2	0.8
Thiamin	Milligrams	1.5	0.5	0.7	1.7
Riboflavin	Milligrams	1.7	0.6	0.8	2.0
Niacin	Milligrams	20	8.0	9.0	20
Vitamin B_4	Milligrams	2.0	0.4	0.7	2.5
Vitamin B_{12}	Micrograms	6.0	2.0	3.0	8.0
Biotin	Milligrams	0.3	0.05	0.15	0.3
Pantothenic acid	Milligrams	10	3.0	5.0	10
Calcium	Grams	1.0	0.6	0.8	1.3
Phosphorus	Grams	1.0	0.5	0.8	1.3
Iodine	Micrograms	150	45	70	150
Iron	Milligrams	18	15	10	18
Magnesium	Milligrams	400	70	200	450
Copper	Milligrams	2.0	0.6	1.0	2.0
Zinc	Milligrams	15	5.0	8.0	15

RECOMMENDED DIETARY ALLOWANCES OF PROTEIN FOR ADOLESCENT AND ADULT MEN AND WOMEN

	Men		Women	
Recommended Amount	Adolescent	Adult	Adolescent	Adult
Grams of protein per kilogram of body mass	0.9	0.8	0.9	0.8
Grams per day based on average weight*	59	56	50	44

* For adolescents, average weight is approximately 65.8 kg (145 lb) for males and 55.7 kg (123 lb) for females. For adult men, average weight is 70 kg (154 lb). For adult women, average weight is 55 kg (120 lb).

Nitrogen balance and imbalance. Nitrogen balance exists when the intake of nitrogen (protein) equals nitrogen excretion. The body is in **positive nitrogen balance** when nitrogen intake is greater than nitrogen excretion, as when new tissue is being synthesized and protein is retained (e.g., during childhood, pregnancy, recovery from illness, or muscle growth through training). A greater output of nitrogen relative to its intake (**negative nitrogen balance**) indicates the use of protein for energy and possible encroachment on the body's available amino acids, primarily those in skeletal muscle.

Organization (WHO). In Canada, the Department of National Health and Welfare has developed the Recommended Nutrient Intakes for Canadians. The FAO/WHO and Canadian standards are similar in scope to the U.S. RDA.

At maturity the body contains about 10 kg of protein most of which is in muscle tissue. With normal food intake, very little body protein is "lost" through metabolism without replacement from dietary sources; consequently, a **protein balance** is maintained. Only during starvation and prolonged semistarvation does the body begin to mobilize its protein "reserves" at the expense of a decrease in lean tissue. Because dieting for many people takes the form of semistarvation, a significant loss of lean body mass is often noted as the weight loss progresses. For this reason, very low calorie diets, as well as those that restrict either protein or carbohydrate intake, are imprudent and counterproductive in achieving both fat loss and a desirable alteration in body composition.

PROTEIN IN FOODS

Proteins that contain the essential amino acids can be found in the cells of both animals and plants. There is nothing "better" about a specific amino acid from an animal compared to the same amino acid of vegetable origin. The proteins contained in food are classified as complete or incomplete, depending on their amino acid content. A complete or **high-quality protein** contains all the essential amino acids in both the quantity and the correct proportion required to maintain nitrogen balance and promote normal growth. An incomplete or **lower-quality protein** lacks one or more of the essential amino acids. Consequently, diets that contain predominantly incomplete protein may eventually hamper the ability of various cells to function properly, even though caloric value and protein quantity are adequate.

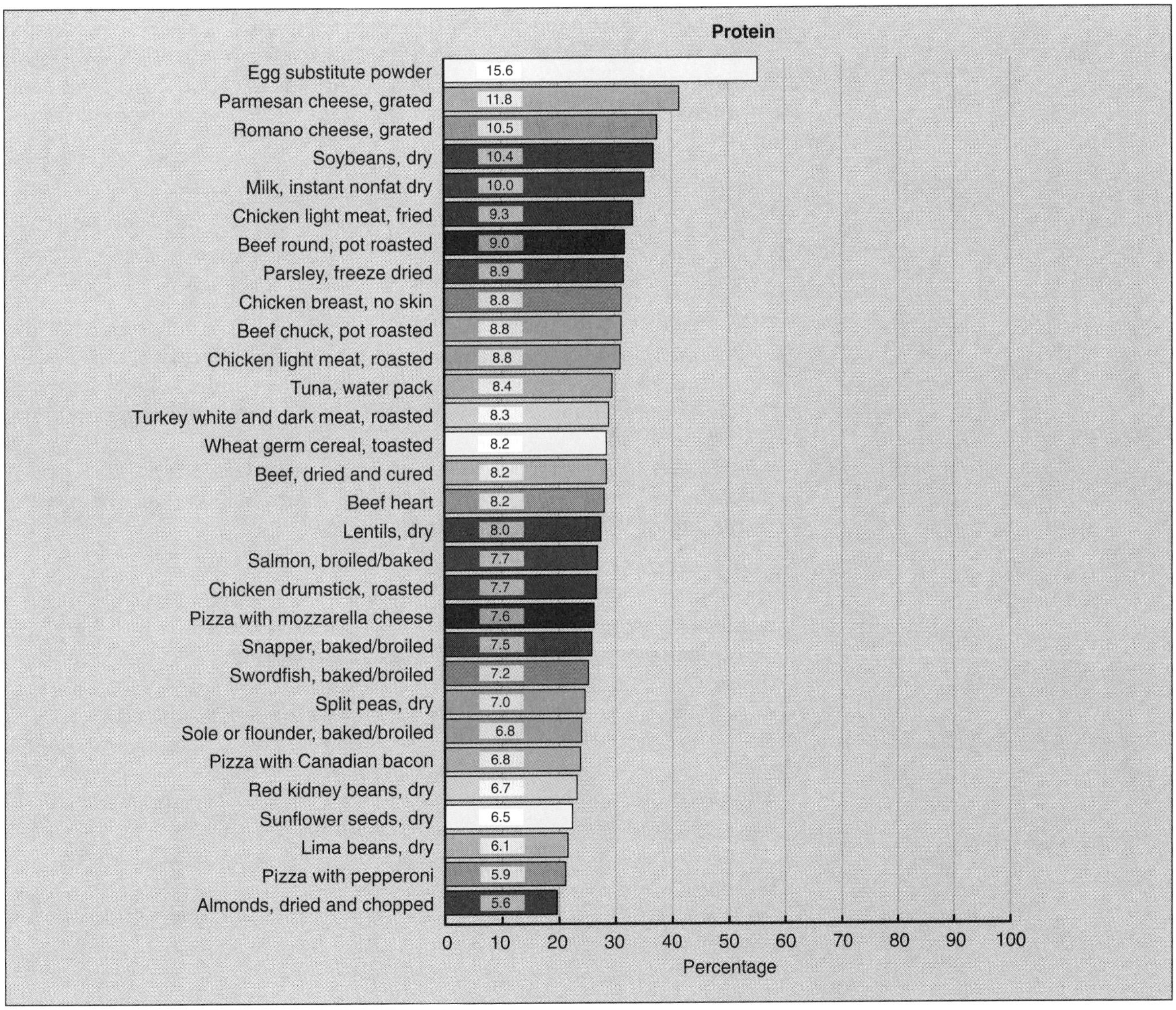

FIG. 5–2. Percentage of protein in commonly served foods. The insert bars display the number of grams per ounce.

The major sources of protein in the American diet are eggs, meat, milk, fish, and poultry. Generally, more than two-thirds of dietary protein comes from animal sources compared to about one-half this amount 75 years ago. The present-day reliance on animal protein is largely responsible for our relatively high intake of cholesterol and saturated fat. Figure 5–2 shows the percentage of protein in commonly served foods.

NUTRIENT DENSITY

The nutritional quality of a particular food can be evaluated by determining its nutrient density. In essence, comparing foods for nutrient density provides a convenient way to determine the better food source for a particular nutrient. This is done by computing a food's **Index of Nutritional Quality,** or INQ. The numerator in determining the INQ is the nutrient amount per 100 g of food divided by the U.S. RDA for that nutrient. The denominator is the number of calories per 100 g divided by the RDA for energy intake. An INQ greater than 1 means the food is an adequate source of that particular nutrient; an INQ lower than 1 indicates an inadequate nutritional source. For convenience in classification, foods with an INQ between 2 and 6 are considered good, while an INQ above 6 denotes an excellent source of the nutrient.

$$\text{INQ} = \frac{(\text{Amount of nutrient per 100 g/U.S. RDA for that nutrient})}{(\text{Calories in 100 g/U.S. RDA for energy intake})}$$

Let's compare, for example, the INQ for protein in whole milk, 1 and 2% low-fat milk, a raw egg, regular vanilla ice cream, chocolate chip cookies, and a McDonald's Big Mac hamburger to determine the best source of protein. The calculations are for an adult male with a daily energy requirement of 2900 calories (from inside covers for U.S. RDA).

First, refer to Appendix B for the protein content for 100 g (100 g = 3.52 oz) of each of the six foods. The following example illustrates the method of computing the INQ for protein in one raw egg.

Step 1.
Compute the amount of protein in 100 g of egg. Appendix B presents the values in 1 oz, or 28.4 g. Since there is 3.52 g of protein per 28.4 g (0.124 per gram of egg), 100 g of egg yields 12.4 g of protein.

Step 2.
Divide Step 1 by 63 g (U.S. RDA for protein for adult males); 12.4 g ÷ 63 g = 0.197.

Step 3.
Compute the number of calories in 100 g of egg. Because there are 40 calories per ounce (1.41 calories per gram of egg), 100 g of egg yields 141 calories.

Step 4.
Divide Step 3 by 2900 (U.S. RDA for energy for adult males): 141 calories ÷ 2900 calories = 0.049.

Step 5.
Divide Step 2 by Step 4.
This is the INQ for the protein in egg: 0.197 ÷ 0.049 = 4.0.

The protein INQ for the other food items is as follows: whole milk, 2.55; 2% milk, 3.09; 1% low-fat milk, 3.57; chocolate chip cookies, 0.58; Big Mac, 0.50. The conclusion is inescapable: the egg ranks first and 1% low-fat milk second as the best protein sources per gram compared to the other food items!

An excellent INQ rating for a single nutrient does not mean that a particular food is also superior for other nutrients. It is almost a certainty that no single food ranks excellent for all of its nutrients. While many foods may rate as good to excellent sources for several nutrients, they will also rate only adequate or below for the remainder. There is no one perfect food, just some that are more nutritious per amount consumed than others.

VEGETARIAN APPROACH TO SOUND NUTRITION

The **"biologic value"** of a food refers to the completeness with which it supplies essential amino acids. Food proteins containing essential amino acids are found in both animal and vegetable sources. *There is nothing "better" about a specific amino acid from an animal compared to one of vegetable origin.* It is simply that high-quality protein comes only from animal sources, whereas vegetable proteins are incomplete in terms of one or more essential amino acids and thus have a lower biologic value. The mixture of essential amino acids present in eggs has been judged to be the best among food sources.

All of the essential amino acids can be obtained by consuming a variety of vegetable foods, each with a different quality and quantity of amino acids. *Plant sources meet nutritional needs for protein provided a sufficient variety of foods such as grains, fruits, and vegetables is incorporated in the diet.*

True vegetarians or **vegans** who obtain all of their nutrients from the plant kingdom and in dietary supplements represent less than 1% of the United States population. There are also numerous individuals, including champion athletes, whose diet consists predominantly of nutrients from varied vegetable sources as well as some dairy products. In fact, two-thirds of the people in the world are adequately nourished on essentially vegetarian diets containing only small amounts of animal protein. Well-balanced vegetarian and vegetarian-type diets provide relatively large amounts of carbohydrates often crucial to the endurance athlete and others involved in regular, strenuous training.

For the active individual, one potential problem with a vegetarian-type diet is the difficulty in consuming sufficient calories to match energy output. With the exceptions of calcium, phosphorus, iron, and vitamin B_{12}, a strict vegetarian's nutritional problem is one of getting ample high-quality protein. This is easily resolved with a **lactovegetarian** diet that allows the addition of milk and related products such as ice cream, cheese, and yogurt. The lactovegetarian approach minimizes the problem of obtaining sufficient protein and increases the intake of calcium, phosphorus, and vitamin B_{12}. By adding an egg to the diet (**lacto-ovovegetarian** diet), an intake of the indispensable essential amino acids is assured. The vegetarian approach has additional positive "spin-offs" because foods from the plant kingdom are (1) rich sources of vitamins and minerals, (2) high in fiber, and (3) generally low in calories and fat, especially saturated fatty acids—and they contain no cholesterol!

For vegetarians, diversity is the key. The essential amino acids can be obtained in a vegan diet if the RDA for protein is consumed with 60% of the protein coming from grain products, 35% from legumes, and the remaining 5% from green leafy vegetables. For a 70-kg person who requires about 56 g of protein, the essential amino acids would be obtained by consuming approximately 1¼ cups of beans, ¼ cup of seeds or nuts, about 4 slices of whole-grain bread, 2 cups of vegetables (half being leafy green), and 2½ cups from various grain sources such as brown rice, oatmeal, and cracked wheat.

Complementary sources of essential amino acids. Grains and legumes are excellent protein sources, but neither provides the full complement of essential amino acids. Grains lack the essential amino acid lysine, while legumes contain lysine but lack the sulfur-containing essential amino acid methionine for which grains are rich sources. Consequently, tortillas and beans, rice and beans, rice and lentils, rice and peas, and peanuts and wheat (bread) are staples in various cultures that provide complementary sources of essential amino acids from the plant kingdom. However, because large quantities of those foods must be eaten to obtain the required quantity of essential amino acids, most people worldwide eat some animal food.

DIGESTION AND ABSORPTION

Figure 2–6 illustrates that the digestion of protein begins in the stomach by the action of the powerful enzyme pepsin. Pepsin is the active form of its precursor pepsinogen, and its release is controlled by the hormone gastrin. Pepsin is particularly effective in the highly acid stomach medium in breaking down the collagenous connective tissue fibers in meat. Once these fibers are digested, other digestive enzymes effectively act on the remaining animal protein.

Gastrin. Gastrin is a peptide hormone secreted by the stomach that stimulates the secretion of gastric acid.

The appearance of **gastrin** is linked to the production of hydrochloric acid, a harsh acidic substance that (1) activates pepsin, (2) helps to keep the stomach free from bacteria, (3) improves absorption of the minerals iron and calcium, and (4) inactivates plant and animal hormones. Specialized stomach cells produce gastrin in response to external environmental cues such as the sight and smell of food, or internal cues such as the thought of food or actual distention of the stomach by its food contents. As gastrin production increases, it stimulates the release of stomach acid. The food mass in the stomach also stimulates acid secretion in proportion to the quantity of food. Stomach enzymes and acids attack the long, complex protein strands. As they uncoil their three-dimensional shape in the process of denaturation, they are degraded to smaller units called polypeptides and peptides.

The final steps in the digestion of protein occur in the small intestine. Here the peptide fragments are further dismantled by alkaline enzymes from the pancreas, most notably **trypsin** from its inactive precursor **trypsinogen,** into tripeptides, dipeptides, and single amino acids. These smaller protein fragments can all be absorbed by active transport and delivered via the hepatic-portal vein to the liver. When amino acids reach the liver, one of three things happens. They are: (1) converted to glucose, (2) converted to fats, or (3) released directly into the bloodstream as plasma proteins such as albumin, or as free amino acids to serve the anabolic requirements of various tissues.

SUMMARY

1. Proteins provide the building blocks for the synthesis of essentially all cellular material (anabolism). Under certain conditions, the amino acids also contribute their "carbon skeletons" for energy metabolism (catabolism).
2. Proteins differ chemically from carbohydrates and lipids in that they contain nitrogen in addition to other elements such as sulfur, phosphorus, and iron.
3. Proteins are formed from their "building block" subunits called amino acids. The body requires 20 different amino acids, each containing an amino radical (NH_2) and an organic acid radical called a carboxyl group (COOH). In addition to NH_2 and COOH, amino acids contain a side-chain molecule that gives each amino acid its particular chemical characteristics.
4. The number of potential combinations for the different amino acids is almost infinite; thus, there is almost an unlimited number of possible protein structures.

5. Eight of the 20 amino acids cannot be synthesized in the body. These are the essential amino acids and must be consumed in the diet. The remaining 12 that can be manufactured by the body are termed nonessential amino acids.
6. Proteins are formed in the cells of all animals and plants. Proteins containing all the essential amino acids are called complete (high-quality) proteins; the others are called incomplete (lower-quality) proteins. Animal proteins such as those found in eggs, milk, cheese, meat, fish, and poultry are examples of high-quality, complete proteins.
7. The Recommended Dietary Allowance (RDA) represents a liberal, yet safe level of nutrient intake to meet the nutritional needs of practically all healthy people. The RDA of protein intake for adults is 0.8 g per kilogram of body mass.
8. The nutritional quality of a particular food can be evaluated by the Index of Nutritional Quality, or INQ. The INQ provides a measure of nutrient density so that various food sources can be rated per unit mass.
9. All of the essential amino acids can be obtained by consuming a variety of plant foods, each with a different quality and quantity of amino acids.
10. The digestion of protein begins in the stomach by the action of the enzyme pepsin. The peptide fragments are further dismantled in the small intestine by alkaline enzymes released from the pancreas. The smaller protein fragments are then absorbed and transported to the liver for further assimilation.

RELATED LITERATURE

Albert, J.K., et al.: Exercise mediated tissue and whole body amino acid metabolism during intravenous feedings in normal men. Clin. Sci., 77:113, 1989.

Åstrand, P.O., and Rodahl, K.: Textbook of Work Physiology. New York, McGraw-Hill, 1986.

Bentivegna, A., et al.: Diet, fitness, and athletic performance. Phys. Sportsmed., 7:99, 1979.

Booth, F.W., and Watson, P.A.: Control of adaptations in protein levels in response to exercise. Fed. Proc., 44:2293, 1985.

Borchers, J., and Butterfield, G. The effect of meal composition on protein utilization following an exercise bout. Med. Sci. Sports Exerc., 24:551, 1992.

Brooks, G.A.: Amino acid and protein metabolism during exercise and recovery. Med. Sci. Sports Exerc., 19:S150, 1987.

Butterfield, G.E.: Whole body protein utilization in humans. Med. Sci. Sports Exerc., 19:S157, 1987.

Carraro, F., and Wolfe, R.R.: High-protein intake alters the response of fasting in normal human subjects. Am. J. Clin. Nutr., 55:959, 1992.

Christensen, H.N.: Role of amino acid transport and counter transport in nutrition and metabolism. Physiol. Rev., 70:43, 1990.

Dohm, G.L., et al.: Protein degradation during endurance exercise and recovery. Med. Sci. Sports Exerc., 19:5166, 1987.

Evans, W.J.: Muscle damage: nutritional considerations. Int. J. Sports Nutr., 1:214, 1991.

Felig, P., and Wahren, J.: Amino acid metabolism in exercising men. J. Clin. Invest., 50:2703, 1971.

Friedman, J.E., and Lemon, P.W.R.: Effect of chronic endurance exercise on retention of dietary protein. Int. J. Sports Med., 10:118, 1989.

Goldberg, A.L., et al.: Mechanism of work-induced hypertrophy of skeletal muscle. Med. Sci. Sports Exerc., 7:185, 1975.

Guthrie, H.A.: Introductory Nutrition, 7th ed. St. Louis, C.V. Mosby, 1988.

Guyton, A.C.: Textbook of Medical Physiology, 7th ed. Philadelphia, W.B. Saunders, 1986.

Horswill, C.A., et al.: Excretion of 3-methylhistidine and hydroxyproline following acute weight training exercise. Int. J. Sports Med., 9:245, 1988.

John-Adler, H.B., et al.: Reduced running endurance in gluconeogenesis-inhibited rats. Am. J. Physiol., 251:R137, 1986.

Konstantin, N., et al.: Effects of dieting and exercise on lean body mass, oxygen uptake, and strength. Med. Sci. Sports Exerc., 17:466, 1985.

Lemon, P.W.R.: Does exercise alter dietary protein requirements? In Advances in Nutrition and Top Sport. Edited by F. Brouns. 32:38–58, Basel, Karger, 1991.

Lemon, P.W.R.: Protein and exercise: update 1987. Med. Sci. Sports Exerc., 19:S179, 1987.

Lemon, P.W.R.: Protein and amino acid needs of the strength athlete. Int. J. Sports Nutr., 1:127, 1991.

McArdle, W.D., et al.: Exercise Physiology: Energy, Nutrition, and Human Performance, 3rd ed. Philadelphia, Lea & Febiger, 1991.

Meridith, C.N., et al.: Dietary protein requirements and food protein metabolism in endurance trained men. J. Appl. Physiol., 66:2850, 1989.

Nieman, D.: Vegetarian dietary practices and endurance performance. Am. J. Clin. Nutr., 48:754, 1988.

Parizkova, J., and Rogozkin, V.A.: Nutrition, Physical Fitness and Health. Baltimore, University Park Press, 1978.

Pivarnik, J.M., et al.: Urinary 3-methylhistidine excretion increases with repeated weight training exercise. Med. Sci. Sports Exerc., 21:283, 1989.

Shils, M.E., and Young, V.R. (Eds.): Modern Nutrition in Health and Disease, 6th ed. Philadelphia, Lea & Febiger, 1988.

Short, S.H., and Short, W.R.: Four-year study of university athletes' dietary intake. J. Am. Diet. Assoc., 82:632, 1983.

Slavin, J.L., et al.: Nutritional practices of women cyclists including recreational riders and elite racers. In: Sport, Health, and Nutrition. Edited by F.I. Katch. Champaign, IL, Human Kinetics Publishers, 1986.

Tarnopolosky, M.A., et al.: Influence of protein intake and training status on nitrogen balance and lean body mass. J. Appl. Physiol., 64:187, 1988.

Walberg, J.L., et al.: Macronutrient content of a hypoenergy diet affects nitrogen retention and muscle function in weight lifters. Int. J. Sports Med., 9:261, 1988.

Wardlaw, G.M., and Insel, P.M.: Perspectives in Nutrition. St. Louis, Times Mirror/Mosby, 1990.

White, T.P., and Brooks, G.A.: [u-^{14}C] glucose-alanine and leucine oxidation in rats at rest and two intensities of running. Am. J. Physiol., 240:E155, 1981.

Williams, M.H.: Nutritional Aspects of Human Physical and Athletic Performance. Springfield, IL, Charles C Thomas, 1985.

Wolfe, R.R., et al.: Isotopic analysis of leucine and urea metabolism in exercising humans. J. Appl. Physiol., 52:458, 1982.

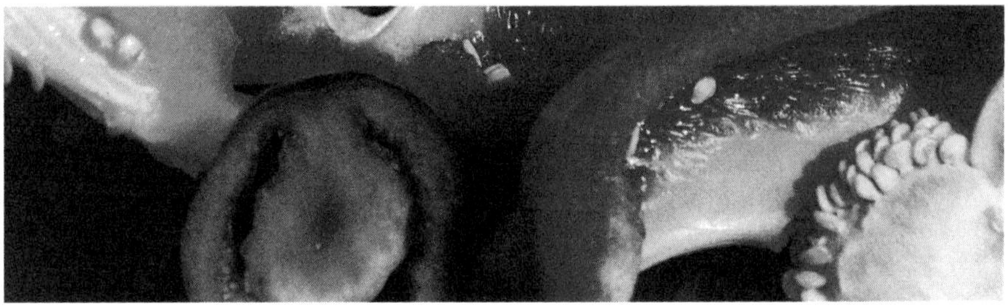

6

VITAMINS

The efficient regulation of metabolic processes requires a delicate blending of food nutrients in the watery medium of the cell. Of special significance in the metabolic mixture are the vitamin micronutrients—the water- and fat-soluble organic substances that play highly specific roles in facilitating energy transfer and tissue synthesis.

WHAT ARE VITAMINS?

Vitamins *are essential organic substances needed in minute amounts by the body to perform a highly specific metabolic function.* The body requires only about 350 g (12 oz) of vitamins from the 820 kg (1820 lb) of food consumed by the average adult during the year. Vitamins are often considered accessory nutrients because they neither supply energy, serve as basic building units for other compounds, nor contribute substantially to the body's mass. Nonetheless, prolonged inadequate intake of a particular vitamin can trigger the symptoms of vitamin deficiency and lead to severe medical complications. For example, symptoms of thiamine deficiency can be observed after only two weeks on a thiamine-free diet, and symptoms of vitamin C deficiency can appear after three or four weeks. At the other extreme, consuming excessive quantities of some fat-soluble vitamins can cause a toxic overdose that is manifested as hair loss, irregularities in bone formation, fetal malformation, hemorrhage, bone fractures, abnormal liver function, and even death.

Essential for energy transfer. Many vitamins serve as **coenzyme** components or precursors of coenzymes that regulate energy metabolism. These coenzymes, when united with a protein compound (apoenzyme), form an active enzyme that accelerates the interconversion of chemical compounds.

When a vitamin is synthesized from existing chemicals in the body, the ingredient necessary to make the conversion is called a precursor or **provitamin.** For vitamin A the precursor is carotene, while tryptophan serves as a precursor for the vitamins D and niacin. When the vitamin is obtained from dietary sources or supplied in synthetic form as a supplement, it is referred to as a **preformed vitamin.** There is no difference or advantage between a vitamin obtained naturally from food and a synthetic vitamin. Even among the various supplements, the huge profit gained by the manufacturer is the only advantage in consuming so-called natural or organically isolated vitamins compared to those synthesized in the laboratory.

Provitamin. Many vitamins are found in food in an inactive or precursor form. In the body, these provitamins are changed to the active form of the vitamin. In this regard, the vitamin content of a specific food is most accurately expressed in terms of the total potential vitamin activity available from both its actual vitamin content and its precursor provitamins.

THE DISCOVERY OF VITAMINS

Before the discovery of vitamins, the importance of such substances was recognized as far back as ancient China, Greece, Rome, and Egypt. The physicians and healers in those civilizations wrote about diseases such as night blindness, scurvy, rickets, pellagra, and neural disorders. As one can imagine, many cures were prescribed and some worked, although it would take several centuries to explain the reasons for their success. In ancient Greece, for example, night blindness could be cured by applying the juice squeezed from cooked liver directly into the patient's eyes. While the Greeks did not know the reason for the cure, we now know that vitamin A, which helps to prevent night blindness, is plentiful in such preparations.

Another serendipitous example was the cure for **scurvy,** a disease whose symptoms often become apparent after only three weeks on a diet lacking vitamin C. Symptoms can include muscle cramps, painful joints, dizziness, loss of appetite, diarrhea, pinpoint hemorrhages around the hair follicles on the arms and legs, excessive bleeding of the gums, skin deterioration, infection, and finally death. Scurvy took its toll when fresh fruits were absent from the diet during long military campaigns and sea voyages when food was scarce. Vasco da Gama, the explorer who forged a trade route to the Indies by sailing around the tip of Africa, lost over half his crew to scurvy during a two-year journey. Another adventurer, Jacques Cartier, was more fortunate; his crew survived a scurvy outbreak by being fed a concoction made from the needles of spruce trees. Several centuries later, in 1742, the British physician **James Lind** experimented to determine the effect of food supplements on scurvy. Sailors who consumed fruits and a supplement of lemon juice thrived, while a "control" group fed supplements without citrus juice became ill and died from scurvy. Based on these results in addition to year-long, citrus-supplemented voyages where scurvy ceased to be a problem, the British Navy required ships to stock adequate supplies of citrus fruits and lime juice. This caused British sailors to be referred to as "Limeys," a term still used today. It was not until 1928, however, that vitamin C, chemically identified as ascorbic acid, was isolated in crystalline form from orange and cabbage juice.

Ascorbic acid. Ascorbic acid is derived from the terms *a-* (meaning without) and *scorb* (meaning scurvy). Because vitamin C is easily destroyed in reactions with oxygen, it is the most unstable of all the vitamins and thus is difficult to preserve in foods.

The existence of vitamins was actually established in the early part of the twentieth century. Sir Frederick Hopkins, a British biochemist, showed that foods contain—in addition to carbohydrates, lipids, and proteins—certain necessary "accessory factors." The discovery of the first vitamin was published in 1911 by a Polish biochemist, **Casimir Funk,** who conducted experiments at the world-famous Lister Institute in London. He observed that an amine substance (an organic compound containing nitrogen) isolated from rice polishings cured beriberi, an affliction resembling degenerative nerve disease. Because this water-soluble substance was essential for life, Funk named the accessory amine factor a **vitamine** (*vita* meaning "life-giving"). The term was changed several years later to *vitamin* when it was discovered that some of the newly identified substances were not amines. Following the discovery of the antiberiberi vitamin (now known as thiamine), four additional vitamins were identified over the next decade. The last vitamin discovery was made in 1941; the compound identified was folic acid, also called folacin or folate. Table 6–1 summarizes the discovery of the vitamins.

TABLE 6–1. DISCOVERY OF THE VITAMINS

SCIENTIST	YEAR*	VITAMIN
Funk	1911	Thiamine (vitamin B_1)
McCollum	1915	Vitamin A (retinol)
Riches, Folkers, et al.	1918	Cobalamin (vitamin B_{12})
McCollum	1922	Vitamin D
Evans and Bishop	1922	Vitamin E
Szent-Gyorgyi	1928	Vitamin C (ascorbic acid)
Kuhn, Gyorgy, and Wagner-Januergy	1933	Riboflavin (vitamin B_2)
Williams	1933	Pantothenic acid
Dam	1935	Vitamin K
Elvehjem	1937	Niacin (nicotinic acid)
Gyorgy and Kuhn	1938	Vitamin B_6 (pyridoxine)
Gyorgy	1940	Biotin
Mitchell et al.	1941	Folacin (folic acid)

* For some vitamins, it is difficult to pinpoint the exact year of the discovery.

CLASSIFICATION OF VITAMINS

Thirteen different vitamins have been isolated, analyzed, and synthesized, and their recommended dietary intakes established. The vitamins also have been classified into one of two groups depending on their particular chemical properties.

Storage of fat-soluble vitamins. Vitamins A and D are stored predominantly in the liver, whereas vitamin E is distributed throughout the body's fatty tissues. Vitamin K is stored only in small amounts, mainly in the liver.

FAT-SOLUBLE VITAMINS

Vitamin A was the first of the vitamins to be classified as fat soluble because they are dissolved in the fat and oil in foods. Daily ingestion of the **fat-soluble vitamins** is unnecessary, as they are stored in the liver and in fat cells of adipose tissue, mainly the subcutaneous tissues. These vitamins are retained in the tissues for a relatively long time because there is no mechanism for them to leave the body other than as by-products of their eventual breakdown. Consequently, it may take years for symptoms of deficiency of a fat-soluble vitamin to become evident. However, because the fat-soluble vitamins are usually obtained in dietary fat, consuming a "fat-free" diet will speed up the development of a vitamin deficiency.

The four fat-soluble vitamins—composed entirely of the elements carbon, hydrogen, and oxygen—are vitamins A, D, E, and K. Each has a different chemical structure and performs different and highly specific functions. Table 6–2 lists the Recommended Dietary Allowance (RDA), food sources, major bodily functions, and symptoms resulting from both excess and deficiency of the fat-soluble vitamins.

Excessive intake of water-soluble vitamins. Existing medical conditions can be aggravated with megadoses of the water-soluble vitamins.

MEDICAL CONDITION	VITAMIN
Diabetes	Niacin, vitamin C
Liver disease	Niacin
Diarrhea	Niacin, vitamin C, pantothenic acid
Kidney stones	Vitamin C
Scurvy	Vitamin C
Heart disease	Niacin
Parkinson's disease	Vitamin B_6
Sensory neuropathy	Vitamin B_6
Central nervous system disorders	Vitamin B_6, thiamine, folic acid
Peptic ulcers	Niacin
Asthma	Niacin

WATER-SOLUBLE VITAMINS

Certain vitamins are classified as water soluble because they are transported throughout the watery medium of the body; thus, they are not stored in the tissues to any appreciable extent. The **water-soluble vitamins** are normally voided in the urine because their amount in plasma exceeds the capacity for reabsorption by the kidneys. Consequently, these vitamins

TABLE 6–2. RECOMMENDED DIETARY INTAKE, FOOD SOURCES, MAJOR BODILY FUNCTIONS, AND SYMPTOMS OF DEFICIENCY OR EXCESS OF THE FAT-SOLUBLE VITAMINS FOR HEALTHY ADULTS (AGE 19–50)*

VITAMIN	RDA FOR MALES AND FEMALES† (MG)	DIETARY SOURCES	MAJOR BODY FUNCTIONS	DEFICIENCY	EXCESS
Vitamin A (retinol)	1.0 0.8	Provitamin A (beta-carotene) widely distributed in green vegetables. Retinol present in milk, butter, cheese, fortified margarine	Constituent of rhodopsin (visual pigment). Maintenance of epithelial tissues. Role in mucopolysaccharide synthesis	Xerophthalmia (keratinization of ocular tissue), night blindness, permanent blindness	Headache, vomiting, peeling of skin, anorexia, swelling of long bones
Vitamin D	0.01‡ 0.01	Cod-liver oil, eggs, dairy products, fortified milk, and margarine	Promotes growth and mineralization of bones. Increases absorption of calcium	Rickets (bone deformities) in children. Osteomalacia in adults	Vomiting, diarrhea, loss of weight, kidney damage
Vitamin E (tocopherol)	10 8	Seeds, green leafy vegetables, margarines, shortenings	Functions as an antioxidant to prevent cell membrane damage	Possibly anemia	Relatively nontoxic
Vitamin K (phylloquinone)	0.08 0.06	Green leafy vegetables. Small amount in cereals, fruits, and meats	Important in blood clotting (involved in formation of active prothrombin)	Conditioned deficiencies associated with severe bleeding; internal hemorrhages	Relatively nontoxic. Synthetic forms at high doses may cause jaundice

* Recommended Dietary Allowances. Revised 1989. Food and Nutrition Board, National Academy of Sciences–National Research Council, Washington, D.C.
† First values are for males.
‡ 0.005 mg for adults 25 and older.

B-complex vitamins. The **B-complex vitamins** generally act as part of coenzymes to participate with enzymes in initiating and regulating a variety of metabolic processes, especially those related to energy metabolism. An enzyme cannot function without its specific coenzyme.

must be consumed regularly—usually daily or at least within a period of several days. The nine water-soluble vitamins include vitamin C (ascorbic acid) and the B-complex group: thiamin (B_1), riboflavin (B_2), niacin, pyridoxine (B_6), cobalamin (B_{12}), pantothenic acid, folic acid, and biotin. These vitamins differ in structure from their fat-soluble counterparts because in addition to carbon, hydrogen, and oxygen, they contain nitrogen (thiamine, riboflavin, vitamins B_6 and B_{12}, folic acid), sulfur (thiamin and biotin), and cobalt (vitamin B_{12}). The RDA, food sources, major bodily functions, and symptoms resulting from both excess and deficiency of the water-soluble vitamins are summarized in Table 6–3.

TOXICITY OF VITAMINS

Once the enzyme systems that are catalyzed by specific vitamins become saturated, the excess vitamins function as chemicals in the body. In excess, these chemicals can be harmful. Although the potential for overdose is considerably less for the water-soluble than for the fat-soluble vitamins, prolonged excess intake of vitamins of either type can produce toxic effects.

WHERE DO VITAMINS COME FROM?

Much of the food we eat contains an abundant quantity of vitamins. With the exception of vitamin B_{12}, which is found only in animals, vitamins are

TABLE 6–3. RECOMMENDED DIETARY INTAKE, FOOD SOURCES, MAJOR BODILY FUNCTIONS, AND SYMPTOMS OF DEFICIENCY OR EXCESS OF THE WATER-SOLUBLE VITAMINS FOR HEALTHY ADULTS (AGE 19–50)*

VITAMIN	RDA FOR MALES AND FEMALES† (MG)	DIETARY SOURCES	MAJOR BODY FUNCTIONS	DEFICIENCY	EXCESS
Vitamin B_1 (thiamin)	1.5 1.1	Pork, organ meats, whole grains, legumes	Coenzyme (thiamine pyrophosphate) in reactions involving the removal of carbon dioxide	Beriberi (peripheral nerve changes, edema, heart failure)	None reported
Vitamin B_2 (riboflavin)	1.7 1.3	Widely distributed in foods	Constituent of two flavin nucleotide coenzymes involved in energy metabolism (FAD and FMN)	Reddened lips, cracks at mouth corner (cheilosis), eye lesions	None reported
Niacin	19 15	Liver, lean meats, grains, legumes (can be formed from tryptophan)	Constituent of two coenzymes in oxidation-reduction reactions (NAD and NADP)	Pellagra (skin and gastrointestinal lesions, nervous, mental disorders)	Flushing, burning and tingling around neck, face, and hands
Vitamin B_6 (pyridoxine)	2.0 1.6	Meats, vegetables, whole-grain cereals	Coenzyme (pyridoxal phosphate) involved in amino acid and glycogen metabolism	Irritability, convulsions, muscular twitching, dermatitis, kidney stones	None reported
Pantothenic acid	4–7§ 4–7	Widely distributed in foods	Constituent of coenzyme A, which plays a central role in energy metabolism	Fatigue, sleep disturbances, impaired coordination, nausea	None reported
Folacin	0.2 0.2	Legumes, green vegetables, whole-wheat products	Coenzyme (reduced form) involved in transfer of single-carbon units in nucleic acid and amino acid metabolism	Anemia, gastrointestinal disturbances, diarrhea, red tongue	None reported
Vitamin B_{12}	0.002 0.002	Muscle meats, eggs, dairy products, (absent in plant foods)	Coenzyme involved in transfer of single-carbon units in nucleic acid metabolism	Pernicious anemia, neurologic disorders	None reported
Biotin	0.03–0.10§	Legumes, vegetables, meats	Coenzymes required for fat synthesis, amino acid metabolism, and glycogen (animal starch) formation	Fatigue, depression, nausea, dermatitis, muscular pains	None reported
Vitamin C (Ascorbic acid)	60‡ 60	Citrus fruits, tomatoes, green peppers, salad greens	Maintains intercellular matrix of cartilage, bone, and dentine. Important in collagen synthesis.	Scurvy (degeneration of skin, teeth, blood vessels, epithelial hemorrhages)	Relatively nontoxic. Possibility of kidney stones

* Recommended Dietary Allowances. Revised 1989. Food and Nutrition Board, National Academy of Sciences–National Research Council, Washington, D.C.
† First values are for males.
‡ 100 for adults who smoke.
§ Because there is less information on which to base allowances, these figures are given in the form of ranges.

Highly sensitive compounds. Vitamins in food are sensitive to heat, light, air, and moisture. Cooking can also cause severe depletion of vitamins. For example, 50 to 70% of vitamin B_6 is lost in processing grains into cereal, and about 75% is lost when wheat is milled into flour. In processing luncheon meats, vitamin B_6 is reduced by 50 to 70%, while up to 56% of its potency is lost in the freezing and 77% in the canning of vegetables; fruits show losses of 15% in freezing and 40% in canning.

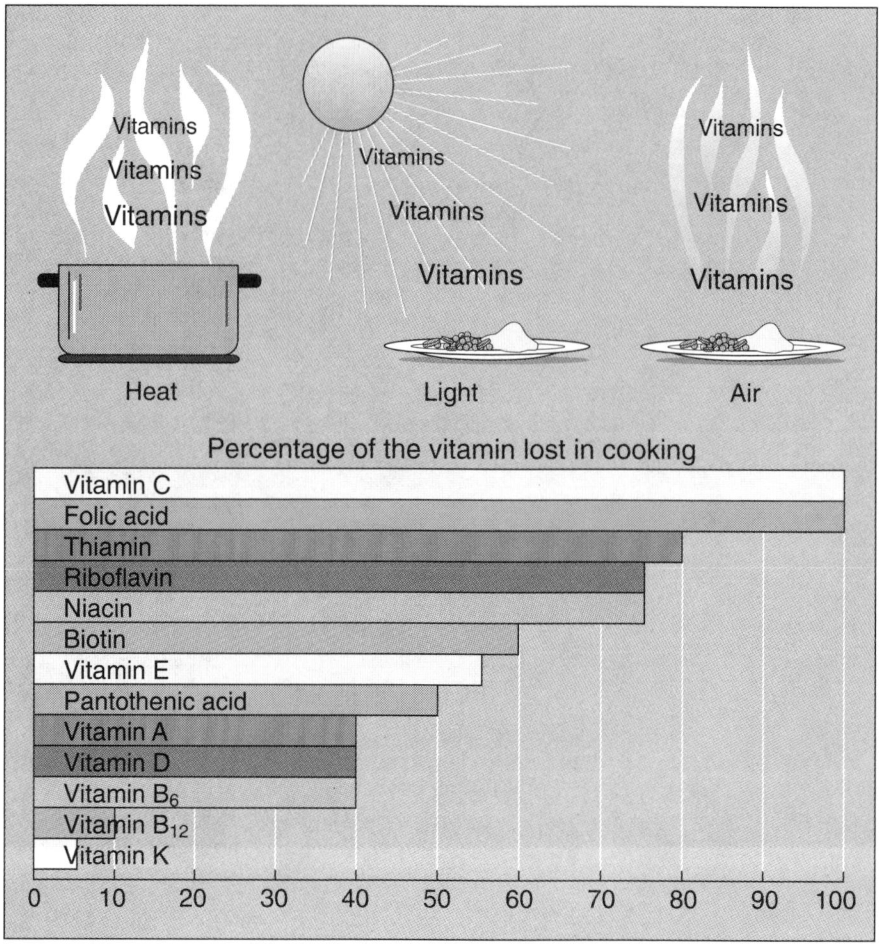

Beta carotene. Beta-carotene is a water-soluble compound found in fruits and vegetables that is transformed into vitamin A in the body. While vitamin A can be toxic if taken in excess, in precursor form as beta carotene the risk of overdose is eliminated. This is because the body makes as much vitamin A as we need—and no more—from beta carotene.

Vitamin A drug, a promising agent for chemoprevention. A synthetic vitamin A drug (Accutane, or 13-CIS retinoic acid) holds promise in preventing precancerous mouth lesions called leukoplakia, common in smokers and smokeless tobacco users, compared to beta carotene.

manufactured in the green leaves and roots of plants by the process of photosynthesis. This **synthesis of vitamins** involves integration of the energy from sunlight with carbon dioxide, water, and minerals in the soil. Animals obtain their vitamins from the plants, seeds, grains, and fruits they eat, or from the meat of other animals that have previously consumed these foods.

Most animals are able to manufacture some of the vitamins within their own cells. Vitamin C, for example, can be synthesized by all animals with the exception of humans, monkeys, guinea pigs, and some species of birds. Several of the vitamins, notably A, D, niacin, and folic acid, are converted to an activated form in the body from precursor provitamins. The best known of the provitamins are the carotenes, the yellow and yellow-orange pigments that give color to vegetables and fruits such as carrots, squash, corn, pumpkins, sweet potatoes, apricots, peaches, and melons. Carotenes, the precursors of vitamin A, are also present in all green plants, but the green pigment chlorophyll masks their color. They are converted to vitamin A in the walls of the intestines and in the liver. Besides playing an important role in the prevention of night blindness and other eye diseases, vitamin A prevents some digestive and urogenital tract diseases. In carotene form, it may protect against several forms of cancer. A provitamin substance in the skin is converted to vitamin D when the skin is exposed to the ultraviolet rays of the sun or to artificial ultraviolet light. Niacin, the B-complex vitamin that prevents pellagra (a skin disease), is converted to an active form by its precursor, the essential amino acid tryptophan, in the small intestine. Although vitamin K cannot be synthesized by the body per se, it is readily formed by bacterial action in the large intestine.

Quantitatively almost inconsequential. Annual adult requirement for 11 vitamins

VITAMIN RDA	ANNUAL ADULT REQUIREMENT Males	Females
Vitamin A, μg RE*	365,000	292,000
Vitamin D, μg	3,650	1,825
Vitamin E, mg α-TE†	3,650	2,920
Vitamin K, μg	29,200	23,725
Vitamin C, mg	21,900	21,900
Thiamine, mg	548	402
Riboflavin, mg	621	475
Folic acid, mg NE‡	6,935	5,475
Vitamin B_6, mg	730	584
Folate, μg	73,000	65,700
Vitamin B_{12}, μg	730	730

* Retinol Equivalents.
† α-Tocopherol Equivalents.
‡ Niacin Equivalents.

RECOMMENDED INTAKE OF VITAMINS

Only a minute amount of a particular vitamin is required to carry out its function in the body. Just 738 g, or 26 oz, of vitamin B_{12} would supply the daily requirement of the entire adult population of the United States! Likewise, for an individual, the projected yearly RDA for the various vitamins is not very high. For example, the adult daily requirement for vitamin B_6 (2 mg) projects to only about three-quarters of a gram over the year. Over an average lifetime, the vitamin B_6 requirement is less than 58 g (2 oz)! For vitamin C, which has the highest daily requirement, the yearly recommended intake would still amount to less than 5 g. For several of the vitamins with much smaller RDAs, the yearly requirement is quantitatively almost inconsequential.

Notwithstanding these minute but crucial dietary requirements, about 50% of American adults regularly supplement with vitamins, often in amounts that exceed the RDA by more than 150%. The annual cost of vitamin and mineral supplements is about $60 per person for a conservative estimate of 70 million people who currently use supplements! Of these individuals, approximately 80% believe that this excess vitamin intake is essential for optimal health and fitness, independent of the quality of their food intake. Of great concern to nutritionists is that some people routinely take **megavitamins,** or doses at least *tenfold* and up to one thousand times the RDA, believing that "supercharging" with vitamins will upgrade their health status and physical fitness, and retard aging. Such nutritional excess is often counterproductive and can produce tragic consequences. For example, from 1985 to 1990, approximately 5000 people a year required medical treatment for poisoning by vitamin supplements.

Heading the list. The most common vitamins supplemented are C, E, and certain B-vitamins—these are also the most commonly used in excess.

In economic terms, **vitamin supplements are big business.** In 1991, vitamin sales exceeded 4.2 billion dollars, an increase of approximately 33% since the printing of the third edition of this book. This volume of business is certainly incentive for the vitamin industry to be overly zealous in promoting its products. The average profit in a single dose of the RDA for all of the vitamins exceeds 1300%. If you doubt such excessive profit margins, the wholesale cost for the RDA of *all* of the vitamins in a single capsule is less than one cent!

Try mangos for vitamin A. Mangos, the oval-shaped tropical fruit, have 20 times more vitamin A and half the vitamin C of navel oranges.

FUNCTIONS OF VITAMINS

Vitamins perform diverse functions. They generally serve as essential links and regulators in the chain of metabolic reactions that release energy within the food molecule. They are also intimately involved in the process of tissue synthesis as well as in many other biologic processes. Figure 6–1 summarizes many of the biologic functions of vitamins in the body.

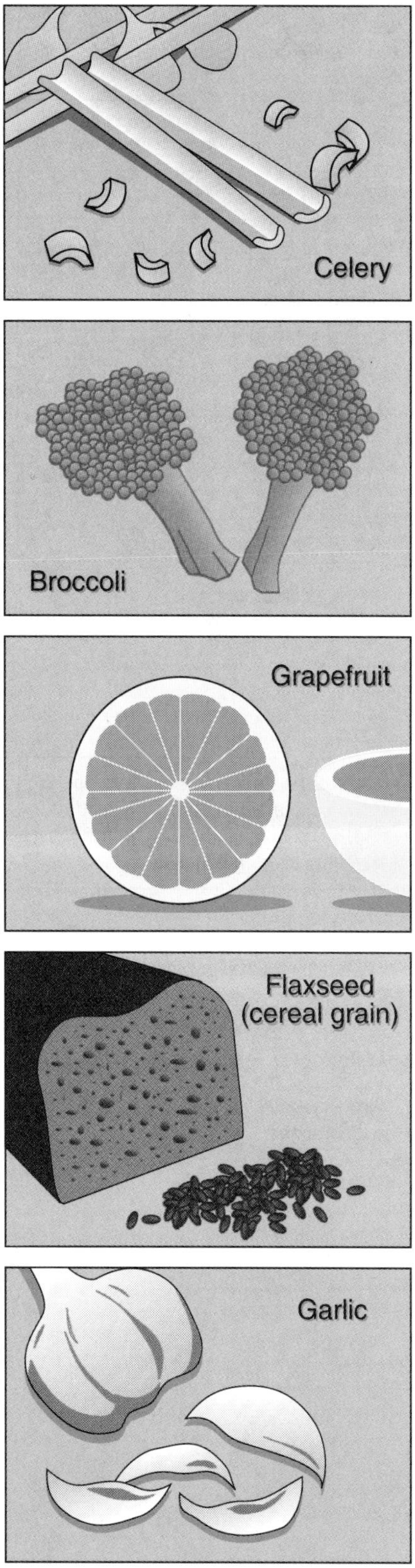

Good food sources of antioxidants

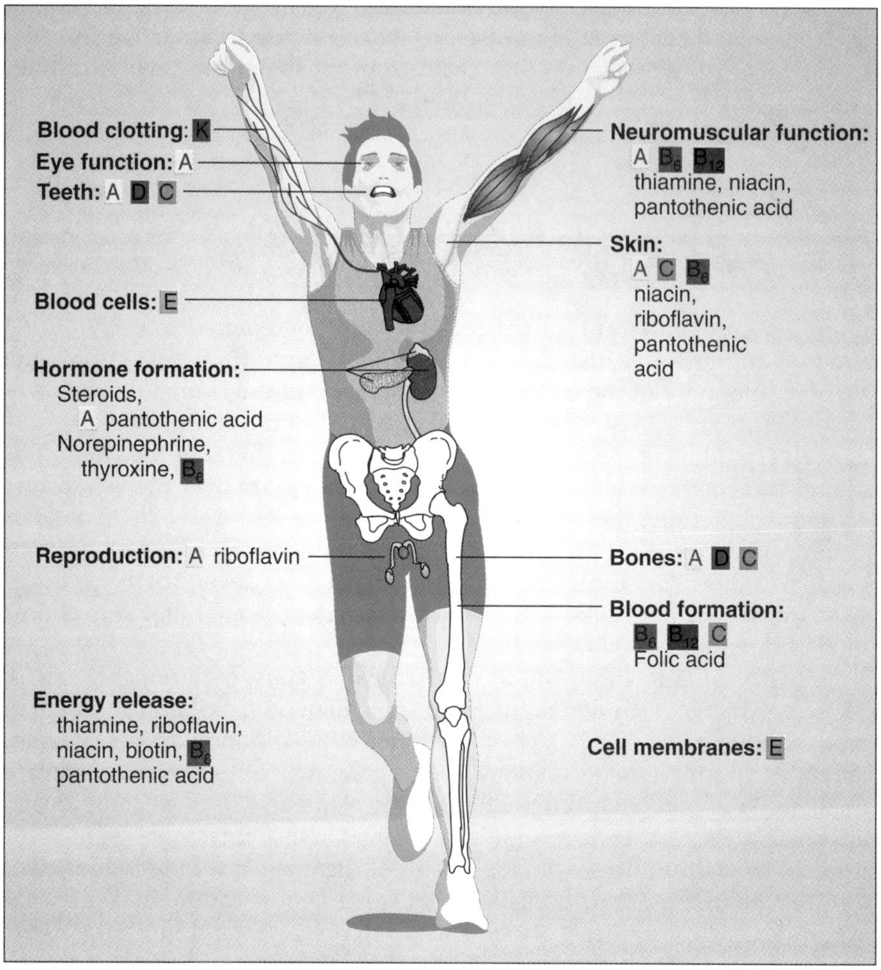

FIG. 6–1. Biologic functions of vitamins in the body.

The water-soluble vitamins play an essential role as part of coenzymes in the complex series of energy-generating reactions that occur within the body's cells. Figure 6–2 presents an overview of the various routes of the food nutrients in metabolism and the role of the water-soluble vitamins in these metabolic pathways.

Because vitamins can be used repeatedly in metabolic reactions, the vitamin needs of physically active individuals are generally no greater than for those who are sedentary. If there is a dietary deficiency in either the vitamin or its precursor, the resulting defect in cellular function manifests itself in a variety of symptoms. Once a nutritional deficiency is cured, supplements do *not* further improve a normal status.

ANTIOXIDANT ROLE OF VITAMINS

Foods that are rich in vitamins C and E along with beta carotene may protect against many cancers and heart disease. They serve as antioxidants to counter the damaging effects of reactive chemicals called free radicals. Free radicals can be acquired from the environment in cigarette smoke or from air pollution, for example, or are formed in the body during metabolism.

They can damage cell membranes, making the cell more vulnerable to carcinogens, or they change potentially harmful chemicals in the body into actual carcinogens. They may also alter circulating cholesterol into the LDL form that facilitates the atherosclerotic process, thus increasing the risk of heart attack and stroke. Rich sources of antioxidants are:

- **Beta carotene:** carrots, dark-green leafy vegetables like spinach, broccoli, turnips, beets, and collard greens, sweet potatoes, winter squash, and apricots, cantaloupe, mangos, and papaya
- **Vitamin C:** citrus fruits and juices, cabbage, broccoli, turnip greens, and cantaloupe
- **Vitamin E:** vegetable oils, wheat germ, whole-grain bread and cereals, dried beans, and green leafy vegetables

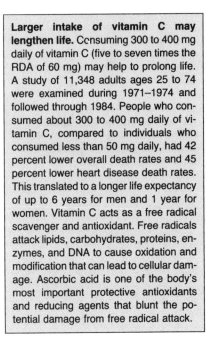

Larger intake of vitamin C may lengthen life. Consuming 300 to 400 mg daily of vitamin C (five to seven times the RDA of 60 mg) may help to prolong life. A study of 11,348 adults ages 25 to 74 were examined during 1971–1974 and followed through 1984. People who consumed about 300 to 400 mg daily of vitamin C, compared to individuals who consumed less than 50 mg daily, had 42 percent lower overall death rates and 45 percent lower heart disease death rates. This translated to a longer life expectancy of up to 6 years for men and 1 year for women. Vitamin C acts as a free radical scavenger and antioxidant. Free radicals attack lipids, carbohydrates, proteins, enzymes, and DNA to cause oxidation and modification that can lead to cellular damage. Ascorbic acid is one of the body's most important protective antioxidants and reducing agents that blunt the potential damage from free radical attack.

VITAMINS AND EXERCISE PERFORMANCE

An adequate quantity of all vitamins is available for individuals who consume well-balanced meals. This is true regardless of gender, age, and level of physical activity. Indeed, there is no need for the physically active person to consume extra vitamins in the form of special foods or supplements. Contrary to popular belief, vitamins themselves contain no usable energy. Thus, they cannot be a source of "quick energy" as touted by some vitamin manu-

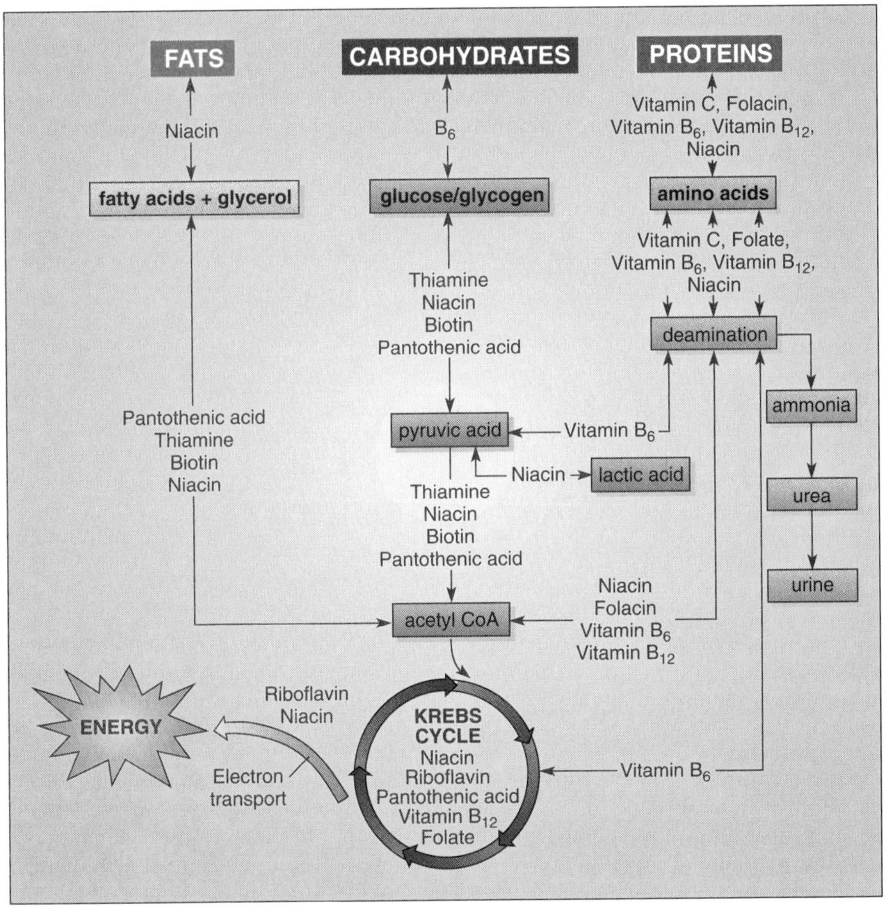

FIG. 6–2. General schema for the role of water-soluble vitamins in food metabolism.

Accuracy of vitamin C intake and usage. A promising new laboratory method called *in situ kinetics* measures the amount of vitamin C actually used by specific body tissues, rather than plasma vitamin C concentration. This new technique will help scientists to determine the optimal requirements of vitamin C needed in the diet for children and adults, rather than relying on the current RDA for this important micronutrient.

facturers. Also, at high levels of physical activity, food intake is generally increased to sustain the added energy requirements of exercise. If this added food is obtained through well-balanced meals, a proportionate increase in micronutrient intake is assured.

The supplementers. The heaviest use of vitamin supplements is among white female college graduates aged 25 to 40 who live in the western region of the United States.

Over 45 years of research has not supported the wisdom of using vitamin supplements to improve exercise performance or the ability to train in nutritionally adequate, healthy people. When vitamin intake is at recommended levels, supplements neither improve exercise performance nor necessarily increase the blood levels of these nutrients. The facts have become clouded by the "testimonials" of some coaches and elite athletes to the effect that their success was due to a particular dietary modification that usually included vitamin supplements.

A COMPETITIVE EDGE?

Figure 6–2 illustrates that the B-complex vitamins play key roles as coenzymes in important energy-yielding reactions during carbohydrate, lipid, and protein breakdown. Consequently, it is tempting to speculate that increasing the intake of these vitamins will "supercharge" energy release and improve physical performance. The belief that "if a little is good, more must be better" has led many coaches, athletes, and fitness enthusiasts to either advocate or use vitamin supplements. This approach, however, is simply not supported by research findings or by the overwhelming majority of professional nutritionists. For example:

- Supplementing with vitamin B_6, an essential cofactor in glycogen and amino acid metabolism, was of no benefit to exercise metabolism during high-intensity aerobic exercise.
- No exercise benefits have been demonstrated for an excess of other water-soluble vitamins including vitamin C. For example, supplements of vitamin C had no effect on endurance performance or on the rate, severity, and duration of injuries compared to treatment with a placebo.
- It has never been firmly established that a deficiency state for vitamin E exists for normal individuals, let alone that vitamin E supplements are beneficial to stamina, circulatory function, energy metabolism, aging, or sexual potency.

Micronutrient deficiencies among athletes. Vitamin and mineral deficiencies are rare among athletes except when caloric intake is restricted in an effort to reduce or maintain a low body weight.

Today's active men and women must focus on sound eating and training practices. The time, energy, and money spent in the quest for the ideal nutritional elixir is not only futile, but potentially counterproductive.

TOXICITY OF FAT-SOLUBLE VITAMINS

Vitamin A. Ingesting an excess of vitamin A above the RDA can produce **toxic accumulations.** For Vitamin A, the normal adult daily requirement is 1000 μg, or 3333 International Units (IU) of retinol.* When taken in excess

* There are basically three interchangeable chemical forms of vitamin A obtained in the diet: retinol, retinal, and retinoic acid. Together, these compounds are known as retinoids. In plants, the most potent source of vitamin A comes from a class of compounds known as carotenoids; the best known of these is beta-carotene, or provitamin A. Vitamin A can be expressed quantitatively in one of three forms: micrograms of retinol, micrograms of retinol equivalents, and international units (IU).

The IU designation is an older method of expressing vitamin A activity. This has been

(7500 to more than 300,000 μg per day) for an extended period, vitamin A accumulates in the liver to levels toxic for both infants and adults. Fetal deformities of internal organs, malformations and abnormalities of the face and brain, and spontaneous abortion can occur during pregnancy from consuming a daily dose of between 5400 and 150,000 μg.

In children aged 1 to 3 years, excessive intake of vitamin A (called **hypervitaminosis A** or vitamin A intoxication) can cause nervous irritability, swelling of bones, weight loss, and dry, itchy skin. In adults, general signs of toxicity are reflected in changes in many important bodily functions. Toxicity can affect the (1) blood (loss of hemoglobin and potassium from red cells, easier induction of bleeding, cessation of menstruation), (2) bone (leaching of calcium from bones causing bone brittleness and decalcification, pains in the joints, severe headache), (3) GI tract (nausea, vomiting, diarrhea, abdominal pain), (4) integumentary system (hair loss, drying and scaling of the skin, itching, cracking of the lips, brittle nails), (5) nervous system (drowsiness, visual impairment, failure to eat, muscle weakness, headache, nausea, general fatigue), and (6) intestinal organs (enlargement of the liver and spleen, liver damage including jaundice, high levels of blood triglyceride). Discontinuing a high intake of vitamin A reverses the symptoms. An acute overdose of vitamin A is also possible. Some Arctic explorers have been poisoned by extremely high concentrations of vitamin A from a meal of polar bear liver.

Poisonous in excess. Excessive intake of specific foods can precipitate vitamin A toxicity. One pound of beef liver contains about 240,000 IU of vitamin A, nearly 10 times a toxic dose of 25,000 IU and about 48 times more than the adult RDA!

Vitamin D. **Excessive intake of vitamin D** above the RDA of 5 to 10 μg per day (200 to 400 IU per day) also can be toxic. In children, regular daily intake of between 50 and 75 μg of vitamin D can induce vomiting, diarrhea, hypertension, and failure to thrive. In adults, prolonged intake of 50 μg a day may trigger marked disturbances in calcium metabolism that lead to hypertension, nausea, and loss of appetite. Extensive kidney damage also is possible because toxicity produces increased reabsorption of calcium with subsequent formation of calcium crystals in the kidneys. This condition of **hypercalcemia** is characterized by general malaise, gastrointestinal distress (vomiting and diarrhea), and copious urine flow. The end result of calcium deposits in the kidneys is local destruction of renal tissues.

Vitamins E and K. Although a toxic "overdose" from vitamins E and K is rare, excessive intake of these vitamins is probably of no benefit and in rare situations produces undesirable side effects such as muscle weakness, fatigue, nausea, diarrhea, and gastrointestinal distress.

TOXICITY OF WATER-SOLUBLE VITAMINS

Vitamin C. There are few potential toxic side effects from consuming up to 2 g (2000 mg) daily of vitamin C. Although the RDA for this vitamin is 60 mg, the amount actually required by the body is considerably less. An intake of 60 mg is equivalent to the vitamin C in ½ cup of broccoli, 2

---

replaced by the **retinol equivalent,** or RE. The RE is a measure of vitamin A activity, and reflects the amount of retinol that one of the vitamin A compounds produces after it is metabolized in the body. The RDA for vitamin A for adults is 1000 RE. In general, to convert from the IU system to the RE system, divide IU by 5. Thus, if you consumed 20,000 IU of vitamin A, it would be equivalent to 4000 RE.

oz of green peppers, one small grapefruit, one orange or ½ cup of orange juice, two large tomatoes, ¾ cup of strawberries, or 1½ cups of spinach. Consuming much more than 60 mg would be "overkill" because the body maintains a total balance of approximately 1500 mg of vitamin C. This quantity remains in the body tissues and fluids without overstressing kidney reabsorption of the vitamin. Once the available pool of vitamin C increases above the 1500 mg level, the kidneys are unable to reabsorb all of the vitamin and the excess is voided in the urine.

In healthy people, consuming a **vitamin C megadose** of 2000 mg or more daily can precipitate diarrhea, nausea, abdominal cramps, headache, fatigue, and hot flashes. In predisposed individuals, excess vitamin C intake contributes to the formation of kidney stones, and can raise serum uric acid levels and trigger gout (formation of crystals of uric acid in the joints). Some racial groups (Sephardic Jews, black Americans and Africans, and Asians) have an inherited enzyme deficiency that is aggravated by high intake of vitamin C. Excessive dosages for these individuals can cause hemolytic anemia or the bursting of red blood cells. Also, in people with sickle-cell anemia, vitamin C excess causes the red blood cells to become further deformed and clump together. In individuals who are iron deficient, megadoses of vitamin C destroy significant amounts of vitamin B_{12}.

Consuming a megadose of vitamin C, sometimes up to twice the yearly amount each day, has been advocated by some for maladies ranging from the common cold to various cancers. Available research indicates that vitamin C supplementation has little effect on the frequency and duration of the common cold, although vitamin C may work as an antihistamine to reduce cold symptoms. We are unaware of rigorously controlled research in humans to support an anticancer effect for excessive vitamin C intake, although administering massive doses to some animals has reduced the size of cancerous tumors. The lack of "hard data" from human research does not exclude the possibility that a vitamin C excess may elicit beneficial effects under certain medical conditions. An intake of 100 mg above the RDA is recommended for smokers and for people who experience unusually high levels of daily stress, the elderly, and those who are institutionalized.

Thiamine and Riboflavin. There is no known toxicity for either vitamin when taken in excess.

Niacin. A fivefold intake of niacin above the 20 mg RDA can increase skin blood flow to cause redness or flushing at the skin surface in the hands, neck, and face. This rush of blood into the dilated capillaries is called the "niacin flush." Symptoms of **niacin excess** also include nausea, headaches, itching, and abdominal cramps. Prolonged excess can interfere with normal liver function and produce higher than normal levels of blood sugar.

Pyridoxine (Vitamin B_6). Many women supplement with this vitamin in the hope of providing relief from premenstrual syndrome (PMS), a malady related to hormonal fluctuations that affects women in different ways. Common PMS symptoms most often occur 7 to 10 days before menstruation and include fatigue, slight weight gain, sleep disorders, mild to severe depression, noticeable irritability, water retention (bloating), breast tenderness, frequent headaches, lower back pain, cravings for high-carbohydrate, high-calorie, and chocolate foods, and constipation. **Pyridoxine**

supplementation has never been objectively shown to benefit symptoms of PMS.

Consuming from 2 to 6 g of pyridoxine daily for only two months has been reported to produce irreversible nerve damage! Two grams of pyridoxine is approximately 1250 times the adult woman's 1.6 mg daily requirement, or more than 100,000% of the RDA! In fact, consuming only 25 mg a day for several months can produce toxic effects that affect the sensory nerves. Symptoms include numbness in the hands and feet and deterioration in coordination while walking. There is widespread but unsubstantiated belief that high doses of pyridoxine can relieve the symptoms of carpal tunnel syndrome, an inflammation and irritation of nerves to the wrist.

Folic Acid. Even though folic acid deficiency is the most common vitamin deficiency in the United States, **excessive folic acid intake** also can precipitate toxic side effects including gastrointestinal distress, nervous irritability, insomnia, and disruption of normal patterns of sleep. Folic acid also negatively affects some anticonvulsant drugs prescribed for epileptic patients. However, therapeutic doses are prescribed to correct a deficiency in vitamin B_{12}. This deficiency can trigger megaloblastic anemia, an abnormality in the maturation of red blood cells that produces enlarged cells containing excessive hemoglobin. During pregnancy, the RDA for folic acid is 400 μg, more than double the 180 μg requirement for nonpregnant adult females. It is now apparent that pregnant women who take folic acid from the time of conception greatly reduce the risk of having babies with common, serious neurological defects.

DIGESTION AND ABSORPTION

A basic difference between the fat- and water-soluble vitamins is how they are absorbed and stored by the body. Up to 90% of fat-soluble vitamins are absorbed with dietary fats along various sections of the small intestine. More specifically, vitamin A (along with vitamin K), is absorbed in the duodenum and jejunum; vitamin D is absorbed in the duodenum, while vitamin E is absorbed along the central portion of the small intestine. Once these vitamins are absorbed, they are transported to the liver and fatty tissues by chylomicrons and lipoproteins.

In contrast, the water-soluble vitamins except for vitamin B_{12} are generally not retained in the tissues to any great extent. Instead, they are excreted in the urine when their concentration in plasma exceeds the renal capacity for reabsorption. Thus, these vitamins must be regularly replenished by daily food intake. Because the ingested B vitamins in food exist as part of coenzymes, they are broken down to the free vitamin form, first in the stomach and then along various sections of the small intestine, before they are absorbed. The sites of absorption for the water-soluble vitamins are as follows:

- **Vitamin C.** About 90% of absorption takes place in the distal portion of the small intestine. Excess intake of vitamin C above a threshold of approximately 1500 mg daily decreases the efficiency of kidney reabsorption, and large amounts are voided in the urine.

- **Thiamine.** Absorption occurs mainly in the jejunum of the small intestine. Symptoms of thiamine deficiency (beriberi, depression, mental confusion, loss of muscle coordination), especially among alcoholics, individuals on extremely low calorie diets, and the confined elderly, often become evident within 10 days because the body's store of thiamine is minuscule.
- **Riboflavin.** Absorption occurs mainly in the proximal portion of the small intestine.
- **Niacin.** Some absorption takes place in the stomach, but most occurs in the small intestine.
- **Pantothenic acid.** This vitamin exists as part of coenzyme A, and thus absorption readily takes place throughout the small intestine when the coenzyme releases it.
- **Biotin.** Absorption occurs mainly in the upper one-third to one-half of the small intestine.
- **Folic acid.** Absorption occurs readily in the liver and small intestine with the help of a specialized intestinal enzyme system called conjugase.
- **Vitamin B_6 (pyridoxine).** Absorption occurs mainly in the intestinal jejunum.
- **Vitamin B_{12}.** This vitamin is first acted on in the stomach by a salivary enzyme. It then combines with a protein called R-protein before entering the small intestine. Here, the pancreatic enzyme trypsin liberates vitamin B_{12} from the R-protein; after the vitamin joins with another protein, up to 70% is absorbed in the ileum of the small intestine.

Not found in the plant kingdom. Vitamin B_{12} is not available in plants because it is produced by bacteria in the digestive tract of animals. Only a small amount of this vitamin is needed (3 μg RDA). Thus, vitamin B_{12} deficiency in nonvegetarians is usually caused by failure in intestinal absorption.

For most of us, the ingestion of a diversity of vitamin-laden nutrients, not their absorption, is a limiting factor in good nutrition. However, vitamin supplementation is often appropriate for those individuals with limitations in intestinal absorption. Such supplementation should be supervised by a physician with a solid background in nutrition.

Focus on well balanced nutrition. Consuming daily vitamin supplements to improve the quality of an unbalanced, nutritionally inadequate diet is both naive and potentially harmful. Simply stated, "A poor diet plus a vitamin pill is still a poor diet."

SUMMARY

1. Vitamins are relatively simple organic compounds that neither supply energy nor contribute to the body's mass, but that serve crucial functions in almost all body processes. Vitamins must be obtained from food or from dietary supplementation.
2. There are 13 known vitamins, classified as either water- or fat-soluble. The fat-soluble vitamins are A, D, E, and K; vitamin C and the B-complex vitamins are water soluble.
3. Vitamins are synthesized by plants and are also found in animals, which produce them from substances known as provitamins.
4. Vitamins regulate metabolism, facilitate energy release, and are important in the process of tissue synthesis.
5. Research generally shows that vitamin supplementation (above that obtained in a well-balanced diet) is not related to improved exercise performance or capacity for training.
6. Fat-soluble vitamins taken in excess accumulate in the tissues and eventually can be toxic. Except in relatively rare and specific instances, ex-

cesses of water-soluble vitamins are generally nontoxic and are eventually excreted in the urine.

7. The major site for vitamin absorption is the small intestine.

RELATED LITERATURE

Antioxidant vitamins and β-carotene in disease prevention. Proceedings of a conference held in London, UK. Am. J. Clin. Nutr., 53 (Suppl.):189S, 1991.

Belko, A.Z.: Vitamins and exercise: an update. Med. Sci. Sports Exerc., 19:S191, 1987.

Boland, R.: Role of vitamin D in skeletal muscle function. Endocrine Rev., 7:434, 1986.

Clinical nutrition: Vitamin C toxicity. Nutr. Rev., 34:236, 1977.

Deuster, P.A., et al.: Nutritional survey of highly trained women runners. Am. J. Clin. Nutr., 44:954, 1986.

Guthrie, H.A.: Introductory Nutrition, 7th ed. St. Louis, C.V. Mosby, 1988.

Haymes, E.M.: Vitamin and mineral supplementation to athletes. Int. J. Sports Nutr., 1:146, 1991.

Herbert, V.: Toxicity of vitamin E. Nutr. Rev., 35:158, 1977.

Herbert, V., et al.: Destruction of vitamin B by vitamin C. Am. J. Clin. Nutr., 30:297, 1977.

Lawrence, J.D., et al.: Effects of α-tocopherol acetate on the swimming endurance of trained swimmers. Am. J. Clin. Nutr., 28:205, 1975.

Manore, M.M., and Leklem, J.E.: Effect of carbohydrate and vitamin B-6 on fuel substrates during exercise in women. Med. Sci. Sports Exerc., 20:233, 1988.

McArdle, W.D., et al.: Exercise Physiology: Energy, Nutrition, and Human Performance, 3rd ed. Philadelphia, Lea & Febiger, 1991.

Percy, E.C.: Ergogenic aids in athletics. Med. Sci. Sports, 10:298, 1978.

Position of the American Dietetic Association: Nutrition for physical fitness and athletic performance for adults. ADA Rep., 81:933, 1987.

Roe, D.A.: Vitamin requirements for increased physical activity. In: Exercise, Nutrition, and Energy Metabolism. Edited by E.H. Horton and R.L. Terjung. New York, Macmillan, 1988.

Schaumberg, H., et al.: Sensory neuropathy from pyridoxine abuse: a new megavitamin syndrome. N. Engl. J. Med., 309:445, 1983.

Schrimshaw, N.S., and Young, V.R.: The requirements of human nutrition. Sci. Am., 235:50, 1976.

Shekelle, R.B., et al.: Dietary vitamin A and risk of cancer in Western Electric study. Lancet, 2:1186, 1981.

Shils, M.E., and Young, V.R. (Eds.). Modern Nutrition in Health and Disease, 6th ed. Philadelphia, Lea & Febiger, 1988.

Singh, A., et al.: Chronic multivitamin-mineral supplementation does not enhance physical performance. Med. Sci. Sports Exerc., 24:726, 1992.

Suter, P.M., and Russell, R.M.: Vitamin requirements of the elderly. Am. J. Clin. Nutr., 45:501, 1987.

Telford, R.D., et al.: The effect of 7 to 8 months of vitamin/mineral supplementation on athletic performance. Int. J. Sport Nutr., 2:135, 1992.

Tremblay, A., et al.: The effects of riboflavin supplementation on the nutritional status and performance of elite swimmers. Nutr. Res., 4:201, 1984.

Use of vitamin and mineral supplements in the United States. Nutr. Rev., 70:43, 1990.

Wardlaw, G.M., and Insel, P.M.: Perspectives in Nutrition. St. Louis, Times Mirror/Mosby, 1990.

Weight, L.M., et al.: Vitamin and mineral supplementation: Effect on the running performance of trained athletes. Am. J. Clin. Nutr., 47:186, 1988.

Williams, M.H.: Vitamin and mineral supplements to athletes: Do they help? Clin. Sports Med., 3:623, 1984.

Williams, M.H.: Nutritional Aspects of Human Physical and Athletic Performance. Springfield, IL, Charles C Thomas, 1985.

Wolf, W., and Lohman, T.G.: Nutritional practices of coaches in the Big Ten. Phys. Sportsmed., 7:112, 1979.

7

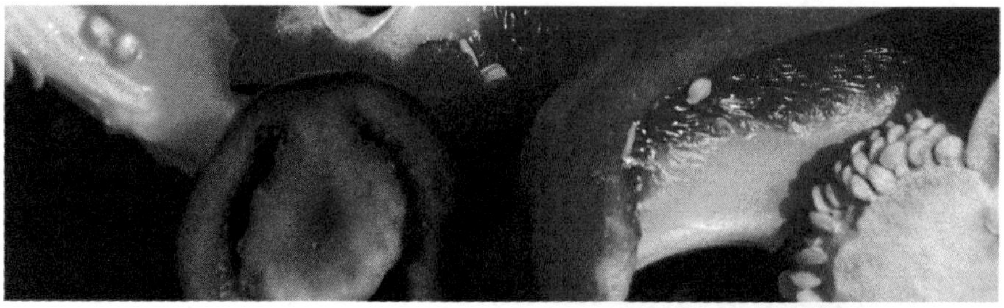

MINERALS

The body is composed of at least 31 known chemical elements of which 24 are considered essential for sustaining life. These essential elements are combined in thousands of different ways to form the various structures of the body. The most abundant nonmetal chemical element is oxygen, which amounts to 65% of our body mass. Three other nonmetal elements constitute 31% of the body mass; these are carbon (18%), hydrogen (10%), and nitrogen (3%). The remainder of the body is composed of a group of elements called minerals. Although the total quantity of minerals in the body is relatively small, each is vital for proper cell functioning. If purchased in a store, however, these elements would cost only about 12 cents!

WHAT ARE MINERALS?

Major Minerals	Trace Minerals
Sodium	Iron
Potassium	Zinc
Calcium	Copper
Phosphorus	Selenium
Magnesium	Iodine
Sulfur	Fluorine
Chlorine	Chromium
	Molybdenum
	Manganese

Research is continuing to discover how these minerals affect the body: boron, nickel, vanadium, arsenic, cobalt, lithium, silicon, tin, and cadmium.

In addition to the elements oxygen, carbon, hydrogen, and nitrogen, approximately 4% of the body's mass is composed of some 22 mostly metallic elements collectively called **minerals.** Most of the minerals are found within living cells, although not all are necessarily essential for life. Important minerals are those found in enzymes, hormones, and vitamins. Minerals also appear in combination with specific compounds, for example, calcium phosphate in bone, or singly, such as free calcium (Ca^{+2}) and sodium (Na^{+2}) in the intracellular fluids.

In the body, minerals are classified as **major minerals** (those required in amounts greater than 100 mg per day) and minor or **trace minerals** (those required in amounts less than 100 mg a day). The total quantity of the body's trace minerals is less than 15 g, or about 0.5 oz. Excess accumulation of minerals is useless to the body and could become toxic if allowed to build up through regular overconsumption.

BIOAVAILABILITY

Bioavailability *refers to the extent that a particular mineral is absorbed by the body and made available for its biologic functions.* Consuming an excess of one mineral can affect the absorption of others because some minerals interact and compete against each other. For example, consuming excess calcium interferes with iron and magnesium absorption; likewise, supplementing with zinc can reduce copper absorption. There can be synergism in consuming some vitamins and minerals together. This is referred to as **vitamin-mineral interaction.** Iron absorption is improved if consumed with vitamin C, and calcium uptake is facilitated if calcium-rich foods are consumed in the presence of vitamin D.

Bioavailability can also be affected by **fiber-mineral interactions.** This is particularly true for fibrous compounds such as **phytate,** an organic compound found in grain fibers and coffee, and **oxalate,** contained in the fibers of vegetables such as spinach and rhubarb and in chocolate, tea, and coffee. Consuming too much fiber (more than 35 g daily) actually decreases the absorption of calcium, zinc, magnesium, and iron because these minerals become bound to dietary phytate and oxalate and are excreted in the urine and feces.

Increase the bioavailability of calcium. Combining foods is important. Combining foods that are rich in vitamin C, such as citrus fruits or tomatoes, with calcium-rich foods increases the body's absorption of calcium.

WHERE DO MINERALS COME FROM?

Minerals occur freely in nature, mainly in the waters of rivers, lakes, and oceans, in topsoil, and beneath the earth's surface. Minerals are found in the root systems of plants and in the body structures of animals that consume these plants and water. The best sources of minerals are animal products. This is because minerals are more highly concentrated in animal tissues than they are in plants.

FUNCTIONS OF MINERALS

Whereas vitamins activate chemical processes without becoming part of the products of the reactions they catalyze, minerals are often incorporated within the structures and working chemicals of the body. Minerals serve three broad roles in the body:

- They provide structure in the formation of bones and teeth
- They are intimately involved in a functional role to maintain normal heart rhythm, muscle contractility, nerve conduction, and the acid-base balance of body fluids
- They play a regulatory role in cellular metabolism and serve as important parts of enzymes and hormones that modify and regulate cellular activity

Figure 7–1 lists the important minerals that participate in catabolic (breakdown) and anabolic (buildup) cellular processes. Minerals serve as essential links to provide a balance between catabolism and anabolism. They are important in activating reactions that release energy during the breakdown of carbohydrates, lipids, and proteins. In addition, minerals are essential for synthesis of the major biologic nutrients: glycogen from glucose, lipids from fatty acids and glycerol, and proteins from amino acids. Minerals also form important constituents of hormones. Inadequate thyroxine production resulting from dietary iodine deficiency could slow the body's resting metabolism. Synthesis of insulin, the hormone that facilitates glucose uptake by the cells, requires the mineral zinc, and hydrochloric acid—the digestive acid—is formed from the mineral chlorine.

Tropical fruits: low in fat and a good source of minerals. Tropical fruits are often overlooked as a good source of nutrients. Like all fruits, they contain no cholesterol and are relatively low in calories and fat content. The sources of most tropical fruits in North America include South Florida, Central America, and the Caribbean. The values in the table are based on a 1 oz portion.

FRUIT	CALORIES	FAT, G	CALCIUM, MG	MAGNESIUM, MG	PHOSPHORUS, MG	POTASSIUM, MG
Breadfruit	29	0.07	5.5	7.2	8.5	124
Cassava	34	0.11	25.8	18.7	19.8	217
Coconut	100	9.5	4.0	8.8	32.1	101
Guava	14.2	0.2	5.7	2.8	7.2	81
Kiwi	17.2	0.1	7.5	8.6	11.2	94
Kumquat	17.9	0	11.9	3.0	6.0	55
Lime	8.5	0.06	9.3	1.6	5.1	29
Lychees	17.7	0.12	0	3.0	8.9	47
Mango	18.5	0.08	2.9	2.5	3.0	44
Papaya	10.9	0.04	6.7	2.9	1.5	73
Passion fruit	28.4	0.21	3.2	7.9	18.9	99
Pummelo	10.6	0.01	1.04	1.8	4.8	61
Tamarind	67.8	0.17	21.0	261	32	178
Taro	30.5	0.06	12.3	9.3	23.7	168
Watercress	3.3	0.03	33.4	6.7	16.7	93

RECOMMENDED INTAKE AND SOURCES OF MINERALS

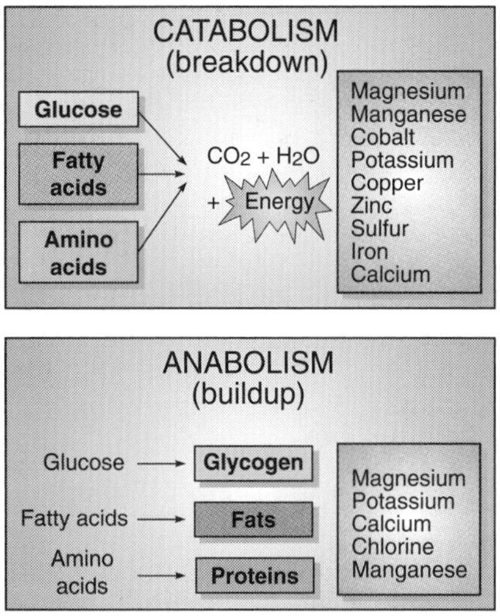

FIG. 7–1. Minerals involved in the catabolism (breakdown) and anabolism (buildup) of nutrients.

Table 7–1 lists the important major and minor minerals and their daily requirements, food sources, functions, and the effects of deficiencies and excesses. *As is the case with vitamins, mineral supplements are generally not needed because most minerals are readily available in foods and the water supply.* Some supplementation may be necessary, however, in geographic regions where the soil or water is poor in a particular mineral. In the basin of the Great Lakes and Pacific Northwest, for example, sources of the mineral **iodine** are scarce. This mineral is absorbed by the thyroid gland to become part of **thyroxine,** the hormone that exerts an accelerating influence on resting metabolism. Deficiency can be easily prevented by adding iodine to the water supply or to table salt. In the latter case, the compound is called **iodized salt.**

Thyroxine. Thyroxine is an iodine-containing amine hormone produced by the thyroid gland located in the neck just below the larynx. The hormone's major effect is to increase the resting metabolic rate by as much as fourfold. Underproduction of thyroxine is usually not a major contributor to obesity, because fewer than 3% of obese people have abnormal thyroid function.

Another common mineral deficiency results from lack of dietary iron. Approximately 30 to 50% of American women of childbearing age suffer some form of **iron insufficiency.** In most instances, appropriate iron intake can be achieved with a diet rich in iron-containing foods such as beans, peas, dried uncooked fruits, leafy green vegetables, egg yolk, and meats, especially liver, kidney, and heart. Further consideration is given to this important mineral in the section on iron later in this chapter.

MINERALS IN FOOD: THEIR RELATION TO PHYSICAL ACTIVITY

The minerals required by the body can be readily obtained from food sources in a well-balanced diet. In the following sections, specific functions are described for several of the more important minerals found in foods, as well as their influence and significance during physical activity. Often, mineral metabolism is influenced by the stress of regular exercise.

CALCIUM

At approximately 1400 g, **calcium** is the body's most abundant mineral, representing between 1.5 and 2.0% of body mass. When combined with phosphorus, it forms **hydroxyapatite**—$Ca_{10}(PO_4)_6(OH)_2$—the crystalline structure of the bones and teeth. In its ionized form, calcium plays an important role in:

- Muscle contraction
- Transmission of nerve impulses
- Activation of enzymes
- Blood clotting
- Fluid movement across plasma membranes

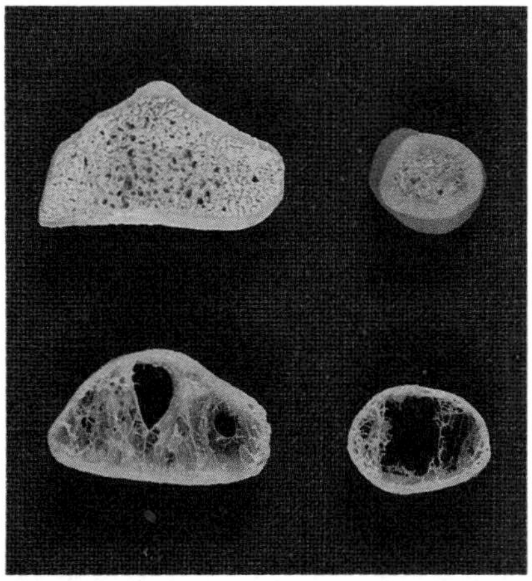

Normal radius and ulna (top), and radius and ulna in a patient with bone loss due to osteoporosis (bottom). Photos courtesy of Dr. Lisbeth Nilas, Department of Clinical Chemistry. Glostrup Hospital, Glostrup, Denmark.

Osteoporosis: Calcium, Estrogen, and Exercise. Although growing children need more calcium per unit body mass on a daily basis than adults do, a significant number of adult men and women are deficient in calcium intake. For example, about 75% of adults in the United States consume less than the Recommended Dietary Allowance (RDA) for calcium, and about 25% of all females consume less than 300 mg on any given day compared to the RDA of between 800 and 1200 mg. When calcium intake is deficient,

TABLE 7–1. THE IMPORTANT MAJOR AND TRACE MINERALS FOR HEALTHY ADULTS (AGE 19–50) AND THEIR DIETARY REQUIREMENTS, FOOD SOURCES, FUNCTIONS, AND THE EFFECTS OF DEFICIENCIES AND EXCESSES*

MINERAL	RDA FOR MALES AND FEMALES† (MG)	DIETARY SOURCES	MAJOR BODY FUNCTIONS	DEFICIENCY	EXCESS
Major					
Calcium	1200‡ 1200	Milk, cheese, dark green vegetables, dried legumes	Bone and tooth formation Blood clotting Nerve transmission	Stunted growth Rickets, osteoporosis Convulsions	Not reported in humans
Phosphorus	1200‡ 1200	Milk, cheese, yogurt, meat, poultry, grains, fish	Bone and tooth formation Acid-base balance	Weakness, demineralization of bone Loss of calcium	Erosion of jaw (phossy jaw)
Potassium	2000	Leafy vegetables, cantelope, lima beans, potatoes, bananas, milk, meats, coffee, tea	Fluid balance Nerve transmission Acid-base balance	Muscle cramps Irregular cardiac rhythm Mental confusion Loss of appetite Can be life-threatening	None if kidneys function normally. Poor kidney function causes potassium buildup and cardiac arrythmias
Sulfur	Unknown	Obtained as part of dietary protein, and is present in food preservatives	Acid-base balance Liver function	Unlikely to occur if dietary intake is adequate	Unknown
Sodium	1100–3300	Common salt	Acid-base balance Body water balance Nerve function	Muscle cramps Mental apathy Reduced appetite	High blood pressure
Chlorine (chloride)	700	Chloride is part of salt-containing food Some vegetables and fruits	Important part of extracellular fluids	Unlikely to occur if dietary intake is adequate	Along with sodium, contributes to high blood pressure
Magnesium	350 280	Whole grains, green leafy vegetables	Activates enzymes Involved in protein synthesis	Growth failure Behavioral disturbances Weakness, spasms	Diarrhea
Minor					
Iron	10 15	Eggs, lean meats, legumes, whole grains, green leafy vegetables	Constituent of hemoglobin and enzymes involved in energy metabolism	Iron deficiency anemia (weakness, reduced resistance to infection)	Siderosis Cirrhosis of liver
Fluorine	1.5–4.0	Drinking water, tea, seafood	May be important in maintenance of bone structure	Higher frequency of tooth decay	Mottling of teeth increased bone density Neurologic disturbances
Zinc	15 12	Widely distributed in foods	Constituent of enzymes involved in digestion	Growth failure Small sex glands	Fever, nausea, vomiting, diarrhea
Copper	1.5–3.0§ 1.5–3.0	Meats, drinking water	Constituent of enzymes associated with iron metabolism	Anemia, bone changes (rare in humans)	Rare metabolic condition (Wilson's disease)
Selenium	0.070 0.055	Seafood, meat, grains	Functions in close association with vitamin E	Anemia (rare)	Gastrointestinal disorders, lung irritation
Iodine (Iodide)	150	Marine fish and shellfish, dairy products, vegetables, iodized salt	Constituent of thyroid hormones	Goiter (enlarged thyroid)	Very high intakes depress thyroid activity
Chromium	0.075–0.25§ 0.05–0.25§	Legumes, cereals, organ meats Fats, vegetable oils, meats, whole grains	Constituent of some enzymes Involved in glucose and energy metabolism	Not reported in humans Impaired ability to metabolize glucose	Inhibition of enzymes Occupational exposures: skin and kidney damage

* *Recommended Dietary Allowances*, Revised 1989. Food and Nutrition Board, National Academy of Sciences–National Research Council, Washington, DC.
† First values are for males.
‡ 800 mg for adults 25 and older.
§ Because there is less information on which to base allowances, these figures are given in the form of ranges.

Menopause. Menopause usually affects women beginning at about age 50. The major biologic change is the cessation of ovulation, although decreases in some reproductive hormones can begin 10 years earlier. Menopause is confirmed when menstruation ceases for at least one year. Following menopause, the ovaries become nonfunctional. There is little or no release of estrogen; this coincides with reduced intestinal calcium absorption, less production of calcitonin (a hormone that inhibits bone demineralization), and an increase in bone resorption. Estrogen is often prescribed to offset the side effects of menopause: atrophy of the sex organs, epidermal (skin) vasodilation and "hot flashes," thinning of the skin, increases in LDL and decreases in HDL cholesterol, changes in mood state, and loss of bone mass.

the body draws on its calcium reserves in bone to replace the deficit. If the imbalance is prolonged, the condition of **osteoporosis** (literally meaning "porous bones") eventually sets in as the bones lose their mineral mass and progressively become porous and brittle. Eventually, they may break under the stress of normal living. Among older individuals, especially women past the age of 60, osteoporosis has reached epidemic proportions. Nearly 25% of women over age 65 will suffer spontaneous bone fractures! The increased susceptibility to osteoporosis is closely related to the decrease in **estrogen** production that accompanies the menopause. The precise manner by which estrogen exerts its protective effect on bone is not known, although it is believed to enhance calcium absorption and limit its resorption (withdrawal) from bone.

A Progressive Disease. Osteoporosis, which affects about 20 million Americans, begins early in life because the average teenager consumes suboptimal calcium to support the growing bones. This imbalance worsens into adulthood, and women by middle age consume only about one-third of the calcium they require for optimal bone maintenance. Starting around age 50, the average man experiences bone loss of approximately 0.4% each year, while females begin to lose twice this amount starting at age 35. For men, the normal rate of bone mineral loss does not usually pose a problem until the eighth decade of life. Women, however, become extremely susceptible to the ravages of osteoporosis during the menopause, when bone loss accelerates to between 1 and 3% per year. At this rate, an average woman loses about 15% of her bone mineral mass in the first decade after menopause; for some women, as much as 30% of the bone mass is lost by age 70! Certain risk factors predispose a person to osteoporosis. These include: white or Asian female of slight build, sedentary life style, early menopause, cigarette and alcohol abuse, long-term dieting, and family history.

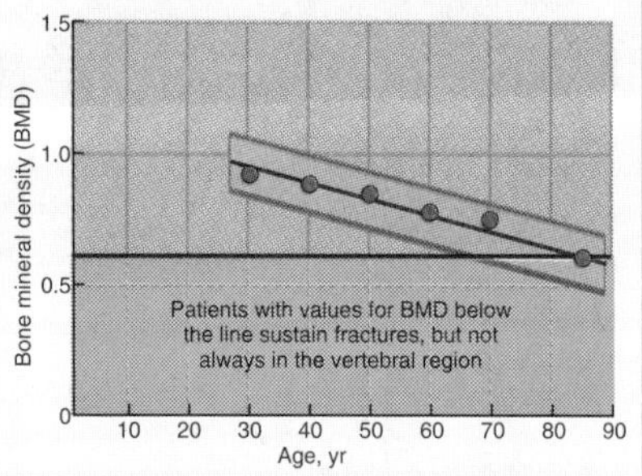

The most dramatic outward change when an adult loses bone mass is an overall shrinkage of the spinal vertebrae. Figure 7–2 illustrates the progressive deterioration in bone mass in the spinal column, and the concomitant reduction in stature, from age 50 to 75. Leg length remains unchanged but the insides of the vertebrae crumble, causing shrinkage and compression of the spinal bones. This occurs because the trabecular bone, also called "spongy bone," loses its mineral content as the bones become even more honeycombed with progressive bone resorption.

A bone disease of epidemic proportions. Osteoporosis accounts for more than 1.2 million fractures yearly, including 500,000 spinal fractures and 230,000 hip fractures. Each year, 1.3 million osteoporotic women will fracture one or more of their bones. About 1 of every 6 older men and 1 of 3 women will eventually sustain a hip fracture. Shockingly, death occurs in as many as 20% of these individuals; those who survive often require long-term nursing care. X-rays cannot detect decreases in bone mass until 30 to 50% of the bone mineral is lost!

Dietary Calcium Is Crucial. The previous 800 mg RDA has recently been upgraded to 1200 mg for males and females aged 11 to 24. Many experts recommend a further increase to between 1200 and 1500 mg for estrogen-deprived women after menopause to assure a positive calcium balance during this period. It is not clear, however, just how beneficial these calcium supplements are in the absence of adequate estrogen. On a per gram basis, one of the richest sources of calcium is canned sardines, followed by pink salmon (with the bones), ricotta cheese made from whole milk, and dried figs. A person would have to consume four times as much creamed cottage cheese or twice as much whole milk to obtain the calcium contained in canned sardines. The calcium content is about the same for whole milk and 1% and 2% milk, followed closely by buttermilk and the various types of chocolate milk.

Extra calcium intake can help correct dietary deficiencies whether this

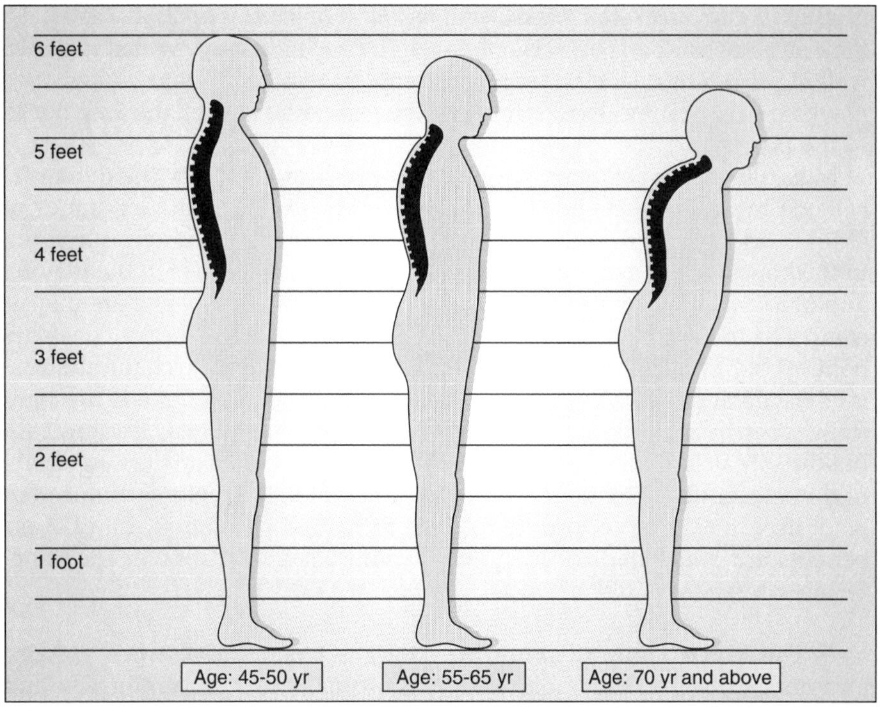

FIG. 7–2. Bone loss in the vertebrae during aging is associated with a reduction in stature.

calcium comes from supplements (calcium carbonate and calcium citrate are recommended) or from food products. *Adequate vitamin D facilitates calcium uptake, while excessive consumption of meat, salt, coffee, or alcohol inhibits calcium absorption.* Although estrogen supplements often serve as a treatment for severe osteoporosis, this therapy must be continued for prolonged periods, thus increasing the risk for cancers of the uterus, breast, and other organs. For this reason, estrogen replacement therapy for osteoporosis is often viewed as a more dramatic approach.

Benefits and Risks of Estrogen Therapy. During the next 10 years, 50 million American women will go through menopause. But are there benefits in replacing the loss of natural estrogen that marks menopause? Recent research shows that estrogen replacement therapy can reduce heart attack risk by 40 to 50% in the first 10 years after menopause. In addition, women receiving estrogen therapy had a 60% reduction in hip fractures because the hormone slows or stops osteoporosis. The down side is that the risk of endometrial cancer is 6 times higher in estrogen users than in nonusers, and long-term estrogen therapy may increase the risk of breast cancer. The benefit-to-risk ratio for estrogen therapy requires assessing each woman's risk for heart disease, osteoporosis, and cancer.

Exercise Is Helpful. Men and women who maintain an active lifestyle have significantly greater bone mass compared to their sedentary counterparts, and this benefit is maintained into the seventh and even eighth decades of life! Even at ages 70 and 80, if former athletes keep physically active, their bone mass will be superior compared to average individuals of the same age. In fact, the decline in vigorous physical activity associated with aging closely parallels the age-related loss of bone mass. *Exercise pro-*

Inadequate calcium intake can lead to porous bones. Research indicates that children who consume more than 1000 mg of calcium daily have denser bones in their arms than children who ingest less calcium. During the adolescent growth spurt, bone mineral content increases at an average rate of about 8.5% a year. Approximately 30% of college women consume only 400 to 500 mg of calcium daily; their bones were significantly less dense than women who consumed close to 1200 mg of calcium daily.

Consuming more calcium makes kids' bones more dense. The results of a 3-year study of 45 sets of identical twins, ages 6 to 14 years, showed that the twin who received an additional 1,000 mg daily of calcium had a 3% increase in wrist and spine bone density compared to the other, who took a placebo. The additional calcium intake did not affect overall growth (mass and stature) through puberty. Continuing studies will evaluate whether the increased bone mass persists into adulthood. If confirmed, this could lead to changes in the calcium RDA in younger children.

Calcium reduces hypertension in pregnancy. About 10% of American women develop hypertension during pregnancy which, if untreated, poses the potential danger of serious organ damage for the mother. The simple nutritional change of increasing the daily calcium intake to 2000 mg during the last half of pregnancy reduces the risk of developing high blood pressure in pregnancy by 34%.

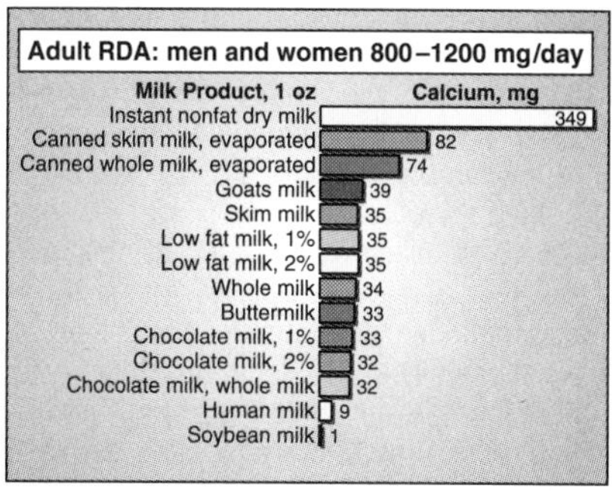

Dietary sources of calcium per oz. of milk products

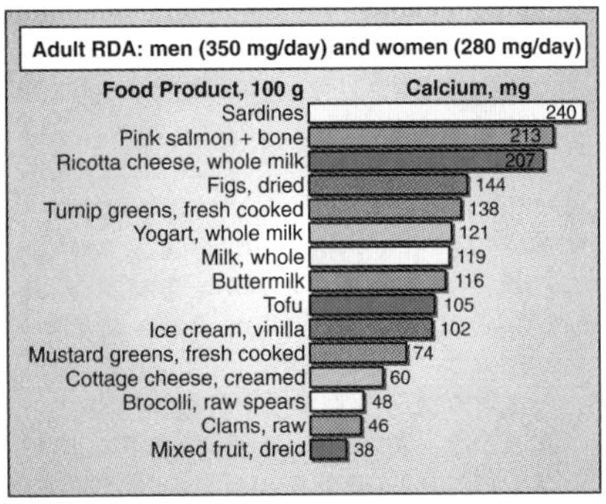

Excellent food sources of calcium expressed per 100 g of food.

vides a safe and potent stimulus to maintain and even increase bone mass in adults. Especially beneficial is exercise of a weight-bearing nature, which includes walking, running, dancing, rope skipping, or resistance-training activities in which significant muscular force can be generated against the long bones of the body.

Muscular forces acting on specific bones appear to modify the dynamics of bone metabolism at the point of stress. For example, the leg bones of older cross-country runners show greater bone mineral content compared to the bones of less active counterparts. Likewise, the bones in the playing arm of a tennis player and the throwing arm of a baseball player are thicker compared to the less used, nondominant arm. Prevailing theory considers bone to behave as a piezoelectric crystal that converts mechanical stress into electrical energy. The electric changes created when bone is mechanically stressed stimulate the activity of bone-forming cells, leading to a buildup of calcium. The quantity of bone buildup depends on the magnitude of the force and its frequency of application. Chemical factors produced in bone itself may also contribute to bone formation. Of course, all of these benefits are predicated on adequate calcium being available for the bone-forming process.

RDA for calcium. As a general guideline, adolescents and young adults need 1200 mg of calcium daily (800 mg for adults past age 24), or about as much calcium as in four 8 oz glasses of milk.

Is Too Much Training Harmful? There is a paradox between exercise and bone dynamics for premenopausal women who train intensely and reduce their body mass and body fat to a point at which the menstrual cycle actually ceases, a condition termed **secondary amenorrhea.** The hormonal imbalances associated with menstrual cessation are likely to remove estrogen's protective effect on bone, making these women vulnerable to calcium loss and possible decrease in bone mass. Concurrently, nutritional factors (e.g., low protein and fat intake) magnify the problem. If amenorrhea persists, then the benefits of exercise on bone mass are negated, the risk of musculoskeletal injuries during exercise increases, and osteoporosis sets in at an early age.

Regular exercise and increased muscle strength slow the aging of the skeleton. Moderate to high intensity aerobic exercise (walking, jogging, aerobic dancing, stair climbing) performed 3 days a week for 50 to 60 minutes a workout, builds bone and retards its rate of loss. Muscle-strengthening exercises are also beneficial. Individuals with greater back strength and those who train regularly with resistance exercise have a greater spinal bone mineral content than weaker and untrained individuals.

PHOSPHORUS

Besides its important function in combining with calcium to give rigidity to bones and teeth, **phosphorus** is an essential component of ATP and CP (adenosine triphosphate and creatine phosphate), the high-energy compounds that supply energy for biologic work. Phosphorus joins with lipids to form phospholipids that become an integral part of cell membranes. Phosphorus plays a key role in the structure of DNA and RNA. The nucleotide of the DNA molecule consists of a phosphate group (the same phosphate that is part of the high-energy phosphates), a nitrogen-containing base, and a five-carbon sugar molecule. Phosphorus also participates in buffering the acid end products of energy metabolism; in the kidneys, hydrogen ions are secreted with the aid of phosphorus, thus helping to regulate fluid pH. Phosphorus is involved in the energy metabolism of proteins, lipids, and carbohydrates, and in the regulation of nerve and muscle function. Approximately 80% of the body's phosphorus resides in the skeleton. The remainder is found in the cells and body fluids. About 40 mg of phosphorus is contained in each 100 ml of blood.

Young, fit women with middle-aged bones. Some amenorrheic young adult females have the bone mass of middle-aged women. In one study, bone density in the lumbar region was 14% lower in amenorrheic athletes who ran nearly twice the mileage compared to athletes with regular menstrual cycles. This is troubling because these amenorrheic athletes were actually losing bone mass during a period of potential bone growth. Further bad news was that intervention did not lead to resumption of normal ovarian function in all of the amenorrheic athletes.

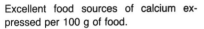

Because of the role of phosphorus in the buffering process, some coaches and trainers recommend the consumption of special "phosphate drinks" prior to strenuous exercising. It is believed that this extra phosphate will improve athletic performance by minimizing the effects of excess hydrogens that build up during "all-out" anaerobic exercise. The wisdom of this procedure has yet to be conclusively supported by careful research. Some studies report a positive effect of phosphate loading (1 g of phosphate administered several times a day for up to a week) on both moderate and all-out treadmill running performance, while other studies conclude there is no significant benefit to performance.

Animal products are a superior source of dietary phosphorus. Phosphorus in grains is present as phytic acid, which is readily catabolized by the enzyme phytase that liberates phosphate from phytic acid. In mammals, however, this enzyme is not present. Thus, phosphorus in the form of sodium phosphate (animal source) is absorbed about two times faster than the phosphate in phytic acid present in grains and soy-based food sources.

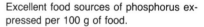

Dietary deficiencies for phosphorus are rare in the United States. This is because most Americans consume nearly twice the 800 mg daily requirement of the mineral. Up to 30% of dietary phosphorus is ingested as food additives in soft drinks, processed meats and baked foods, and various cheeses. Excellent food sources of phosphorus include bran and granola cereals, foods made with baking powder and whole-wheat flour, cheeses, almonds, liver, evaporated and whole milk, and fish. On a per gram basis, 1% and 2% lowfat milk and plain yogurt contain less than one-half of the phosphorus content of baked fish.

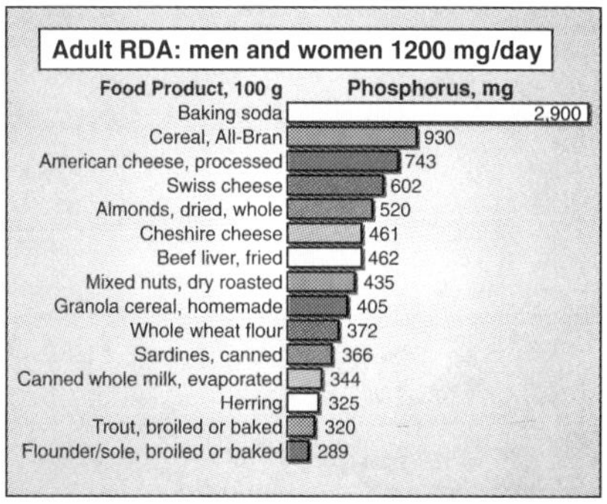

Excellent food sources of phosphorus expressed per 100 g of food.

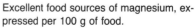

MAGNESIUM

Magnesium is the fourth most abundant mineral in the body. About 60% of the body's 25 g of magnesium is in the skeletal mass. The remainder is located in the intracellular spaces (mostly in muscle tissues), except for a minute amount that circulates in plasma. Magnesium plays an important role in the following:

- Formation of muscle and liver glycogen from blood-borne glucose
- Breakdown of glucose, fatty acids, and amino acids
- Conduction of nerve impulses and muscle contraction
- Function of hormones
- Synthesis of protein

Emphasizing good dietary sources of magnesium is especially important for women who consume additional calcium to combat osteoporosis. This is because high calcium intake can depress magnesium absorption. The daily RDA for magnesium is 280 mg for women and 350 mg for men. Excellent food sources of magnesium include whole-grain products, popcorn, sunflower seeds, legumes, and vegetables. Approximately 50% of the magnesium in plants can be lost in the cooking water if a vegetable is prepared by boiling.

SODIUM, POTASSIUM, AND CHLORINE

The minerals **sodium, potassium,** and **chlorine** are collectively termed **electrolytes** because they are dissolved in the body as ions. *The major function of the electrolytes is to modulate fluid exchange within the body's various fluid compartments.* This allows for a well-regulated exchange of nutrients and waste products between the cell and its external fluid environment. Sodium and chlorine are the chief minerals in blood plasma and extracellular fluid, while potassium is the chief intracellular mineral.

Another important function of sodium and potassium is to establish the proper electrical gradient across cell membranes. This electrical difference between the interior and exterior of the cell is required for transmission of nerve impulses, stimulation and contraction of muscle, and proper functioning of glands. The mineral electrolytes are also important in maintaining

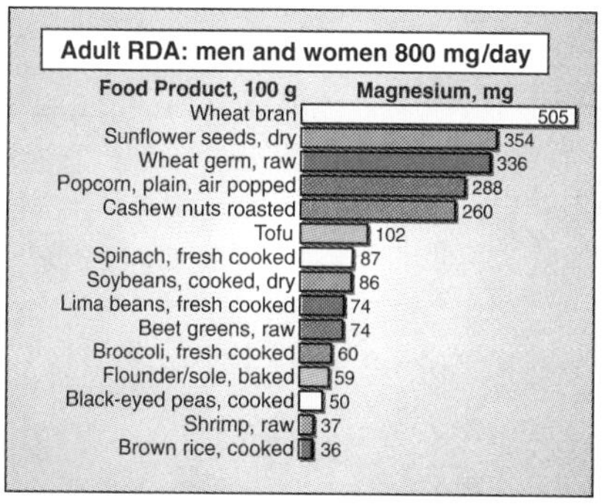

Excellent food sources of magnesium, expressed per 100 g of food.

A relook at magnesium's role. Magnesium, an essential mineral, has not been viewed as playing a major role in nutritionally-related health problems. Recent research, however, indicates that magnesium deficiency may be more prevalent than previously realized, and that adequate magnesium intake may protect in heart disease, high blood pressure, and diabetes, as well as attenuate the effects of chronic fatigue syndrome and premenstrual syndrome. Magnesium is important in the synthesis of body protein, it facilitates energy metabolism, heart and skeletal muscle function, and nerve impulse transmission; it is also important in temperature regulation and in maintaining tooth enamel.

Recommendations for magnesium intake

Age:	Magnesium intake (mg)
To 6 months	50
6 months–1 year	70
Children	
1–3 years	150
4–6	200
7–10	250
Males	
11–14	350
15–18	400
19 and over	350
Females	
11–18	300
19–50	300
51 and over	300
Pregnant	450
Nursing	450

Good sources of magnesium

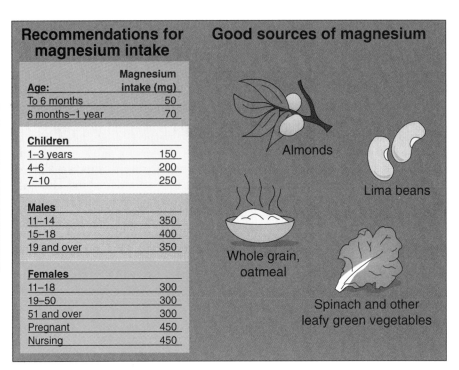

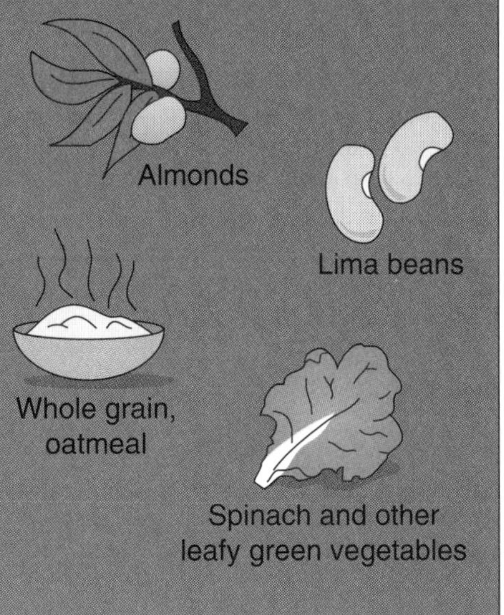

FDA requirements for labeling of sodium in foods.

IF SODIUM LABEL READS:	FDA REQUIREMENT IS:
Reduced sodium	75% less sodium after reduction
Low sodium	149 mg or less per serving
Very low sodium	35 mg or less per serving
Sodium free	5 mg or less per serving
Unsalted	No salt used in processing, but salt can occur naturally in the food

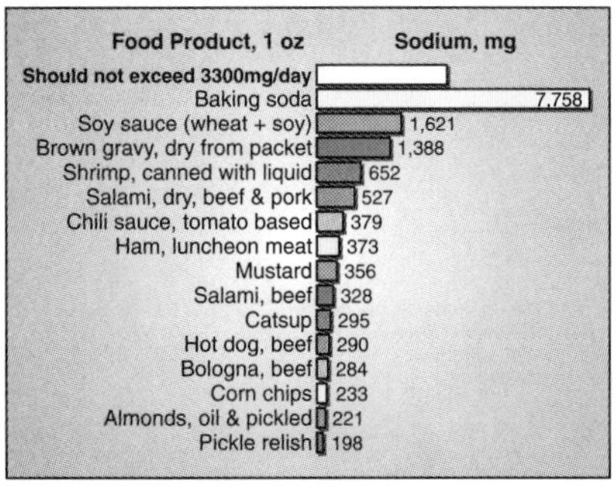

Foods high in sodium content. Values expressed per oz of the food.

the permeability of cell membranes and the acid-base quality of the body fluids, especially blood.

Sodium: How Much is Enough? In general, if sodium intake is low, the hormone **aldosterone** acts on the kidneys to conserve sodium. Conversely, if sodium intake is high, the excess is excreted in the urine. Consequently, a normal balance for this electrolyte is usually maintained throughout a wide range of intakes. For certain *susceptible individuals,* however, this is not always the case and excessive sodium intake is not adequately regulated. A chronic excess of sodium can raise fluid volume and possibly increase peripheral vascular resistance because of heightened arteriolar sensitivity to sodium; both of these factors could elevate blood pressure to levels that pose a health risk. This **sodium-induced hypertension** occurs in about one-third of hypertensive people in the United States and Japan. In these countries, sodium intake regularly exceeds the safe and adequate level for adults of between 1100 and 3300 mg per day.

For decades, one low-risk first line of defense to treat high blood pressure has been to eliminate all excess sodium from the diet. By decreasing sodium intake, it is believed that sodium and fluid levels in the body will be concomitantly reduced to lower blood pressure favorably. If dietary constraints are ineffective, drugs that induce water loss (diuretics) are the next line of defense. In addition to reducing sodium and fluid in the body, however, diuretics also cause loss in other minerals, particularly potassium. For a patient using diuretics, a potassium-rich diet is a must. Although the effectiveness of sodium restriction for controlling hypertension in the general population is presently debated among medical specialists, it does appear that certain individuals are "salt sensitive": they respond favorably to salt restriction, and blood pressure is lowered.

A person who consumes the typical Western diet ingests about 3000 to 7000 mg of sodium each day. This value is 6 to 14 times the 500 mg of sodium the body actually requires on a daily basis. Thus, the National Research Council recommendation of 1100 to 3300 mg per day is liberal in terms of actual sodium requirements. Our large sodium intake results primarily from the heavy reliance placed on table salt in processing, curing, cooking, seasoning, and storing foods. Aside from table salt, common sodium-rich dietary sources are monosodium glutamate (MSG), soy sauce, condiments, canned foods, baking soda, and baking powder. Because table salt is composed of 40% sodium and 60% chloride, this translates to a typical daily salt intake of 7.5 to 18 g. In some Asian countries, heavy reliance on soy sauce and MSG increases sodium intake to as much as 40 g a day!

IRON

The total **iron** content of the human body is largely a function of body size and physiologic and nutritional status. Pregnancy, for example, usually depresses total body iron, while iron stores increase following menopause. Likewise, monthly menstruation and resulting blood loss cause a slight decrease in total iron, while eating iron-rich foods increases the body's iron content. On average, males have about 50 mg of iron per kilogram of body mass and females have 38 mg. Thus, total body iron content is 3.5 g (50 mg × 70 kg) for a 70 kg male and 2.3 g for a 60 kg female. At greater extremes for body mass, a 123 kg male offensive football lineman stores about 6.2 g of iron, whereas the body of a 38.5 kg female jockey contains only about 1.5 g.

A dietary iron boost. Cooking with iron pots adds additional dietary iron to the foods cooked in them, especially if the foods are acidic, such as tomato sauce.

Primarily Related to Energy Metabolism. About 80% of the body's iron is part of a functionally active molecule called heme. The structural configuration of heme makes it crucial to cell function. At the center of the heme molecule is ferrous iron (Fe^{+2}), which attaches to six other atoms including four nitrogens that are part of a protein structure which combines readily with oxygen. It is ferrous iron that makes heme chemically reactive to permit its rapid attachment and detachment with oxygen. Heme, when combined with the protein globin, forms **hemoglobin,** the major constituent of red blood cells. This iron-protein compound increases the oxygen-carrying capacity of blood about 65 times.

Iron serves other important functions aside from its role in oxygen transport by the red blood cells. Heme iron constitutes an important component of **myoglobin,** a compound similar to hemoglobin that aids in the storage and transport of oxygen within muscle cells. About 5% of the body's total iron is bound in the form of myoglobin. A third depot of heme iron is in specialized chains of enzymes called **cytochromes** whose function is to catalyze energy transfer within the mitochondria. Cytochromes, in conjunction with iron, operate by transferring electrons (hydrogens) during energy-generating oxidation-reduction cellular reactions. When cytochromes become reduced, their iron atoms are in the ferrous state; when they are oxidized, the iron is changed to the ferric (Fe^{+3}) state. This transfer of electrons in the aerobic process generates significant energy for cellular function and ultimately allows hydrogen and oxygen to combine to form water. In essence, iron plays a pivotal role in oxygen transport and utilization in processes that power all forms of biologic work. Chapter 11 focuses more specifically on the reactions of energy metabolism.

Vegetarian athletes at greater risk. Research indicates that vegetarian athletes have a poorer iron status than their counterparts who consume the same quantity of iron from predominantly animal sources.

Iron Stores. Approximately 20% of iron in the body is not combined in functionally active compounds. This iron is stored in the liver, spleen, and

Iron deficiency is a universal problem. More than 550 million people worldwide suffer from iron deficiency, making it the most common nutritional deficiency in the world.

TABLE 7–2. RECOMMENDED DIETARY ALLOWANCES FOR IRON*

	AGE	IRON (MG)
Children	1–10	10
Males	11–18	12
	19+	10
Females	11–50	15
	51+	10
	Pregnant	30†
	Lactating	15†

* Recommended Dietary Allowances, Revised 1989. Food and Nutrition Board, National Academy of Sciences–National Research Council, Washington, DC.

† Generally, this increased requirement cannot be met by ordinary diets; therefore, the use of 30 to 60 mg of supplemental iron is recommended.

bone marrow and is known as hemosiderin and ferritin. It is these storage reserves that replenish the iron lost from the functional compounds and provide the "backup" iron reserves in periods of dietary insufficiency. Unfortunately, this is all too frequent for those consuming the typical Western diet, where iron content averages only about 6 mg per 1000 calories of food intake. Thus, a young adult female who typically consumes 1700 calories daily takes in only about 10.2 mg of iron. Without supplementation, iron intake would remain at about 30% below her RDA of 15 mg.

Individuals who consume insufficient iron or who have limited iron absorption or high rates of iron loss often develop reduced concentrations of hemoglobin in the blood. In an extreme condition of iron insufficiency, commonly called **iron deficiency anemia,** hemoglobin is reduced to levels characterized by general sluggishness, loss of appetite, and reduced capacity for sustaining even mild exercise. With "iron therapy," both blood hemoglobin content and physiologic responses generally return to normal levels. Table 7–2 lists the RDA for iron for children and adults.

The Source of Iron Is Important. While iron absorption from the intestines varies with iron need, a considerable difference in the bioavailability of iron occurs in relation to the composition of the diet. *For example, only between 2 to 20% of the iron obtained from the plant kingdom is absorbed, compared with 10 to 35% of animal or heme iron.* Research indicates that vegetarian athletes have poorer iron status than their counterparts who consume the same quantity of iron from predominantly animal sources. Iron bioavailability from plants can be improved by consuming iron from both heme and nonheme sources. Thus, consuming red meat with grain and vegetable products increases overall iron absorption. Iron absorption also can be increased by adding foods rich in vitamin C, which convert the ferric form of iron to the ferrous state and make it available for absorption at the alkaline pH of the intestines. For example, drinking one glass of orange juice or adding 1 oz of sesame seeds to a salad or 1 oz of toasted wheat germ to cereal stimulates a two- to three-fold increase in nonheme iron absorption. In a practical sense, people who are taking an iron supplement should drink a large glass of orange juice with it.

Excessive iron intake is risky. In children, accidental poisoning deaths from iron supplement tablets are second only to poisonings from aspirin overdose.

Females: A Population At Risk. Inadequate iron intake frequently occurs among young children, teenagers, and females of childbearing age, including groups of physically active women. A moderate iron deficiency anemia is common during pregnancy, when iron demand is increased for both mother and fetus. In addition, females usually lose between 5 and 45 mg of iron during the menstrual cycle. This menstrual iron loss is the main source of variation in the iron requirements of menstruating women. This, in turn, is governed mainly by genetic factors.

Taking an additional 5 mg of iron a day would increase a woman's average monthly intake by about 150 mg. Because an average of about 15% of the iron ingested in food is absorbed (depending on a person's iron status, the form of iron intake, and composition of the meal), the woman would then have available to her each month an additional 15 to 25 mg of iron for synthesis of red blood cells lost during menstruation. This need for extra iron, coupled with a generally poor dietary intake of iron, accounts for the fact that 30 to 50% of American women exhibit significant dietary iron insufficiencies.

Bioavailability of iron. Two main factors influence iron absorption from the gut: present iron status and the composition of the diet, especially in terms of heme and nonheme iron. On average, about 17% of iron consumed in the typical American diet is absorbed.

Exercise-induced Anemia: Fact or Fiction? Because of the great interest in endurance activities combined with the increased participation of women in such sports, research has focused on the influence of hard training on the body's iron status. The term "**sports anemia**" is sometimes used to describe an assumed effect of training on reductions in hemoglobin to levels approaching **clinical anemia,** defined as 12 g per 100 ml of blood for women and 13 g for men. Some researchers maintain that prolonged exercise training creates an added demand for iron that outstrips its intake. As a result, iron reserves are taxed and eventually cause a fall in hemoglobin levels or reduction in iron-containing compounds within the cell's energy transfer system; both may occur. Of concern is the possibility that active women who would be most susceptible to an "iron drain" may suffer reduced exercise capacity due to the crucial role of iron in energy metabolism.

It is postulated that heavy training creates an augmented iron demand because of iron loss in sweat (probably minimal) and loss of hemoglobin in urine resulting from actual destruction of red blood cells with increased temperature, spleen activity, and rapid blood flow. Iron loss may also occur from mechanical trauma during weight-bearing activity caused by repetitive pounding of the feet on the ground surface. There may even be some gastrointestinal bleeding following long-distance running that is unrelated to age, gender, or performance time. Such increases in iron loss would certainly stress the body's iron reserves needed for the synthesis of new red blood cells.

To support the possibility that exercise can induce anemia, some studies indicate that suboptimal hemoglobin concentration and hematocrit are more prevalent among endurance athletes. On closer scrutiny, however, it appears that any reduction in hemoglobin concentration is transient and occurs in the early phase of training, and hemoglobin then returns to pretraining values. This general response is illustrated in Figure 7–3 for a group of high school female cross-country runners during a competitive season. The decrease in hemoglobin early in training generally parallels the disproportionately large expansion in plasma volume. For example, just four days of submaximal exercise training increases plasma volume by 20%, whereas the red blood cell volume remains unchanged. Consequently, total hemoglobin may actually increase with training, yet its concentration in plasma decreases. Despite this apparent dilution of hemoglobin, aerobic capacity and exercise performance consistently increase during training. Although there may be some mechanical destruction of red blood cells with vigorous exercise and some loss of iron in sweat, it has yet to be verified whether these factors are of sufficient magnitude to strain an athlete's iron reserves and precipitate anemia if iron intake is normal.

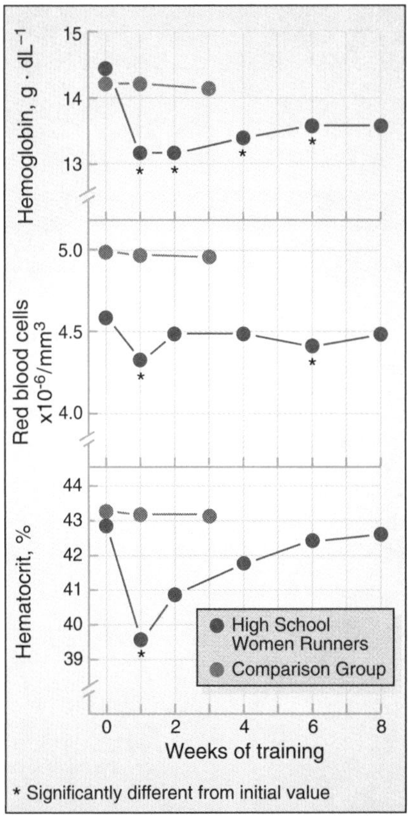

FIG. 7–3. Hemoglobin, red blood cells, and hematocrit during the competitive season. (From Puhl, J. L., et al.: Erythrocyte changes during training in high school women cross-country runners. Res. Q. Exerc. Sport, 54:484, 1981.)

MINERALS AND EXERCISE PERFORMANCE

An important consequence of long-duration exercise, especially in hot weather, is the loss of water and mineral salts, primarily sodium and some potassium chloride in sweat. These losses impair heat tolerance and exercise performance, and can lead to severe dysfunction related to heat disorders. The yearly toll of heat-related deaths during spring and summer football practice provides a tragic illustration of the importance of fluid and electrolyte replacement. It is not uncommon for an athlete to lose anywhere from 1 to 5 kg of water each practice session or during a game as a result

The RDA is sufficient for mineral salts. For most individuals who consume the RDA for minerals, there is no evidence that supplementation benefits exercise performance.

of sweating. This fluid loss also corresponds to a depletion of 1.5 to 8.0 g of salt, because each kilogram (1 liter) of sweat generally contains about 1.5 g of salt. *The crucial and immediate need in these situations, however, is to replace the water lost through sweating.* The three important heat disorders can be described as follows:

Heat disorders. If the normal signs of heat stress—thirst, tiredness, grogginess, and visual disturbances—are not heeded, cardiovascular compensation begins to fail and a series of disabling complications of heat illness can result.

- **Heat cramps.** Involuntary muscle spasms that occur during or after intense physical activity and are easily observed in the specific muscles exercised. This form of heat illness is probably caused by an imbalance in the body's fluid and electrolyte concentrations.
- **Heat exhaustion.** Usually characterized by a weak, rapid pulse, low blood pressure in the upright position, headache, dizziness, and general weakness. Sweating may be reduced, but body temperature is not elevated to dangerous levels. It is caused by ineffective circulatory adjustments compounded by depletion of extracellular fluid, especially blood volume, owing to excessive sweating. The person should stop exercising and move to a cooler environment, and fluids should be administered.
- **Heat stroke.** This is the most serious and complex of the heat maladies and requires immediate medical attention. Heat stroke is a failure of the body's heat-regulating mechanisms caused by excessively high body temperature. When thermoregulation fails, sweating usually ceases, the skin becomes dry and hot, body temperature rises to dangerous levels, and excessive strain is placed on the circulatory system. If left untreated, the disability progresses and death ensues from circulatory collapse and eventual damage to the central nervous system. Immediate aggressive steps to lower body temperature while awaiting medical treatment include alcohol rubs, ice packs, and whole-body immersion in cold or even ice water.

Vigorous exercise triggers a rapid and coordinated release of the hormones vasopressin, renin, and aldosterone, which reduce sodium and water loss through the kidneys. Even under extreme conditions, such as marathon running in warm weather, in which sweat output may reach 2 liters per hour, electrolyte conservation by the kidneys increases. Any salt loss can usually be replenished by adding a slight amount of table salt to the fluid ingested or to the normal food intake. In one study of runners during a 20-day road race in Hawaii, plasma minerals were maintained at normal levels when the athletes consumed an unrestricted diet without mineral supplements. Research indicates that ingesting so-called athletic drinks is of no special benefit in replacing mineral loss through sweating when individuals maintain a well-balanced diet. In fact, most people unconsciously consume more salt when the need exists. For fluid losses in excess of 4 or 5 kg and during prolonged work in the heat, salt supplementation may be necessary. This can be achieved with a 0.1 to 0.2% salt solution made by adding about 0.3 teaspoon of table salt to a liter of water. Although a potassium deficiency may occur with prolonged and intense exercise, for most active people appropriate potassium levels are assured by consuming a diet containing normal amounts of this mineral. A glass of orange or tomato juice replaces almost all of the calcium, potassium, and magnesium lost in about 3 liters (3.2 kg) of sweat.

Exercise Effects on Other Trace Minerals. Strenuous exercise may place a drain on the body's content of chromium and zinc (and perhaps copper and selenium), essential trace minerals required for normal carbohydrate and lipid metabolism. In one study, urinary losses of zinc and chromium were 1.5- and 2-fold higher, respectively, on the day of a strenuous 6-mile run compared to a rest day. Although this loss does not mean that athletes should supplement these micronutrients, it is possible that for people with marginal zinc and chromium intakes, any further exercise-induced loss should be replaced to prevent an overt deficiency. More research is needed in the fascinating area of trace mineral metabolism in general, and the effects of exercise and training on mineral requirements in particular.

DIGESTION AND ABSORPTION

Both extrinsic (dietary) and intrinsic (cellular) factors control the eventual fate of ingested minerals. In general, when the dietary intake of a particular mineral falls below the body's requirement, intestinal absorption increases to preserve the preciously small quantities of the micronutrients. The converse also occurs: when mineral supplies are adequate or in excess, there is little need for increased absorption. Overall, however, mineral absorption by the body is generally poor. This simplv means that for most people, minerals are available in fairly generous amounts in the diet. Except for many women's need to supplement iron and calcium intake, there is little

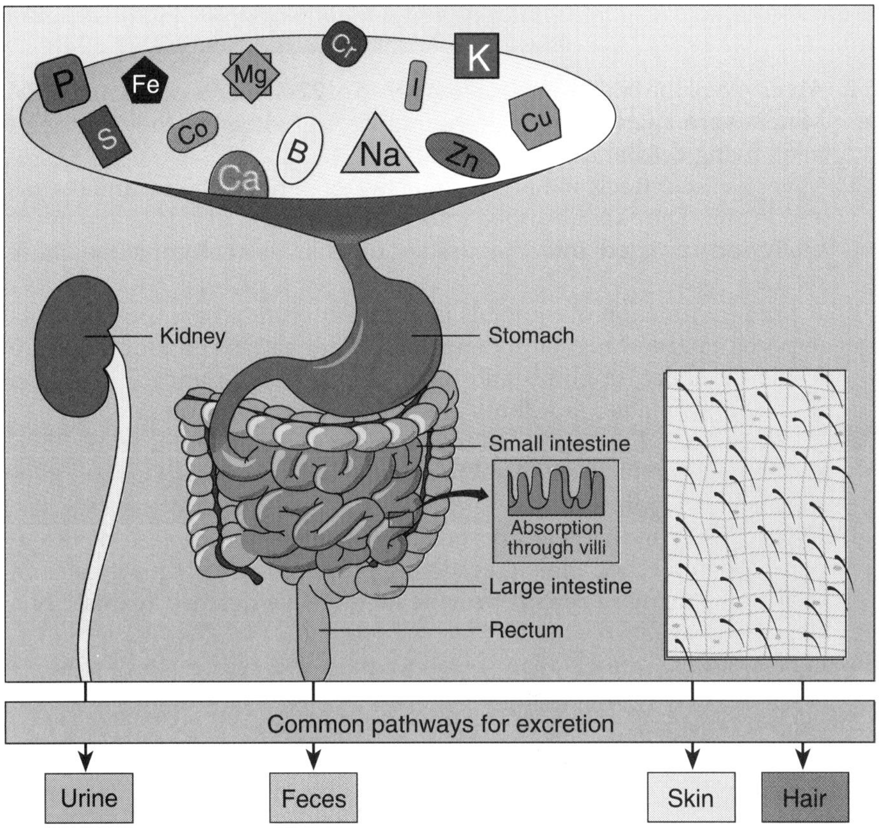

FIG. 7–4. Absorption of minerals and common pathways of excretion.

Vitamin and mineral "scorecard" for veggies. Consuming a variety of vegetables provides a good source of vitamins (vitamins A and C, folic acid) and minerals (magnesium, phosphorus, potassium). Nutrient values are for a 1 oz portion.

ITEM	VIT A, µG RE	VIT C, MG	FOLIC ACID, MG NE	MAGNESIUM, MG	PHOSPHORUS, MG	POTASSIUM, MG
Artichokes	4.08	2.1	12.6	11.1	16.9	74.6
Asparagus	25.9	9.3	29.8	4.9	14.7	85.5
Green beans	18.9	4.6	10.3	7.0	10.8	59.3
Beets	0.4	1.6	16.3	10.3	8.7	88.7
Broccoli	43.7	26.5	20.0	7.1	18.6	92.0
Brussels sprouts	24.8	24.0	17.3	6.4	19.3	110
Cabbage	3.6	13.4	16	4.1	6.5	69.7
Carrots	797	2.6	4.0	4.3	12.6	91.7
Cauliflower	0.5	20.3	18.8	4.0	13.0	101
Celery	3.5	1.8	2.6	3.4	7.1	80.8
Corn	8.0	2.0	13.0	10.5	25.4	76.6
Cucumber	1.3	1.3	3.9	3.1	4.8	42.2
Eggplant	2.0	0.5	5.0	3.1	9.4	62.2
Garlic	0	8.8	0.9	7.1	43.5	113
Kale	252	34	8.3	9.7	16	127
Leeks	2.7	3.4	18.2	7.9	9.8	51.0
Lettuce	9.4	1.1	15.9	2.6	5.7	44.8
Mushrooms	0	1.0	6.0	2.8	29.5	105
Onions	0	2.4	5.7	2.8	8.1	43.9
Peppers	15	36.3	4.8	3.8	6.1	55.2
Potatoes	0	3.7	3.1	7.7	16.1	118
Radishes	0.2	6.5	7.7	2.5	5.0	65.5
Romaine	73.9	6.8	38.5	1.7	12.7	82.0
Spinach	227	8.0	56.2	22.4	13.9	158
Squash, summer	5.6	4.2	7.3	6.5	10.0	55.2
Zucchini	9.6	2.4	6.5	5.9	9.2	60.2

† RE = retinol equivalent, NE = niacin equivalent.

advantage for the body to stockpile minerals. This is particularly true for heme iron, with an absorptive rate of about 15%, compared to nonheme iron absorption which ranges from 2 to 20%. There is also considerable variation in the absorption of other minerals, even between genders. Males, for example, absorb calcium better than females, yet total calcium absorption rarely exceeds about 35% of the quantity ingested. Approximately two-thirds of ingested calcium is excreted in the feces; of the calcium absorbed, half is voided in the urine. A somewhat different picture is seen for phosphorus, of which two-thirds, or about 13 mg per kilogram of body mass, is excreted daily in the urine, while one-third, or 7 mg/kg, is excreted in the feces. Magnesium is also poorly absorbed (20 to 30%), as are the trace minerals zinc (14 to 41%) and chromium (less than 2%). Additional research is needed to pinpoint absorption rates for the other minerals. Figure 7–4 presents a generalized schema for absorption of the major and minor minerals, including the four common pathways of excretion.

The small intestine serves as the major site for mineral absorption, particularly of calcium, phosphorus, magnesium, and the trace minerals. Intrinsic factors that affect absorption include bioavailability, transit time from the source (diet) to the site of absorption, quantity of digestive juices in the intestines that influence nutrient absorption, the presence of receptor sites in the mucosal lining and brush border of the intestine, and availability of substances that combine with the minerals as they are transported to the gut and across cell membranes to carry out their functions.

SUMMARY

1. About 4% of the body's mass is composed of 22 elements called minerals. Minerals are a part of enzymes, hormones, and vitamins; they are found in all living cells and all body fluids.
2. Minerals occur freely in nature, in the water of rivers, lakes, and oceans and in soil. They are absorbed into the root system of plants and eventually incorporated into the tissues of animals that consume these plants.
3. A primary function of minerals is in metabolism, where they serve as important parts of regulatory enzymes. Minerals also provide structure in the formation of bones and teeth, and are important for synthesis of the biologic macronutrients glycogen, lipid, and protein.
4. With a balanced diet, mineral intake is generally adequate except perhaps in geographic locations where there is an absence of certain minerals such as iodine.
5. Among older individuals, particularly women, the disease of osteoporosis has reached almost epidemic proportions. Adequate calcium intake and regular exercise provide an effective defense against bone loss at any age.
6. Paradoxically, women who train intensely and reduce body mass to the point where menstruation is adversely affected often show advanced bone loss.
7. Evidence indicates that about 30 to 50% of women of childbearing age in the United States suffer some form of iron insufficiency. This could lead to iron deficiency anemia, a condition that significantly affects the capacity for aerobic metabolism and exercise performance.

8. It is not clear whether regular physical activity creates a significant drain on the body's iron reserves. If this proves to be the case, females—who as a group have the greatest iron requirements and lowest intake—could be at risk of developing anemia.
9. Assessment of the body's iron status should include an evaluation of both hematologic characteristics and iron reserves.
10. Excessive sweating caused by exercise results in large losses of body water and related minerals. While water should be replaced during and following exercise, in most instances specific mineral supplementation is not required if sound nutritional practices are followed.
11. The small intestine is the main site for mineral absorption. Both intrinsic and extrinsic factors influence the bioavailability of these micronutrients.

RELATED LITERATURE

American College of Sports Medicine: Position statement on prevention of heat injuries during distance running. Med. Sci. Sports Exerc., 16:ix, 1984.

Anderson, R.A.: New insights on the trace elements, chromium, copper and zinc, and exercise. In Advances in Nutrition and Top Sport. Edited by F. Brouns. Basel, Karger, 32:38, 1991.

Anderson, R.A., and Guttman, H.N.: Trace minerals and exercise. In: Exercise, Nutrition and Energy Metabolism. Edited by E.H. Horton and R.L. Terjung. New York, Macmillan, 1988.

An update on calcium: applications for the 90's. Proceedings of a symposium held in Chantilly, VA. Am. J. Clin. Nutr., 54 (Suppl):177S, 1991.

Balban, E.P., et al.: The frequency of anemia and iron deficiency in the runner. Med. Sci. Sports Exerc., 21:643, 1989.

Block, J.E., et al.: Determinants of bone density among athletes engaged in weight-bearing and non-weight-bearing activity. J. Appl. Physiol., 67:1100, 1989.

Blum, S.M., et al.: The effect of fitness-type exercise on iron status in adult women. Am. J. Clin. Nutr., 43:456, 1986.

Bothwell, T.H., et al.: Iron Metabolism in Man. Boston, Blackwell, 1979.

Broun, E.R. Excessive zinc ingestion. JAMA, 264:1441, 1990.

Cann, E.C.: Decreased spinal mineral content in amenorrheic women. JAMA, 251:626, 1984.

Clarkson, P.M.: Minerals: exercise performance and supplementation in athletes. J. Sports Sci., 9:91, 1991.

Clarkson, P.M.: Vitamins and trace minerals. In: Ergogenics: enhancement of performance in exercise and sport. Perspect. Exer. Sci. Sports Med., 4:123, 1991.

Clarkson, P.M., et al.: Nutritional ergogenic aids: chromium, exercise, and muscle mass. Int. J. Sports Nutr., 1:289, 1991.

Clement, D.B., and Sawchuck, L.L.: Iron status and sports performance. Sports Med., 1:65, 1984.

Costill, D.L., et al.: Dietary potassium and heavy exercise: effects on muscle water and electrolytes. Am. J. Clin. Nutr., 36:266, 1982.

Dalsky, G.P., et al.: Weight-bearing exercise training and lumbar bone mineral content in postmenopausal women. Ann. Inter., Med., 108:824, 1988.

Dalsky, G.P., et al.: Effect of exercise on bone: permissive influence of estrogen and calcium. Med. Sci. Sports Exerc., 22:281, 1990.

DeSouza, M.J., et al.: Menstrual status and plasma vasopressin, renin activity, and aldosterone exercise responses. J. Appl. Physiol., 67:736, 1989.

Dressendorfer, R.H., et al.: Plasma mineral levels in marathon runners during a 20-day road race. Phys. Sportsmed., 10:113, 1982.

Drinkwater, B.L., et al.: Bone mineral content of amenorrheic and eumenorrheic athletes. N. Engl. J. Med., 311:277, 1984.

Frederickson, L.A., et al.: Effects of training on indices of iron status of young female cross-country runners. Med. Sci. Sports Exerc., 15:271, 1983.

Gardner, G.W., et al.: Cardiorespiratory, hematological and physical performance responses of anemic subjects to iron treatment. Am. J. Clin. Nutr., 28:982, 1975.

Green, H.J., et al.: Training induced hypervolemia: lack of an effect on oxygen utilization during exercise. Med. Sci. Sports Exerc., 19:202, 1987.
Grisso, J.A., et al.: Risk factors for falls as a cause of hip fracture in women. N. Engl. J. Med., 324:1326, 1991.
Guthrie, H.A.: Introductory Nutrition, 7th ed. St. Louis, C.V. Mosby, 1988.
Gutin, B., and Kasper, M.J.: Can vigorous exercise play a role in osteoporosis prevention? A review. Osteo. Int., 2:55, 1991.
Haliova, L., and Anderson, J.J.B.: Lifetime calcium intake and physical activity habits: independent and combined effects on the radial bone of healthy premenopausal Caucasian women. Am. J. Clin. Nutr., 49:534, 1989.
Heaney, R.P., et al.: Calcium nutrition and bone health in the elderly. Am. J. Clin. Nutr., 36:986, 1982.
Johnson, H.L., et al.: Effects of electrolyte and nutrient solutions on performance and metabolic balance. Med. Sci. Sports Exerc., 20:26, 1988.
Johnston, C.C., et al.: Clinical use of bone densitometry. N. Engl. J. Med., 324:1105, 1991.
Klingshirn, L.A., et al.: Effect of iron supplementation on endurance capacity in iron-depleted female runners. Med. Sci. Sports Exerc., 24:819, 1992.
Lamanca, J.J., et al.: Sweat iron loss of male and female runners during exercise. Int. J. Sports Med., 9:52, 1988.
Lukaski, H.C., et al.: Physical training and copper, iron, and zinc status of swimmers. Am. J. Clin. Nutr., 51:1093, 1990.
Lynch, S.R., et al.: Iron status of elderly Americans. Am. J. Clin. Nutr., 36:1032, 1982.
Marcus, R., et al.: Osteoporosis and exercise in women. Med. Sci. Sports Exerc. 24:S301, 1992.
McArdle, W.D., et al.: Exercise Physiology: Energy, Nutrition, and Human Performance, 3rd ed. Philadelphia, Lea & Febiger, 1991.
McCabe, M.E., et al.: Gastrointestinal blood loss associated with running a marathon. Dig. Dis. Sci., 31:1229, 1986.
National Dairy Council: Food vs pills vs fortified foods. Dairy Counc. Dig. 58:7, 1987.
O'Toole, M.L., et al.: Hemolysis during triathlon races: its relation to race distance. Med. Sci. Sports Exerc., 20:172, 1988.
Owen, R.A., et al.: The national cost of acute care of hip fractures associated with osteoporosis. Clin. Orthop., 150:172, 1980.
Pate, R.: Sports anemia: a review of the current literature. Phys. Sportsmed., 11:115, 1983.
Puhl, J.L., et al.: Erythrocyte changes during training in high school women cross-country runners. Res. Q. Exerc. Sport, 52:484, 1981.
Riis, B., et al.: Does calcium supplementation prevent postmenopausal bone loss? A double-blind controlled clinical study. N. Engl. J. Med., 36:173, 1987.
Risser, W.L., et al.: Iron deficiency in female athletes: Its prevalence and impact on performance. Med. Sci. Sports Exerc., 20:116, 1988.
Robertson, J.O., et al.: Fecal blood loss in response to exercise. Br. Med. J., 295, 303, 1987.
Schrimshaw, N.S., and Young, V.R.: The requirements of human nutrition. Sci. Am., 235:50, 1976.
Schoene, R.B., et al.: Iron repletion decreases maximal exercise lactate concentrations in female athletes with minimal iron-deficiency anemia. J. Lab. Clin. Med., 102:306, 1983.
Selby, G.B.: When does an athlete need iron? Phys. Sportsmed. 19:97, 1991.
Shils, M.E., and Young, V.R. (Eds.): Modern Nutrition in Health and Disease, 6th ed. Philadelphia, Lea & Febiger, 1988.
Snyder, A.C., et al.: Importance of dietary iron source on measures of iron status among female runners. Med. Sci. Sports Exerc., 21:7, 1989.
Spencer, H., and Kramer, L.: NIH Consensus Conference: Osteoporosis. J. Nutr., 116:316, 1986.
Terblanche, S., et al.: Failure of magnesium supplementation to influence marathon running performance or recovery in magnesium-replete subjects. Int. J. Sport Nutr., 2:154, 1992.
Tobian, L.: Dietary salt and hypertension. Am. J. Clin. Nutr., 32:2659, 1979.
Use of vitamin and mineral supplements in the United States. Nutr. Rev., 70:43, 1990.
Wardlaw, G.M., and Insel, P.M.: Perspectives in Nutrition. St. Louis, Times Mirror/Mosby, 1990.

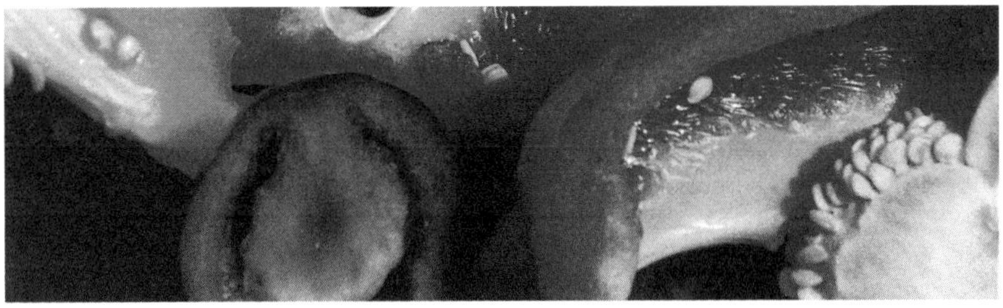

8

WATER

Water is a substance made up of the elements hydrogen and oxygen that can exist in a gaseous, liquid, or solid state. As shown in Chapter 1, a water molecule consists of two hydrogen atoms, each linked by a single chemical bond to an atom of oxygen. **Water** is one of the most plentiful and essential compounds vital to life. In essence, water is involved in virtually every bodily process.

Although water does not contribute to the nutrient value of food per se, it is still important in describing food composition and energy balance. For example, the energy content of a particular food tends to be inversely related to its water content. As a general rule, foods that are high in water are low in calories. For this reason, the energy content of a food is often expressed per "dry weight" of the food.

WATER IN THE BODY

Water represents almost 75% of a newborn's body mass. In adults, **differences in total body water** among individuals are largely the result of variations in body composition (amount of lean vs. fat tissue), and these differences are linked to gender. Males typically have a water content that ranges between 57 and 65% of total body mass; for females, water content ranges from 46 to 53%. **Gender differences** in the body's water content are primarily attributable to differences in body fat. Compared to males, females have a larger quantity of body fat (15.3 kg, or 25% of body mass, vs. 10.5 kg, or 15%) and a smaller lean body mass component (48 kg vs. 62 kg). Water constitutes 65 to 75% of the weight of muscle, while body fat is the least hydrated of the tissues, being made up of 20 to 30% water. Surprisingly, bone also contains about the same amount of water as body fat. In relation to body composition, individuals who are lean and muscular have a larger water content than their fatter counterparts with the same body mass. Changes in the body's water content with aging are also closely linked to age-related variations in body composition.

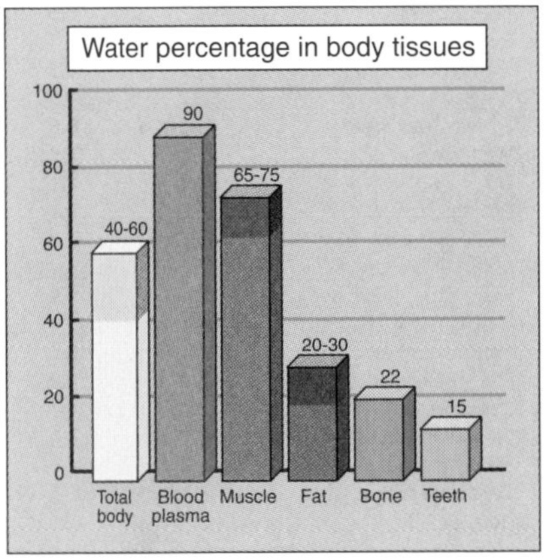

FLUID COMPARTMENTS

The body has two main water "compartments": ***intracellular fluid (ICF),*** referring to the fluids within the cell, and ***extracellular fluid (ECF),*** referring to all water outside of the cell. ECF includes the blood plasma, or fluid portion of the blood, and the interstitial fluid that occupies the spaces between the various tissue components. The blood plasma serves as the common connection between the internal (ICF) and external (ECF) cellular environments. Other examples of ECF include lymph, saliva, and fluids in the eyes and joints (synovial fluid), fluids secreted by glands and the intestines, fluids that bathe the nerves of the spinal cord, and fluids excreted from the skin and kidneys. The ICF and ECF each are associated with specific electrolytes, particularly Na^+, Cl^-, and K^+. The ICF contains relatively low concentrations of Na^+ and Cl^- and a high concentration of K^+. In contrast, the interstitial fluids and blood plasma have high concentrations of Na^+ and Cl^- but a very low amount of K^+. Differences in electrolyte concentration in the fluid compartments affect the exchange of chemicals through the permeable cell membrane, especially the soluble proteins, nonelectrolyte molecules such as cholesterol, phospholipids, and fats, minerals (e.g., Mg^{+2} and Ca^{+2}), and other dissolved solutes.

Water compartments. Of the total water content of the body, about 62% exists as ICF and 38% as ECF. For a 70 kg person, total body water is about 42 liters. Thus, ICF volume is 26 liters (0.62 × 42) and ECF volume equals 16 liters (0.38 × 42). Blood plasma accounts for 20% of the ECF, or a volume of about 3 liters. Much of the fluid lost through sweating is ECF, predominantly from the blood plasma.

FUNCTIONS OF BODY WATER

Water is truly a remarkable substance; without it, death occurs within days. Water serves as the body's transport and reactive medium. Diffusion of gases always takes place across surfaces moistened by water. Nutrients and gases are transported in aqueous solution, and waste products leave the body through the water in urine and feces. Water has tremendous heat-stabilizing qualities because it absorbs a considerable quantity of heat with only a small change in temperature. Water is part of the fluids that lubricate the joints, keeping bony surfaces from grinding against each other. Because it is essentially noncompressible, water provides structure and form to the body through the turgor it gives body tissues.

Aqueous solutions. The body utilizes aqueous solutions such as blood, cytoplasm, and digestive juices as the mediums in which all biologic processes take place.

FOODS HIGH IN WATER CONTENT

Food Item, 1 oz	Water Content, %	Total Calories
Iceberg lettuce, leaf	95.8	3.7
Tomato, fresh	93.7	5.5
Summer squash	93.7	5.7
Pumpkin, cooked fresh	93.7	5.8
Cabbage, raw	92.2	6.5
Strawberries, fresh	91.5	8.6
Watermelon	91.2	8.9
Grapefruit, fresh	90.8	9.1
Broccoli spears, raw	90.5	3.7
Canteloupe, fresh	89.8	10.0
Milk, 1% low fat	87.7	11.9
Honeydew melon, fresh	89.4	9.9
Milk, whole	87.7	17.4
Peach, fresh	87.7	12.0
Orange, fresh	86.6	13.2
Pears, fresh	83.8	16.7
Blueberries, fresh	84.5	16.0
Pizza, cheese	45.8	68.5
Chocolate fudge	8.1	115
Corn oil	0	251

WATER BALANCE: INTAKE VERSUS OUTPUT

The body's water content remains relatively stable over time. Although water output frequently exceeds intake, the imbalance is quickly adjusted with appropriate ingestion of fluid. The **sources of water intake and output** at normal ambient temperatures are shown in the top panel of Figure 8–1. The bottom portion of the figure indicates that fluid balance can change dramatically during exercise, especially in a hot, humid environment.

WATER INTAKE

Normally, about 2.5 liters (2.7 quarts) of water are required each day for a sedentary adult living within the normal range of environmental temperatures. Naturally, there can be considerable variation in total water consumption because of differences in the composition and size of meals, external temperature and humidity, and extent of participation in physical activity. Water is obtained from three sources: liquids, foods, and metabolism.

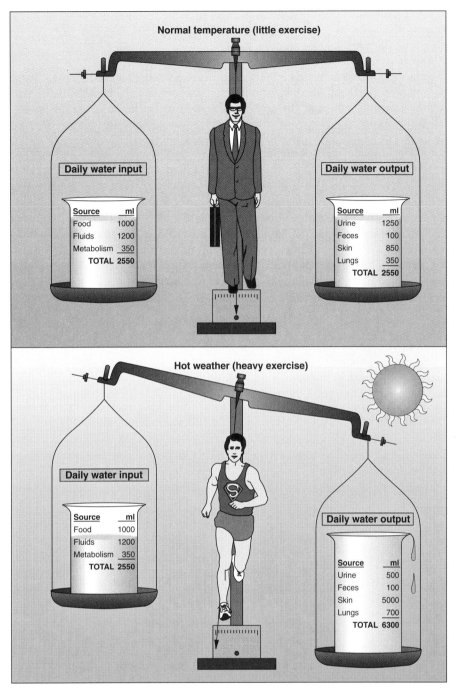

FIG. 8–1. Water balance in the body. Top: Exercise in normal ambient temperature and humidity. Bottom: Moderate to heavy exercise in a hot, humid environment.

Soft drinks, the beverage of choice. In 1990, the average American consumed 1 gallon of soft drinks each week! Total consumption was 1.3 billion gallons, a 2.6% increase over 1989. Coca Cola Classic was the most popular soft drink, with about one-third of all sodas sold being of the diet variety. The total consumption of bottled water and fruit drinks was 3 million gallons.

Water from Liquids. The typical individual normally consumes about 1200 ml of water daily. This amount changes drastically during exercise and thermal stress, when total fluid intake can increase five or six times above normal. There is a report of a male endurance runner who lost 13.6 kg (30 lb) of water weight during a 55-mile run across Death Valley, California, that took 2 days, 17 hours. This highly conditioned athlete was able to maintain fluid intake, so weight loss at the completion of this unusual accomplishment was only 1.4 kg. Fluid loss and replenishment amounted to between 3.5 and 4 gallons of liquid!

Water in Foods. Foods contain different quantities of water. Fruits and vegetables (lettuce, pickles, green beans, broccoli) are generally high in water content, whereas the water contained in butter, oils, dried meats, and chocolate, cookies, and cakes is quite low. Generally, about 1000 ml of water is contained in the foods consumed in the daily diet.

Metabolic Water. Carbon dioxide and water are formed in varying amounts when food nutrients are degraded for energy. This **metabolic water** provides about 25% of the daily water requirement for a sedentary person. For example, the complete breakdown of 100 g of carbohydrate produces 55 g of metabolic water and protein produces 100 g, while the combustion of a similar quantity of lipid produces 107 g of water. Because each gram of glycogen is hydrated with 2.7 g of water, this water also becomes available when glycogen is used as the fuel for biologic work. For a sedentary person, about 350 ml of water is provided through the daily metabolic processes.

> **Facts about urine.** Urine pH ranges from about 4.5 to 8.0, depending on the composition of the diet. High-protein diets produce an acidic urine, while a carbohydrate-rich, vegetarian diet produces an alkaline urine. The specific gravity of urine exceeds 1.0 (the value for distilled water) because its solute components exceed the density of distilled water. The color of urine is normally clear to deep yellow because of the pigment urochrome, an end product of hemoglobin breakdown. Urine normally has a slightly pungent odor, although some drugs and disease states dramatically affect its odor. In diabetes mellitus, for example, the urine has a fruitlike smell caused by the chemical acetone. A routine urinalysis can detect abnormalities in urine composition; the presence of solutes such as glucose (glycosuria), red blood cells (hematuria), white blood cells (pyuria), proteins (proteinuria and albuminuria), bile pigments (bilirubinuria), and ketones (ketonuria) can help to pinpoint suspected medical conditions.

WATER OUTPUT

Water is lost from the body in urine, through the skin, as water vapor in expired air, and in feces.

Water Loss in Urine. Urine is composed of approximately 95% water, with the remainder being various soluble and insoluble solids. Under normal conditions, the kidneys reabsorb about 99% of the 140 to 160 liters of filtrate formed each day. Consequently, the daily urine volume excreted by the kidneys ranges between 1000 and 1500 ml, or about 1.5 quarts.

Water is always being lost from the body via urine formation. About 15 ml of water is required to eliminate 1 g of solute by the kidneys. This portion of water in urine is "obligated" to rid the body of metabolic by-products such as urea (an end product of protein breakdown), uric acid (a breakdown product of nucleic acids), the electrolytes sodium and potassium, sulfate ions, and creatinine. The ingestion and subsequent energy metabolism of large quantities of protein (as would occur with a high-protein diet) facilitates water loss through urea production and subsequent excretion. This increased urine flow could actually speed up the body's dehydration.

Water Loss through the Skin. A small quantity of water, perhaps 350 ml, continually seeps from the deeper tissues through the skin to the body's surface. This loss of water is called *insensible perspiration.*

Water is also lost through the skin in the form of sweat produced by the approximately 2 to 4 million specialized sweat glands located beneath the skin. ***Evaporation** of **sweat** provides the refrigeration mechanism to cool the body.* This effect is termed "evaporative cooling." Under normal conditions, 500 to 700 ml of sweat is secreted each day. This by no means reflects sweating capacity, because from 8 to 12 liters of sweat (about 10 kg) at a rate of 1 liter per hour can be produced during prolonged exercise in a hot environment.

> **The cooling effect of evaporation.** Evaporation is what cools. It provides the major physiologic defense against overheating. The evaporative loss of 1 liter of sweat from the body's surface releases about 600 kcal of heat energy from the body to the environment.

Water Loss as Water Vapor. The amount of insensible water loss through small water droplets in exhaled air is about 250 to 350 ml per day.

Exercise significantly affects this source of water loss. For physically active persons, about 3.5 ml of water is lost from the respiratory passages each minute during strenuous exercise. This amount varies considerably with climate, being less in hot, humid weather and greater at cold temperatures where the inspired air contains little moisture, or at high altitudes where ventilatory volumes are significantly elevated both at rest and during exercise.

Electrolyte concentrations in blood serum and sweat. Values are expressed in milliequivalents per liter (mEq/L).

	Na^+	K^+	Cl^-	Mg^{+2}
Blood serum	140	4.0	110	1.5–2.1
Sweat	40–45	3.9	39	3.3

Water Loss in Feces. Between 100 and 200 ml of water is lost through **intestinal elimination** because approximately 70% of fecal matter is water. The remainder is composed of nondigestible material; this includes bacteria from the digestive process and the residues of digestive juices from the intestines, stomach, and pancreas. With diarrhea or vomiting, water loss can increase to 1500 to 5000 ml. This can create significant **dehydration** and electrolyte loss.

WATER REQUIREMENTS IN EXERCISE

The most serious consequence of profuse sweating is loss of body water. During a vigorous workout, sweating will frequently cause a person to lose between 1 and 2 kg of body fluid. For endurance athletes, a fluid loss equivalent to 4% of body mass is not uncommon in a training session. Of course, the amount of water lost depends on the severity and duration of physical activity as well as environmental conditions. Quite important is the **relative humidity** of the ambient air, as this greatly affects the cooling efficiency of sweating. The term relative humidity refers to the water content of the air. During conditions of 100% relative humidity, the air is completely saturated with water vapor. Thus, evaporation of fluid from the skin is impossible, and this important avenue for body cooling is closed. Under such conditions, sweat beads on the skin and eventually rolls off. On a dry day, the air can hold considerable moisture, and fluid evaporates rapidly from the skin. This enables the sweating mechanism to function at optimal efficiency and body temperature is more easily controlled. However, even moderate loss of fluid through sweating is not without consequences. Blood volume becomes reduced when sweating causes a fluid loss of about 2% of body mass. This places a strain on circulatory function that ultimately impairs our capacity for both exercise and thermoregulation.

Defend against dehydration. Water that beads and drips off the skin is of no benefit to body cooling. It is only when sweat evaporates that a cooling effect is noted. The only effective way to prevent dehydration is to drink water regularly during exercise. As a practical guide, it is a good idea to wear loose-fitting white workout clothes during hot-weather exercise (a loose fit permits air circulation between skin and environment, and white reflects heat more effectively than other colors). Also, do not remove soaked clothing: changing to dry clothes hinders evaporative cooling.

PRACTICAL RECOMMENDATIONS FOR FLUID REPLACEMENT

The primary aim of fluid replacement is to maintain plasma volume so that circulation and sweating progress at optimal levels. Ingesting "extra" water prior to exercising in the heat provides some thermoregulatory protection. It delays the development of dehydration, increases sweating during exercise, and brings about a smaller rise in body temperature compared to exercising without prior fluids. In this regard, it is wise to consume 400 to 600 ml (13 to 20 oz) of cold water 10 to 20 minutes before exercising. Doing this does not eliminate the need for continual fluid replacement during exercise, however.

Fluid replacement is critical. Sweat loss during a marathon run at world record pace (2 hr, 6 min, 50 s) averages about 5.3 liters (12 lb), depending on environmental conditions. This fluid loss corresponds to an overall reduction of about 6 to 8% in body mass. To avoid exercise-induced dehydration, it is important to consume fluids regularly during physical activity.

Speed up gastric emptying. To obtain a high rate of gastric emptying, the stomach should remain partially filled with fluid and the ingested fluid should be at the relatively cold temperature of 5° C (41° F).

When it's hot, drink water with only small amounts of glucose and electrolytes. During exercise in the heat, when the need for water greatly exceeds the need for carbohydrate supplementation, highly concentrated sugar and salt solutions hinder water replenishment and impair temperature regulation.

Athletes are often at greatest risk. Athletes involved in long-term endurance activities generally replace only 20 to 30% of their fluid sweat loss.

Dehydration, an undesirable bodily state. Dehydration occurs when there is depletion of the extracellular fluid volume as the body goes into negative water balance. In such cases, water loss exceeds water intake and there is a corresponding loss of electrolytes. Dehydration commonly occurs with prolonged vomiting and diarrhea, hemorrhage, severe burns, water restriction, medical conditions such as diabetes mellitus or diabetes insipidus, and during exercise, especially when performed in hot, humid environments.

Water "intoxication," too much of a good thing. Under normal conditions, a maximum of about 9.5 liters (10 quarts) of water can be consumed daily without unduly straining the kidneys or diluting important chemicals. Consuming more than this volume can produce **hyponatremia,** or water intoxication, a condition related to significant dilution of the body's normal sodium concentration. Early symptoms include headache, blurred vision, excessive sweating, and vomiting. In extreme cases, the person can develop cerebral edema and can even become delirious, convulsive, comatose, and eventually die. Although uncommon, water intoxication has been reported in experienced athletes. For example, an ultramarathoner was hospitalized after consuming nearly 20 liters of fluid during a 62-mile nonstop, 8½ hour run!

GASTRIC EMPTYING

Fluids must be emptied from the stomach before being absorbed in the small intestine. There are several **factors that influence gastric emptying.**

- **Fluid temperature.** Cold fluids (5° C; 41° F) are emptied from the stomach at a faster rate than fluids at body temperature.
- **Fluid volume.** Gastric emptying speeds up for each 100 ml increase in gastric volume up to 600 ml. Ingesting a volume of about 250 ml (8.5 oz) at 15-minute intervals is a realistic goal for fluid intake during exercise because larger volumes tend to produce feelings of a "full stomach."
- **Fluid osmolarity.** Gastric emptying is slowed when the ingested fluid is concentrated with simple sugars, whether in the form of glucose, fructose, or sucrose. For example, a 40% sugar solution is emptied from the stomach at a rate only one-fifth that of plain water.

On the other hand, during exercise in a cold environment, fluid loss from sweating may not be so great. Here, a reduction in gastric emptying and subsequent fluid uptake can be tolerated and a more concentrated sugar solution (15 to 30 g per 100 ml of water) may be beneficial. The trade-off between the composition of the ingested fluid and the rate of gastric emptying must be evaluated on the basis of both environmental stress and energy demands. *In terms of survival, fluid replacement is the primary concern during prolonged exercise in the heat.*

ADEQUACY OF REHYDRATION

Preventing dehydration and its consequences, especially a dangerously elevated body temperature, or **hyperthermia,** can be achieved only with an adequate water replacement schedule. This is often "easier said than done" because some individuals feel that ingesting water hinders exercise performance. For wrestlers, dehydration is a way of life, as young boys and men will lose considerable fluid so they can wrestle in a lower weight class. This is also the case for many ballet dancers, who are continually preoccupied with their weight so as to appear thin. Many individuals on weight loss programs incorrectly believe that by restricting fluid intake, body fat loss will in some way occur at a more rapid rate.

Changes in body mass before and after exercising should be used to indicate water loss during exercise and the adequacy of rehydration in subsequent recovery. Coaches often have their athletes "weigh in" before and after practice, and insist that weight loss be minimized by periodic water breaks during activity. The thirst mechanism is an imprecise guide to water needs. In fact, if rehydration were left entirely to a person's thirst, it could take several days to reestablish fluid balance, especially after severe dehydration.

USE OF GLUCOSE POLYMERS

The negative effects of simple sugar solutions on gastric emptying can be greatly reduced by drinking a solution of **polymerized glucose** such as maltodextrins. These solutions have one-fifth the osmolarity of an equivalent carbohydrate-containing solution of simple sugars. In effect, polymerized glucose solutions provide water and carbohydrate at a more rapid rate than a drink of similar carbohydrate content composed of monosaccharides and disaccharides.

SUMMARY

1. Water makes up 45 to 65% of the total body mass. Muscle is about 70% water by weight, whereas water represents only about 20 to 30% of the weight of adipose tissue.
2. Of the total body water, roughly 62% is located intracellularly and 38% extracellularly in the plasma, lymph, and other fluids outside the cell.
3. Food and oxygen are always supplied in aqueous solution, and waste products always leave via a watery medium. Water also helps to give structure and form to the body and plays a vital role in temperature regulation.
4. Normal daily water intake of about 2.5 liters is supplied from liquid intake (1.2 liters), food (1.0 liter), and metabolic water produced during energy-yielding reactions (0.35 liter).
5. For a sedentary person, water is lost from the body each day in the urine (1.0 to 1.5 liters), through the skin as sweat and insensible perspiration (0.70 to 1.0 liter), as water vapor in expired air (0.25 to 0.35 liter), and in feces, as about 70% of fecal matter is water (0.15 liter).
6. Exercise in hot weather greatly increases the body's water requirement. In extreme conditions where outside ambient temperature and humidity increase markedly, the fluid needs can increase five or six times above normal because water output far exceeds usual water intake.
7. Several factors affect the rate of fluid absorption: cold fluids are emptied from the stomach more rapidly than fluids at body temperature; when the stomach is partially filled with fluid, the rate of gastric emptying increases; and concentrated sugar solutions impair gastric emptying and fluid replacement.
8. The primary aim of fluid replacement is to maintain plasma volume so that circulation and sweating progress at optimal levels. For the ideal replacement schedule during exercise, fluid intake should match fluid loss. The effectiveness of this replacement can be evaluated by monitoring changes in body mass before, during, and following workouts.
9. Beverages of moderate glucose-polymer content provide a ready source of carbohydrate and do not impair fluid uptake and thermoregulation.

Sports drinks with polymerized carbohydrates. Polymerization links 10 to 15 glucose molecules together to maximize carbohydrate content while minimizing the osmolarity of a solution. This facilitates the delivery of water and carbohydrate to the body.

RELATED LITERATURE

American College of Sports Medicine: Position statement on prevention of heat injuries during distance running. Med. Sci. Sports Exerc., 16:ix, 1984.

Coyle, E.F., and Montain, S.J.: Carbohydrate and fluid ingestion during exercise: are there trade-offs? Med. Sci. Sports Exerc., 24:671, 1992.

Gisolfi, C.V., and Duchman, S.M.: Guidelines for optimal replacement beverages for different athletic events. Med. Sci. Sports Exerc., 24:679, 1992.

Guthrie, H.A.: Introductory Nutrition, 7th ed. St. Louis, C.V. Mosby, 1988.

Guyton, A.C.: Textbook of Medical Physiology, 7th ed. Philadelphia, W.B. Saunders, 1986.

Meyer, F., et al.: Sweat electrolyte loss during exercise in the heat: effects of gender and maturation. Med. Sci. Exerc. Sports., 24:776, 1992.

Mitchel, J., et al.: Respiratory weight loss during exercise. J. Appl. Physiol., 32:474, 1972.

Robinson, S.: Cardiovascular and respiratory reactions to heat. In Physiological Adaptations. Edited by M.K. Yosef, et al. New York, Academic Press, 1972.

9

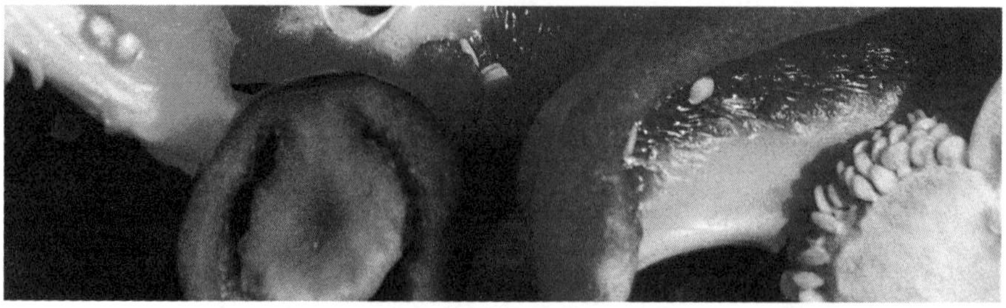

FOOD ADVERTISING, PACKAGING, AND LABELING, AND PATTERNS OF FOOD CONSUMPTION

The food, nutrition, and health scene has changed continually, often dramatically, over the past 25 years. In many instances, information "fed" to us concerning nutritional quality and potential health benefits of particular foods are prepared by individuals and companies more concerned about sales and profit than about our well-being. Although many "watchdog" organizations and governmental agencies attempt to upgrade quality control in the food and nutrition marketplace, for the consumer, the caveat "buyer beware" is all too apropos!

FOOD ADVERTISING AND PACKAGING

In the late 1970s, renewed interest in nutrition and healthful eating was sparked by media attention concerning the contribution of cholesterol-rich diets to high blood cholesterol, a primary risk factor for heart disease. This was followed by the revelation that many forms of cancer are intimately related to diet, if not caused by it. Superimposed on the diet–heart disease and diet-cancer connections was the emerging fitness craze that swept North America. Health clubs and spas flourished, and newspaper and magazine articles were filled with the latest tips on how to improve fitness and health by eating well and exercising regularly.

Choices, choices, choices! Each year, approximately 13,200 new foods are introduced, yet many of these items never take their place on supermarket shelves. Despite the difficulty in mainstreaming new products, the average supermarket stocks about 16,500 products—often a decision-making nightmare for the consumer.

ADVERTISING'S GOAL IS TO SHAPE BEHAVIOR

Advertising and media blitzes are designed to create, shape, and alter our perceptions about what we eat and how we exercise. For example, the amount of **money spent by the food industry** to lure customers in 1990 exceeded $40 billion:

$10 billion devoted to advertising and $30 billion spent on packaging! In the physical fitness marketplace, consumer research indicates that the American public spends more than $1 billion annually on exercise equipment, and sales of fitness products will soon exceed $2.1 billion. Given the number of people jogging, joining health clubs, or working out at the local gym, we might conclude that Americans are quite physically active. That, however, is the illusion: when we take a closer look at the evidence, it is apparent that while many people may begin an exercise program, few actually stick with it.

There is no question that advertising plays an extremely important role in shaping the consumer's image of a particular product or service. Consider popular magazines such as *Vogue, Shape, Muscle and Fitness, Gentlemen's Quarterly,* and *Mademoiselle.* Do you think the cover on any of these magazines would ever feature someone who was obese, or even slightly overweight? Would wrinkles, misshapen teeth, a crooked nose, flabby midsection, or less than shapely thighs or hips ever grace advertising pages, much less the cover? The answer is a resounding "no" because such images do not sell! And if the images do not sell, say the advertising agencies, then neither will the products they are meant to promote. Product imagery is intimately linked to what the consumer buys, and that is what advertising and promotion are all about. The whopping sums of money spent by the food industry on advertising and packaging are intended to influence what consumers purchase and what we eat. Food manufacturers, for example, often pay a supermarket to locate and display their products where the consumer is most likely to notice them. The practice is not illegal—it's just "good business" because increased sales lead to increased profits! And in business, that *is* the bottom line.

Governmental agencies try their best to police the food industry by establishing rules and guidelines for manufacturers and advertisers. However, health claims made for products often try to persuade the consumer that a particular item will produce certain health-related effects, when in fact it may not. Unfortunately, no state or federal guidelines require that *all* the facts be presented for a given health claim. Manufacturers are relatively free to interpret the "facts" as they see them. The consumer is then left to decipher what exactly is meant by the advertising and what is the precise meaning of the material printed on a food label.

GOVERNMENTAL WATCHDOG AGENCIES

Four **governmental agencies** are responsible for the rules, regulations, and legal requirements concerning advertising, packaging, and labeling of foods and alcoholic beverages.

Federal Trade Commission (FTC). The FTC is directly responsible for regulating the advertising of food products in the various media (TV, radio, newsprint). The FTC can pursue legal action against manufacturers who advertise unsubstantiated claims. For example, if a label reads "This cereal will reduce your chances of colon cancer," the FTC can require the manufacturer to document clearly that a particular food in fact does what the advertising claims. The FTC can remove a product from the marketplace for advertising unsubstantiated claims.

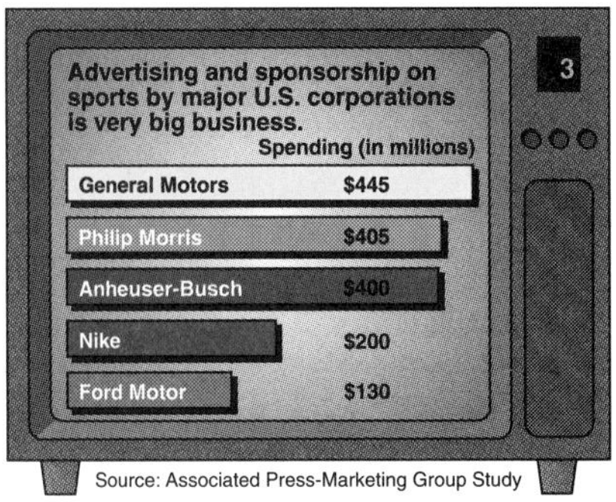

Source: Associated Press-Marketing Group Study

It's sales, not quality, that counts. Soft drink manufacturers spend about $500 million a year to advertise their products compared to $60 million spent by the dairy industry. Small wonder the average American drinks 45.9 gallons of soft drinks yearly compared to only 20.9 gallons of milk!

Just say, "Charge it." To stimulate sluggish growth in the fast-food industry, large chains such as Arby's, Burger King, and McDonald's are test marketing credit card use, even for a purchase as small as fries or a cup of coffee.

Dietary supplements: an unregulated industry. An estimated 25% of Americans consume $3.3 billion worth of dietary supplements each year. For many, the FDA has no idea whether or not they are safe, let alone effective. These supplements range from ordinary vitamin and mineral capsules to more exotic potions such as bee pollen, royal jelly, germanium, coenzyme Q10, evening primrose oil, Maximum Memory, and Cardio-Endurance. When injury or illness is traced to a supplement, the FDA will step in. This occurred in 1990 when the agency banned the sale of the amino acid L-tryptophan after 38 deaths and 1500 illnesses were associated with taking this supplement.

Zapping food with radiation requires the irradiation logo. Treating food by irradiation is a newly approved process that sterilizes food to kill micro-organisms such as salmonella, combats insect infestation, and delays spoilage by slowing growth of mold. Irradiated foods must be labeled "treated with radiation" or "treated by irradiation," and the irradiation logo must be clearly shown on the label.

Food and Drug Administration (FDA). With the exception of poultry and meat products, the FDA is directly responsible for regulating what manufacturers state on food labels. The FDA also decides what additives can be added to foods. Furthermore, it deals with matters related to potential hazards with food additives such as contaminants, food-borne infections, toxicants, artificially constituted foods, and pesticide residue.

United States Department of Agriculture (USDA). The USDA is directly responsible for regulating the material that appears on food labels for poultry and meat products.

Bureau of Alcohol, Tobacco and Firearms (BATF). This regulatory agency is responsible for the material that appears on labels for alcoholic beverages.

DEFINITIONS USED IN ADVERTISING

The following legal definitions pertain to common terms prevalent in food labeling. These definitions are subject to changes in the rules and regulations established by the specific governing federal agency.

- **Organic.** This term has no legal meaning and can be used at the discretion of the manufacturer.
- **Natural.** Refers to a product as it occurs in nature, without additives, artificial flavoring, synthetic ingredients, preservatives, or coloring.
- **Sugar-free.** The product is devoid of all simple sugars. These include sucrose (table sugar), fructose, maltose, galactose, molasses, honey, and fruit juice.
- **Low-calorie, diet, reduced-calorie, or dietetic.** The product contains no more than 40 calories in a single serving or a maximum of 0.4 kcal per gram, or one-third fewer calories than the regular product.
- **Light or "lite."** Currently, there are no laws governing the use of these terms and they can mean anything the manufacturer wishes.
- **Imitation.** The product has been changed from the regular recipe. For example, a substance can be added to a product to reduce its percentage of fat or other nutrients. A good example is the addition of water to margarine to reduce its caloric content. If the word imitation is used, it means that the product is a substitute for and resembles another food but is nutritionally inferior, according to government regulations, to the food it imitates.
- **Sodium-free.** A serving contains less than 5 mg of sodium.
- **Low-sodium.** A serving has no more than 140 mg of sodium.
- **Very-low-sodium.** A serving has no more than 35 mg of sodium.
- **Reduced sodium.** Sodium is reduced by 75% compared with the product it replaces.
- **Fortified.** Vitamins and minerals have been added to the product if they were missing previously (milk to which vitamins A and D have been added; table salt to which iodine is added).
- **Enriched.** Vitamins (riboflavin, niacin, and thiamine) and the mineral iron are added to the product because they were missing previously or were destroyed during the food's processing.

Fewer calories, or simply less of the product? Buyer beware—some "lite" breads are 50% lower in calories simply because each slice is 50% thinner!

Enriched. Enriched means that nutrients lost during the refining process have been added back. For example, enriched flour contains the iron and B vitamins in amounts originally present in the whole grain prior to processing.

Plants contain no cholesterol. Unless a plant food is cooked in lard, the label "no cholesterol" on foods made from vegetables can be misleading because cholesterol comes only from animal products. The more relevant consideration is the vegetable food's level of saturated and unsaturated fatty acids.

- **No cholesterol.** There is no cholesterol in the product.
- **Cholesterol-free.** There is less than 2 mg of cholesterol per serving.
- **Low-fat.** For meat, fat content does not exceed 10% fat by weight; for milk, the fat content can range from 0.5 to 2%.
- **Fat-free.** When a product is "fat free" it generally has less than 0.5 g of fat per serving.
- **New.** The product has been changed substantially within the prior six months or is completely new.
- **No artificial flavoring.** The product can contain flavors only from naturally occurring products. Currently, about 2000 flavoring agents are permitted in foods. One of the most common flavor-enhancing agents is the sodium-rich amino acid compound monosodium glutamate, or MSG. The trade name for MSG is Accent.
- **No artificial coloring.** The product does not contain one or more of the 33 coloring agents that are permitted in food products. Naturally occurring colors come from products such as carrot oils, grape skin, or beet juice.
- **Wheat.** Wheat is part of the product, but it does not necessarily include whole wheat.

FOOD LABELING

The Fair Packaging and Labeling Act approved by Congress requires that food labels include the name of the product; name and address of the manufacturer; serving or portion size; ingredients, listed in descending order by weight; calorie content per serving; weight (in grams) of protein, carbohydrate, and lipid; protein, vitamin, and mineral content as a percentage of the U.S. RDA*; and weight of the product. If a label contains a nutritional claim, there must be an accompanying statement concerning the specific nutritional value of that claim.

A manufacturer does not have to list the ingredients for a product if the food is prepared according to a specific recipe that is filed with the FDA. This is referred to as a ***standard of identity.*** Examples have included ice cream, mustard, mayonnaise, and ketchup. In such cases the manufacturer is legally protected from disclosing the ingredients, although many now list them on the label in response to consumer demand. The level of detail contained in labels is not standard; some manufacturers provide relatively complete nutritional information, while others present only the minimums specified by current law. Figure 9–1 displays sample food labels from three manufacturers that illustrate a wide range in nutrient information provided for a cereal, a frozen vegetable, and cookies.

A new law makes labeling on processed foods mandatory by 1993, and there will be a major effort for voluntary labeling of fruits, vegetables, and seafood. The new law requires that labels contain the following information: *number of calories per serving, number of calories from fat per serving, total fat,*

* The **U.S. RDA** refer to a single set of values taken from tables of the RDA (Recommended Dietary Allowances). The U.S. RDA are the same as the RDA for adult men; for women, the values from the tables of the RDA are used for the U.S. RDA because of the woman's greater need for iron. If a label states that a serving supplies 15% of the U.S. RDA for protein, this means the food will supply 15% of the protein RDA for the typical male and female. These generalized standards are quite robust and apply to almost all individuals, regardless of gender or age. No consideration is given, however, to variability in overall body size.

Complete truth in advertising? Fleishman's margarine has touted its product as being low in cholesterol and indicates that a low-cholesterol diet can reduce the risk of heart disease. What is not mentioned is that margarines are high in trans fatty acids that may *increase* heart disease risk. Stouffer Foods Corp. extols that its Lean Cuisine never contains more than a gram of sodium—failing to mention that this one "little" gram is the equivalent of 1000 mg, probably all the body needs for the entire day!

It's tough to comparison shop. The FDA says that an average serving of fish or seafood weighs 4 oz. It is the USDA, however, that has jurisdiction over meat and poultry, and this organization fails to require nutrition labels on serving sizes equivalent to those of the FDA. Thus, Perdue uses a 1 oz serving size to list its nutritional information and "show" the consumer how low in calories and saturated fat its chickens are. Buyer beware, because the customary serving size for chicken is about 5 oz!

Experts give this food label high marks. The FDA has rated this food label as its No. 1 choice. The example illustrates the likely design for a can of condensed soup.

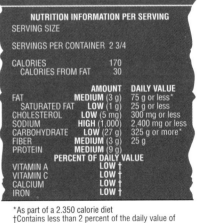

NUTRITION INFORMATION PER SERVING

SERVING SIZE		
SERVINGS PER CONTAINER 2 3/4		
CALORIES	170	
CALORIES FROM FAT	30	
	AMOUNT	**DAILY VALUE**
FAT	**MEDIUM** (3 g)	75 g or less*
SATURATED FAT	**LOW** (1 g)	25 g or less
CHOLESTEROL	**LOW** (5 mg)	300 mg or less
SODIUM	**HIGH** (1,000)	2,400 mg or less
CARBOHYDRATE	**LOW** (27 g)	325 g or more*
FIBER	**MEDIUM** (3 g)	25 g
PROTEIN	**MEDIUM** (9 g)	
	PERCENT OF DAILY VALUE	
VITAMIN A	**LOW** †	
VITAMIN C	**LOW** †	
CALCIUM	**LOW** †	
IRON	**LOW** †	

*As part of a 2.350 calorie diet
†Contains less than 2 percent of the daily value of this nutrient
INGREDIENTS: XXXXXXXXXXXXXXXXXXXXXXXXX
XXXXXXXXXXXXXXXXXXXXXXXXXXXXXXXXXX
XXXXXXXXXXXXXXXXXXXXXXXXXXXXXXXXXX
STARNES' SOUP COMPANY
BLOUNTVILLE, TN U.S.A. 37617

California Fresh Cut Broccoli

NUTRITION INFORMATION PER SERVING:
SERVING SIZE: 1/2 CUP
SERVING PER CONTAINER: 3

CALORIES	16	CHOLESTEROL	0mg
PROTEIN	2g	SODIUM	95mg
CARBOHYDRATE	3g	POTASSIUM	140mg
FAT	0g		

PERCENTAGE OF U.S. RECOMMENDED DAILY ALLOWANCES (U.S. RDA) PER SERVING:

PROTEIN	2	NIACIN	*
VITAMIN A	10	CALCIUM	2
VITAMIN C	60	IRON	*
THIAMINE (B1)	*	PHOSPHORUS	4
RIBOFLAVIN (B2)	4		

*CONTAINS LESS THAN 2% OF THE U.S. RDA OF THESE NUTRIENTS.

INGREDIENTS: CUT BROCCOLI, WATER, SALT, BAKING SODA

DIST. BY THE STARNES FRESH FARM PRODUCE, SALINAS, CA, MFG. IN U.S.A.

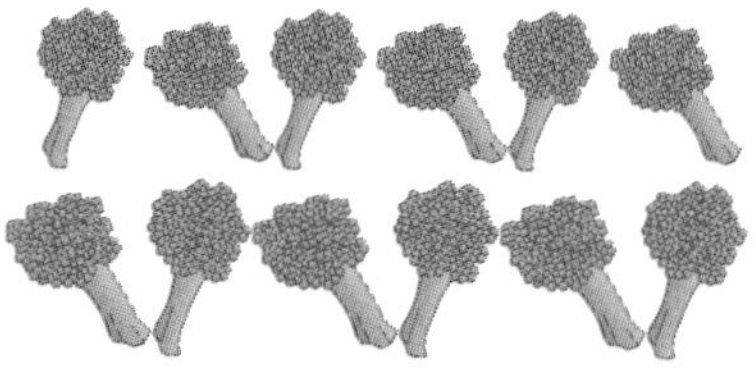

KERRY'S COOKIE COLLECTION

Low Fat • Low Cholesterol • Low Sodium

ELLEN'S COOKIE — MONOUNSATURATED FAT 2 GRAMS

NUTRITION INFORMATION PER SERVING

SERVING SIZE	2 COOKIES	FAT	7 GRAMS
SERVINGS PER CONTAINER	2 1/2	POLYUNSATURATED	1 GRAM
CALOREIS	130	SATURATED	2 GRAMS
PROTEIN	1 GRAM	CHOLESTEROL	0 mg
CARBOHYDRATE	14 GRAMS	SODIUM	50 mg

CONNIE'S COOKIE — MONOUNSATURATED FAT 3 GRAMS

NUTRITION INFORMATION PER SERVING

SERVING SIZE	2 COOKIES	FAT	6 GRAMS
SERVINGS PER CONTAINER	2	POLYUNSATURATED	0 GRAMS
CALOREIS	120	SATURATED	2 GRAMS
PROTEIN	1 GRAM	CHOLESTEROL	5 mg
CARBOHYDRATE	15 GRAMS	SODIUM	45 mg

JENNIFER'S COOKIE — MONOUNSATURATED FAT 3 GRAMS

NUTRITION INFORMATION PER SERVING

SERVING SIZE	1 COOKIE	FAT	5 GRAMS
SERVINGS PER CONTAINER	3	POLYUNSATURATED	1 GRAM
CALOREIS	90	SATURATED	1 GRAM
PROTEIN	1 GRAM	CHOLESTEROL	Less than 5 mg
CARBOHYDRATE	10 GRAMS	SODIUM	30 mg

MISSY'S COOKIE — MONOUNSATURATED FAT 2 GRAMS

NUTRITION INFORMATION PER SERVING

SERVING SIZE	2 COOKIES	FAT	5 GRAMS
SERVINGS PER CONTAINER	2	POLYUNSATURATED	0 GRAMS
CALOREIS	110	SATURATED	2 GRAMS
PROTEIN	1 GRAM	CHOLESTEROL	0 mg
CARBOHYDRATE	13 GRAMS	SODIUM	65 mg

THERESA'S COOKIE — MONOUNSATURATED FAT 3 GRAMS

NUTRITION INFORMATION PER SERVING

SERVING SIZE	3 COOKIES	FAT	5 GRAMS
SERVINGS PER CONTAINER	1 5/8	POLYUNSATURATED	0 GRAMS
CALOREIS	80	SATURATED	1 GRAM
PROTEIN	0 GRAMs	CHOLESTEROL	5 mg
CARBOHYDRATE	9 GRAMS	SODIUM	30 mg

ERNIE'S CHOCOLATE CHIP — MONOUNSATURATED FAT 2 GRAMS

NUTRITION INFORMATION PER SERVING

SERVING SIZE	3 COOKIES	FAT	6 GRAMS
SERVINGS PER CONTAINER	1 5/8	POLYUNSATURATED	0 GRAMS
CALOREIS	90	SATURATED	2 GRAMS
PROTEIN	0 GRAMS	CHOLESTEROL	0 mg
CARBOHYDRATE	11 GRAMS	SODIUM	30 mg

KERRY's COOKIES CONTAIN LESS THAN 2% OF THE U.S. RDA OF PROTEIN, VITAMIN A, VITAMIN C, THIAMINE, RIBOFLAVIN, NIACIN, CALCIUM AND IRON.

MADE FROM: UNBLEACHED WHEAT FLOUR, SWEET CHOCOLATE (WITH SOY LECITHIN ADDED AS AN EMULSIFIER), SUGAR, PARTIALLY HYDROGENATED VEGETABLE SHORTENING (COTTONSEED AND/OR CANOLA OILS), NONFAT MILK, EGG WHITES, WALNUTS, WHOLE EGGS, OATMEAL, CORNSTARCH, INVERT SYRUP, BUTTER, SALT, LEAVENING (BAKING SODA, CREAM OF TARTAR), SOY LECITHIN, VANILLA EXTRACT, PECANS AND PECAN EXTRACT.

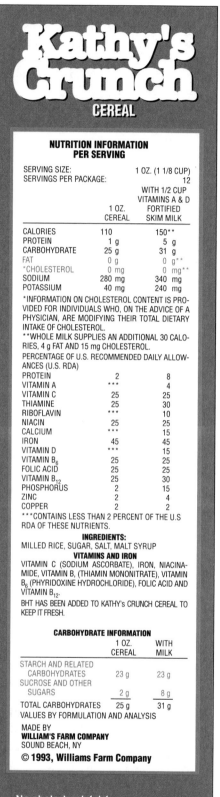

Kathy's Crunch CEREAL

NUTRITION INFORMATION PER SERVING

SERVING SIZE: 1 OZ. (1 1/8 CUP)
SERVINGS PER PACKAGE: 12

	1 OZ. CEREAL	WITH 1/2 CUP VITAMINS A & D FORTIFIED SKIM MILK
CALORIES	110	150**
PROTEIN	1 g	5 g
CARBOHYDRATE	25 g	31 g
FAT	0 g	0 g**
*CHOLESTEROL	0 mg	0 mg**
SODIUM	280 mg	340 mg
POTASSIUM	40 mg	240 mg

*INFORMATION ON CHOLESTEROL CONTENT IS PROVIDED FOR INDIVIDUALS WHO, ON THE ADVICE OF A PHYSICIAN, ARE MODIFYING THEIR TOTAL DIETARY INTAKE OF CHOLESTEROL.

**WHOLE MILK SUPPLIES AN ADDITIONAL 30 CALORIES, 4 g FAT AND 15 mg CHOLESTEROL.

PERCENTAGE OF U.S. RECOMMENDED DAILY ALLOWANCES (U.S. RDA)

PROTEIN	2	8
VITAMIN A	***	4
VITAMIN C	25	25
THIAMINE	25	30
RIBOFLAVIN	***	10
NIACIN	25	25
CALCIUM	***	15
IRON	45	45
VITAMIN D	***	15
VITAMIN B_6	25	25
FOLIC ACID	25	25
VITAMIN B_{12}	25	30
PHOSPHORUS	2	15
ZINC	2	4
COPPER	2	2

***CONTAINS LESS THAN 2 PERCENT OF THE U.S RDA OF THESE NUTRIENTS.

INGREDIENTS:
MILLED RICE, SUGAR, SALT, MALT SYRUP

VITAMINS AND IRON
VITAMIN C (SODIUM ASCORBATE), IRON, NIACINAMIDE, VITAMIN B, (THIAMIN MONONITRATE), VITAMIN B_6 (PHYRIDOXINE HYDROCHLORIDE), FOLIC ACID AND VITAMIN B_{12}.

BHT HAS BEEN ADDED TO KATHY's CRUNCH CEREAL TO KEEP IT FRESH.

CARBOHYDRATE INFORMATION

	1 OZ. CEREAL	WITH MILK
STARCH AND RELATED CARBOHYDRATES	23 g	23 g
SUCROSE AND OTHER SUGARS	2 g	8 g
TOTAL CARBOHYDRATES	25 g	31 g

VALUES BY FORMULATION AND ANALYSIS

MADE BY
WILLIAM'S FARM COMPANY
SOUND BEACH, NY

- No cholesterol, fat-free
- Excellent source of complex carbohydrates
- Low in sugar and no artificial flavoring

FIG. 9–1. Examples of food labels that show nutrient information of the food.

saturated fat, and *cholesterol, sodium, sugars, dietary fiber, protein, carbohydrates and complex carbohydrates*, and important *vitamins and minerals*.

Food Additives. If a manufacturer wishes to include an additive in a food, specific FDA guidelines must be followed. The manufacturer must perform chemical tests to ensure that the additive is effective (i.e., that it does what it is supposed to). The FDA also requires that the additive can be detected and measured in the product and that it produces no undesirable health effects, such as cancer or birth defects, when given in large doses to animals (mainly rodents and dogs). Once the FDA approves an additive, there are strict guidelines for its use. The FDA tells the manufacturer what foods may contain the additive and in what amounts.

Approximately 700 additives were initially included on a list of additives *generally recognized as safe* (GRAS). The **GRAS list** has expanded substantially and currently includes approximately 2000 flavoring agents and 200 coloring agents. The substances on this list do not receive permanent approval but are reviewed periodically. Additives include emulsifiers, stabilizers, thickeners (to provide texture, smoothness, and consistency), nutrients such as vitamin C added to fruit juice or potassium iodide added to salt (to improve nutritive value), flavoring agents (to enhance taste), leavening agents (to make baked goods rise, or to control acidity or alkalinity), preservatives, antioxidants, sequestrants, and antimycotic agents (to prevent spoilage, rancidity of fats, and microbial growth), coloring agents (to increase attractiveness), bleaches (to whiten foods and speed up the maturing of cheese), and humectants and anticaking agents (to retain moisture and keep other foods free flowing, such as salts and powders).

Commonly used additives	Additives are used in these foods	Function
Acetic acid (vinegar) Citric acid Lactic acid Phosphoric acid	Fresh and cooked sausage	Acidifiers increase acid levels in products to improve flavor and texture
BHA/BHT Butylated hydroxyanisole/ Butylated hydroxytoluene TBHQ (tertiary butylhydroquinone) Propyl gallate	Fresh pork, beef, and Italian sausages: some beef patties: margarine and oleomargarine	Antioxidants prevent rancidity
Isolated soy protein Dry whey Sodium caseinate Algin	Sausage, imitation sausage, some meat loaves, soups and stews Breading mix and sauces	Binders thicken ingredients and extend the products
Sodium nitrite Sodium ascorbate	Frankfurters, salami, bacon, bologna, and other cured meat and poultry products	Curing agents improve color and taste
Corn syrup Dextrose	Sausage, frankfurters, meat loaf, luncheon meat, chopped and pressed ham	Flavoring agents impart desired flavor

USDA standards for popular meat and poultry products. The US Department of Agriculture's Food Safety and Inspection Service approves labels for all products that contain at least 2% poultry or 3% meat. For example, beef stew must contain at least 25% beef and turkey pie must contain at least 14% cooked turkey meat. Labels for other products are approved by the US Food and Drug Administration.

PRODUCT NAME	STANDARD
Beef stew	Must contain at least 25% beef
Chili con carne	At least 40% meat
Chicken soup	Ready to Eat—at least 2% chicken meat; Condensed—at least 4% chicken meat
Frankfurter, bologna and similar cooked sausage	May contain only skeletal meat; no more than 30% fat, 10% added water, and 2% corn syrup; no more than 15% poultry meat
Frankfurter or bologna "with by-products" or "with variety meats"	Same limitations on fat, added water, and corn syrup as products without variety meats; must contain at least 15% skeletal meat, and the terms "Variety Meats" or "Byproducts" must be part of the product name and in the ingredients list
Ham—water added, cooked, or cooked and smoked	Must be from the hind legs of a hog; picnic hams are from the front legs; both must contain at least 17% meat protein (fat-free)
Hamburger, ground beef, or chopped beef	No more than 30% fat; no extenders or other added substances except seasonings
Nuggets	Bite-size, solid pieces of meat and poultry; usually breaded and deep fat fried
Nuggets, chopped and formed	Meat or poultry chopped and shaped into nuggets; "Chopped and Formed" must be part of the product name
Pizza with sausage	At least 12% cooked sausage or 10% dry sausage, such as pepperoni
Turkey pie	At least 14% cooked turkey meat
Turkey ham	Cured turkey thigh meat

Standards for over 200 popular meat and poultry products are listed in USDA's publication, "Meat and Poultry Products—A Consumer Guide to Content and Labeling Requirements" (Home and Garden Bulletin No. 236, July, 1981). For further information, contact: FSIS Publications Office, USDA, Rm. 1165-S, Washington, D.C. 20250.

DETERMINING THE PERCENTAGE OF A NUTRIENT IN A FOOD

While food labels must indicate the amount of a nutrient, there is no requirement to list its percentage in a food. Such information can be quite revealing—and embarrassing—to manufacturers who extol their "commitment to consumers to promote healthy products." Consider several popular franchise chains that tout their hamburgers for providing quality nutrition: McDonald's informs consumers that a "Big Mac" contains 35 g of fat, Burger King lists the fat content of a "Whopper" as 42 g, and Roy Rogers lists its cheeseburger as having 37.3 g of fat. What these food retailers fail to promote is the different picture that emerges when the fat content is expressed as a percentage of total calories in the food. For the Big Mac, 35 g of fat amounts to 315 calories from fat (35 g × 9 calories/g). Because a Big Mac contains a total of 570 kcal, (315 ÷ 570) × 100 translates to a food containing 55.2% fat! Burger King's "Whopper" is a whopping 57.7% fat, and the cheeseburger from Roy Rogers tops out at 59.6% fat. Should it occasion little surprise that manufacturers prefer *not* to reveal such information?

Learn to Read Food Labels. To illustrate the importance of understanding the content of a food label, four popular products from the Hershey Foods company are compared in Table 9–1 for their protein, carbohydrate, and fat content. The comparison includes caloric value and amount of the nutrient (expressed in grams), based on information provided by the manufacturer. Note that the percentage of the nutrient in relation to total caloric content, not provided by the manufacturer, can be easily uncovered with a simple computation as illustrated in the footnote to Table 9–1. In Hershey's nutrition brochure, widely distributed to consumers, one question about their chocolate products is, "How many calories are there in a Hershey's Miniature Bar?" The answer: "There are 40 calories in a Hershey's Miniature Bar. This same calorie count applies for all the Hershey's Miniature Bars—Milk Chocolate, Special Dark, Mr. Goodbar, and Krackel." What the bro-

TABLE 9–1. CONSUMER BEWARE! LEARN TO INTERPRET THE NUTRITIONAL LABEL TO DETERMINE THE PERCENTAGE OF A PARTICULAR NUTRIENT IN RELATION TO A FOOD'S TOTAL CALORIE CONTENT

			PROTEIN		CHO		FAT	
ITEM	AMOUNT	CALORIES (kcal)	g	%, kcal*	g	%, kcal*	g	%, kcal*
Hershey's Chocolate milk (2% low fat)	1 cup (8 oz)	190	8	16.8	29	61.0	5	23.7
Hershey's Chocolate Kisses	9 pieces (1.5 oz)	220	3	5.5	23	41.8	13	53.0
Hershey's Reese's Peanut Butter Cup	2 cups (1.8 oz)	280	6	8.6	26	37.1	17	54.6
Hershey's New Trail Granola Snack Bars, chocolate covered cocoa creme	1.3 oz	190	2	4.2	24	50.5	9	42.6

* Note the percentage (%) column; this column, which represents the percentage of total calories for each of the macronutrients, was not provided by the manufacturer. To compute the percentage contribution of a particular nutrient, multiply the caloric value for the nutrient (protein and carbohydrate = 4 kcal/g; fat = 9 kcal/g) times the number of grams. Express the value in relation to the total number of calories. For example, to compute the percentage of fat in Hershey's Chocolate Kisses (last column), we multiplied 9 (kcal/g) × 13 (number of grams) and obtained 117 kcal. Then (117 ÷ 220) × 100 = 53%, which is the percentage of total calories supplied by fat!

Source: Data from Nutrition Information for Consumers. Hershey Foods, Consumer Relations Department, P.O. Box 815, Hershey, PA 17033-0815. The percentage values were computed from the nutrient information listed in the table provided by Hershey's; data on percentages were not included as part of their table.

chure does not reveal is that, like its larger-size chocolate bars, the fat content of the chocolate is approximately 50%!

A consumer does not need the skills of a Sherlock Holmes to revel in such discoveries. All that is required for any food is to perform the same computations as done for the Hershey products listed in Table 9–1.

PATTERNS OF FOOD CONSUMPTION

Numerous factors influence the quantity, quality, and **pattern of food consumption** in the United States. These factors include level of income and education, racial and ethnic background, and geographic locale and personal interests.

The USDA's Economic Research Service maintains records of annual per capita food consumption in the United States. During 1990, Americans spent $546 billion on food and $79.7 billion for alcoholic beverages. On a worldwide basis for 1988, $1044 was spent by each American for food and beverages consumed at home, which ranked well below Japan where the average was $4814; it was $3099 in Switzerland, $2087 in Norway, $2079 in West Germany (before unification), and $1284 in Canada. As expected, the lowest was spent in the economically poor and underdeveloped countries of Zimbabwe ($37), India ($107), Ecuador ($150), Sierra Leone ($285), and Sudan ($369). In these countries, approximately 50% of total income was spent on food, while in the countries that spent the most on food, the cost accounted for about 17% of total income.

Differences in economic affluence impact on what a country's people choose to eat or what is available for them to eat. In poorer countries, lack of modern farming practices—including efficient channels for transportation and distribution—as well as other socioeconomic and political factors dictate the type of diet a person consumes. In essence, the majority of these people eat what is available. When relatively affluent people have numerous alternatives in food selection, as in the more developed countries, they must learn to make intelligent choices to maximize good health. But this does not always occur. If it did, there would be better adherence to consuming less total fat and salt in the diet, and reducing consumption of cholesterol-rich and sugar-laden foods.

If relative affluence coincided with general knowledge and good decisions about health and fitness, then as a nation Americans would be exercising more and at an appropriate intensity, eating less and better-quality food, and saying no to drugs, alcohol, and cigarettes! But we apparently are not, and therein lies the dilemma. How does a nation extricate itself from the cycle of using automated devices instead of its own muscle power, of relying less on restaurants and fast-food joints and returning to cooking and eating well at home, and of learning how to moderate many of life's stressors instead of being driven by them?

Average amount spent on food in the largest metropolitan areas.

	Annual food bill	Percent of household income
Nassau-Suffolk, NY	$5,752	14%
New Orleans	4,673	23
San Antonio	4,665	22
Newark	4,307	12
Anaheim-Santa Ana	4,290	12
Milwaukee	4,253	15
Dallas	4,210	16
Phoenix	4,195	16
Houston	4,910	18
Orlando	4,157	17
San Francisco	4,123	12
Washington DC	4,038	11
Philadelphia	4,031	14
Boston	4,020	12
Seattle	3,963	12
Miami	3,939	9
San Jose	3,973	16
Oklahoma City	3,815	19
Atlanta	3,746	13
Cincinnati	3,743	15
San Diego	3,632	12
Pittsburg	3,604	15
Denver	3,563	13
Cleveland	3,459	14
Detroit	3,453	13
St. Louis	3,429	13
Baltimore	3,405	12
Louisville	3,367	15
Chicago	3,223	11
New York City	3,074	13
Nashville	2,871	11

Groceries and your pocketbook. In 1988, the average American household of 2.7 people spent $3,736 of their income on food products. Laredo, Texas, with an average of 3.7 people per household to feed, spent $8,034 and was highest in the nation. Check out the food bills of the large metropolitan areas in the chart.

WHAT ARE WE EATING?

The panels in Figure 9–2 display patterns in the United States over a 20-year period for the consumption of red meat, fish, and poultry; whole, low-fat, and nonfat milk; eggs; fats and oils from animal and vegetable sources;

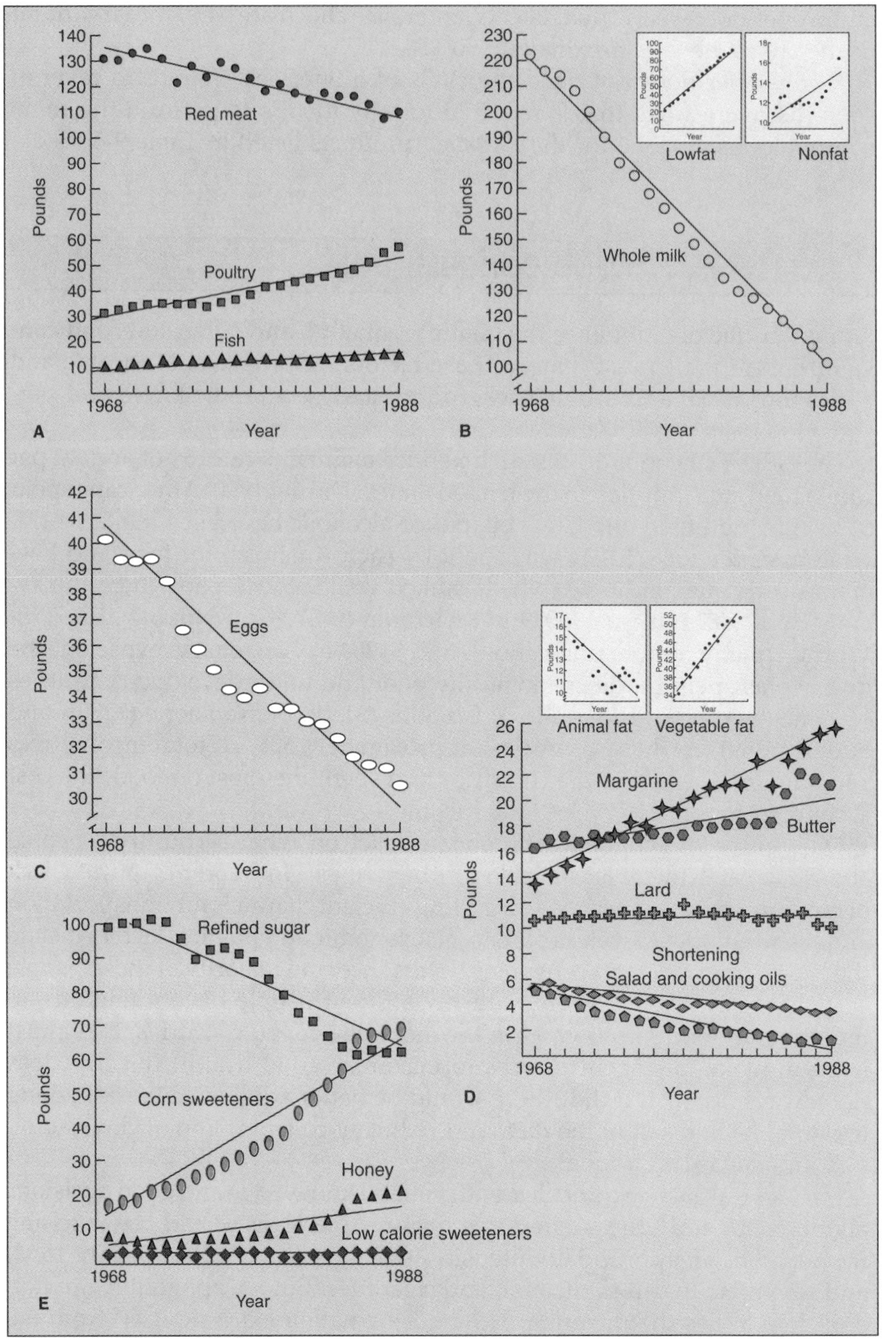

FIG. 9–2. Patterns of food consumption over a 20-year period. A. Red meat, fish, and poultry. B. Whole, lowfat, and nonfat milk. C. Egg consumption. D. Fats and oils from animal and vegetable consumption. E. Consumption of refined sugars, corn sweeteners, honey, and low-calorie sweeteners. Data from Putnam, J.J. Food consumption, prices, and expenditures, 1967–1988. United States Department of Agriculture. Commodity Economics Division. Economic Research Service. Statistical Bulletin No. 804. Washington, D.C., May 1990.

and refined sugars, corn sweeteners, honey, and low-calorie sweeteners. For some classes of foods, the scorecard on a health basis would rate as improved; for most other items, we still have a considerable way to go.

The meaningful trends in the data can be summarized as follows:

Eating out is a way of life. As many as 60 to 70% of the meals eaten in the United States are now prepared outside of the home.

The impact of the fast food in restaurants has been dramatic. Consider these facts for McDonald's only:

- Ninety-six percent of people in the U.S., ages 16 to 65, have eaten at McDonald's at least once.
- One in four people in the United States who eat breakfast out will eat breakfast at McDonald's.
- Almost 20 million people in the U.S. will eat at McDonald's every day; 5 million people outside of the U.S. eat in McDonald's each day.
- On an average day, almost 10% of the U.S. population eats at McDonald's; 64% of adults will eat there once a month.
- 80 billion McDonald's burgers consumed since 1967 translates to the equivalent of about 40 trillion calories, or the amount of fat equal to the total body weight of 6,534,000 people (or 105,000 people who attend Michigan's football stadium for 62 consecutive games)!

- There is an inverse relation between the consumption of red meat versus poultry and fish. Over the 20-year period Americans now consume, on a yearly per person basis, 8.2 kg less red meat, 13.2 kg more poultry, and about 1 kg more fish and shellfish. The relatively small increase in fish consumption may be due to fears of contamination. Unlike red meat and poultry, seafood does *not* as yet require federal inspection! The United States was twenty-seventh in fish and shellfish consumption compared to 45 other countries ranked by the Food and Agricultural Organization of the United Nations. For example, the per capita fish intake in Japan (86.2 kg) and Iceland (180.5 kg) was about 5 and 11 times, respectively, higher than in the United States (16.6 kg).
- There has been a marked increase in drinking of low-fat and nonfat milk compared to whole milk. Since the late 1960s, this represents a 54% decline in consumption of whole milk and over a 300% increase in low-fat and skim milk consumption (from 18.6 kg in 1968 to 56.2 kg per person in 1989).
- Americans consume fewer eggs purchased in shells (285 per capita in 1968 compared to 184 in 1990), but eggs consumed in products such as pasta have correspondingly increased by 40.6% (14.5 kg in 1968 to 20.5 kg in 1989). The steady decline in shell egg consumption is tied to media attention given to cholesterol and its link to coronary heart disease.
- Since 1968 the consumption of fats and oils has increased 19.5% from 23.1 to 27.6 kg per person yearly. The proportion of vegetable to animal fats consumed in 1989 (22.9 kg ÷ 4.8 kg = 4.77) is tenfold higher than

Current		Recommended
• 86% kids eat 36.4% of calories as total fat	→	reduce to 30% or less
• 91.5% kids get 14.1% of calories from saturated fat	→	reduce to 10% or less
• 90% of kids had daily cholesterol intakes of 143.5 mg/1000 calories	→	reduce to 100 mg/1000 calories
• 85.9% of kids had sodium intakes averaging 2861 mg	→	reduce to 1800 mg
• Carbohydrate intake averaged 50% of total kcal	→	increase to 55%
• Fiber intake averaged 11.5 g/day	→	increase to 20-30 g/day
• Children from poor families were deficient in vitamins and minerals	→	school lunches should conform to U.S. Dietary Guidelines

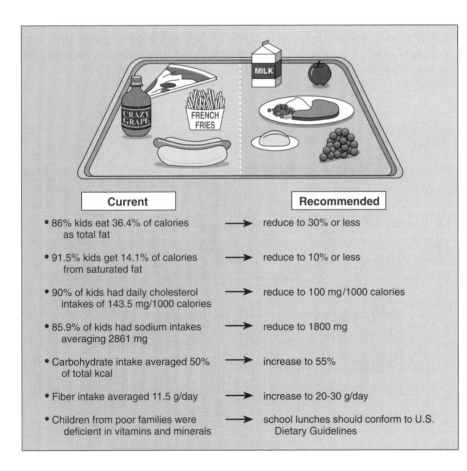

Put into practice what we preach. Advocacy groups concerned with upgrading school lunch programs are urging the U.S. government to upgrade federal standards for kids' nutrition as shown in the accompanying graphic.

the ratio in 1968 (7.45 kg ÷ 15.7 kg = 0.475). Animal fat accounted for 17% of total fat consumption in 1989, compared to 32% in 1968. Vegetable fat and oil represented 68% of total fat consumption in 1968; the corresponding value was 83% in 1989. This shift from animal to vegetable sources of fats and oils reflects the consumer's health preference for reduced cholesterol and unsaturated rather than saturated fatty acids. Of potential concern, however, is the increase in total fat consumption from a greater intake of fried foods (reliance on fast-food restaurants) from various food outlets and the increased consumption of salad oils. The use of salad and cooking oils has doubled, shortening increased by one-third, yet there was a decrease in the use of whole-lard shortening, butter, and margarine. Of the 6.6 billion kilograms of oils consumed in 1988, 4%—or 250 million—were highly saturated tropical oils (palm oil, palm kernel oil, and coconut oil).

- The per capita consumption of sweeteners has increased steadily from 56.8 kg in 1968 to a high of 69.5 kg in 1988. Since 1968, high-fructose corn syrup has increased from 0.23 kg to 22.2 kg per person in 1990! The dramatic rise in our use of low-calorie sweeteners reflects the introduction in 1981 of aspartame, a sugar substitute almost 200 times as sweet as sucrose.

HOW MUCH ARE WE EATING?

Figure 9–3 shows that, over a 20-year span, the average American increased total yearly food consumption from about 680 kg (1495 lb) in 1967 to 732 kg (1610 lb) in 1988. It is reasonable to surmise that this 7.6% or 52.3 kg rise in overall food intake represented a higher caloric intake that was unmatched by an equivalent increase in caloric expenditure, because the average American has become about 9 kg heavier (and fatter) over the same period. Part of this corpulence can be accounted for by a 6.1 kg increase

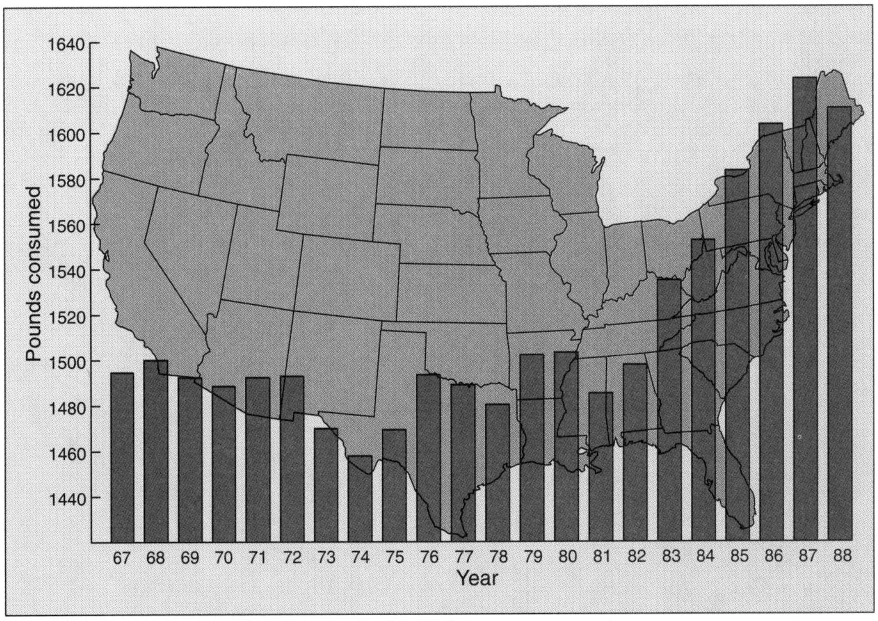

FIG. 9–3. Trends in 20-year food consumption for the average American.

in fat and oil consumption, the yearly equivalent of an additional 47,250 calories. To balance this added energy input, the same number of calories would have to be expended by increased caloric output through exercise. This would be equivalent to very slow jogging for about 473 miles over the 20-year period. While this might seem at first glance to be a heroic amount of exercise, it is actually slightly less than one-half mile a week!

When increased caloric expenditure through exercise is viewed from this broader, longer-term perspective, we can appreciate that only a small change in lifestyle truly makes a difference. College students who make modest increases in their daily activity starting at age 20 probably can avoid the statistically expected 9.1 kg (20 lb) increase in body mass by age 40! That's because the typical 20-year-old American will gain, over the next two decades, about 0.45 kg (1 lb) of weight per year. The specifics of weight control are discussed in Chapter 16.

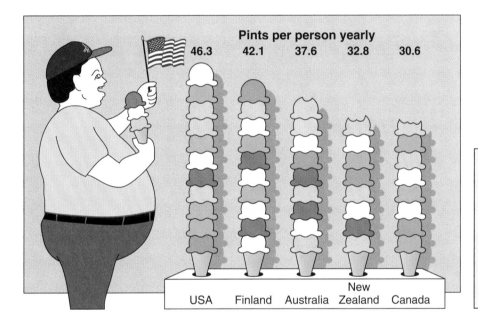

We're still No. 1! The United States leads the world in ice cream consumption with Sunday being our national ice cream day. What's your favorite flavor? According to the International Ice Cream Association, 816 million gallons, or $9.3 billion worth, of ice cream was consumed in the United States in 1990—and a third of it was vanilla, making this the number one choice among consumers. You guessed it, chocolate was second.

SUMMARY

1. The past 25 years have seen a tremendous increase in public awareness of the health benefits of good nutrition. Concurrently, advertisers have linked all types of food products to health maintenance and enhancement.
2. Various governmental agencies continually monitor the food industry to provide some degree of "truth in advertising" in the packaging of foods and alcoholic beverages. Despite this input from government, an educated consumer is the most effective defense against potential "flim-flam" in advertising.
3. A variety of terms are used in advertising. Many have specific legal definitions that are subject to rules and regulations established by the appropriate governmental watchdog agency.

4. Although food labels must indicate the amount of a particular nutrient, there is no requirement to list its relative percentage in a food. Consequently, a food may be advertised as "low in fat" (absolute quantity) when, in reality, its percentage of fat might exceed 50%!
5. Numerous factors influence the amount, type, and quality of food consumed by a particular group or individual in the group. These include level of income and education, racial and ethnic background, and geographic locale and personal interests.
6. Significant changes have been noted in food consumption over the past 20 years. Partly this reflects heightened public awareness of the relationship between diet and health. Unfortunately, our increased reliance on eating out may impact negatively on the quality of nutrition.
7. A major defense against the national trend for weight gain in adults would be a small but regular increase in daily energy expenditure through physical activity.

RELATED LITERATURE

American Dietetic Association Timely Statement: Nutrition information on food labels. J. Am. Diet. Assoc., *89*:266–268, 1989.

Annual Editions. Nutrition 91/92: 4th ed. Edited by C.C. Cook-Fuller, Guilford, Connecticut, Dushkin Publishing Group, 1991.

Food and Drug Administration. Food labeling health messages and label statement: reproposed rule. Fed. Reg., *55*:5176–5192, 1990.

Food Consumption, Prices, and Expenditures, 1968–1990: Edited by J.J. Putnam. Commodity Economics Division, Economic Research Service, U.S. Department of Agriculture. Statistical Bulletin No. 825. Washington, DC.

Hegarty, V.: Decisions in Nutrition. St. Louis, Times Mirror/Mosby College Publishing, 1988.

McGinnis, J.M.: The public health burden of a sedentary lifestyle. Med. Sci. Sports Exerc., *24*:S196, 1992.

Nieman, D.C., et al: Nutrition. Rev. 1st ed. Dubuque, 1992.

Shils, M.E. and V.R. Young: Modern Nutrition in Health and Disease. 7th ed. Philadelphia, Lea & Febiger, 1988.

Truswell, A.S.: Evolution of dietary recommendations, goals, and guidelines. Am. J. Clin. Nutr., *45*:1060–1072, 1987.

Wardlaw, G.M., and Insel, P.M.: Perspectives in Nutrition. St. Louis, Times Mirror/Mosby College Publishing, 1990.

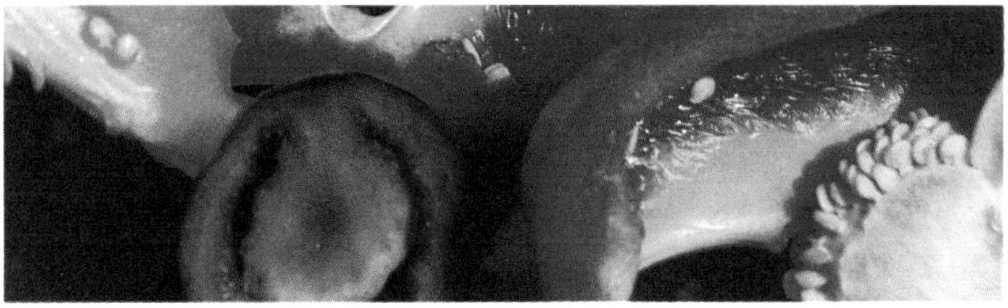

10

OPTIMAL NUTRITION FOR EXERCISE AND GOOD HEALTH

In an **optimal diet,** the supply of required nutrients is adequate for tissue maintenance, repair, and growth. Nutritionists generally agree that active men and women do not require additional nutrients beyond those obtained in a balanced diet. For example, people who eat well-balanced, calorically adequate meals of meats, cereals, vegetables, fruits, and milk consume more than enough nutrients to meet daily needs. Because vitamins can be used repeatedly in metabolic reactions, the vitamin needs of athletes and other active people are generally no greater than those of sedentary people. Also, because the level of daily energy expenditure increases significantly when exercising, the amount of food consumed increases to maintain body mass. Competitive endurance athletes, for example, consume as much as 4,000 to 5,000 calories per day simply to supply the energy required for daily training. This augmented level of food consumption will increase vitamin and mineral intake provided the person maintains a well-balanced diet. This means that nutritional guidelines must be followed in planning and evaluating food intake. In essence, however, the requirements for sound nutrition are similar for both the active person and the competitive athlete.

Consuming more of a well-balanced diet provides additional nutrients. Active people, including those involved in exceptional endurance activities, consume typical diets that are remarkably similar in composition to the diets of their more sedentary counterparts. The main difference is that they eat more food to provide the extra energy required by training. This results in a larger total nutrient intake.

The backbone of a healthful diet. Foods that are low in cholesterol, total fat, saturated fat, salt, and sugar should be consumed with regularity.

Five a day for better health—even for athletes. The National Cancer Institute is helping to sponsor a program that attempts to get people to eat five or more servings of fruits and vegetables daily. The "five a day for better health" program dovetails with the USDA Dietary Guidelines that recommend two to four servings of fruits and three to five servings of vegetables daily. A slice of tomato on a hamburger or peppers and olives on a subway sandwich doesn't qualify as a serving. Examples of a serving of fruit include one medium piece of fresh fruit or one half cup of cooked or raw fruit; for vegetables, an example is one cup of raw leafy greens.

RECOMMENDED NUTRIENT INTAKE

Figure 10–1 illustrates the general percentage contributions of the major macronutrients in a balanced diet for active people in which caloric intake is sufficient to meet energy expenditure. For a more specific breakdown in terms of gram composition of specific food, Figure 10–2 shows the carbohydrate, lipid, and protein components of food sources in a balanced diet assuming only a 1200 calorie daily intake. To meet the necessary vitamin, mineral, and protein requirements for most people, only about 252 g (9 oz) of a blend of the pure food macronutrients is actually required daily! Based on this 1200 calorie minimum, the gram and percentage requirements of total caloric intake would be 43 g of fat (~30%), 147 g of

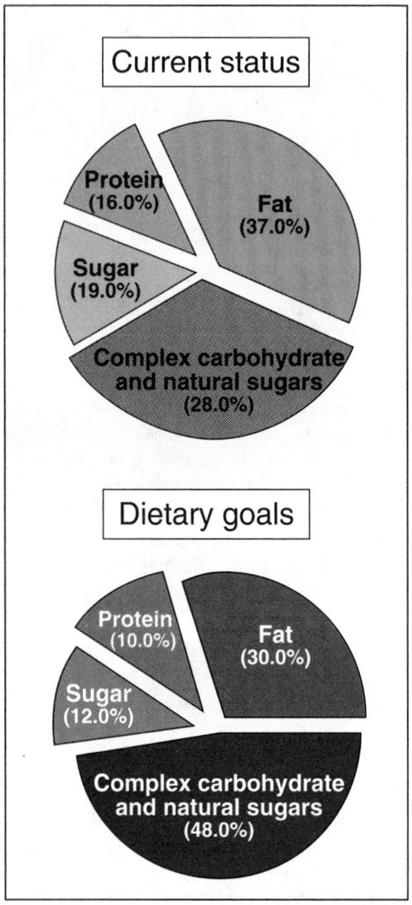

U.S. Dietary Goals.

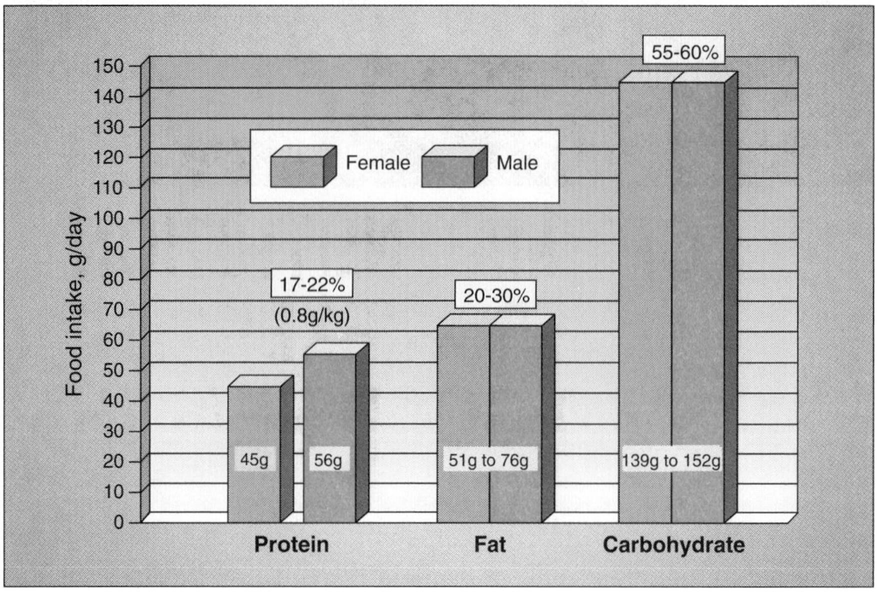

FIG. 10–1. Recommended percentage contribution of the major macronutrient components in a balanced diet.

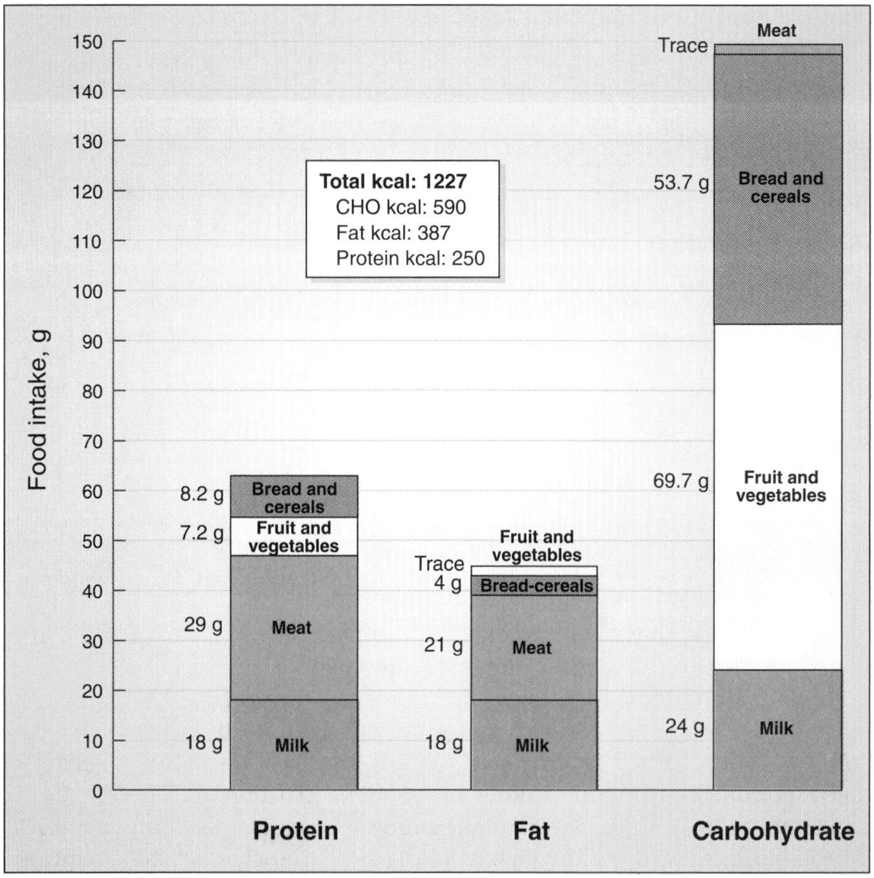

FIG. 10–2. Basic recommendations for carbohydrate, lipid, and protein components as well as the general categories of food sources in a balanced diet.

carbohydrate (~50%), and 62 g of protein (~20%). *Once the minimum nutrient requirements are met, a person's extra energy needs can be obtained from a variety of food sources based on individual preference.* This extra energy would amount to between 900 and 1500 calories for the typical person.

PROTEIN

As discussed in Chapter 5, the standard recommendation for protein intake is 0.8 g of protein per kilogram of body mass. This amounts to approximately 12% of the total calories in the average American diet. A person who weighs 77 kg (170 lb) would require about 62 g, or 2.2 oz, of protein daily. This quantity of protein is contained in three 8 oz glasses of whole milk and a piece of pizza with beef topping from Pizza Hut, or two lamb chops (10 oz) and a large cup of cream of vegetable soup, or one Burger King "Whopper," two glasses of whole milk, and two scrambled eggs. As you can see, not much food is required to supply the daily protein requirement.

On an average day, the typical American consumes nearly twice the protein requirement. For athletes, many of whom consume considerable quantities of food, the diet may contain more than two to four times the protein RDA! These additional protein calories are either used for energy or tissue synthesis, or converted to fat and stored in the subcutaneous depots. Clearly, one can become fat by eating protein! Furthermore, excessive protein intake may be harmful because the metabolism of large quantities of this nutrient can place an excessive strain on liver and renal function.

Excess protein does not make muscle. In terms of body composition, there is no benefit from consuming excessive protein. Muscle mass is not increased simply by eating high-protein foods.

Preparations of Simple Amino Acids. The practice among some weight lifters and body builders of consuming protein in the form of liquids, powders, or pills that have been chemically "predigested" in the laboratory to **simple amino acids** is a waste of money and may actually be counterproductive in terms of desired outcome. The sales pitch is that the simple amino acid molecule is absorbed more easily by the body and, in some magical way, becomes rapidly available to "power" exercise and facilitate the expected muscle growth brought on by resistance training. But nothing could be farther from the truth! For one thing, carbohydrates and fats, not protein, are the primary energy macronutrients to power exercise. In addition, the body absorbs dietary proteins during digestion when they are part of more complex dipeptide and tripeptide molecules as well as in simple amino acid form. To complicate matters, a concentrated amino acid solution draws water into the intestines. This process can cause irritation, cramping, and diarrhea.

Let your body digest the protein. Consuming "purified" or "predigested" amino acids is not the way to add muscle mass or to improve strength, power, and vigor for heavy training.

LIPID

Standards for optimal lipid intake have not been firmly established because relatively little is known about the human requirement for this nutrient. The amount of dietary lipid varies widely according to personal taste, money spent on food, and the availability of lipid-rich foods. For people living in Asia, only about 10% of the energy in the average diet is furnished by lipid; in contrast, lipids account for 40 to 50% of caloric intake for people living in the United States, Canada, Scandinavia, Germany, and France. *Many nutritionists believe that to promote optimal health, lipid intake should not exceed 30% of the energy content of the diet.* Of this, less than one-third of dietary lipids should be in the form of saturated fats. Even the 30% value for total calories as lipids may be too high, especially for individuals who suffer from gallbladder disease or are predisposed to cancer or diseases of the cardiovascular system.

To attempt to eliminate all lipids from the diet, however, is imprudent as well as potentially detrimental to exercise performance. With low-fat diets, it is difficult to increase carbohydrate and protein intake to furnish sufficient energy to maintain a stable body mass during strenuous training. Because the major essential fatty acid, linoleic acid, and many vitamins gain entrance to the body through dietary lipids, a "fat-free" diet could eventually lead to a relative state of malnutrition! Fifteen to 25 g of dietary fat per day is probably a **minimal level of fat** consumption. It does not take much to consume this amount: 2 oz of bologna has 16 g, one pork chop has 21 g, and 10 chicken nuggets from McDonald's contain 34 g of fat. The typical American consumes over 100 g (3.5 oz) of lipid every day!

Don't be fooled by "cholesterol-free," "fiber-rich" muffins! Check out the fat content and total calories before you eat just any type of muffin.

Type of muffin	Size, oz	Calories	Fat, g	Fat, %
Sara Lee Banana Nut Bran	2.5	230	9	35.2
Dunkin' Donuts Blueberry	3.1	263	10	34.2
Keebler Banana Elfin Loaves	2.0	190	7	33.2
Dunkin' Donuts Bran	3.5	353	13	33.1
Entenmann's Fruit & Fiber Honey Raisin Bran	2.5	248	9	32.7
Sara Lee Oat Bran	2.5	220	8	32.7
Sara Lee Raisin Bran	2.5	220	7	28.6

CARBOHYDRATE

Active men and women need carbohydrate. Stored muscle glycogen and blood-borne glucose are prime contributors of energy when the oxygen supplied to muscles is insufficient in relation to oxygen needs. In addition to this anaerobic role of carbohydrate, glycogen also provides substantial energy during high levels of aerobic exercise. Consequently, dietary carbohydrate is of utmost importance to individuals maintaining a physically active lifestyle.

It is difficult to state precisely how much carbohydrate should be consumed in the diet. Like lipids, the prominence of dietary carbohydrates varies widely throughout the world, depending upon factors such as the availability and relative cost of lipid- and protein-rich foods. Carbohydrate-rich foods such as grains, starchy roots, and dried peas and beans are usually the cheapest in relation to their energy value. In the Far East, carbohydrates (rice) make up 80% of total caloric intake, whereas in the United States only about 40 to 50% of daily energy comes from this macronutrient. For a sedentary 70-kg person, for example, this would amount to approximately 250 g of carbohydrate per day.

Most research evidence suggests there is no health hazard in subsisting chiefly on complex carbohydrates, provided that the essential amino acids, minerals, and vitamins are also present in the diet. In fact, this type of high-carbohydrate, high-fiber diet may offer health benefits to those who partake of it. The diet of the relatively primitive Tarahumara Indians of Mexico is high in complex carbohydrates (75% of calories) and fiber, and correspondingly low in cholesterol (71 mg/day), fat (12% of calories), and saturated fat (2% of calories). These people are noted for their remarkable physical endurance; they reportedly run distances of up to 200 miles in competitive soccer-type sporting events that often last several days. Particularly notable among the Tarahumaras is the virtual absence of hypertension, obesity, and death from cardiac and circulatory complications.

Cruciferous veggies may offer cancer protection. The chemical sulforaphane, recently discovered by scientists, is present in vegetables of the cruciferous family such as Brussels sprouts, cabbage, kohlrabi, mustard, radishes, rutabagas, turnips, and broccoli. This chemical may offer protection against certain types of cancers by blocking tumor formation.

For a physically active person, the ***"prudent" diet*** *should contain about 60% of its calories in the form of carbohydrates, predominantly unrefined starches.* Be-

Nutrition Information Per Serving	
One medium potato (1/3 lb; 150 g)	
Calories	110
Protein	3 g
Carbohydrates	23 g
Fat	0 g
Dietary fiber	2.7 g
Sodium	10 mg
Potassium	750 mg

Percentage of U.S. RDA			
Protein	6	Folic acid	8
Vitamin A	*	Phosphorus	8
Vitamin C	50	Magnesium	8
Thiamin	8	Zinc	2
Riboflavin	2	Copper	8
Niacin	10	Pantothenic acid	4
Calcium	*	Iodine	15
Iron	8		
Vitamin B_6	15		

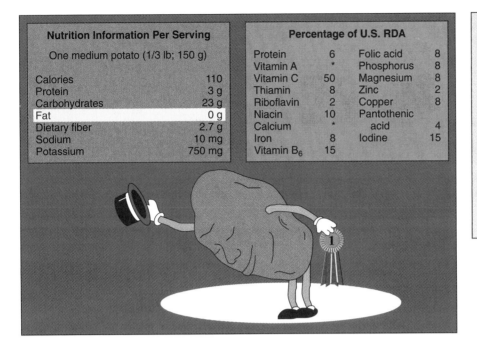

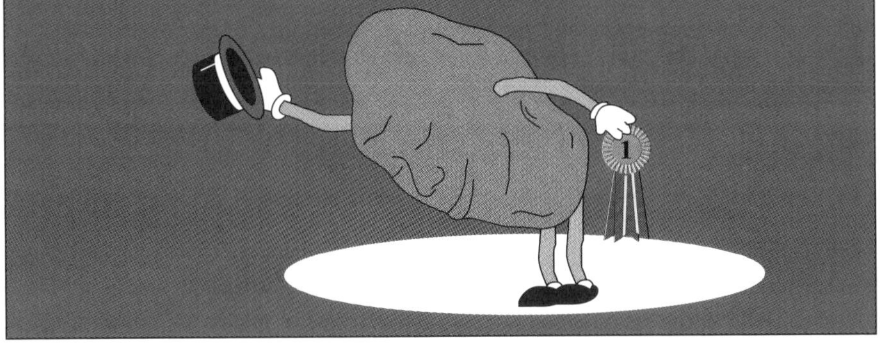

The potato is America's favorite vegetable, and it's good eating for carbo loading. Over the past 5 years, the per capita consumption of potatoes in the United States has averaged about 126 pounds a year, or the equivalent of eating one medium-sized potato daily. Potatoes come from a variety of sources: canned (2 pounds), frozen (45 pounds), chips and shoestring (18 pounds), dehydrated (11 pounds), and farm fresh (50 pounds). Ireland in the 1600–1700s was one of the first European countries to farm the potato as a major crop. The potato was introduced to America in the early 1700s with the arrival of Scottish-Irish immigrants.

cause glycogen synthesis in liver and muscle is related to dietary carbohydrate, some researchers in exercise physiology recommend increasing the daily carbohydrate intake to 70% of total calories (400 to 600 g) to prevent gradual depletion of glycogen stores with successive days of hard training. The specific dietary-exercise techniques for facilitating glycogen storage are discussed in a later section.

THE FOUR-FOOD-GROUP PLAN: THE ESSENTIALS OF GOOD NUTRITION

A practical approach to sound nutrition is to categorize foods that make similar nutrient contributions and then provide servings from each category in the daily diet. A key to achieving success with such an approach is variety. This can be readily achieved by use of the **Four-Food-Group Plan** described in Table 10–1. Adequate nutrition will be assured as long as the recommended number of servings from the variety provided in each group is supplied and cooking and handling are proper. More of these and other foods can be used as needed for growth, for activity, and for maintaining desirable weight. For individuals on meatless diets, a small amount of milk, milk products, or eggs should be included because vitamin B_{12} is available only in foods of animal origin. In fact, if milk and eggs are included in a vegetarian diet ("lacto-ovovegetarian" diet), nutritional quality will equal the typical recommended diet that contains meat, fish, and poultry.

Sound framework, even when calorie intake is low. The Four-Food-Group Plan guidelines provide for the necessary vitamin, mineral, and protein requirements even though the energy content of the diet may be as low as 1200 calories per day. The average daily caloric intake of adult Americans is about 2100 calories for women and 2700 to 3000 calories for men.

Table 10–2 presents examples of three daily menus formulated from the guidelines of the basic diet plan shown in Table 10–1. These menus can serve as nutritional models for reducing diets. For active individuals whose daily energy requirements may be as great as 5000 calories, all that need be done once the essentials are provided is to increase the quantity of food consumed; this is achieved by increasing either the size of portions, the

Eating smart. To get a broad rating of the diversity of your diet, complete the Eating Smart Quiz in the *Study Guide*.

TABLE 10–1. THE FOUR-FOOD-GROUP PLAN: THE FOUNDATION FOR A GOOD DIET

FOOD CATEGORY	EXAMPLES	RECOMMENDED DAILY SERVINGS‡
I. Milk and milk products*	Milk, cheese, ice cream, sour cream, yogurt	2‖
II. Meat and high-protein†	Meat, fish, poultry, eggs—with dried beans, peas, nuts, or peanut butter as alternatives	2
III. Vegetables and fruits§	Dark green or yellow vegetables, citrus fruits or tomatoes	4
IV. Cereal and grain food	Enriched breads, cereals, flour, baked goods, or whole-grain products	4

* If large quantities of milk are normally consumed, *fortified* skimmed milk should be substituted to reduce the quantity of saturated fats.

† Fish, chicken, and high-protein vegetables contain significantly less saturated fats than other protein sources.

‡ A basic serving of meat or fish is usually 100 g, or 3.5 oz, of edible food; 1 cup (8 oz) milk; 1 oz cheese; ½ cup fruit, vegetables, juice; 1 slice bread; ½ cup cooked cereal or 1 cup ready-to-eat cereal.

§ One should be rich in vitamin C; at least one every other day rich in vitamin A.

‖ Children, teenagers, and pregnant and nursing women—4 servings.

frequency of meals or snacks, or the variety of nutritious food consumed at each meal.

The Eating-Right Pyramid. The Four-Food-Group Plan developed in 1958 by the U.S. Department of Agriculture (USDA) was greatly influenced by lobbyists of the beef and dairy industries. Based on findings from research in cancer, heart disease, and nutrition over the past 35 years, the shortcomings of the "basic four" (with its overemphasis on meat and milk products) as a guide to healthful eating became apparent. To reflect the current state of nutritional knowledge more clearly, the USDA began to develop a new model for good nutrition as illustrated in Figure 10–3. The result was the **"eating-right pyramid,"** which keeps the concept of the basic four food groups but refocuses emphasis on grains, vegetables, and fruits as the basis of the diet and downplays food sources high in animal protein, lipids, and dairy products.

EXERCISE AND FOOD INTAKE

For individuals who engage regularly in moderate to intense physical activity, it is relatively easy to match food intake with the daily level of energy expenditure. Lumbermen, for example, who expend about 4500 calories daily, unconsciously adjust their caloric intake in relation to energy output. Consequently, body mass remains stable despite an extremely large food consumption. The balancing of food intake to meet a new level of energy output takes about a day or so, during which time a new energy equilibrium is attained. This balance between energy expenditure and food intake observed in physically active individuals is often not maintained in sedentary people. Here, caloric intake somewhat exceeds daily energy expenditure.

TABLE 10–2. THREE DAILY MENUS FORMULATED FROM GUIDELINES ESTABLISHED BY THE FOUR-FOOD-GROUP PLAN*

3 MEALS A DAY	5 MEALS A DAY	6 SMALL MEALS A DAY
Breakfast	**Breakfast**	**Breakfast**
½ cup unsweetened grapefruit juice	½ grapefruit	½ cup orange juice
1 poached egg	⅔ cup bran flakes	¾ cup ready-to-eat cereal
1 slice toast	1 cup skimmed or low-fat milk or other beverage	½ cup skimmed milk
1 teaspoon butter or margarine	**Snack**	tea or coffee, black
½ cup skimmed milk	1 small package raisins	**Mid-Morning Snack**
tea or coffee, black	½ bologna sandwich	½ cup low-fat cottage cheese
Lunch	**Lunch**	**Lunch**
2 oz lean roast beef†	1 slice pizza	2 oz sliced turkey on 1 slice white toast
½ cup cooked summer squash	carrot sticks	1 teaspoon butter or margarine
1 slice rye bread	1 apple	2 canned drained peach halves
1 teaspoon butter or margarine	1 cup skimmed or low-fat milk	½ cup skimmed milk
1 cup skimmed milk	**Snack**	**Mid-Afternoon Snack**
10 grapes	1 banana	1 cup fresh spinach and lettuce salad
Dinner	**Dinner**	2 teaspoons oil + vinegar or lemon
3 oz poached haddock†	baked fish with mushrooms (3 oz)†	3 saltines
½ cup cooked spinach	baked potato	**Dinner**
tomato and lettuce salad	2 teaspoons margarine	1 cup clear broth
1 teaspoon oil + vinegar or lemon	½ cup broccoli	3 oz broiled chicken breast†
1 small biscuit	1 cup tomato juice or skimmed or low-fat milk	½ cup cooked rice with 1 teaspoon butter or margarine
1 teaspoon butter or margarine		¼ cup cooked mushrooms
½ cup canned drained fruit cocktail		½ cup cooked broccoli
½ cup skimmed milk		½ cup skimmed milk
		Evening Snack
		1 medium apple
		½ cup skimmed milk
Total Calories: about 1200	**Total Calories: about 1400**	**Total Calories: about 1200**

* Each menu provides *all* essential nutrients; the energy or caloric value of the diet can easily be raised by increasing the size of portions, the frequency of meals, or the variety of foods consumed at each sitting.

† Cooked weight.

On a long-term basis, this lack of precision in regulating food intake at the low end of the physical activity spectrum contributes to the "creeping obesity" commonly observed in highly mechanized and technically advanced societies.

CALORIC INTAKE AMONG ATHLETES

The daily food intake of competitors in the 1936 Olympics reportedly averaged more than 7000 calories, or roughly three times the average daily intake. These values are often quoted to justify what appears to be an enormous food requirement for athletes in training. However, the results were based on self-reports of food intake rather than more objective dietary data. In all likelihood, the results are inflated estimates of the actual energy expended (and required) by the athletes. For example, distance runners who train upward to 160 km (100 miles) per week (pace of 6 min/mile at about 15 calories per minute) probably do not expend more than 800 to 1300 "extra" calories each day above their normal energy requirement. For

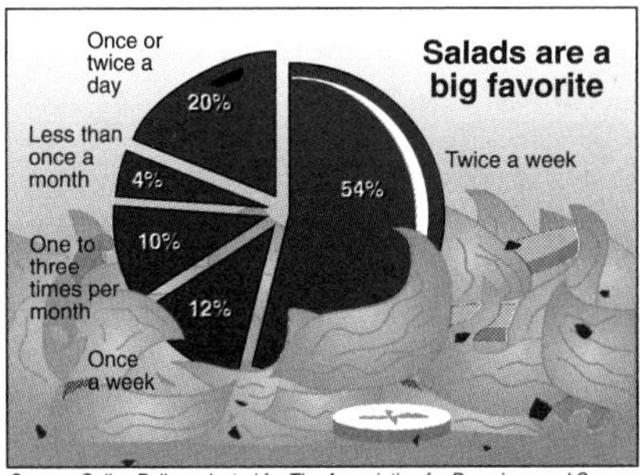

Source: Gallop Poll conducted for The Association for Dressings and Sauces

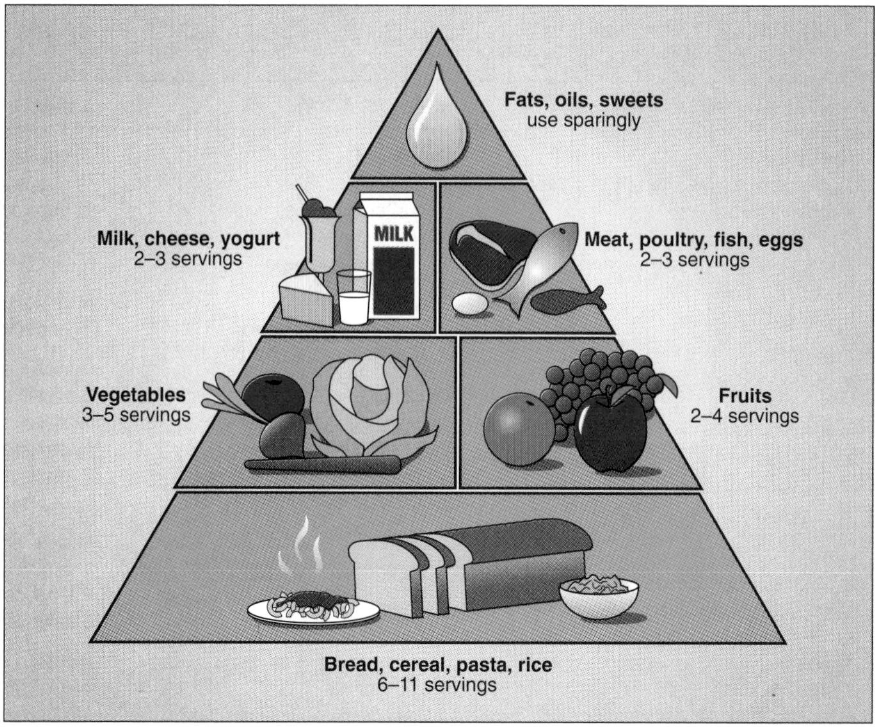

FIG. 10–3. A new proposal: the eating-right pyramid.

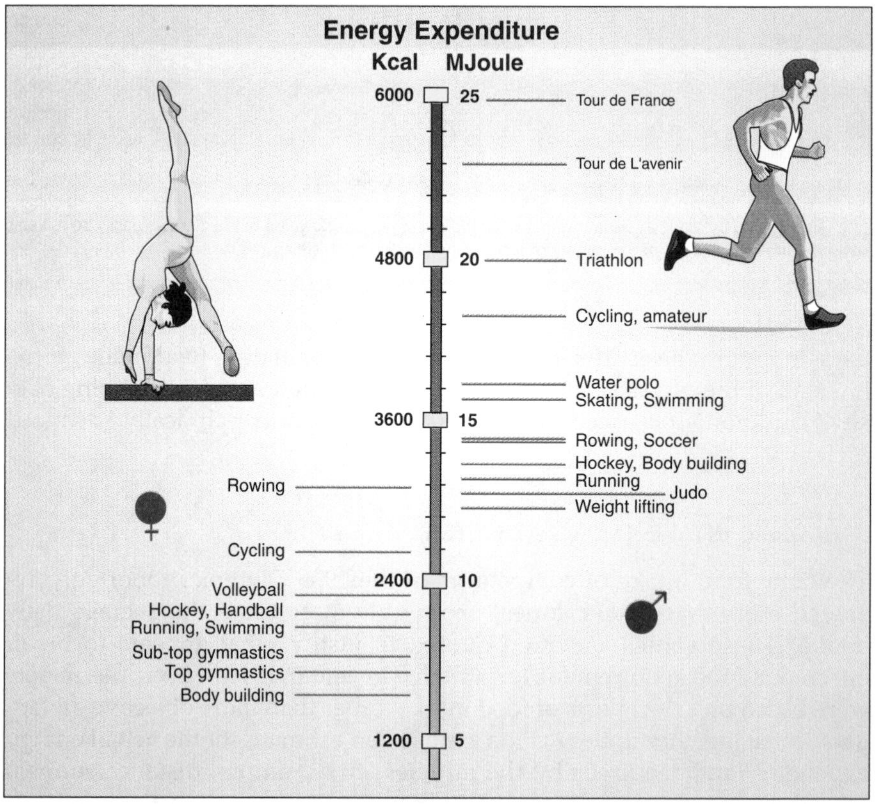

FIG. 10–4. Daily energy intake in Mjoule and kcal per day in elite male and female endurance, strength, and team sport athletes. (From van Erp-Baart, A.M.J., et al.: Nationwide survey on nutritional habits in elite athletes. *Int. J. Sports Med.* 10:53, 1989.)

these endurance athletes, the daily food intake should supply about 4000 calories to balance the increased energy expenditure. Figure 10–4 presents data on energy intake from a large sample of elite male and female endurance, strength, and team sport athletes in the Netherlands. For male athletes, energy intake ranged between 2900 and 5900 calories a day, while the daily intake of female competitors ranged between 1600 and 3200 calories.

Caloric intake of athletes. With the exception of the relatively high daily energy intake of athletes at extremes of performance and training, such as triathletes and Tour de France cyclists (5880 kcal), daily caloric intake for athletes generally does not exceed 4000 kcal for men and 3000 kcal for women.

EAT MORE, WEIGH LESS

Table 10–3 shows that the daily caloric intake of 61 middle-aged men and women who ran an average of 60 km each week amounted to between 40 and 60% more calories per kilogram of body mass than sedentary counterparts. This larger caloric intake resulted from the extra energy required to run between 8 and 10 km daily. Paradoxically, the active men and women who ate considerably *more* on a daily basis weighed considerably *less* than the runners who were less active. Such data are generally consistent with other studies of active people and add further evidence to the strong argument that regular exercise provides an effective means for weight control, so that a person can actually **"eat more, yet weigh less"** and maintain a lower percentage of body fat. *Active people maintain a lighter, leaner body and a healthier heart disease risk profile despite an increased intake of the typical American*

TABLE 10–3. COMPARISON OF CARBOHYDRATE, FAT, PROTEIN, AND CALORIC INTAKE OF MIDDLE-AGED MALE AND FEMALE RUNNERS AND SEDENTARY CONTROLS[a]

	RUNNERS	SEDENTARY CONTROLS
Males		
Calories (kcal/day)	2959*	2361
Protein (g/day)	102.1	93.6
Protein (%)	13.8*	15.8
Fat (g/day)	134.4*	109.0
Fat (%)	40.8	41.5
Carbohydrate (g/day)	294.6*	225.7
Carbohydrate (%)	39.8	38.6
Cholesterol (mg/1000 kcal)	175.0	190.0
Saturated fat (g/1000 kcal)	16.2	16.0
Polyunsaturated fat (g/1000 kcal)	9.0	9.3
Females		
Calories (kcal/day)	2386*	1871
Protein (g/day)	82.2	76.7
Protein (%)	14.2*	17.4
Fat (g/day)	110.7*	83.0
Fat (%)	41.1	40.3
Carbohydrate (g/day)	234.3*	174.7
Carbohydrate (%)	39.5	39.1
Cholesterol (mg/1000 kcal)	190.0	205.0
Saturated fat (g/1000 kcal)	16.8	16.5
Polyunsaturated fat (g/1000 kcal)	8.5	7.9

[a] % calories do not total 100% because alcohol calories constitute the difference.
* Values for runners are significantly different from controls.
(From: Blair, S.N., et al.: Comparisons of nutrient intake in middle-aged men and women runners and controls. *Med. Sci. Sports. Exerc.*, 13:310, 1981.)

diet. The important role of exercise for weight control is discussed more fully in Chapter 16.

COMPUTERIZED MEAL PLANS

Nutritionists and exercise specialists have applied computer technology for formulating well-balanced meals and prudent exercise programs for weight control. The creation of daily menus is based on the Four-Food-Group Plan and dietary exchange method developed by the American Dietetic Association. Rather than prescribing a particular food plan, the computerized dietary plan allows a person to make specific selections from a basic list of the most common foods. Foods can be exchanged among food groups, and meals can be exchanged for breakfast, lunch, and dinner on other days. Combined with age, body mass and stature, weight loss desired, and current level of physical activity, the computer prepares nutritious meals for breakfast, lunch, and dinner for a 14-day period. The menu varies from day to day, and the meals are balanced for nutrient intake of carbohydrate, lipid, protein, and vitamins and minerals. The daily meals are designed so the individual can reduce excess weight (fat) at a safe but steady level. The 15- to 18-page printout includes a weight loss curve, daily meal plans, and a beginner, intermediate, or advanced aerobic walk/jog/run, cycle, or swim program. Appendix D shows examples of the nutrition and exercise computer printout as well as the questionnaire, which can be completed and mailed for your own use.

DIET AND EXERCISE PERFORMANCE

The glycogen supply is limited. High-intensity exercise for an hour can decrease liver glycogen by about 55%. A 2-hour strenuous workout can just about deplete the glycogen content of the liver and specifically exercised muscles.

The specific nutrient fuel for muscle contraction depends on the intensity and duration of exercise and, to some degree, on the fitness and nutritional status of the individual. During continuous moderate exercise, the energy for muscle contraction is provided predominantly from the body's fat and carbohydrate reserves. As exercise continues and glycogen stores in the liver and muscles become reduced, an even greater percentage of energy for exercise must be supplied by the breakdown of lipid. This energy nutrient is mobilized from storage sites such as adipose tissue and delivered via the circulation to working muscles. If exercise is performed to the point where the glycogen stored in specific muscles is severely lowered, the performer may tire easily. Endurance athletes commonly refer to this sensation of fatigue as "bonking" or **"hitting the wall."** Interestingly, glycogen is reduced *only* in the muscles that are actively involved in performing the exercise. This occurs because enzymes are not present to aid the release and transfer of glycogen between muscles. Thus, the relatively nonactive muscles retain their glycogen supply.

The phosphatase enzyme is a "gatekeeper" for glucose. Liver cells contain the enzyme **phosphatase** that can change glycogen back to glucose, which then exits the cell; muscles do not have this enzyme.

Fatigue can occur during prolonged exercise even though sufficient oxygen is available to the muscles; similarly, the potential energy from the body's storehouse of lipids remains almost unlimited. This fatigue occurs because the limited amount of muscle glycogen becomes depleted—and without some carbohydrate available to muscle, the body cannot generate sufficient energy in strenuous aerobic exercise from lipid breakdown alone. If a solution of glucose and water is ingested at the point of fatigue, exercise may be prolonged for an additional period, but for all practical purposes the muscles' "fuel tank" becomes "empty." This imposes severe limitations for continuing a high level of energy production for exercise.

CARBOHYDRATE NEEDS IN INTENSE TRAINING

Repeated days of strenuous endurance workouts for activities such as distance running, swimming, cross-country skiing, and cycling can induce a state of fatigue in which continued hard training becomes progressively more difficult. Often referred to as **"staleness,"** this physiologic state is caused by gradual depletion of the body's glycogen reserves, even though the person's diet may contain the typical percentage of carbohydrate. Figure 10–5 shows that after three successive days of running 16.1 km (10 miles) a day, runners had nearly depleted the glycogen in the thigh muscles although their diet contained about 45% carbohydrates. By the third day, the quantity of glycogen used during the run was less than on the first day because the energy for exercise was supplied predominantly from lipid breakdown. However, no further glycogen depletion occurred when daily dietary carbohydrate was increased to 500 to 600 g (70% of caloric intake).

Optimizing glycogen reserves. Gradually reducing or tapering the intensity of workouts several days prior to competition while maintaining a high carbohydrate intake is sound nutrition for establishing optimal energy reserves.

Glycogen is not rapidly replenished when it becomes severely depleted. At least 48 hours are needed to restore muscle glycogen levels after prolonged, exhaustive exercise, and some individuals may require more than five days if the diet contains only a moderate amount of carbohydrate. *Unmistakably, during periods of heavy training, daily carbohydrate allowances must be increased to balance glycogen utilization and permit optimal **glycogen resynthesis.*** At least two days of rest and high carbohydrate intake are required to reestablish an optimal level of muscle glycogen.

Glycogen replenishment. The most important time for glycogen resynthesis is during the first few hours immediately after exhaustive exercise. It is at this time that a high-carbohydrate diet is most effective for replenishing liver and muscle glycogen.

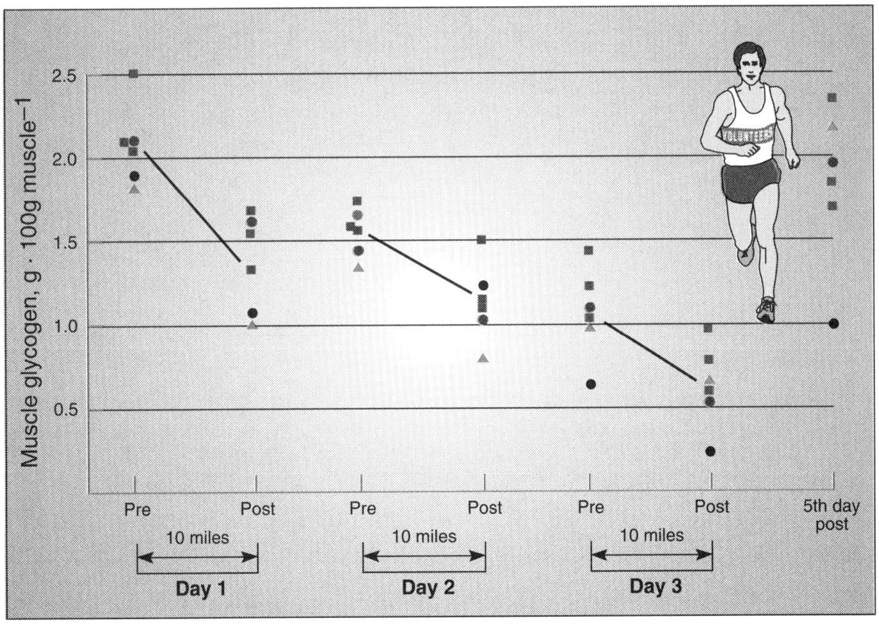

FIG. 10–5. Changes in muscle glycogen concentration for 6 male subjects before and after each 16.1 km run performed on three successive days. Muscle glycogen was measured five days after the last run and is referred to as "5th day post." (From Costill, D.L., et al.: Muscle glycogen utilization during prolonged exercise on successive days. *J. Appl. Physiol.*, 31:834, 1971.)

DIET, GLYCOGEN STORES, AND ENDURANCE

In the late 1930s, scientists observed that endurance performance was significantly improved simply by consuming a carbohydrate-rich diet for three days prior to exercising. Conversely, endurance was drastically reduced if the diet consisted predominantly of lipids. Researchers have evaluated different methods to increase the glycogen content of muscle because of the crucial relationship between diet composition and optimal physical performance. In one series of experiments, subjects consumed one of three diets. The first maintained normal caloric intake but supplied the major quantity of calories from lipids and only 5% of calories from carbohydrate. The second diet was normal for calories and contained the recommended percentages of macronutrients. The third diet provided 80% of calories as carbohydrates. The results, illustrated in Figure 10–6, reveal that the glycogen content of leg muscles, expressed as grams of glycogen per 100 g of muscle, averaged 0.6 for subjects fed the high-fat diet, 1.75 for the normal diet, and 3.75 for the high-carbohydrate diet. Furthermore, the subjects' endurance capacity varied greatly depending on the pre-exercise diet. When the subjects were fed the high-carbohydrate diet, endurance was more than three times greater than when they consumed the high-fat diet! *These findings highlight the important role that nutrition plays in establishing appropriate energy reserves for exercise.* A diet deficient in carbohydrate rapidly depletes muscle and liver glycogen. This subsequently affects performance in both maximal, short-term anaerobic exercise and in lower intensity, prolonged aerobic activities. These observations are pertinent for the athlete as well as for moderately active people who modify their diets and consume less than the recommended quantity of carbohydrate.

Dieting can hinder exercise performance and optimal nutrition. Reliance on starvation diets or other potentially harmful practices such as high-fat, low-carbohydrate diets, "liquid-protein" diets, or water diets is counterproductive for weight control, exercise performance, and optimal nutrition for good health. Reliance on low-carbohydrate diets compromises the energy supply required for vigorous physical activity or regular training.

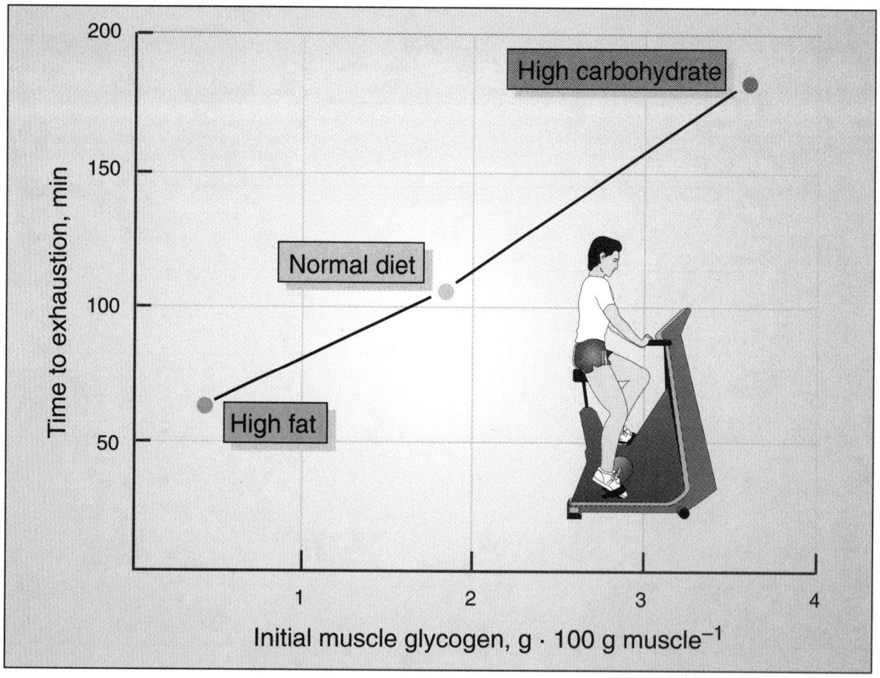

FIG. 10–6. Effects of a low-carbohydrate diet, a mixed diet, and a high-carbohydrate diet on glycogen content of the quadriceps femoris and duration of exercise on a bicycle ergometer. (From Bergstrom, J., et al.: Diet, muscle glycogen and physical performance. *Acta Physiol. Scand.*, 71:140, 1967.)

Although research has firmly established the important role of carbohydrate during various intensities of physical activity, carbohydrate supplements are not always beneficial.

During Exercise. *Performance during high-intensity aerobic exercise is improved by consuming carbohydrate-laden drinks at regular intervals.* Supplementary carbohydrate may spare muscle glycogen because the ingested glucose is used as fuel, or it helps to maintain a more optimal level of blood glucose that prevents headache, light-headedness, nausea, and other symptoms of central nervous system distress. Maintaining a status quo for blood glucose also supplies the needs of muscles when glycogen reserves become depleted in the later stages of prolonged exercise. During less intensive exercise, the beneficial effect of carbohydrate feeding is negligible because moderate exercise is fueled mainly by the breakdown of lipid with little drain on carbohydrate reserves.

Sugar drinks are beneficial during exercise. The benefits of sugar drinks occur only when they are consumed during exercise. Intestinal absorption of glucose may also facilitate both sodium and water absorption.

What to Drink? Commercially available carbohydrate drinks are not necessarily more effective than a liquid mixture of glucose or sucrose. Such a drink (5% solution) can be prepared by adding 50 g of either glucose, fructose, or sucrose to 1 liter of water. For prolonged, high-intensity aerobic exercise, a practical recommendation is to ingest a strong, 50% sugar solution (70 g of sugar in 140 ml of water) 20 to 30 minutes after the start of exercise, followed by less concentrated solutions that contain about 24 g of carbohydrate (8 oz of a 5% solution every 15 minutes) over 30-minute intervals during exercise.

Sports drink recommendations. Although the contents of the optimal "sports drink" have yet to be determined, drinks containing between 2 and 8% carbohydrate are probably as effective as pure water in providing fluid replenishment—and the extra carbohydrate could be beneficial if glycogen reserves become low.

Glucose Feedings and Water Uptake. An important property of sugar drinks is their *potential* negative effect on water absorption from the digestive tract. This is because the emptying of fluid from the stomach into the small intestine, where it is absorbed, is inhibited by the concentration of particles in solution. This effect could be detrimental during exercise in the heat, when adequate fluid intake *and* absorption are crucial to the athlete's health and safety. Researchers have devised a strategy to counter the negative effects of sugar molecules on gastric emptying so that plasma volume is preserved during exercise in the heat. This is accomplished by formulating the drink with **glucose polymers,** which greatly reduce the number of particles in solution. Polymerized glucose facilitates the movement of water and glucose from the stomach to the small intestine for absorption. Once glucose is in the intestine, its presence stimulates both sodium and water absorption.

Glucose polymers in sports drinks. Adding glucose polymers to **sports drinks** links 10 to 15 simple sugar molecules together to provide increased carbohydrate content for equivalent osmolarity compared to solutions of simple sugars. Maltodextrins are common glucose polymers in sports drinks.

Before Exercise. *Drinking a strong sugar solution 30 to 60 minutes prior to exercise actually hinders endurance capacity.* For example, the riding time of young men and women on an exercise bicycle was reduced nearly 20% when they consumed a 25% glucose solution 30 minutes before exercising, compared to similar exercise preceded by drinking the same volume of plain water. Consuming concentrated sugar drinks before exercising causes blood sugar to rise dramatically within 5 to 10 minutes. This leads to an overshoot in insulin release from the pancreas that actually produces a decline in blood sugar (hypoglycemia) as glucose moves rapidly into the muscle cells. At the same time, insulin inhibits the mobilization of lipids for energy. Consequently, carbohydrate is metabolized during subsequent exercise to a much greater degree than under normal conditions. The effect of glycogen depletion causes fatigue to occur sooner than would normally be the case.

Fructose is absorbed more slowly from the gut than either glucose or sucrose, and causes only a minimal insulin response with essentially no decline in blood glucose. This has prompted some to suggest that fructose would be beneficial for immediate pre-exercise carbohydrate feeding. Although the theoretical rationale for this use of fructose appears sound, the ergogenic benefits are inconclusive concerning such feedings. What is important, however, is that consuming high-fructose beverages is often accompanied by significant gastrointestinal distress that in itself can negatively affect exercise performance.

CARBOHYDRATE LOADING: A WAY TO INCREASE GLYCOGEN RESERVES

TABLE 10–4. TWO-STAGE DIETARY PLAN FOR INCREASING MUSCLE GLYCOGEN STORAGE

STAGE 1—DEPLETION
Day 1: Exhausting exercise performed to deplete muscle glycogen in specific muscles Days 2, 3, 4: Low-carbohydrate food intake (high percentage of protein and fat in the daily diet)
STAGE 2—CARBOHYDRATE LOADING
Days 5, 6, 7: High-carbohydrate food intake (normal percentage of protein in the daily diet)
COMPETITION DAY
Follow high-carbohydrate pre-event meal outlined in Table 10–5

Strategy for carbohydrate loading. Because carbohydrate loading occurs only in the specific muscles exercised, the person must engage the muscles involved in his or her sport during the depletion phase of the loading procedure. In preparation for a marathon, a 15- or 20-mile run is usually necessary; for swimming and bicycling, 90 minutes of moderately intense exercise in the specific activity would be required.

Research has shown that a particular combination of diet and exercise results in significant "packing" of muscle glycogen. This procedure is termed **carbohydrate loading** and is commonly used by endurance athletes. The end result of carbohydrate loading is an even greater increase in muscle glycogen than would occur with simply consuming a carbohydrate-rich diet.

The classic procedure for carbohydrate loading, outlined in Table 10–4, is accomplished as follows: First, the glycogen stores are reduced with a period of relatively long, aerobic exercise. Second, muscle glycogen is further depleted by maintaining a high-fat, low-carbohydrate diet (60 to 120 g carbohydrate) for several days while continuing a moderate exercise program. Third, the activity level is reduced for the next several days; at the same time, a switch is made to a carbohydrate-rich diet (400 to 600 g carbohydrate). With this procedure, the muscle glycogen increases to a new, higher level. Of course, adequate protein, minerals and vitamins, and abundant water must also be part of the daily diet.

The combination of diet and exercise to produce glycogen packing or "supercompensation" should be of considerable interest to the serious endurance athlete, whose success can be influenced by the body's carbohydrate reserves. For nonathletes or those involved in activities lasting less than 75 minutes, normal levels of muscle glycogen are more than adequate to sustain exercise. Normal levels of glycogen can be assured by ingesting approximately 60% of the daily caloric intake as carbohydrates. This should be increased if the energy requirements are consistently high, as occurs during periods of intensive training.

Table 10–5 lists sample meal plans for carbohydrate depletion (Stage 1) and carbohydrate loading (Stage 2) that precede the endurance event.

Negative Aspects. The wisdom of repeated bouts of carbohydrate loading has yet to be verified. A severe carbohydrate overload interspersed with periods of high lipid or protein intake may increase blood cholesterol and urea nitrogen levels and could pose problems in people susceptible to adult diabetes or heart disease, or for those who have certain muscle enzyme deficiencies or kidney disease. During the low-carbohydrate phase of the loading procedure, the potential exists for a marked ketosis that is often observed among individuals who exercise in the carbohydrate-depleted

TABLE 10–5. SAMPLE MEAL PLAN FOR CARBOHYDRATE DEPLETION AND CARBOHYDRATE LOADING DIETS PRECEDING AN ENDURANCE EVENT*

MEAL	STAGE 1 DEPLETION	STAGE 2 CARBOHYDRATE LOADING
Breakfast	½ cup fruit juice 2 eggs 1 slice whole-wheat toast 1 glass whole milk	1 cup fruit juice hot or cold cereal 1 to 2 muffins 1 tsp butter coffee (cream/sugar)
Lunch	6 oz hamburger† 2 slices bread salad 1 tbsp mayonnaise or salad dressing 1 glass whole milk	2–3 oz hamburger† with bun 1 cup juice 1 orange 1 tbsp mayonnaise pie or cake
Snack	1 cup yogurt	1 cup yogurt, fruit, or cookies
Dinner	2 to 3 pieces chicken, fried 1 baked potato with sour cream ½ cup vegetable iced tea (no sugar) 2 tbsp butter	1–1½ pieces chicken, baked 1 baked potato with sour cream 1 cup vegetable ½ cup sweetened pineapple iced tea (sugar) 1 tsp butter
Snack	1 glass whole milk	1 glass chocolate milk with 4 cookies

* During stage 1, the intake of carbohydrate is approximately 100 g or 400 calories; in stage 2, the carbohydrate intake is increased to 400 to 625 g or about 1600 to 2500 calories.

† Cooked weight.

state. Failure to eat a balanced diet may eventually lead to deficiencies in some minerals and vitamins, particularly water-soluble vitamins. Furthermore, the glycogen-depleted state certainly reduces a person's capability to engage in hard training and may result in an actual detraining effect. The elimination of dietary carbohydrate for three days could also set the stage for loss of lean tissue because the muscles' amino acids are used in gluconeogenesis to maintain blood glucose. For this reason, the less stringent modified approach to carbohydrate loading is an attractive option.

MODIFIED LOADING PROCEDURE

Many negative aspects of the classic carbohydrate loading sequence can be eliminated by following the less stringent, **modified carbo-loading** dietary protocol outlined in Figure 10–7. This six-day protocol is achieved without prior exercise to exhaustion. The athlete trains at a high aerobic intensity for 1.5 hours and gradually reduces or tapers the duration of exercise on successive days. Carbohydrates represent about 50% of total calories during the first three days, then are increased to about 70% of total calories for the last three days before competition. This results in an increase in glycogen reserves to about the same level as is achieved with the classic protocol.

A better way to "carboload." Glycogen stores can be increased by 30 to 40% above normal levels by following the modified diet and exercise protocol for carbohydrate loading.

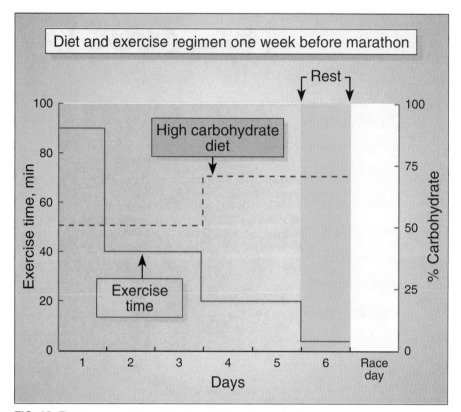

FIG. 10–7. Recommended combination of diet and exercise for overloading muscle glycogen stores during the week before an important contest. Exercise is gradually reduced during the week, and the carbohydrate content of the diet is increased for the last three days. (From Sherman, W.M., et al.: Effect of exercise-diet manipulation on muscle glycogen and its subsequent utilization during performance. *Int. J. Sports Med.* 2:114, 1981.)

THE PRECOMPETITION MEAL

Carbohydrate is favored as the main nutrient source for intense exercise, and is also crucially important as an energy source in prolonged exercise. The precompetition meal must therefore provide adequate quantities of this nutrient to assure normal levels of blood glucose and sufficient glycogen "energy reserves." This, of course, presumes that the person has maintained a nutritionally sound diet throughout training. As a general rule, foods high in lipid and protein content should be eliminated from the diet on the day of competition. These foods are digested slowly and remain in the digestive tract for a longer time than carbohydrate-rich foods of similar energy content. Furthermore, with the increased stress and tension that usually accompany competition, there may be significant diversion of blood from the intestines and an accompanying decrease in absorption from the digestive tract. A three-hour period generally is adequate for the meal to be digested and absorbed by the body.

High Protein Is Not the Best Choice. Many athletes are psychologically accustomed to and even depend on the "classic" pregame meal of steak and eggs. Although this meal may be satisfying to the athlete, coach, and restauranteur, its benefits have never been demonstrated in terms of improved exercise performance. In fact, a meal so low in carbohydrate may actually hinder optimal performance. For one thing, carbohydrates are digested and absorbed more rapidly than either proteins or lipids. Thus, carbohydrates are available for energy faster and may also reduce the feeling of fullness following a meal. A high-protein meal can also elevate the resting metabolism more than a high-carbohydrate meal. This added heat production may place a further strain on temperature regulation that could be detrimental to exercise performance in hot weather. Concurrently, the breakdown of protein for energy facilitates dehydration because the by-products of amino acid breakdown demand water for urinary excretion.

What to eat before competing. The main purpose of the precompetition or pregame meal is to provide the athlete with adequate food energy and assure optimal hydration.

LIQUID MEALS

Commercially prepared **liquid meals** offer an alternative and seemingly effective approach to pre-event feeding. These foods are generally well balanced in nutritive value; they are high in carbohydrate, yet contain enough lipid and protein to contribute to a feeling of satiety. Because they are in liquid form, they also contribute to the athlete's fluid needs. Another advantage is more rapid digestion, leaving essentially no residue in the intestinal tract. The liquid meal approach to nutrition on the day of competition is especially effective during day-long swimming and track meets or tennis and basketball tournaments. In these situations, an athlete may have relatively little time for or interest in food. Liquid meals are also practical for supplementing the caloric intake of athletes who have difficulty maintaining their body mass or who wish to increase it.

SUMMARY

1. Many dietary options are available for obtaining the required nutrients for tissue maintenance, repair, and growth. Within rather broad limits, the nutrient requirements of athletes and other individuals engaged in training can be achieved with a balanced diet.
2. With well-planned menus, the necessary vitamin, mineral, and protein requirements can be met with a food intake of about 1200 calories a day. Additional food can then be consumed to meet energy needs that fluctuate depending on the daily level of physical activity.
3. The RDA for protein is 0.8 g per kilogram of body mass. For the average man and woman, this is a liberal requirement and represents about 12% of the normal daily caloric intake.
4. Athletes generally consume two to four times the recommended protein intake because their greater caloric intake usually provides proportionately more protein.
5. Precise recommendations for lipid and carbohydrate intake have not been established. A prudent recommendation is that no more than 30% of daily calories be obtained from lipids; of this, the majority should be as unsaturated fatty acids. For people who are physically active, 60% or more of calories should come from carbohydrates, particularly polysaccharides. This generally represents between 400 and 600 g on a daily basis.
6. Because sustained, vigorous exercise can greatly increase energy expenditure, the most important factor determining the daily caloric re-

quirement is a person's level of physical activity. In all likelihood, the caloric requirements of most athletes do not exceed 4000 calories per day unless body mass is considerable. This high caloric intake usually greatly exceeds the RDA for protein, vitamins, and minerals.

7. Successive days of hard training can gradually deplete the body's glycogen reserves, even if the recommended carbohydrate intake is maintained. This could lead to training "staleness" because muscle glycogen takes several days to be fully replenished following a single session of prolonged exercise.
8. The optimal pre-event meal includes foods that are readily digested and contribute to the energy and fluid requirements of exercise. Consequently, it should be high in carbohydrate and relatively low in fat and protein. Clearly, the typical low-carbohydrate "steak-and-eggs" meal does not meet the pre-event nutrition requirements.
9. Commercially prepared liquid meals offer a practical approach to pre-event nutrition and caloric supplementation. These "meals" are well balanced in nutritive value, contribute to fluid needs, are absorbed rapidly, and leave practically no residue in the digestive tract.
10. Two or three hours is sufficient time to permit digestion and absorption of the pre-event meal.

RELATED LITERATURE

Applegate, E.A. Nutritional consideration for ultra-endurance performance. Int. J. Sports Nutr., 2:118, 1991.

Barnett, D.W., and Conlee, R.K.: The effects of a commercial dietary supplement on human performance. Am. J. Clin. Nutr., 40:586, 1984.

Berning, J.R., et al.: The nutritional habits of young adolescent swimmers. Int. J. Sports Nutr., 1:240, 1991.

Blair, S.N., et al.: Comparison of nutrient intake in middle-aged men and women and controls. Med. Sci. Sports Exerc., 13:310, 1981.

Blom, P.C.S., et al.: Effect of different post-exercise sugar diets on the rate of muscle glycogen synthesis. Med. Sci. Sports Exerc., 19:491, 1987.

Brouns, F., et al.: Eating, drinking, and cycling. A controlled Tour de France simulation study, Part I. Int. J. Sports Med., 10:532, 1989.

Brouns, F., et al.: Eating, drinking, and cycling. A controlled Tour de France simulation study, Part II. Effect of diet manipulation. Int. J. Sports Med., 10:541, 1989.

Burke, L.M., et al.: Dietary intakes and food use of groups of elite Australian male athletes. Int. J. Sport Med., *1*:378–394, 1991.

Candas, V., et al.: Hydration during exercise: effects on thermal and cardiovascular adjustments. Eur. J. Appl. Physiol., 55:113, 1986.

Carter, J.E., and Gisolfi, C.V.: Fluid replacement during and after exercise in the heat. Med. Sci. Sports Exerc., 21:532, 1989.

Coggan, A.R., and Coyle, E.F.: Effect of carbohydrate feedings during high-intensity exercise. J. Appl. Physiol., 65:1703, 1988.

Coggan, A.R., and Coyle, E.F.: Metabolism and performance following carbohydrate ingestion late in exercise. Med. Sci. Sports Exerc., 21:59, 1989.

Coggan, A.R., et al.: Plasma glucose kinetics in a well-trained cyclist fed glucose throughout exercise. Int. J. Sports Nutr., 1:279, 1991.

Conner, W.E., et al.: The plasma lipids, lipoproteins and the diet of the Tarahumara Indians of Mexico. Am. J. Clin. Nutr., 31:1131, 1978.

Costill, D.L., et al.: Effects of repeated days of intensified training on muscle glycogen and swimming performance. Med. Sci. Sports Exerc., 20:249, 1988.

Coyle, E.F., and Coggan, A.R.: Effectiveness of carbohydrate feeding in delaying fatigue during prolonged exercise. Sports Med., 1:446, 1984.

Coyle, E.F., et al.: Muscle glycogen utilization during prolonged strenuous exercise when fed carbohydrate. J. Appl. Physiol., 61:165, 1986.

Davis, J.M., et al.: Fluid availability of sports drinks differing in carbohydrate type and concentration. Am. J. Clin. Nutr., 51:1054, 1990.
Deuster, P.A., et al.: Nutritional survey of highly trained women runners. Am. J. Clin. Nutr., 44:954, 1986.
Erp-Baart, A.M.J. van, et al.: Nationwide survey on nutritional habits in elite athletes, Part I. Energy, carbohydrate, protein, and fat intake. Int. J. Sports Med., 10:53, 1989.
Foster, C., et al.: Effects of pre-exercise feedings on endurance performance. Med. Sci. Sports Exerc., 11:1, 1979.
Grandjean, A.C.: Macronutrient intakes of U.S. athletes compared with the general population and recommendations made for athletes. Am. J. Clin. Nutr., 49:1070, 1989.
Hargreaves, M., and Briggs, C.A.: Effect of carbohydrate ingestion on exercise metabolism. J. Appl. Physiol., 65:1553, 1988.
Hargreaves, M., et al.: Effect of fructose ingestion on muscle glycogen usage during exercise. Med. Sci. Sports Exerc., 176:360, 1985.
Hargreaves, M., et al.: Effect of pre-exercise carbohydrate feedings on endurance cycling performance. Med. Sci. Sports Exerc., 19:33, 1987.
Hickson, J.F., et al.: Nutritional profile of football athletes eating from a training table. Nutr. Rev., 7:27, 1987.
Horton, E.S., and Terjung, R.L. (Eds.): Exercise, Nutrition, and Energy Metabolism. New York, Macmillan, 1988.
Horwitt, M.D.: Interpretations of requirements for thiamin, riboflavin, niacin-tryptophan, and vitamin E plus comments on balance studies and vitamin B-6. Am. J. Clin. Nutr., 44:973, 1986.
Jandrain, B., et al.: Metabolic availability of glucose ingested three hours before prolonged exercise in humans. J. Appl. Physiol., 56:1314, 1984.
Katch, F.I., and Katch, V.L.: Computer technology to evaluate body composition, nutrition, and exercise. Prev. Med., 12:619, 1983.
Knapit, J.J., et al.: Influence of a 3.5 day fast on physical performance. Eur. J. Appl. Physiol., 56:583, 1987.
Koivisto, V.A., et al.: Glycogen depletion during prolonged exercise: influence of glucose, fructose, or placebo. J. Appl. Physiol., 58:731, 1985.
Lamb, D.R., et al.: Muscle glycogen loading with a liquid carbohydrate supplement. Int. J. Sports Nutr., 1:28, 1991.
Lindeman, A.K.: Eating for endurance or ultraendurance. Phys. Sports Med., 20:87, 1992.
Mayer, J., et al.: Relation between caloric intake, body weight, and physical work in an industrial male population in West Bengal. Am. J. Clin. Nutr., 4:169, 1956.
Mitchell, J.B., et al.: Effects of carbohydrate ingestion on gastric emptying and exercise performance. Med. Sci. Sports Exerc., 20:110, 1988.
Murray, R., et al.: The effects of glucose, fructose, and sucrose ingestion during exercise. Med. Sci. Sports Exerc., 21:275, 1989.
Neufer, P.D., et al.: Effects of exercise and carbohydrate composition on gastric emptying. Med. Sci. Sports Exerc., 18:658, 1986.
Nieman, D., et al.: Running endurance in 27-hr-fasted humans. J. Appl. Physiol., 63:2502, 1987.
Reed, M.J., et al.: Muscle glycogen storage post-exercise: effect of mode of carbohydrate administration. J. Appl. Physiol., 67:720, 1989.
Roberts, K.M., et al.: Simple and complex carbohydrate-rich diets and muscle glycogen content of marathon runners. Eur. J. Appl. Physiol., 57:70, 1988.
Ryan, A.J., et al.: Gastric emptying during prolonged exercise in the heat. Med. Sci. Sports Exerc., 21:51, 1989.
Scott, C.B., et al.: Effect of macronutrient composition of an energy-restrictive diet on maximal physical performance. Med. Sci. Sports Exerc., 24:814, 1992.
Seiple, R.S., et al.: Gastric emptying characteristics of two glucose polymer-electrolyte solutions. Med. Sci. Sports Exerc., 15:366, 1986.
Sherman, W.M., and Costill, D.L.: The marathon: dietary manipulation to optimize performance. Am. J. Clin. Nutr., 12:44, 1984.
Sherman, W.M., and Wimer, G.S.: Insufficient carbohydrate during training: does it impair performance? Int. J. Sports Nutr., 1:28, 1991.
Sherman, W.M., et al.: Effect of exercise-diet manipulation on muscle glycogen and its subsequent utilization during performance. Int. J. Sports Med., 1:114, 1981.
Sherman, W.M., et al.: Effect of carbohydrate in four pre-exercise meals. Med. Sci. Sports Exerc., 20:S157, 1988.

Sole, C.C., and Naokes, T.D.: Faster emptying for glucose-polymer and fructose solutions than for glucose in humans. Eur. J. Appl. Physiol., 58:605, 1989.
Stare, F.J., and McWilliams, M.: Health and nutrition throughout the life cycle. Med. Exerc. Nutr. Health., 1:16, 1992.
Storlie, J.: Nutrition assessment of athletes: a model for integrating nutrition and physical performance indicators. Int. J. Sports Nutr., 2:118, 1991.
Tarnopolsky, M.A., et al.: Influence of protein intake and training status on nitrogen balance and lean body mass. J. Appl. Physiol., 64:187, 1988.
Werblow, J.A.: Nutritional knowledge, attitudes, and food patterns of women athletes. J. Am. Diet. Assoc., 73:242, 1978.
Yannick, C., et al.: Oxidation of corn starch, glucose, and fructose ingested before exercise. Med. Sci. Sports Exerc., 21:45, 1989.

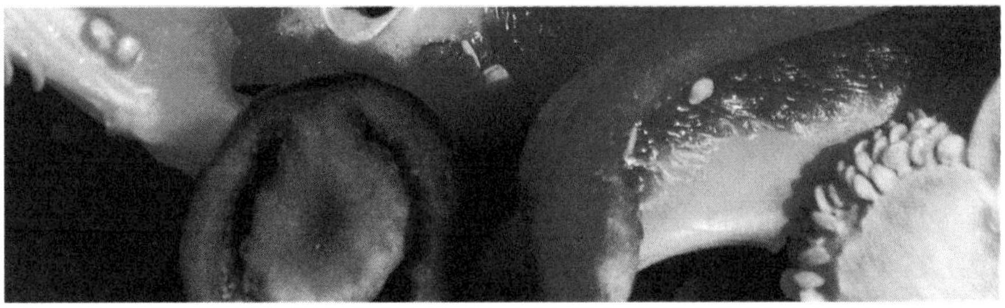

11

ENERGY FOR EXERCISE

In an automobile engine, the proper mixture of gasoline with oxygen ignites to provide the necessary energy to drive the pistons. Various gears and linkages harness this energy to turn the wheels, and increasing or decreasing the energy supply either speeds up or slows down the engine. Similarly, the human body must continuously be supplied with its own form of energy to perform its many complex functions. Aside from the energy required for muscle contraction, the body expends considerable energy for other forms of **biologic work.** This includes the energy required for digestion, absorption, and assimilation of food nutrients, for the function of various glands that secrete special hormones at rest and during exercise, for establishment of the proper electrochemical gradients along cell membranes to permit transmission of signals from the brain via the nerves to the muscles, and for synthesis of new chemical compounds such as the protein in muscle tissue that becomes enlarged from specialized strength training. The story of how the body maintains its continuous supply of energy begins with the energy currency, ATP.

ENERGY PRODUCTION IN THE BODY

THE ENERGY CURRENCY, ADENOSINE TRIPHOSPHATE

Energy. From a broad perspective, **energy** can be viewed as the capacity or ability to do work.

Our cells do not use the nutrients in the diet for their immediate energy supply. Instead, the energy-rich compound **adenosine triphosphate,** or simply ATP, is the "fuel" for *all* the energy-requiring processes of the cell. In turn, the energy in food is extracted to rebuild more ATP. The potential energy stored within the ATP molecule represents chemical energy made in the body as it is needed. As discussed in Chapter 1, molecules are composed of atoms held together by bonds. It is the breaking of these bonds that releases energy. Figure 11–1 illustrates a simplified structure of an ATP molecule.

ATP consists of one molecule of adenine and ribose, called adenosine,

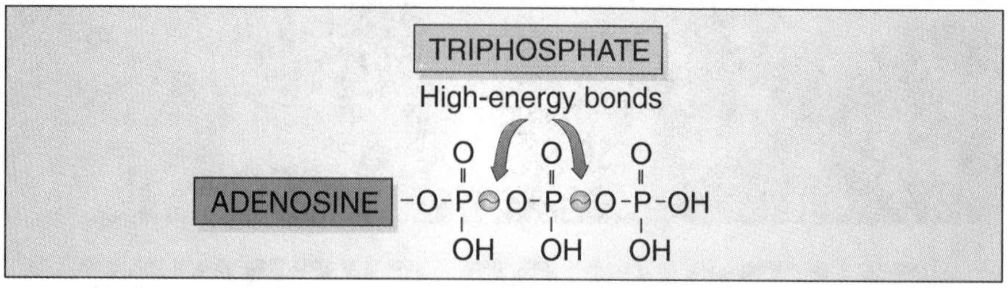

FIG. 11–1. Simplified structure of ATP, the energy currency of the cell. The symbol (~) represents the high-energy bonds.

combined with three phosphates, each consisting of phosphorus and oxygen atoms. A considerable quantity of energy is stored in the ATP molecule at the bonds that link the two outermost phosphate groups with the remainder of the molecule. These bonds, symbolized by (~), represent the high-energy phosphate bonds. When the outermost bond is broken, it releases energy to power biologic work. The remaining molecule with one high-energy bond is known as **adenosine diphosphate,** or ADP.

Energy released from the breakdown of ATP activates other energy-requiring molecules. For example, phosphate-bond energy is transferred to the molecules that make up the contractile elements in muscle tissue. Once activated, these elements slide past each other, causing the muscle to shorten. Because the energy released from ATP is harnessed to power all forms of biologic work, ATP is considered the "energy currency" of the cell (Figure 11–2).

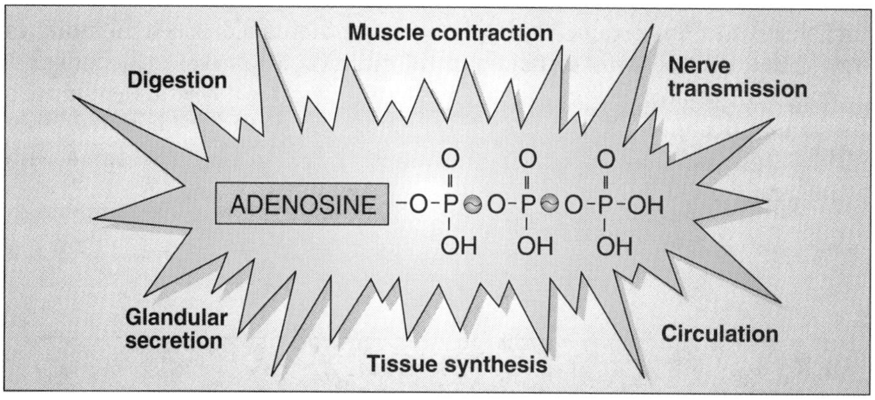

FIG. 11–2. ATP is the energy currency for all forms of biologic work.

Rapid energy release. Anaerobic energy release can be viewed as an emergency or back-up power source that is called upon when the body requires energy in excess of what can be generated aerobically.

Aerobic and Anaerobic Energy Release. Energy-releasing reactions that depend on a constant supply of oxygen are **aerobic.** For example, if the flow of oxygen through the carburetor of an automobile engine is restricted, the energy supply is reduced and the engine will lose power and eventually stall. This is not the case, however, with the breakdown of ATP. Instead, the ATP molecule releases its energy *without* utilizing oxygen. This is an **anaerobic** energy-releasing reaction. The capacity to provide energy anaerobically enables the cell to generate energy for immediate use. Such immediate energy would not be available if oxygen were required at all times. For this reason we can sprint for a bus, lift considerable weight without taking a breath, and survive submersion under water for a minute or more.

THE ENERGY RESERVOIR, CREATINE PHOSPHATE

Although ATP serves as the energy currency for all cells, its quantity is limited. In fact, only about 85 g (3 oz) of ATP is stored in the body at any one time. This would provide only enough energy for running all-out for several seconds. Consequently, ATP must constantly be resynthesized to provide a continuous supply of energy. Some of the energy for ATP resynthesis is supplied directly and rapidly by the anaerobic splitting of a phosphate molecule from another energy-rich compound, **creatine phosphate** or CP. This molecule is similar to ATP because a large amount of energy is released when the bond between its creatine and phosphate molecules is split. Figure 11–3 presents a schematic illustration of the release and use of the phosphate-bond energy in ATP and CP.

In the bottom panel of Figure 11–3, the arrows point in opposite directions to indicate that the reactions are reversible: that is, creatine (C) and phosphate (P) can be joined again to form CP. This is also true for ATP, shown in the top panel, where the union of ADP and P reforms ATP. Resynthesis of ATP occurs if sufficient energy is available to rejoin an ADP molecule with one P molecule. The breakdown of CP can supply this energy, as illustrated in the second panel of the figure. Cells store CP in considerably larger quantities than ATP. Its mobilization for energy is almost instantaneous and does not require oxygen. For this reason, CP is considered the "reservoir" of high-energy phosphate.

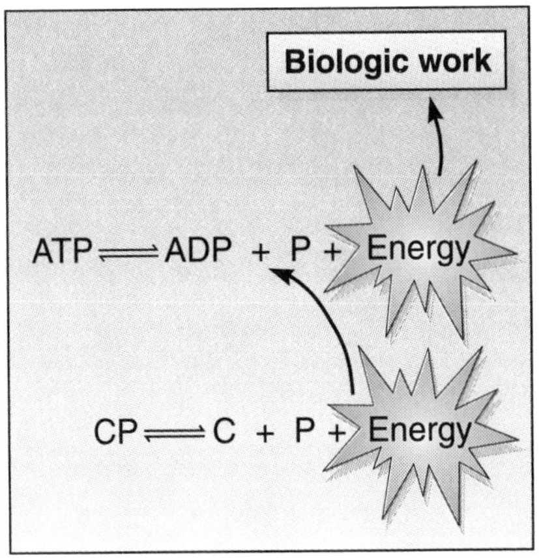

FIG. 11–3. ATP and CP are anaerobic sources of phosphate-bond energy. The energy from the breakdown of CP is used to rebond ADP and P to form ATP.

THE ATP-CP ENERGY SYSTEM

The energy released from the breakdown of the energy-rich phosphates ATP and CP can sustain all-out exercise, such as running or swimming, for approximately 5 to 8 seconds. In the 100-yard dash, the body cannot maintain maximum speed for longer than this. During the last few seconds of the sprint, the runners are actually slowing down, and the winner is the one who slows down least! Thus, as illustrated in Figure 11–4, mobilization of energy from the phosphate pool (ATP + CP), and the size of the pool, are important factors that determine one's ability to maintain maximum speed over a short distance.

The high-energy phosphates. To appreciate the importance of the high-energy phosphates in exercise, consider activities in which short, intense bursts of energy are crucial to success. Football, tennis, track and field, golf, volleyball, field hockey, baseball, weight lifting, and wood chopping are examples of activities that often require maximal effort for up to 8 seconds.

In almost all sports, the capacity of the ATP-CP energy system plays a role in the success or failure of some phase of performance. If all-out effort must continue beyond 8 seconds, however, or if moderate exercise is to continue for much longer periods, an additional source of energy is required to resynthesize ATP. If this does not happen, our "fuel" would be depleted and movement would cease. *The foods we eat and store for ready access in the body provide the energy for continually recharging the supply of ATP and CP.*

Identification of the predominant sources of energy required for a particular sport or physical activity provides the basis for an effective physiologic conditioning program. A person who desires an improved capacity for sustained effort such as hiking or distance swimming, for example, would find it unprofitable to train specifically to increase ATP-CP reserves. On the other hand, a highly developed ATP-CP energy system is of considerable importance in sports such as football and baseball.

Training the immediate energy system. Sprint-type, heavy training requiring repeat intervals of 6 to 10 seconds of all-out exercise in a specific activity increases the muscles' quantity of high-energy phosphates. This will enhance subsequent sprint performance.

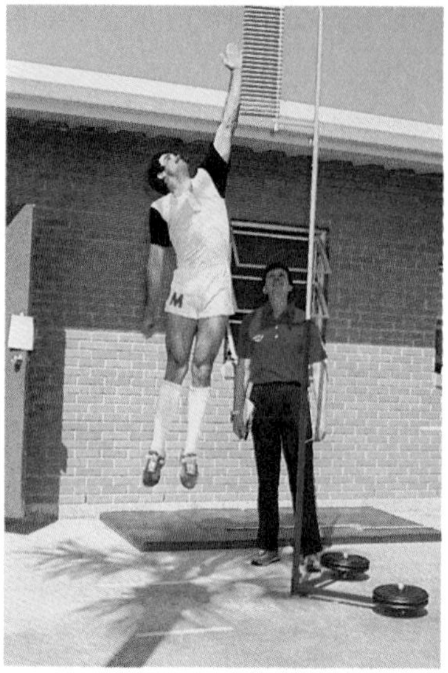

A

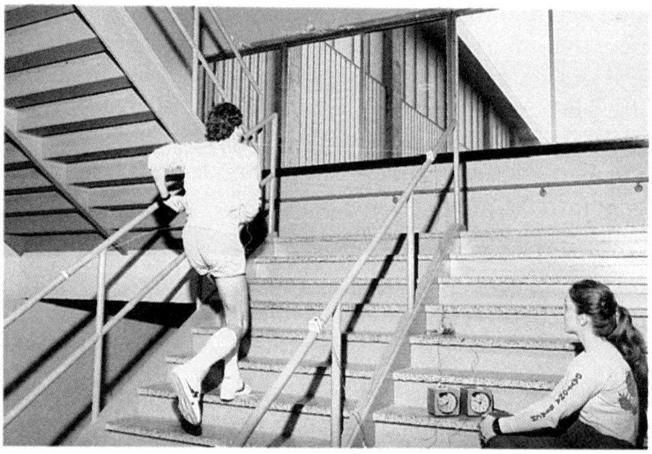

B

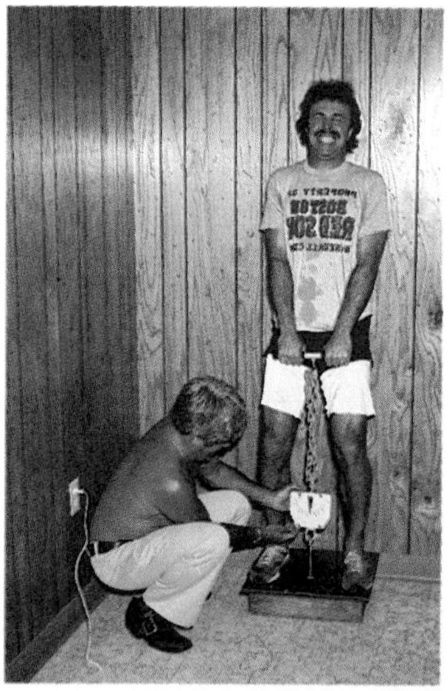

C

FIG. 11–4. The high-energy phosphates ATP and CP are important during many forms of all-out, intense bursts of physical activity. A. Vertical jump test. B. All-out test of power during a 6-meter sprint. C. Test of maximum strength.

ENERGY FROM FOOD

As shown in Figure 11–5, the body extracts the potential energy within the structures of the carbohydrate, lipid, and protein molecules consumed in the diet or stored in the body. *This energy is harnessed for one purpose: to combine ADP and phosphate to reform the energy-rich compound ATP.*

Heat Energy Cannot Be Used for Biologic Work. A flaming steak on a barbecue grill illustrates the potential energy contained in food. The flame from the barbecue ignites the fat in the meat, causing it to suddenly release its stored energy in the form of heat. In the cells of the body, however, energy is not released suddenly at some kindling temperature and then dissipated as heat. On the contrary, the energy produced by the breaking of chemical bonds is released gradually, at a constant, fairly low temperature, through a series of chemical reactions controlled by highly specific

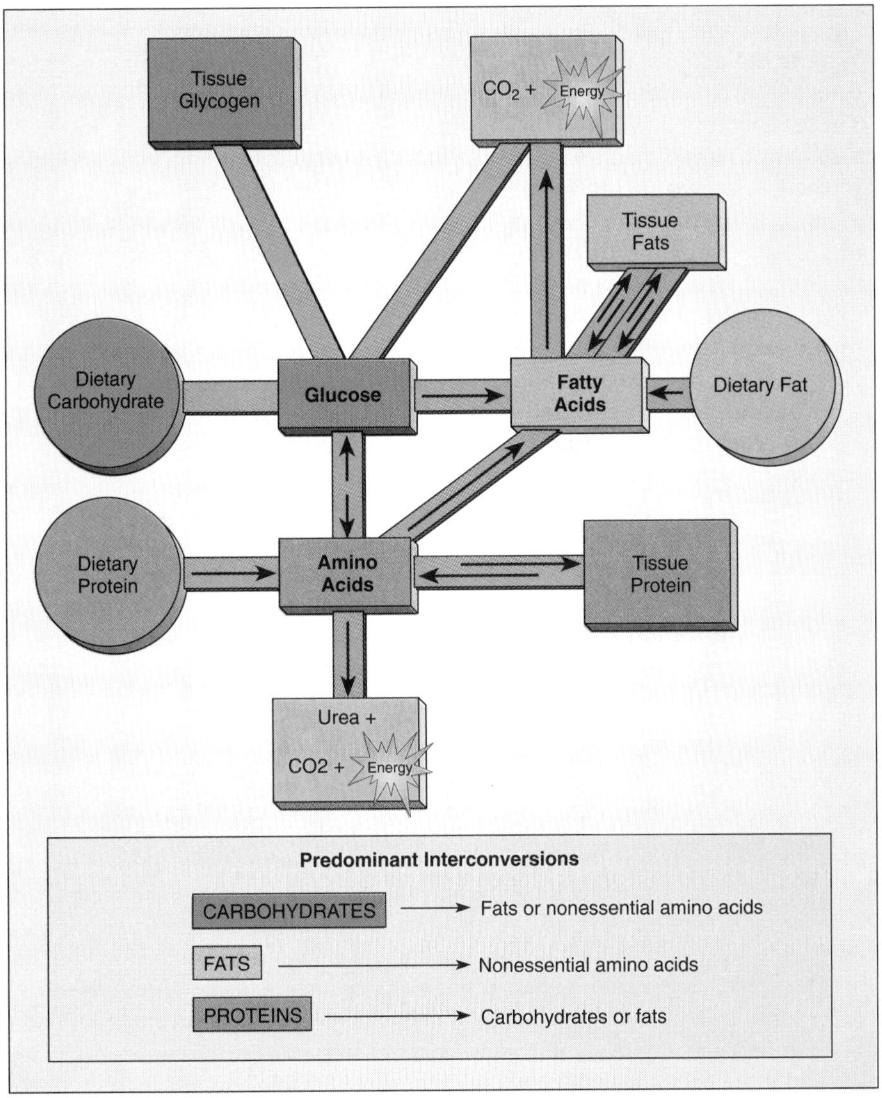

FIG. 11–5. The metabolic mill: interconversions between carbohydrates, lipids, and proteins.

enzymes. As pointed out in Chapter 1, enzymes regulate the speed of reactions by helping to bring molecules together so they interact with one another. The end result of the breakdown of foods is liberation of energy, of which approximately 40% is captured and stored for later use as **chemical energy** in the bonds of ATP. This efficiency is quite impressive compared with machines such as the steam engine, which transforms its fuel into useful energy with an efficiency of only about 30%. The remaining energy is dissipated in the form of heat.

The metabolism of glucose illustrates the ways cells extract and capture the chemical energy contained in food. This example is used for several reasons. First, carbohydrate is the only macronutrient that provides energy anaerobically to form ATP. Second, under conditions of rest and low to moderate exercise in well-nourished individuals, carbohydrate supplies between 30 and 60% of the body's energy requirements. Third, during carbohydrate breakdown certain compounds are formed so the lipid and protein nutrients can be continually metabolized for energy.

ANAEROBIC ENERGY FROM FOOD

When a molecule of glucose enters a cell to be used for energy, it immediately undergoes a series of chemical reactions collectively termed **glycolysis.** These reactions do not require oxygen and are referred to as anaerobic. As a result of enzyme action, the original 6-carbon glucose molecule is transformed into two 3-carbon molecules of pyruvic acid. The breakdown of glucose to pyruvic acid occurs in the watery medium of the cell. Three important events occur during glycolysis: first, the bonds that chemically bind glucose are broken; second, hydrogen atoms are stripped from the glucose molecule; and third, two new molecules of ATP are generated.

The anaerobic macronutrient. During high-intensity, fatiguing exercise in which anaerobic reactions predominate, carbohydrates are the main source of energy supply.

The extraction of usable energy in the form of two ATP molecules during glycolysis represents only about 5% of the total ATPs produced when glucose is completely degraded to carbon dioxide and water in subsequent aerobic reactions. Nevertheless, *ATP production during glycolysis is important because it provides a rapid source of energy for muscular activity.* The anaerobic energy from glucose can be thought of as a reserve of "rapid" food energy for resynthesis of ATP. For example, this energy reserve is utilized by the athlete "kicking" the last part of a 1- or 2-mile race, or the basketball team employing a full-court press during the final minutes of a close game. In other short-duration but high-intensity activities such as a 440-yard run or 100-yard swim, the predominant supply of energy for ATP production also comes from the anaerobic reactions of glycolysis.

Glycolysis is for rapid energy release. The cells' capacity for glycolysis is crucial during physical activities requiring all-out effort for periods of up to 90 seconds.

AEROBIC ENERGY FROM FOOD

Because the anaerobic reactions of glycolysis release only 5% of the energy in a glucose molecule, an additional means is available to extract the remainder. This takes place when pyruvic acid molecules are converted to a 2-carbon form of acetic acid, **acetyl CoA.** This process releases hydrogen atoms and carbon dioxide. Acetyl CoA then passes into the **mitochondria,** highly specialized structures within the cell that serve as its "powerhouses" or "energy factories," where over 90% of the total ATP is produced. Figure 11–6 shows a simplified diagram of the release of hydrogen atoms during the complete breakdown of glucose in both anaerobic and aerobic reactions. In the cytoplasm, hydrogen atoms are released as glucose is degraded to

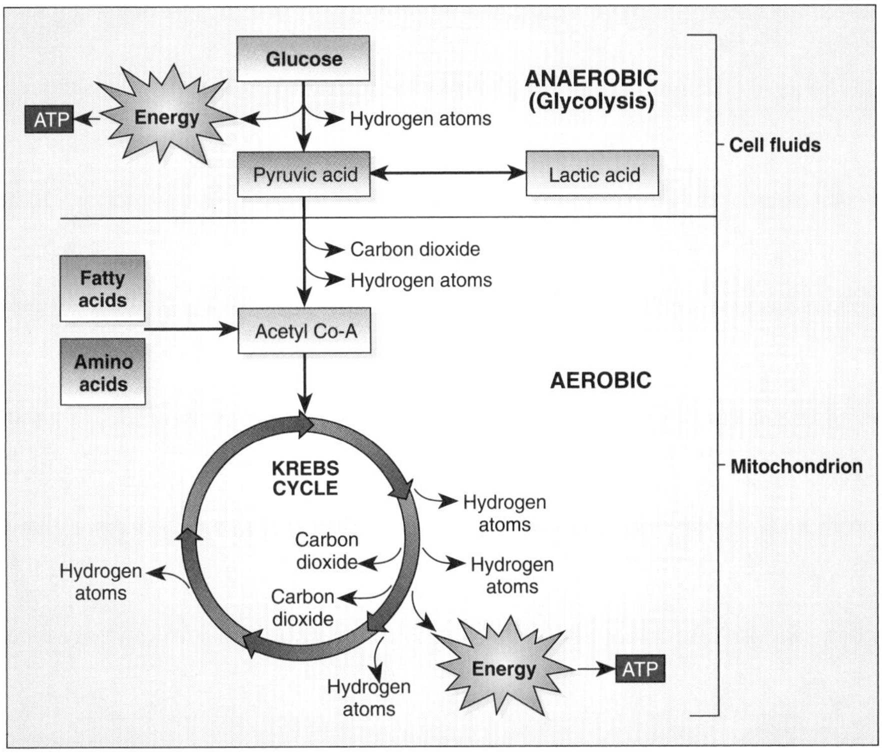

FIG. 11–6. Extraction of hydrogen during the complete breakdown of glucose. Note the energy release during glycolysis and Krebs cycle oxidation. Also indicated are the pathways for utilization of lipids and amino acids at the level of acetyl CoA during aerobic reactions.

pyruvic acid in glycolysis and during the subsequent transformation of pyruvic acid to acetyl CoA. In the mitochondria, carbon and hydrogen atoms are stripped from the molecules of acetyl CoA. The process generates two molecules of ATP, 16 additional hydrogen atoms are set free, and four molecules of carbon dioxide are formed. In similar fashion, this "metabolic mill" also extracts hydrogen from fragments of lipid and protein (amino acid) breakdown. This aspect of the chemical breakdown of acetyl CoA is known as the **Krebs cycle.**

Named for a Nobel laureate. The Krebs cycle was named after the chemist Hans Krebs, who was awarded the Nobel Prize in 1953 for his pioneering studies of these vital metabolic processes.

The freeing of hydrogen atoms from carbohydrate, lipid, and protein molecules during the Krebs cycle is one of the most important chemical events in the cell. The right-hand portion of Figure 11–7 shows the transport of hydrogen through another series of chemical reactions in which the atoms are changed into electrically charged particles. Like a bucket brigade, the electrons from hydrogen are then passed by special carrier molecules through a funneling chain of reactions until they reach "the end of the line" where they combine with oxygen to form water. *This process of aerobic metabolism is the most crucial phase of energy metabolism; it is during the transfer of electrons from hydrogen to oxygen that energy is produced to drive the rebonding of P to ADP to reform ATP.* While the rapid anaerobic release of energy from glucose during glycolysis largely determines maximum, short-term exercise performance, it is an individual's capacity for aerobic resynthesis of ATP that is crucial to performance in physical activities that last beyond 2 minutes.

The diagram of the various pathways of metabolism shown in Figure 11–5 also depicts possible interconversions between the foods and potential

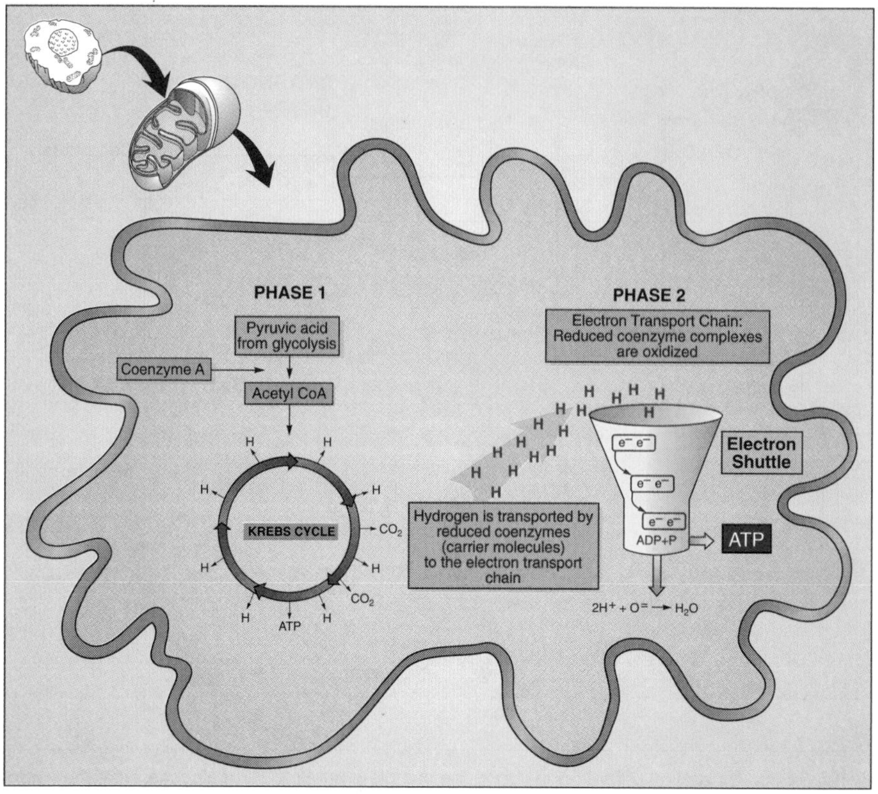

FIG. 11–7. In the mitochondria, the Krebs cycle generates hydrogen atoms during the breakdown of acetyl-CoA (PHASE 1). These hydrogens are then oxidized by the aerobic process of electron transport–oxidative phosphorylation that regenerates significant quantities of ATP (PHASE 2).

Carbohydrate intake is crucial. Although gluconeogenesis provides a metabolic option for making glucose from noncarbohydrate sources, this process cannot maintain glycogen stores unless carbohydrates are consumed in the diet.

routes for nutrient synthesis. Excess carbohydrates, for example, provide the fragments for lipid synthesis and can also donate their "carbon skeleton" for some protein synthesis. Likewise, certain amino acids can be used to synthesize glucose (gluconeogenesis). Because the conversion of carbohydrate to lipid is not reversible (notice the one-way arrow), fatty acids cannot be used to synthesize glucose. This makes dietary sources of carbohydrate crucial for maintaining glycogen reserves.

OXYGEN UPTAKE DURING EXERCISE

Although the rapid energy release from anaerobic metabolism is of considerable importance in certain situations where energy is required immediately to perform a task, the total amount of ATP resynthesized in this manner is relatively small. In contrast, during aerobic metabolism, chemical energy stored in the molecules of carbohydrates, lipids, and to a lesser degree proteins provides a continual supply of ATP.

STEADY STATE

The curve in Figure 11–8 illustrates the amount of oxygen utilized by the body during a relatively slow, steady jog for 20 minutes. The usage of

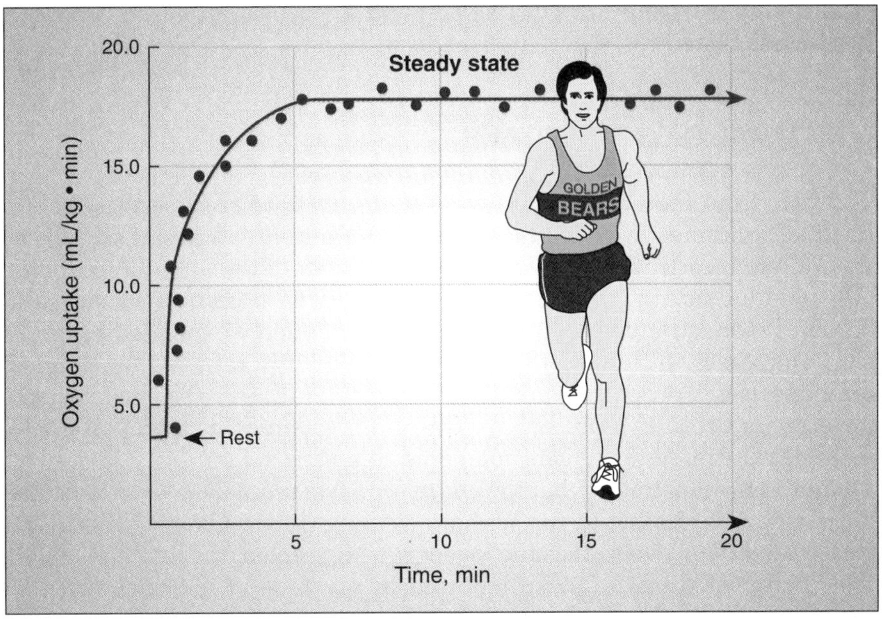

FIG. 11–8. Time course of oxygen uptake during continuous jogging at a relatively slow pace for 20 minutes. The dots along the curve represent measured values of oxygen uptake determined by open-circuit spirometry described in Chapter 13.

Oxygen uptake and body size. To adjust for the effects of **variations in body size on oxygen uptake** (that is, bigger people consume more oxygen), oxygen uptake is often expressed in terms of body mass, as milliliters of oxygen per kilogram of body mass per minute, or ml/kg/min. At rest, the average person's oxygen uptake is between 3.0 and 4.0 ml/kg/min, or about 250 ml/min (one-fourth of a liter).

oxygen by the cells, referred to as **oxygen uptake,** is indicated on the vertical axis (Y-axis) of the graph; the horizontal or X-axis shows exercise time. Oxygen uptake during any minute can easily be determined by locating the time on the X-axis and its corresponding point for oxygen uptake on the Y-axis.

During the first 3 minutes of exercise, oxygen uptake rises steeply above the resting level. The curve then begins to level off during minutes 4 and 5, and remains essentially unchanged during the last 15 minutes of jogging. The horizontal or flat part of the curve is referred to as **steady state.** The steady state, or plateau, in oxygen uptake represents a balance between the energy required by working muscles and the aerobic energy-releasing reactions. Theoretically, once a steady state is attained, exercise could go on indefinitely if the individual so desired. However, factors other than motivation place a limit on the duration of steady-state work. These include loss of important body fluids in sweat and depletion of essential nutrients, especially blood glucose and glycogen stored in the liver and muscles.

The rapid attainment of steady state. An individual who is trained by predominantly aerobic exercise reaches a steady state more rapidly compared to someone who is untrained. This facilitated level of aerobic metabolism early in exercise may be the result of training-induced cellular adaptations that are known to increase the capacity of muscle to generate ATP aerobically.

There Are Many Levels of Steady State. Steady-state exercise for the athlete could be exhausting for an untrained person. For some of us, lying in bed, working around the house, and playing an occasional round of golf represent the spectrum of activity for which adequate oxygen can be utilized to maintain a steady state. A champion marathon runner, on the other hand, can run 26 miles in slightly more than 2 hours and still be in steady state. This 5-minute-per-mile pace is a magnificent accomplishment in terms of the many physiologic functions involved. One of these important functions is delivering adequate oxygen to the exercising muscles. Another is the cells' ability to utilize this oxygen in the aerobic process of energy metabolism. Clearly, training programs to develop endurance must emphasize improvement in both *transport* and *utilization* of oxygen. Chapter 19 discusses how this is accomplished.

MAXIMAL OXYGEN UPTAKE

Consider from the previous example of steady-state exercise that the individual continues to jog at a comfortable pace until a series of six hills is encountered, each steeper than the next. The jogger's goal is to run up the hills without slowing down, although with each successive hill the task becomes more strenuous. Thus, the amount of energy expended progressively increases. In terms of oxygen uptake, energy release from aerobic reactions rises in proportion to exercise severity. As the hills become steeper, the exercise becomes more severe. This is accompanied by a proportionate and linear increase in oxygen uptake up to a certain limit.

Figure 11–9 illustrates what the curve for oxygen uptake would look like if the jogger were able to run without slowing down. Oxygen uptake increases and then levels off as the jogger runs up each of the first three hills. This increased oxygen uptake followed by leveling-off indicates that the runner has reached a progressively higher level of steady state. On the next two hills, oxygen uptake does not increase by the same amount compared to the first three hills. In fact, notice that oxygen uptake does not increase at all during the run up the steepest hill, even though the jogger was just able to make it to the top without slowing down! What occurs is that the runner attains a maximum capacity to generate energy aerobically and cannot increase it further. The region where work continues to become more difficult, yet oxygen uptake fails to increase, is referred to as the **maximal oxygen uptake,** or *max* $\dot{V}O_2$. It represents a person's maximum capacity to utilize oxygen during exercise.

Criterion for max $\dot{V}O_2$. Max $\dot{V}O_2$ is measured as the region where work continues to increase but oxygen uptake levels off or even declines slightly.

An important endurance component. The max $\dot{V}O_2$ is important in determining a person's capacity to sustain high-intensity exercise for longer than 4 to 5 minutes.

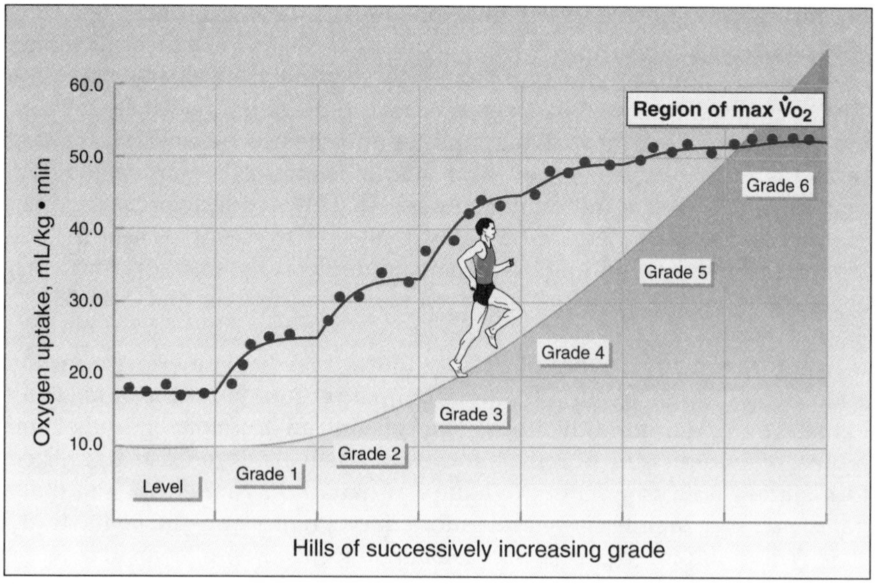

FIG. 11–9. Oxygen uptake while running up hills of increasing slope until the maximal oxygen uptake is reached. This occurs in the region where a further increase in exercise intensity is not accompanied by an additional increase in oxygen uptake. The dots represent measured values of oxygen uptake during each phase of running up the hills.

If a person exercises at an intensity above max $\dot{V}O_2$, as occurred when the jogger ran up the last hill, anaerobic metabolism must supply the additional energy for this work. This form of energy metabolism is crucial, because the energy from aerobic reactions is insufficient to meet the total requirements of the exercise. Because energy can be maximally supplied from anaerobic sources for only about 60 seconds, the runner soon would become exhausted and unable to continue.

Figure 11–10 compares the maximal oxygen uptake of male and female athletes with untrained, sedentary counterparts. The results show that the

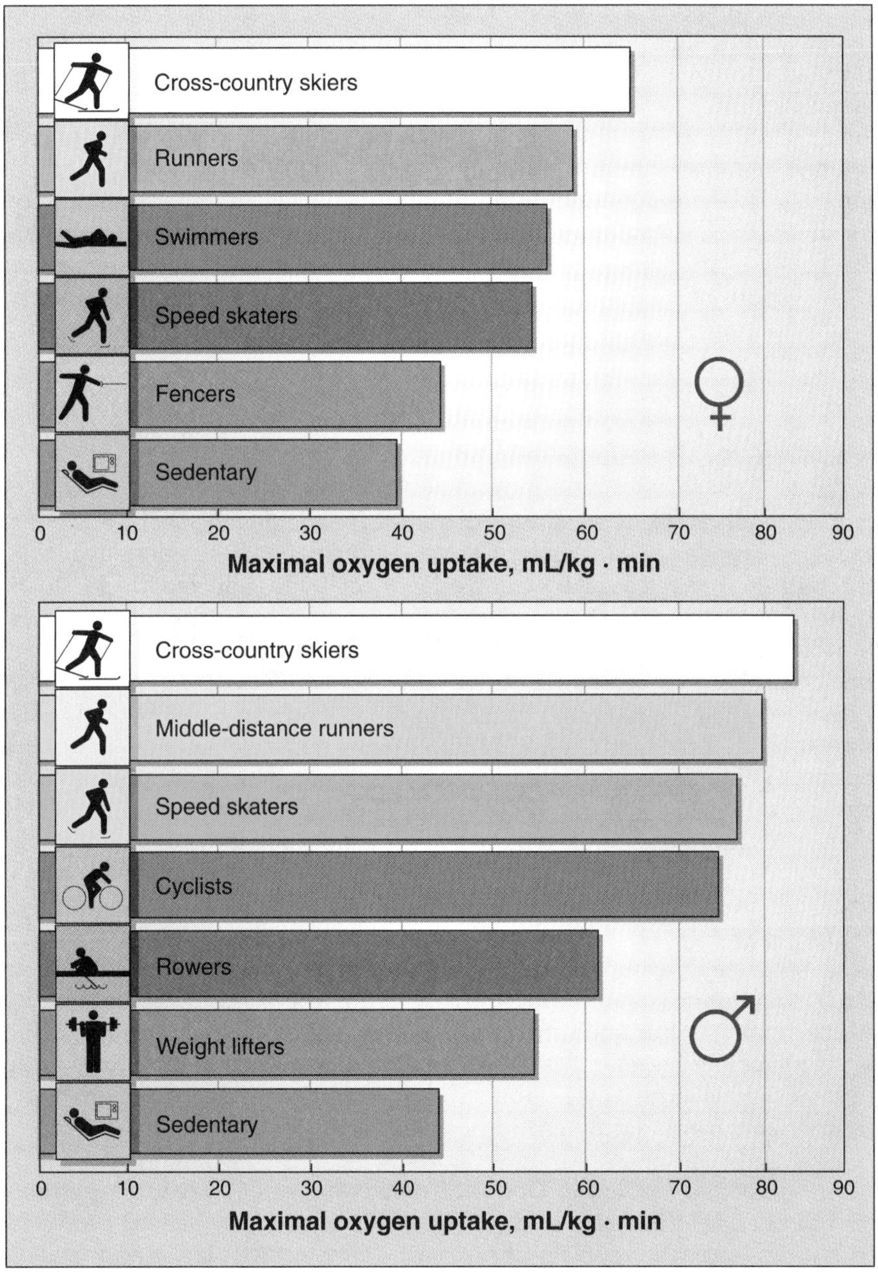

FIG. 11–10. Maximal oxygen uptake of male and female Olympic-caliber athletes and comparison to healthy sedentary subjects.

Additional body fat in women. The difference in body composition between genders is primarily attributable to the additional 5 to 9% of body mass that is essential fat in females. More than likely, this sex-specific fat is biologically important for childbearing and other hormone-related functions.

endurance athletes have nearly twice the aerobic capacity of the sedentary group. The finding that women have a 15 to 30% lower max $\dot{V}O_2$ than men of essentially equal training status is accounted for primarily by women possessing relatively more body fat (and less muscle mass and hemoglobin) than men. In fact, when a woman's max $\dot{V}O_2$ is expressed in relation to "fat-free" body mass, the difference between the genders becomes smaller. The additional fat tissue, although serving important biologic purposes, acts as "dead weight" in most physical activities.

Heritability is the controlling factor. While a vigorous program of physical training will enhance a person's level of fitness regardless of genetic background, it is clear that the limits for developing fitness capacity are also linked to natural endowment.

Is Fitness Capacity Inherited? An interesting question concerns whether inherited characteristics influence the max $\dot{V}O_2$ values presented in Figure 11–10. Although the answer is far from complete, heredity exerts a significant impact on the differences between individuals in fitness capacity. For example, in one study of 15 pairs of identical twins (same heredity) and 15 pairs of fraternal twins (separate fertilization of two eggs) raised in the same city and whose parents were of similar socioeconomic backgrounds, heredity alone accounted for up to 93% of observed differences in aerobic fitness! In addition, there is a high degree of heritability for muscle fiber type, maximum heart rate, anaerobic capacity, as well as the ability to improve fitness with training. Subsequent investigations of larger groups of brothers, fraternal twins, and identical twins have shown a significant but smaller effect of **inherited factors on aerobic capacity** and endurance performance.

LACTIC ACID PRODUCTION

Lactic acid formation permits glycolysis to continue. The temporary storage of hydrogen with pyruvic acid to form lactic acid is a unique aspect of energy metabolism because it allows glycolysis to continue to generate ATP anaerobically.

During moderate exercise, energy demands are adequately met by reactions that use oxygen. In biochemical terms, sufficient ATP is made available through energy released by the oxidation of hydrogen, mainly in slow-twitch muscle fibers (fast- and slow-twitch muscle fibers are explained later in this chapter). Figure 11–8 shows that under these conditions, a steady rate of aerobic metabolism can be comfortably maintained for a considerable time. As demands for energy become more severe, oxygen utilization by the working muscles must increase. During strenuous work, shown in Figure 11–9, oxygen uptake reaches a maximum value because aerobic energy-transfer reactions can no longer increase their energy output. Further increases in exercise intensity require proportionately more anaerobic energy metabolism through activation of a larger number of fast-twitch fibers. *At about 50 to 60% of max $\dot{V}O_2$, release of hydrogen through the anaerobic reactions of glycolysis begins to exceed its subsequent oxidation by aerobic pathways.* A steady state is no longer maintained because more hydrogen is produced than can combine with oxygen to form water. These excess hydrogens begin to accumulate in the active muscles, but their concentration does not build up significantly because the excess hydrogens combine temporarily with pyruvic acid. Figure 11–11 shows that joining two hydrogen atoms with pyruvic acid forms a new chemical called **lactic acid.**

An Important Metabolic Option. The advantage of converting pyruvic acid to lactic acid is that a ready "sump" is provided so the end products of glycolysis can temporarily disappear. Once formed, lactic acid (called **lactate** in its buffered form in blood) diffuses rapidly from muscle into the bloodstream and away from the site of metabolism. In this way, glycolysis

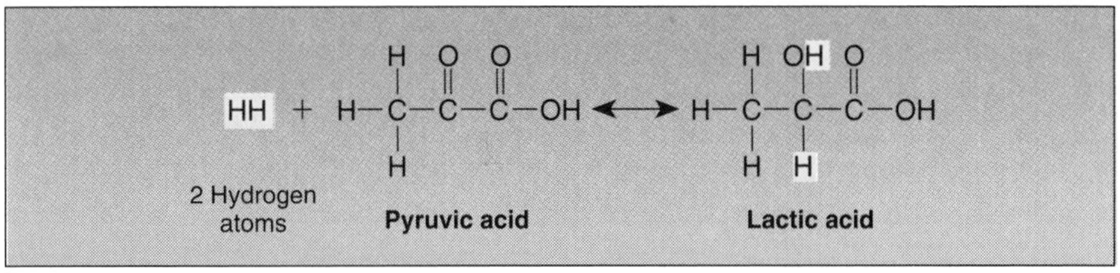

FIG. 11–11. Excess hydrogen molecules unable to combine with oxygen are passed by special carrier molecules to combine temporarily with pyruvic acid. This forms a new chemical, lactic acid. Note that the reaction is reversible.

can continue to supply additional energy anaerobically to resynthesize ATP. Consequently, exercise progresses despite an inadequate level of aerobic metabolism. However, this avenue for extra energy release is only temporary, because the level of circulating lactate increases rapidly as a plateau is reached for aerobic resynthesis of ATP. Lactate accumulation raises the acidity of the cellular environment and causes fatigue.

Training Enhances Lactate-Forming Tolerance. Studies of well-trained sprint athletes show that they become exhausted after strenuous exercise at blood lactate levels 20 to 30% higher than in untrained subjects under similar circumstances. An athlete's ability to tolerate high levels of blood lactate during competition may account in part for superior performance, especially in relatively short and intense physical activities such as sprint running and swimming.

BLOOD LACTATE ACCUMULATION DURING EXERCISE

Figure 11–12 compares the relationship between oxygen uptake and blood lactate accumulation during light, moderate, and heavy exercise in untrained subjects and endurance athletes. Oxygen uptake is expressed as a percentage of an individual's max $\dot{V}O_2$. For an untrained person with a max $\dot{V}O_2$ of 40 ml/kg/min, for example, exercise at 50% of maximum represents an exercise level requiring 20 ml/kg/min; for the trained counterpart with a 60 ml/kg/min aerobic capacity, the 50% level represents somewhat greater exercise at 30 ml/kg/min.

During light and moderate exercise, the blood lactate level remains fairly constant for both groups even though oxygen uptake is increased. Each of the two exercise intensities is maintained in steady state as the ATP for muscle contraction is generated by aerobic metabolism. During exercise that involves approximately 55% of the untrained subjects' max $\dot{V}O_2$, the blood lactate level in the blood begins to rise. The increase is even greater as exercise becomes more intense and the body cannot fully meet the additional energy demands aerobically. This pattern is essentially similar for trained athletes except that the threshold for lactate buildup, termed the **blood lactate threshold,** occurs at a higher percentage of aerobic capacity. This favorable response could result from the athletes' genetic endowment (type of muscle fiber) or more localized physiologic adaptations that occur with training (increased capillaries and aerobic enzymes, and larger and more numerous mitochondria). Such changes favor less lactic acid formation during more intense levels of exercise.

Blood lactate threshold. For both men and women, exercise intensity at the point of lactate accumulation, termed the *blood lactate threshold*, is a powerful predictor of performance in aerobic exercise. In one study of competitive race walkers, the walking speed at which blood lactate began to build up predicted race performance to within 0.6% of the actual time!

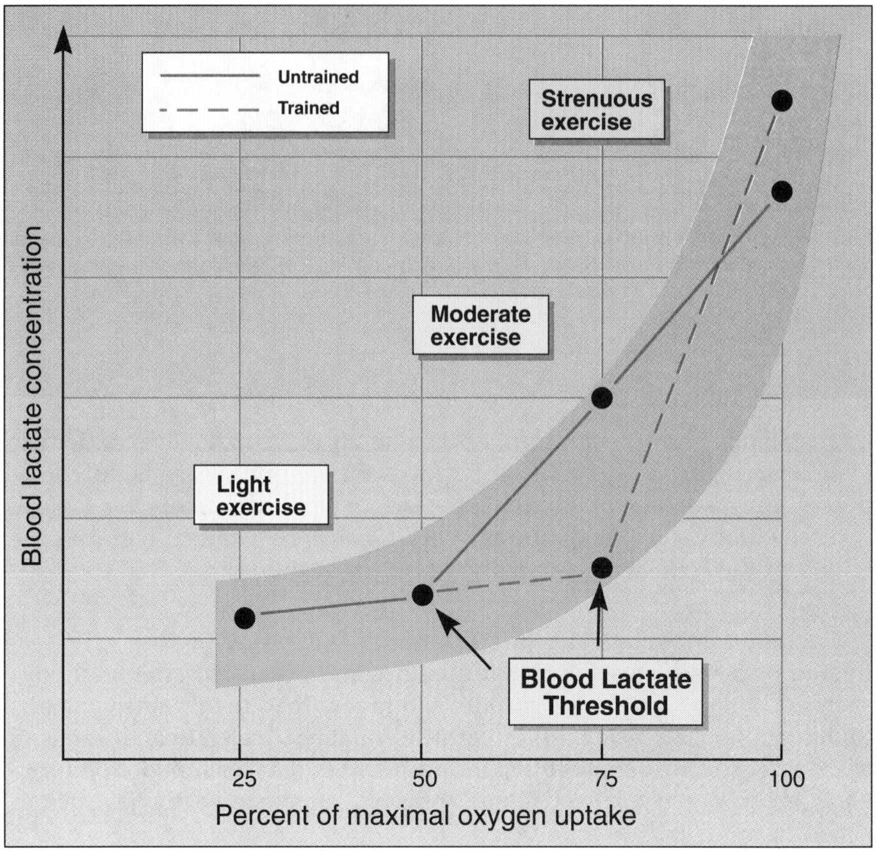

FIG. 11–12. Increases in blood lactate concentration at different levels of exercise expressed as a percentage of maximal oxygen uptake for trained and untrained subjects.

The muscle biopsy. Small fragments of muscle tissue about the size of a grain of rice are removed by means of surgical biopsy. Muscle fibers are then analyzed with chemical and microscopic techniques to determine their specific contractile and metabolic characteristics.

FAST- AND SLOW-TWITCH MUSCLE FIBERS

Biochemists and exercise physiologists are interested in the functional as well as structural differences in muscle fibers. Two distinct types of fibers have been identified in human skeletal muscle.

Fast-twitch Fiber. This muscle fiber, also called a *type II fiber,* possesses a high capacity for anaerobic production of ATP during glycolysis. The contraction speed of these fibers is rapid. **Fast-twitch muscle fibers** are activated in short-term, sprint activities that depend almost entirely on anaerobic metabolism for energy. The metabolic capabilities of fast-twitch fibers are also important in stop-and-go or change-of-pace sports such as basketball, soccer, lacrosse, or field hockey, which at times require rapid energy that can only be supplied through anaerobic metabolism.

Fast-twitch fibers. Subdivisions of type II fast-twitch fibers are present in humans. The *type IIa* fiber is considered intermediate because its fast contraction speed is combined with a moderately well developed capacity for both aerobic and anaerobic metabolism. The type *IIb* fiber is also fast contracting and possesses the greatest anaerobic capacity.

Slow-twitch Fiber. The **slow-twitch muscle fiber** has a contraction speed about half as fast as its fast-twitch counterpart. Slow-twitch fibers possess numerous mitochondria and a high concentration of the enzymes required to sustain aerobic metabolism. Their capacity to generate ATP aerobically is much greater than that of fast-twitch fibers. Hence, slow-twitch fibers are active in endurance activities that depend almost exclusively on aerobic metabolism. Middle-distance running or swimming, or sports such as basketball, field hockey, or soccer, require a blend of both aerobic and anaerobic capacities, and they activate both types of muscle fibers.

SOME QUESTIONS CONCERNING MUSCLE FIBER TYPES

In terms of exercise training and performance, several interesting questions arise concerning fast- and slow-twitch muscle fibers. First, does the distribution of each fiber differ significantly among people, especially those who are successful in various sports? Second, can the metabolic capacity of each fiber be improved through a specific program of physiologic conditioning? Third, can fast-twitch fibers be changed into slow-twitch fibers through aerobic training, and conversely, would anaerobic training develop predominantly fast-twitch fibers?

The answer to the first question is a definite yes. The average percentage of slow-twitch fibers in men and women is about 45 to 50%, but the variation is great. It seems logical that people with a large proportion of slow-twitch fibers in the leg muscles would be successful in endurance running, while those with a distribution favoring fast-twitch fibers would excel in sprinting. As shown in Figure 11–13, muscle biopsies from trained athletes support this contention. Successful endurance runners and cross-country skiers possess on average between 65 and 80% slow-twitch fibers in their leg

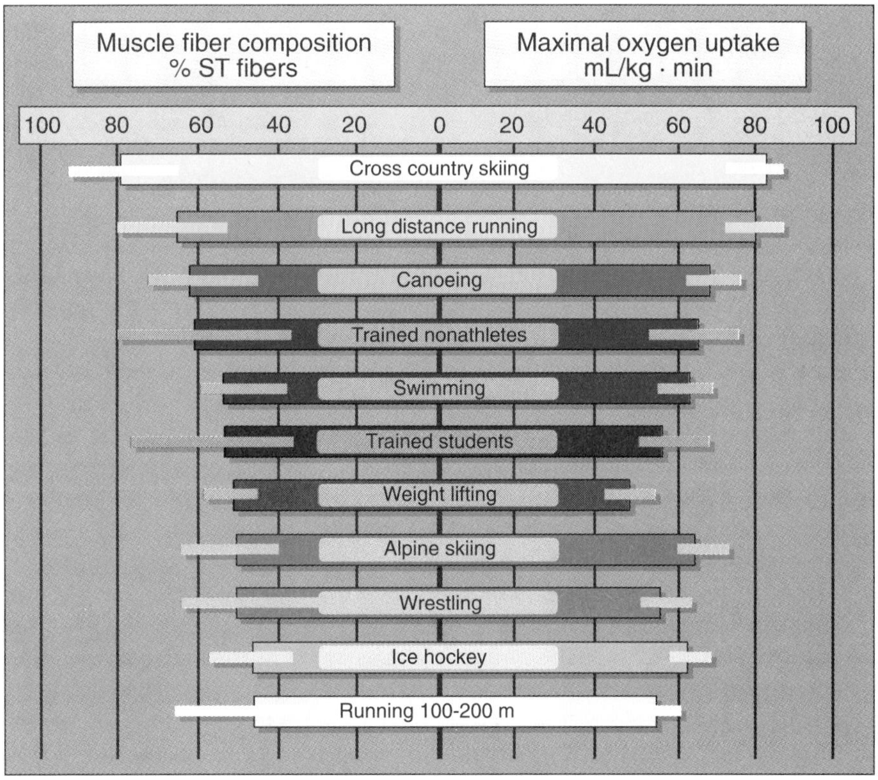

FIG. 11–13. Muscle fiber composition (percent slow-twitch [ST] fibers; left side) and maximal oxygen uptake (right side) in athletes representing different sports. (From Bergh, U., et al.: Maximal oxygen uptake and muscle fiber types in trained and untrained humans. *Med. Sci. Sports Exerc.* 10:151, 1978)

muscles, while sprint-type athletes possess a predominance of fast-twitch fibers. As might be expected, athletes who perform in middle-distance events have an approximately equal percentage of the two fiber types.

In an experiment designed to determine whether fiber type can be changed with training, six men were trained for 1 hour a day, 4 days a week for 5 months, at an exercise intensity between 75 and 90% of their max $\dot{V}O_2$. Fiber type determinations from the leg were made before and after training. Although the work capacity of all subjects increased, training did not change the relative distribution of fast- and slow-twitch muscle fibers. Additional studies with both humans and animals suggest the possibility of change in fiber type with specific and chronic exercise training. More research needs to be done in this intriguing area before definitive statements can be made concerning the fixed nature of a muscle's fiber composition.

In summary, the percentage distribution of fast- and slow-twitch muscle fibers differs significantly from one person to another and among various muscles in the same person. This distribution is probably determined by the genetic code and largely fixed before birth or early in life, and it cannot be greatly changed through physical conditioning. It also appears that a certain percentage of each fiber type is associated with success in sport activities, depending on their specific energy requirements. Although this suggests an obvious genetic predisposition for athletic success, training *can* significantly improve the metabolic capacity of both slow- and fast-twitch muscle fibers independent of an actual change in fiber type.

RECOVERY OXYGEN UPTAKE

After exercise ceases, breathing, pulse rate, and other bodily processes do not immediately return to resting levels. If the exercise is not too strenuous, recovery is fast and proceeds unnoticed. If the activity is strenuous, such as sprinting for a bus or swimming 100 yards as fast as possible, it takes considerable time to return to resting conditions. Recovery from both moderate and intense physical activity is associated largely with the specific metabolic processes involved in the particular form of exercise.

Figure 11–14 shows two curves for oxygen uptake during exercise and recovery. The exercise portion of the top curve is similar to the curve in Figure 11–8 and illustrates the change in oxygen uptake during the transition from rest to moderate, steady-state exercise. Oxygen uptake during the first 3 to 4 minutes of exercise increases progressively until metabolism reaches a steady state. At this point, oxygen-consuming reactions supply the energy for exercise. Little or no lactic acid accumulates in the muscles or blood under these aerobic conditions.

Not surprisingly, oxygen uptake does not increase instantaneously to the steady-state level because the immediate energy for muscular work is *always* provided directly by anaerobic breakdown of ATP. Oxygen is used only in subsequent reactions, when it combines with hydrogen atoms released during glycolysis and in the reactions of the Krebs cycle. Thus, there is a temporary **oxygen "deficit"** during the first few minutes of exercise. The amount of the deficit is shown to the left of the upward-trending curve of oxygen uptake. The anaerobic energy provided during the deficit phase of exercise represents energy that is "borrowed," so to speak, until the steady

Oxygen deficit. Quantitatively, the oxygen deficit represents the difference between the amount of oxygen actually consumed during exercise and the amount that would have been consumed had a steady state been immediately achieved as soon as exercise began.

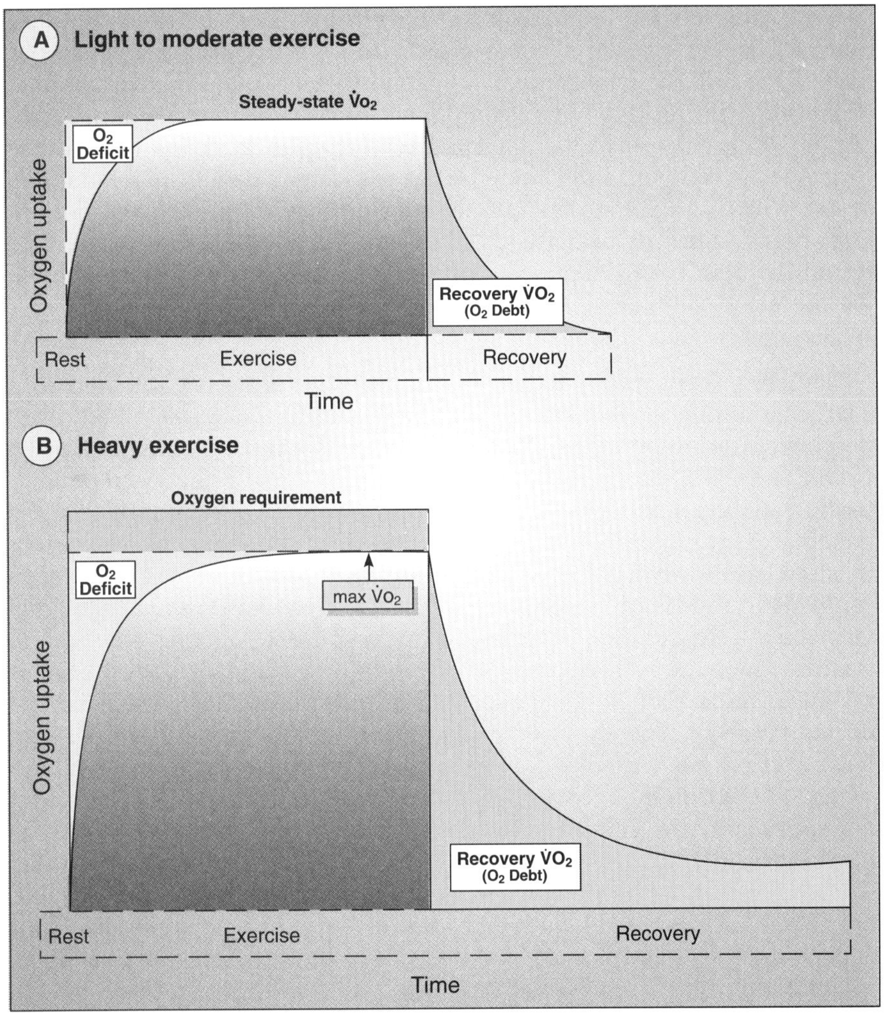

FIG. 11–14. Oxygen uptake during and in recovery from (A) light to moderate, steady-state exercise and (B) exhaustive exercise. There are two components to the recovery curve following exhaustive exercise. The first phase occurs quickly; the second phase is much slower and takes considerable time to return to resting conditions. Note that in exhaustive exercise, the oxygen requirement of the exercise is greater than the curve of oxygen uptake (symbolized as $\dot{V}O_2$).

state is reached. Once exercise stops, any deficit incurred during exercise is "repaid" at the expense of an elevated oxygen uptake in recovery (labeled as recovery $\dot{V}O_2$ in the figure). During light exercise, when steady state is reached quickly, the deficit is relatively small and recovery is rapid. During the transition from moderate to heavy exercise, on the other hand, the oxygen deficit can be quite large.

For exhaustive exercise, illustrated in the bottom curve, a steady state cannot be reached and anaerobic reactions provide considerable energy with an accompanying buildup of lactic acid. *The oxygen in excess of the resting value consumed during recovery from exercise, whether it is small from light exercise or large from heavy or exhaustive exercise, is called the recovery oxygen uptake.* In Figure 11–14, the deficit and recovery oxygen uptake are indicated by shaded areas. The curves for recovery illustrate several important characteristics of recovery oxygen uptake.

Recovery from Moderate Exercise. In recovery from light and moderate exercise, oxygen uptake declines rapidly to resting values when exercise stops. One-half the total recovery oxygen uptake is repaid within the first 30 seconds during this "fast" component of recovery, and within 1 to 2 minutes oxygen uptake has returned to resting level. The extra oxygen consumed in recovery from moderate exercise is associated with restoration of the ATP and CP high-energy phosphates that were depleted and not resynthesized during exercise. A small amount of oxygen is also used to reload the blood, and to supply the slightly elevated energy demands of the heart and ventilatory muscles.

Recovery oxygen uptake. The oxygen consumed in excess of the resting value during recovery from exercise has been called the "oxygen debt." This term was used because the excess oxygen was thought to represent the metabolic cost of repaying the stored energy (glycogen) used during the deficit, or anaerobic, phase of exercise. We now know that a large portion of the oxygen used in recovery is required for a variety of physiologic processes (circulation, ventilation, hormonal and temperature effects) that are actually elevated during recovery. Hence, the term **recovery oxygen uptake** more accurately describes the dynamics of the recovery process.

Recovery from Heavy Exercise. Strenuous exercise is associated with a large accumulation of blood lactate and significant increase in body temperature. In addition to the fast component of the recovery oxygen uptake curve, there is a second, less rapid phase termed the "slow" component. Lactic acid during this phase of recovery is reconverted to pyruvic acid and metabolized for energy through the Krebs cycle; some may also be resynthesized back to glycogen in the liver. A considerable amount of the oxygen consumed in recovery is not directly related to the level of anaerobic metabolism during exercise. For example, the respiratory muscles require considerably more oxygen for the work of breathing during recovery than at rest. The heart also works harder and requires a greater oxygen supply during recovery. The elevation of body temperature brought on by strenuous exercise has a direct stimulating effect on metabolism, and hence, a *significant effect* on the recovery oxygen uptake. In fact, all physiologic systems activated to meet the demands of exercise increase their own particular need for oxygen during recovery.

There are important distinguishing features of the fast and slow components of recovery oxygen uptake. If exercise is not too strenuous, so it is performed in steady state, or if it is heavy but of short duration (10 to 15 seconds), lactic acid will not accumulate to any appreciable extent. Recovery will be rapid (fast component), and exercise can begin again without the hindering effects of fatigue. If intense exercise must continue beyond a 20-second period—as in wrestling, sprint swimming or running, soccer, or ice hockey—energy is supplied predominantly from the anaerobic reactions of glycolysis. This carries a price in the form of disruption of bodily processes and significant lactate buildup in the blood and exercising muscles. In such cases, recovery takes much longer (slow component) and may be incomplete even with short rest periods such as time-outs, or even with longer rest periods such as half-time breaks.

Blood lactate not a waste product. Lactic acid has often been called a metabolic "waste product." To the contrary, lactic acid is not treated as an unwanted chemical and then excreted from the body. Instead, it is a valuable potential source of energy that is retained at relatively high concentrations during intense exercise. When there is sufficient oxygen during recovery, lactic acid is readily converted back to pyruvic acid and then used for energy. This is the way the body preserves about 90% of energy from the original glucose molecule for later use as an aerobic energy source.

Keep Active during Recovery. ***Lactic acid removal** is accelerated by active aerobic exercise in recovery.* While just about any level of submaximal aerobic exercise facilitates the recovery process, the most rapid recovery usually occurs with continuous moderate exercise that can be comfortably maintained. Lactate removal with active recovery is the result of increased blood flow through the liver, heart, and muscles, because these tissues can use lactate and oxidize it for energy during recovery. If, however, recovery exercise is too intense and is performed above the blood lactate threshold, it will be of little benefit and may even prolong recovery by increasing the formation of lactic acid.

THE ENERGY SPECTRUM OF EXERCISE

The relative contributions of the anaerobic and aerobic energy systems differ markedly depending on the exercise performed. Performances of short duration and high intensity, such as the 100-yard dash, long jump or pole vault, volleyball spike, golf swing, or maximum resistance-type exercise, require an immediate energy supply. This energy is provided almost exclusively from anaerobic sources, specifically the high-energy phosphate compounds ATP and CP stored within the specific muscles used in exercise. In strenuous exercise that lasts a minute or two, the major source of energy comes from the anaerobic process of glycolysis with resulting formation of lactic acid. Intense exercise of intermediate duration, performed for 5 to 10 minutes, as in middle-distance running, swimming, basketball, or water polo, represents a blend of metabolic energy demands. Under these conditions, it is desirable to possess a high capacity for both aerobic and anaerobic metabolism. Performances of long duration, such as marathon running, distance swimming, cycling, recreational jogging, or hiking, require a fairly constant energy supply with little or no reliance on the mechanism of lactic acid production.

Figure 11–15 illustrates the relative contribution of anaerobic and aerobic energy sources during maximal physical activity of various durations. These data were originally obtained from running and cycling experiments, although they can easily be applied on a time basis to other activities that

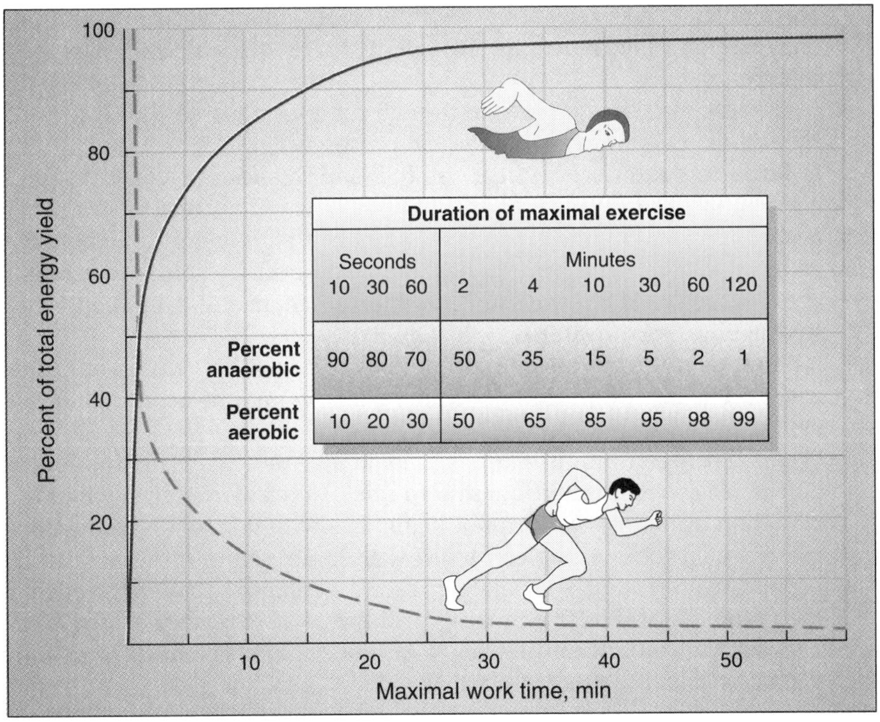

FIG. 11–15. Relative contribution of aerobic and anaerobic energy during maximal physical activity of various durations. It should be noted that 1.5 to 2 minutes of maximal effort requires 50% of the energy from both aerobic and anaerobic processes. (Adapted from Åstrand, P. O., and Rodahl, K.: Textbook of Work Physiology. New York, McGraw-Hill Book Company, © 1977.)

It's difficult to excel in all sports. An understanding of the energy requirements of various activities provides some explanation why a world record holder in the 1-mile run is not necessarily a noted distance runner. Conversely, premier marathoners are generally unable to run a mile in less than 4 minutes.

involve large muscle groups. For example, a 40- to 60-yard sprint of 5 to 8 seconds closely approximates a long pass pattern in football, while a 440-yard run of 60 to 70 seconds would be similar in duration to a 100-yard swim, and possibly a full-court press at the end of a basketball game.

At one extreme, the total energy for exercise is supplied entirely by anaerobic sources. In middle-distance events or in other intense activities that last from 2 to 4 minutes, the ATP-CP and lactic acid energy systems generate approximately 50% of the energy while aerobic reactions supply the remainder. World-class marathoners, on the other hand, derive essentially all their energy from aerobic metabolism. As discussed in Chapters 18 and 19, the scientific approach to training is to identify the predominant energy system (or systems) activated in a given activity, and then to gear training toward improving the capacity of that system.

SUMMARY

1. When the terminal phosphate bond of the ATP molecule is broken, the energy liberated is harnessed to power all forms of biologic work. Thus, ATP is considered the body's energy currency, although its quantity is limited.
2. Creatine phosphate interacts with ADP to form ATP and thus serves as an energy reservoir to replenish ATP rapidly.
3. The energy contained within the chemical structure of the macronutrients is not released in the body suddenly at some kindling temperature; rather, it is released slowly in small amounts during complex enzyme-controlled reactions. This allows for greater efficiency in energy transfer.
4. In the reactions of glycolysis in the cell cytoplasm, some ATP is formed by non-oxygen-requiring anaerobic processes.
5. Cellular oxidation occurs in the mitochondria and involves transfer of electrons from hydrogen to molecular oxygen. This results in release and transfer of chemical energy to form the high-energy phosphates.
6. In the aerobic resynthesis of ATP, oxygen's primary role is to serve as the final electron acceptor in the respiratory chain and to combine with hydrogen to form water.
7. Numerous interconversions are possible among the various food nutrients. The exception are fatty acids, which cannot be used for glucose synthesis.
8. When hydrogen atoms are oxidized at the rate they are formed, a biochemical "steady state" is said to exist. In heavy exercise, when the oxidation of hydrogen does not keep pace with its rate of production, pyruvic acid temporarily combines with hydrogen to form lactic acid.
9. A steady rate of oxygen uptake represents a balance between the energy requirements of working muscles and the aerobic resynthesis of ATP. The difference between oxygen requirement and actual oxygen consumed is called the oxygen deficit.
10. The maximum capacity for aerobic resynthesis of ATP is quantitatively measured as the maximum oxygen uptake, or max $\dot{V}O_2$. This is one of the important indicators of a person's capability for sustained exercise.
11. At about 55% of an average person's max $\dot{V}O_2$, the production of hydrogens through the anaerobic reactions of glycolysis begins to exceed

their subsequent oxidation in aerobic metabolism and lactic acid begins to build up. This blood lactate threshold can be improved with aerobic training; it is a powerful predictor of exercise performance.

12. Humans possess two types of muscle fibers, each with unique metabolic and contractile properties. Type I fibers are low glycolytic–high oxidative, slow-twitch fibers; Type II fibers are low oxidative–high glycolytic, fast-twitch fibers. A person's basic muscle fiber composition probably cannot be changed to any large extent.
13. Following exercise, oxygen uptake remains elevated above the resting level. This recovery oxygen uptake reflects the metabolic characteristics of the preceding exercise as well as the physiologic alterations caused by that exercise.
14. Moderate exercise performed during recovery (active recovery) facilitates the recovery process compared to passive procedures. In most situations, this recovery is reflected in faster removal of lactic acid.
15. The major energy pathway for ATP production differs depending on the intensity and duration of exercise. In intense exercise of short duration (100-yard dash, weight lifting), the energy is derived from already present stores of intramuscular ATP and CP (immediate energy system). For intense exercise of longer duration (1 to 2 min), energy is generated mainly from the anaerobic reactions of glycolysis (short-term energy system). As exercise progresses beyond several minutes, the aerobic system predominates and oxygen supply and utilization (long-term energy system) become important factors.
16. By understanding the energy spectrum of exercise, it is possible to train for specific improvement of the appropriate energy system.

RELATED LITERATURE

Bergh, U., et al.: Maximal oxygen uptake and muscle fiber types in trained and untrained humans. *Med. Sci. Sports Exerc.*, 10:151, 1978.

Bouchard, C., et al.: Genetics of aerobic and anaerobic performances. In Exercise and Sport Science Reviews. Vol. 20. Edited by J.O. Holloszy. Baltimore, Williams &Wilkins, 1992.

Brooks, G.A.: Anaerobic threshold: review of the concept and directions for future research. Med. Sci. Sports Exerc., 17:22, 1985.

Brooks, G.A., and Fahey, T.D.: Exercise Physiology: Human Bioenergetics and Its Applications. New York, Wiley, 1984.

Coggan, A.R., et al.: Endurance training decreases plasma glucose turnover and oxidation during moderate-intensity exercise. *J. Appl. Physiol.*, 68:990, 1990.

Coyle, E.F.: Blood lactate threshold in some well-trained ischemic heart disease patients. *J. Appl. Physiol.*, 54:18, 1983.

Dodd S., et al.: Blood lactate disappearance at various intensities of recovery exercise. *J. Appl. Physiol.*, 57:1462, 1984.

Franklin, B.A.: Exercise testing, training and arm ergometry. Sports Med., 2:109, 1985.

Gladden, L.B.: Lactate uptake by skeletal muscle. In: Exercise and Sport Sciences Reviews, vol. 17. Edited by K.B. Pandolf. New York, Macmillan, 1980.

Hickson, R.C., et al.: Faster adjustment of O_2 uptake to the energy requirement of exercise in the trained state. *J. Appl. Physiol.*, 44:877, 1978.

Holloszy, J.O., and Coyle, E.F.: Adaptations of skeletal muscle to endurance training and their metabolic consequences. *J. Appl. Physiol.*, 56:831, 1984.

Horton, E.S., and Terjung, R.L. (Eds.): Exercise, Nutrition, and Energy Metabolism. New York, Macmillan, 1988.

Jacobs, I., et al.: Sprint training effects on muscle myoglobin, enzymes, fiber types, and blood lactate. *Med. Sci. Sports Exerc.*, 19:368, 1987.

Katz, A., and Sahlin, K.: Regulation of lactic acid production during exercise. *J. Appl. Physiol.*, 65:509, 1988.
Katz, A., and Sahlin, K.: Role of oxygen in regulation of glycolysis and lactate production in human skeletal muscle. In: Exercise and Sport Sciences Reviews, vol. 18. Edited by K.B. Pandolf. Baltimore, Williams & Wilkins, 1990.
Lehninger, A.L.: Principles of Biochemistry. New York, Worth Publishers, 1982.
McArdle, W.D., et al.: Exercise Physiology: Energy, Nutrition, and Human Performance, 3rd ed. Philadelphia, Lea & Febiger, 1991.
Minotti, J.R., et al.: Training-induced skeletal muscle adaptations are independent of systemic adaptations. *J. Appl. Physiol.*, 68:289, 1990.
Saltin, B.: Physiological effects of physical conditioning. *Med. Sci. Sports Exerc.*, 1:50, 1969.
Shepherd, R.E., and Bah, M.D.: Cyclic AMP regulation of fuel metabolism during exercise: regulation of adipose tissue lipolysis during exercise. *Med. Sci. Sports Exerc.*, 20:531, 1988.
Stainsby, W.N., and Brooks, G.A.: Control of lactic acid metabolism in contracting muscles and during exercise. In: Exercise and Sport Sciences Reviews, vol. 18. Edited by K.B. Pandolf. Baltimore, Williams & Wilkins, 1990.
Stryer, L.: Biochemistry, 2nd ed. San Francisco, Freeman, 1988.
Tan, M.H., et al.: Muscle glycogen repletion after exercise in trained normal and diabetic rats. *J. Appl. Physiol.*, 57:1404, 1984.
Vander, A.J., et al.: Human Physiology, 2nd ed. New York, McGraw-Hill, 1985.
Vogel, J.A., et al.: An analysis of aerobic capacity in a large United States population. *J. Appl. Physiol.*, 60:494, 1986.
Wells, C.L., and Plowman, S.A.: Sexual differences in athletic performance: biological or behavioral? *Phys. Sportsmed.*, 11:52, 1983.
Weltman, A., et al.: The lactate threshold and endurance performance. *Adv. Sports Med. Fitness*, 2:91, 1989.

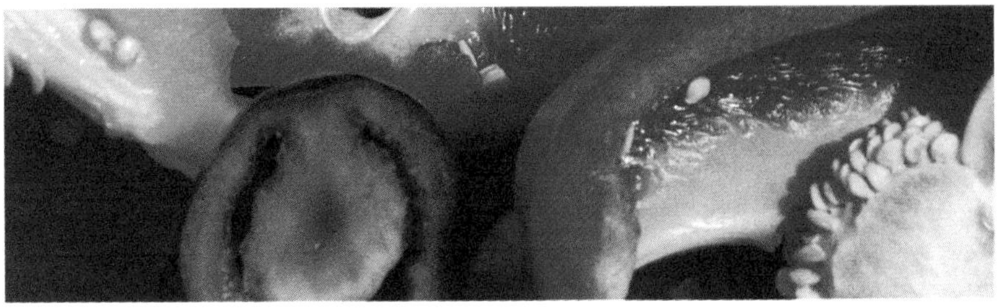

12

VENTILATION AND CIRCULATION: THE OXYGEN DELIVERY SYSTEMS

Most sport, recreational, and occupational activities require a relatively steady and sustained energy supply. This energy for resynthesis of ATP (adenosine triphosphate) is provided by the aerobic breakdown of carbohydrate and lipid and, to a minor degree, protein. Unless a steady state is achieved between energy-yielding reactions and the energy requirements of activity, an anaerobic-aerobic energy imbalance develops, lactic acid accumulates, and fatigue quickly ensues. The ability to sustain physical activity, therefore, depends largely on the capacity and integration of the body's two major **oxygen delivery systems,** the ventilatory and circulatory systems.

PULMONARY VENTILATION

The lungs provide the surface so oxygen can move from the external environment into the body and carbon dioxide produced in the tissues can exit to the outside. The **lung volume** of an average-sized adult varies between 4 and 6 liters, about the amount of air contained in a basketball. If the lung tissue were spread out like a carpet, it would cover a surface about 35 times greater than the person's body surface area, or the equivalent of half a tennis court! Such a large surface provides a tremendous interface for aeration of blood with the environment.

LUNG STRUCTURE AND FUNCTION

A general view of the **ventilatory system** is presented in Figure 12–1. As air moves into the lungs through the nose and mouth, it is filtered, humidified, and adjusted to body temperature. This air-conditioning process continues as inspired air passes down the trachea into the bronchi, two large tubes that serve as primary conduits into each of the lungs. The bronchi further subdivide into many smaller bronchioles that conduct air into the

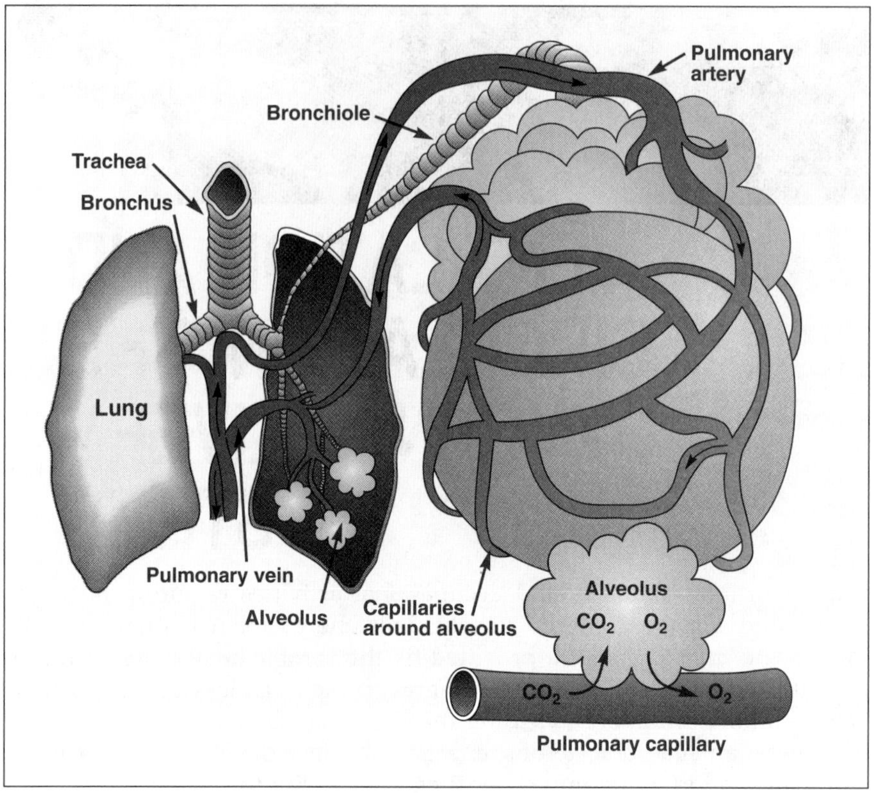

FIG. 12–1. A general view of the ventilatory system that shows the respiratory passages, the alveoli, and the function of an alveolus in gas exchange.

respiratory tract's terminal branches, the **alveoli.** These are the microscopic, thin-walled elastic sacs that serve as the surface for gas exchange between the lungs and blood. Millions of tiny, thin-walled blood vessels, the capillaries, lie side-by-side with the alveoli, with air moving on one side and blood on the other. Only two thin membranes, that of the alveolus and that of the capillary, provide the barrier to exchange of gases between the internal and external environments.

Mechanics of Breathing. A large, dome-shaped sheet of muscle, the **diaphragm,** serves the same purpose as the rubber membrane attached to the bottom of the jar illustrated in Figure 12–2. This muscle makes an airtight seal that separates the lower chest from the upper abdominal cavity. When air enters the lungs—a process called **inspiration**—the diaphragm contracts, flattens out, and moves down toward the abdominal cavity. As a result, the chest cavity enlarges, air rushes in through the nose and mouth, and the lungs inflate. **Expiration**—the process of air movement from the lungs—is predominantly passive; during rest and light exercise, it occurs from relaxation of the inspiratory muscles and the natural recoil of the stretched lung tissue. This action reduces the size of the chest cavity, and air moves out of the lungs.

Lung-chest interaction. In contrast to the balloons that are attached to the jar, the lungs are not merely suspended in the chest cavity. Rather, the pressure differential between the air within the lungs and the lung–chest wall interface causes the lungs to adhere to the chest wall and literally follow its every movement.

During vigorous exercise, muscles that act on the ribs and sternum as well as the abdominal musculature contribute to rapid change in the dimension of the chest cavity, and airflow within the lungs increases dramatically. This flow of air, termed **pulmonary ventilation,** can increase in

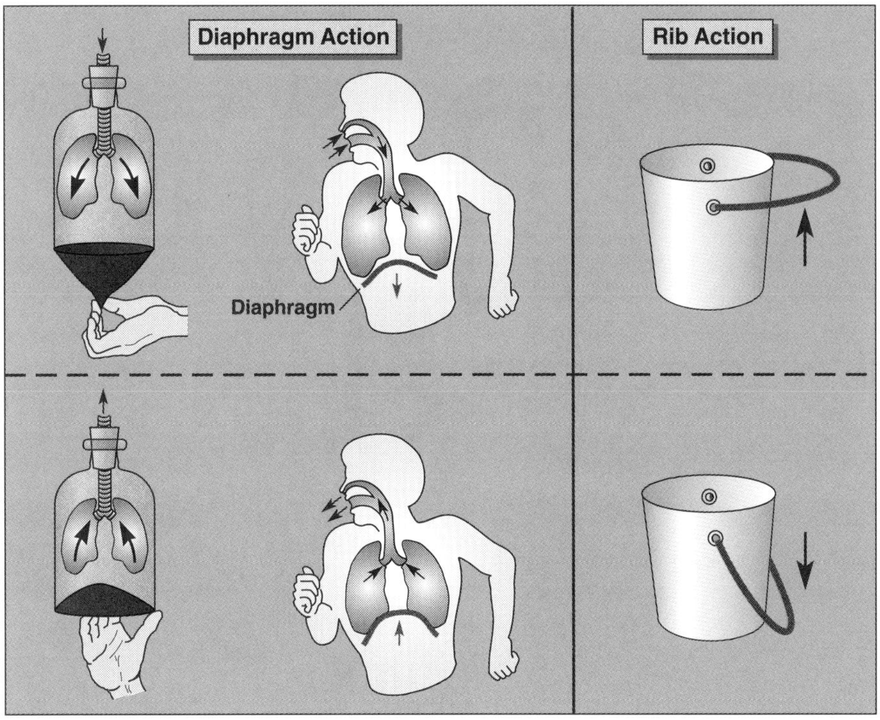

FIG. 12–2. Mechanics of breathing. During inspiration, the chest cavity increases in size because of raising of the ribs and lowering of the muscular diaphragm. During exhalation, the ribs swing down and the diaphragm returns to a relaxed position. This reduces the volume of the thoracic cavity and air rushes out. The movement of the rubber bottom of the jar, causing air to enter and leave the two balloons, simulates the action of the diaphragm; the movement of the bucket handle simulates the action of the ribs.

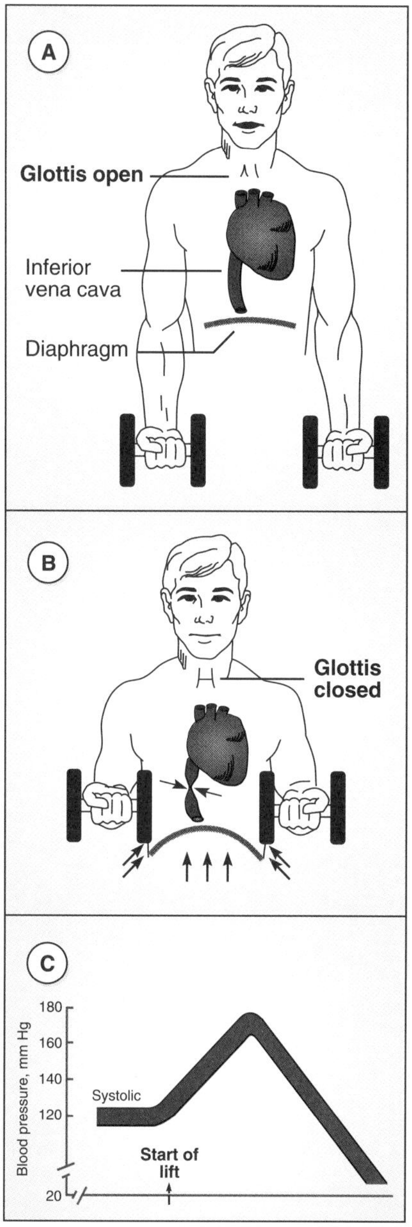

FIG. 12–3. The Valsalva maneuver significantly reduces return of blood to the heart because the increase in intrathoracic pressure collapses the vein that passes through the chest cavity. (A) Normal breathing. (B) Straining exercise with accompanying Valsalva. (C) Blood pressure response prior to and during straining-type exercise.

well-conditioned endurance athletes from about 6 liters of air per minute at rest to 160 to 220 liters in response to maximum metabolic demands. Even such strenuous exercise does not fully tax a healthy individual's ability to breathe because a breathing reserve still remains.

Breathe Normally during Exercise. The expiratory muscles play an important role during coughing and sneezing, as well as in stabilizing the abdomen and chest when lifting a heavy object. During normal breathing, only small changes in pressure within the chest cavity bring about a smooth flow of air within the alveolar chambers. If, however, the **glottis** is closed following a full inspiration, and the expiratory muscles are maximally activated, pressure increases tremendously within the chest cavity. This forced exhalation against a closed glottis, termed the **Valsalva maneuver,** occurs commonly in weight lifting and other straining-type activities that require rapid, near-maximal application of force.

As shown in Figure 12–3, the increase in pressure during the Valsalva is transmitted through the thin walls of the veins that pass through the chest. Because venous blood is under relatively low pressure, these veins are compressed and blood flow is greatly reduced as it returns to the heart. A reduction in venous return can diminish blood supply to the brain, which frequently produces dizziness, "spots before the eyes," and even fainting. *The best way to minimize such consequences is to breathe normally throughout exercise and refrain from breath-holding when straining to lift a heavy object.*

Glottis. The glottis is the narrowest part of the larynx where air passes into and out of the trachea. Normally, its action covers the trachea during swallowing to prevent food from entering the "windpipe."

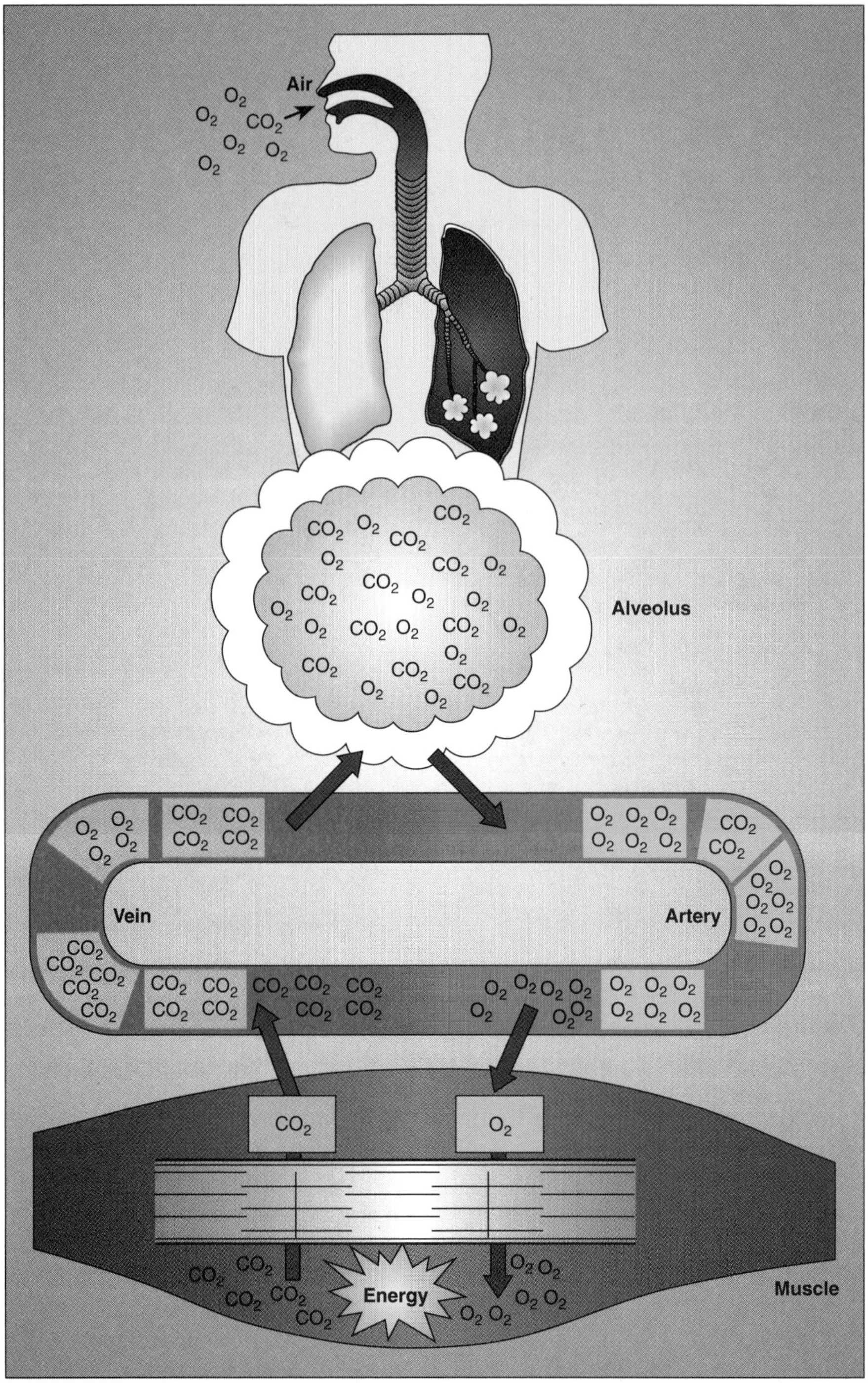

FIG. 12–4. Exchange of oxygen and carbon dioxide at rest between alveoli and the blood and between the blood and tissues. During exercise, alveolar and arterial oxygen and carbon dioxide values remain almost the same as at rest. In the muscles, however, the increased demands for energy cause oxygen values to drop precipitously with a corresponding increase in carbon dioxide. Therefore, venous blood varies considerably in oxygen and carbon dioxide content, depending on a person's level of physical activity.

GAS EXCHANGE IN THE LUNGS

The movement of gas molecules that enter or leave the lungs and body tissues occurs by the process of *diffusion* as the gas moves from an area of higher concentration to one of lower concentration. Figure 12–4 illustrates the exchange of oxygen and carbon dioxide between the lungs and blood, and subsequent diffusion of these gases in the tissues. Gas exchange is entirely the result of **pressure differentials** between gases in various parts of the body. The pressure exerted by oxygen molecules is considerably greater in the alveoli than in the returning venous blood. Thus, oxygen is "forced" through the alveolar membrane into the blood. Carbon dioxide, on the other hand, is under greater pressure in returning venous blood than in the alveoli. Consequently, carbon dioxide diffuses into the lungs.

Gas exchange occurs rapidly. The process of diffusion in the healthy lung is so rapid that an equilibrium of blood gas with alveolar gas takes less than 1 second.

The pressure of oxygen and carbon dioxide gas in arterial blood differs considerably from their pressure in the cells. This is because, in the tissues, oxygen is used continuously during metabolism to produce an almost equal quantity of carbon dioxide. This creates pressure gradients that cause gas to diffuse rapidly between the blood and tissues. Oxygen leaves the blood and moves toward the metabolizing cell, while carbon dioxide flows from the cell into the blood. After leaving the tissues, the blood travels in the veins to the heart and subsequently is pumped to the lungs, where diffusion again takes place.

During exercise, as energy demands increase, large amounts of oxygen diffuse from the alveoli into deoxygenated blood returning from the active muscles. Simultaneously, considerable quantities of carbon dioxide produced in the muscles and carried in the blood move into the lungs. Pulmonary ventilation increases to maintain the proper concentrations of alveolar gases to supply oxygen and remove carbon dioxide. With the normal adjustment of ventilation to the body's metabolic demands, the composition of alveolar air remains remarkably constant, even during strenuous physical activity.

Enhanced oxygen transport. Hemoglobin increases the oxygen-carrying capacity of blood about 65 times above what is normally dissolved in the plasma.

OXYGEN TRANSPORT

Figure 12–5 displays the percentage **composition of centrifuged blood** for plasma and red blood cells **(hematocrit)** as well as representative values for the amount of oxygen carried in each component. By far, the greatest quantity of oxygen in the blood is carried in "piggyback" fashion by combining with **hemoglobin,** the iron-containing protein compound in red blood cells. The iron atoms in each hemoglobin molecule "capture" oxygen molecules loosely and temporarily, thus enabling oxygen to be released readily in response to tissue needs. It is the oxygenation of hemoglobin that gives arterial blood its characteristic red color. When the hemoglobin content of red blood cells decreases significantly, as in certain types of **anemia,** the amount of oxygen carried by the blood also decreases. As discussed in Chapter 7, anemia often results in reduced performance and early fatigue in aerobic activities.

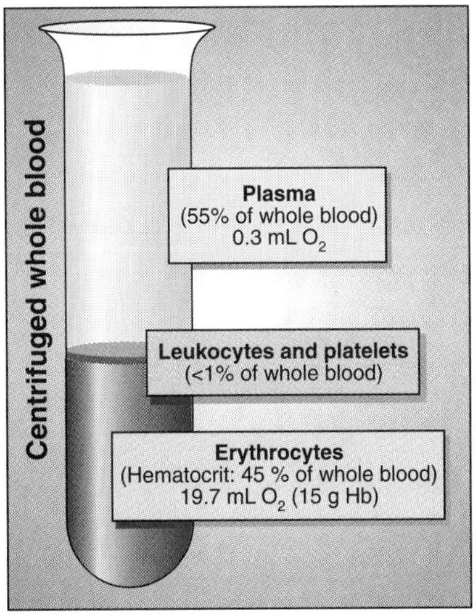

FIG. 12–5. Major blood components and oxygen carried in 100 ml of whole blood. (Hb = hemoglobin.)

Breathing Oxygen-enriched Gas. The nature of the ventilatory adjustments in pulmonary ventilation in a healthy person, as well as the specific chemical characteristics of hemoglobin, are such that even during vigorous exercise hemoglobin carries nearly its full complement of oxygen.

Thus, breathing mixtures of concentrated oxygen, as is often practiced by football players during time-outs, at half-time, or following strenuous exercise, contributes little to the quantity of oxygen already carried in the blood. As one moves to moderate or high altitude and barometric pressure falls accordingly, the pressure of oxygen in air is reduced and the hemoglobin molecule is not fully saturated with oxygen. Oxygen breathing would be of benefit under these circumstances, particularly during endurance exercise, in which oxygen delivery is of utmost importance.

Oxygen breathing. Breathing oxygen-enriched mixtures prior to or in recovery from exercise may give a psychological lift, but its physiological contribution is trivial at best.

PULMONARY VENTILATION DURING EXERCISE

Pulmonary ventilation in the early stages of submaximal exercise rises rapidly to a steady level similar to the pattern for oxygen uptake illustrated in Figure 11–8. As exercise intensity increases, rapid adjustments in the rate and depth of breathing raise ventilation to a new steady level. The curves in Figure 12–6 illustrate the relationship between **pulmonary ventilation and oxygen uptake** for the untrained and trained individual. Each point represents the average ventilation value for a particular oxygen uptake during successive increments in exercise intensity.

During moderate exercise, ventilation volume increases linearly with the quantity of oxygen consumed by the tissues. As a result, the pressures of oxygen and carbon dioxide in the alveoli remain near resting values and blood flowing through the lungs is completely oxygenated. During vigorous exercise, ventilation volume increases disproportionately compared with oxygen uptake; that is, *more* air is breathed per quantity of oxygen consumed than during moderate exercise. If ability to breathe were inadequate for metabolic demands (as occurs in obstructive pulmonary diseases such as asthma and emphysema), the relation between pulmonary ventilation and oxygen uptake would curve in the opposite direction, indicating failure of ventilation to keep pace with the need for oxygen. If this were the case,

An added stimulus to breathing. Overbreathing occurs in heavy exercise because the lactic acid produced places an added demand on pulmonary ventilation. This happens when lactic acid is buffered to produce the weaker carbonic acid. In the lungs, carbonic acid splits into its components, water and carbon dioxide. Carbon dioxide provides an additional stimulus to increase ventilation.

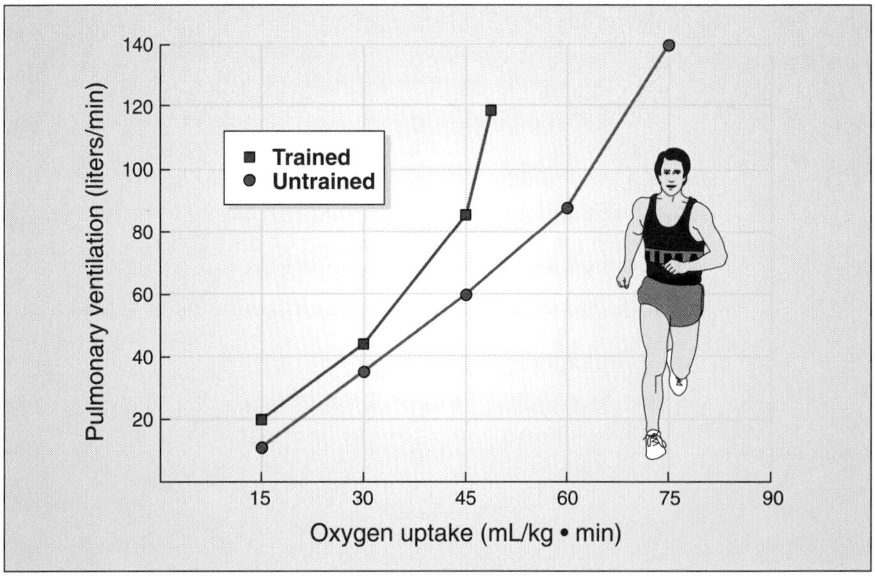

FIG. 12–6. Relationship between pulmonary ventilation and oxygen uptake for trained athletes and untrained subjects.

we would truly run out of air during exercise. Obviously, this does not happen, but overbreathing does occur during heavy exercise.

The Trained Breathe Less. The shape of the curve relating pulmonary ventilation to oxygen uptake during exercise of increasing intensity is essentially similar between trained and untrained individuals. The exception occurs during any level of submaximal exercise, where ventilation volumes are *lower* for the trained person. This adaptation occurs rapidly with training and is beneficial for two reasons: it reduces the fatiguing effects of exercise on the ventilatory muscles, and any oxygen freed from use by the ventilatory muscles becomes available to the exercising muscles.

The lungs of healthy people are more than adequate to maintain proper alveolar gas pressures, even during the most severe exercise when circulation is maximally stressed. For most people, the blood leaving the lungs to flow throughout the body during exercise is loaded with virtually the same amount of oxygen it carries during rest. The bottom line is this: *the capacity to breathe and ventilate the lungs does not limit a healthy person's performance during physical activity.*

Even the fit have asthma. A high level of fitness does not confer immunity from exercise-induced bronchospasm. About 12% of U.S. athletes in the 1984 Olympics suffered from this ailment. The 1984 Olympic marathon champion Joan Benoit Samuelson experienced breathing problems during several marathon races in 1991 that led to the discovery of her asthmatic condition. Despite experiencing breathing difficulties during the 1991 New York Marathon, she still finished with a time of 2:33:40!

Exercise and the Asthmatic. **Asthma** affects about 10 million Americans, most of them children. The disease is characterized by hyperirritability of the pulmonary airways that is usually manifested by coughing, wheezing, or shortness of breath. For many asthmatics, exercise is a potent stimulus for the airway constriction associated with an asthma attack. The movement of large volumes of air during exercise has a cooling effect on the pulmonary system as incoming air is warmed and humidified. This cooling during exercise and abrupt rewarming in recovery triggers spasms of the smooth muscle that lines the walls of the respiratory passages, greatly increasing resistance to airflow. This effect becomes apparent with exercise in a cool, dry environment, where considerable moisture evaporates from the respiratory passages (with subsequent cooling effect) as incoming air is warmed and moistened. However, the **exercise-induced asthmatic response** is blunted when exercise is performed in a humid environment, where there is little loss of fluid and cooling of the airways. This is why walking or jogging on a warm, humid day or swimming in an indoor pool is usually well tolerated by asthmatics, whereas exercise in the cold, dry air of winter often triggers an attack. For the asthmatic who wants to exercise regularly regardless of environmental conditions, medications are available to limit the degree of airway constriction.

Exercise-induced bronchospasm. One technique for diagnosing an exercise-induced asthmatic response is simply to provide progressive increments of exercise. After each exercise bout, breathing function is evaluated during a 10- to 20-minute recovery period. Generally, a 15% reduction in pre-exercise values confirms the diagnosis of exercise-induced asthma.

Post-exercise Coughing. Exercise for the normal person is frequently associated with dryness in the throat and coughing during the recovery period, especially following exercise in cold weather. **Post-exercise coughing** results from water loss and subsequent drying of the respiratory passages associated with the large air volumes breathed during exercise.

Cigarette Smoking. *Evidence is overwhelming that long-term cigarette smoking causes a variety of severe pulmonary and cardiovascular diseases including emphysema, chronic bronchitis, hypertension, coronary heart disease, and several types of cancer.* While these diseases usually take years to become manifest, the immediate **effects of smoking** are of significance to the exercise enthusiast. Airway resistance to breathing is increased as much as threefold following 15 puffs on a cigarette, and the effect lasts an average of 35

Rapid rewards for abstinence. The increased cost of breathing with smoking is substantially reversed in chronic smokers with only one day of abstinence. Thus, if athletes are unable to eliminate smoking completely, they should at least stop on the day of competition.

minutes. This residual effect of smoking on the "cost" of breathing could add significantly to the oxygen required to maintain adequate ventilation during vigorous exercise.

CIRCULATION

The highly efficient ventilatory system is complemented by a rapid transport and delivery system consisting of the blood, the heart, and over 60,000 miles of blood vessels that integrate the body as a unit. The circulatory system serves four important functions during physical activity:

- It delivers blood to the exercising muscles, where oxygen is exchanged for almost equal amounts of carbon dioxide
- It returns blood to the lungs, where metabolic gases are exchanged with the ambient environment
- It transports heat, a by-product of cellular metabolism, from the body's core to the skin, where it then dissipates to the environment
- It delivers the glucose and lipid nutrients to the active tissues to serve as fuel to power exercise

THE CARDIOVASCULAR SYSTEM

Figure 12–7 presents a schematic view of the circulatory system.

The Heart. Within the confines of the closed circulatory system, the force to propel blood is provided by the **heart.** This four-chambered organ, a fist-sized pump, beats at rest about 70 times a minute, 100,800 times a day, and 36.8 million times a year.

> **The heart is a remarkable pump.** At rest, the heart's output of blood is equivalent to 1400 gallons a day, or about 37 million gallons over a 72-year lifetime. When this remarkable organ pumps at its maximum capacity during exercise, it puts out more blood than the fluid coming from a household faucet turned wide open!

Figure 12–8 shows details of the heart as a pump. The two hollow chambers that make up the *right side* of the heart serve two important functions: to receive oxygen-depleted blood returning from all parts of the body, and to pump blood to the lungs for aeration. The *left side* of the heart receives oxygen-rich blood from the lungs and pumps it into the aorta, the main conduit of the arterial system. From it branch other main channels that route oxygen-rich blood to the organs and tissues.

The Arteries. The arterial system eventually branches into smaller blood vessels called arterioles. Nerves and local metabolic conditions act on the smooth muscle bands in the arteriole walls to enable these vessels to alter their internal diameter. The dilation and constriction of arterioles permit rapid redistribution of blood in various body regions. The arterioles end in a network of microscopically thin walled, small blood vessels called **capillaries.** *It is only in the capillaries that nutrient and gas exchange takes place between the slow-moving blood and the tissues.*

The Veins. Deoxygenated blood leaves the capillaries, one cell at a time, to enter the venules or small veins, and eventually flow into the **veins** that return blood to the heart. Spaced at short intervals within the veins are thin, membranous, flaplike valves. Figure 12–9 illustrates that the valves permit **one-way flow of blood** back to the heart. Because venous blood is

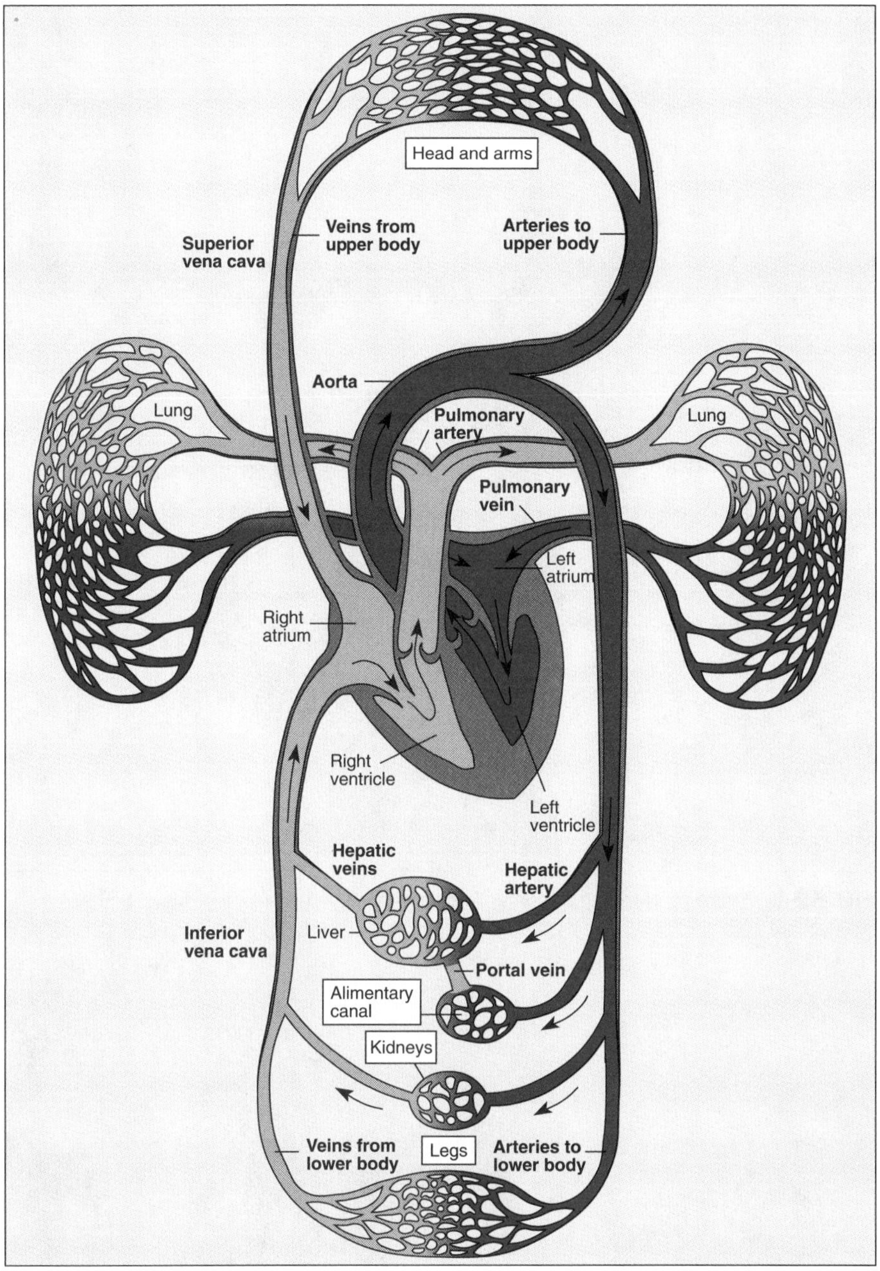

FIG. 12–7. General view of the circulatory system. The arterial system is a darker shade.

under relatively little pressure, the veins are easily compressed by the smallest muscular contractions or even by minor pressure changes in the chest cavity during breathing. *The alternate compression and relaxation of the veins and the one-way action of the valves provide a **"milking" action*** for the steady flow of venous blood back to the heart.

During heavy weight lifting or other activities that often involve sustained, static muscular contractions, neither the muscle nor ventilatory pumps contribute significantly to venous return. In such situations, blood flow to the heart can be impaired to the point that dizziness and even fainting occur as blood flow to the brain is reduced.

Varicose veins. Sometimes the valves within a vein become defective and fail to maintain the one-way flow of blood. This condition, called **varicose veins,** usually occurs in the superficial leg veins owing to the force of gravity that retards blood flow in the upright posture. Blood gathers in these veins, they become excessively distended and painful, and circulation from the affected area is actually impaired.

Help for varicose veins. New chemical methods are replacing the major surgery of "vein stripping" to help the estimated 80 million Americans with blocked veins (including "spider" veins and varicose veins). With sclerotherapy, a chemical is injected into the vein that causes it to collapse and eventually disappear. In some cases, lasers and thin incisions also are used to eliminate blocked veins.

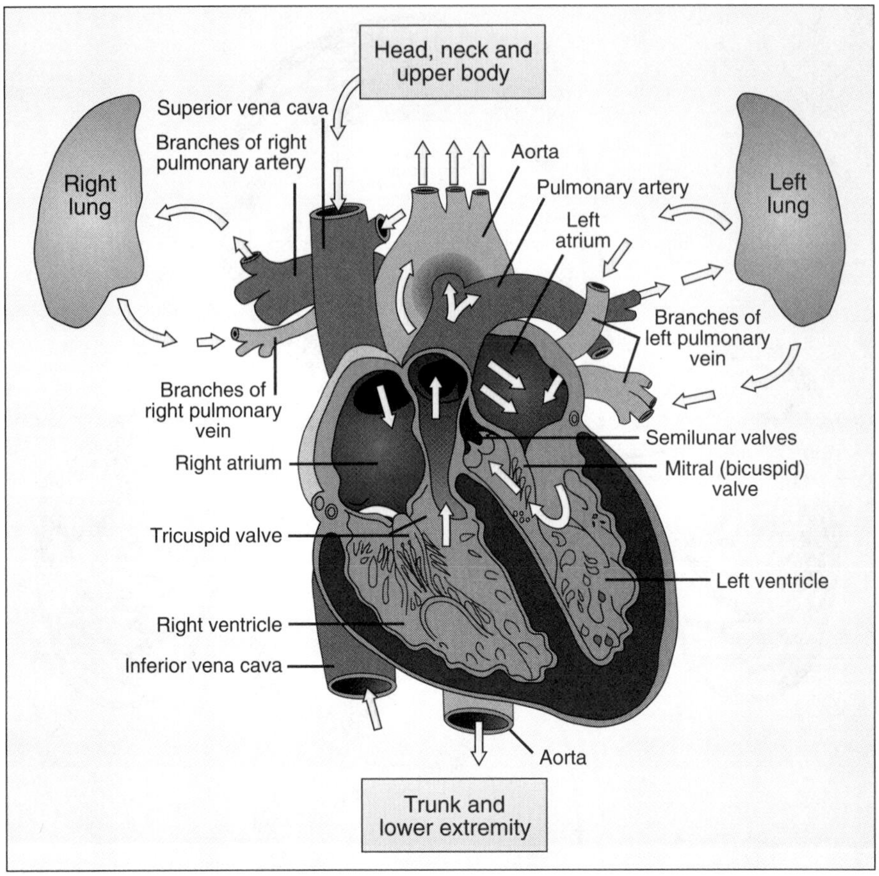

FIG. 12–8. Structure of the heart pump. Arrows indicate the direction of blood flow.

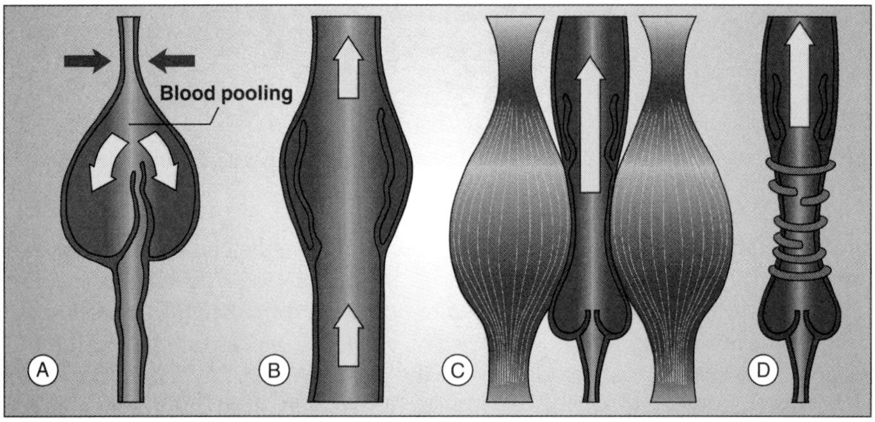

FIG. 12–9. Valves in the veins (A) prevent backflow of returning blood but (B) do not hinder the normal flow very much. Blood can be pushed through veins (C) by nearby active muscle or (D) by the contraction of smooth muscle bands within the veins themselves.

BLOOD PRESSURE

A surge of blood enters the aorta with each contraction of the left ventricle, distending the vessel and creating pressure within it. The stretch and subsequent recoil of the vascular wall travels as a wave through the entire arterial system. This wave of pressure can readily be felt as the characteristic **pulse** in the superficial radial artery on the thumb side of the wrist, in the temporal artery (on the side of the head at the temple), or at the carotid artery along the side of the trachea (near the "Adam's apple") in the neck. Each site is convenient for counting the heart rate at rest and following exercise because in healthy persons the pulse rate and heart rate are identical. Figure 12–10 illustrates the pulse taken at these three convenient locations.

Blood pressure. Blood pressure represents the forces exerted by the blood against the walls of the arteries during a cardiac cycle and is written as systolic/diastolic or, for example, 120/80 mm Hg (stated as 120 over 80).

At Rest. Figure 12–11 illustrates the measurement of **blood pressure** by the ***auscultatory method.*** At rest, the highest pressure generated by the heart to move blood through a healthy, resilient vascular system is usually about 120 mm Hg during contraction of the left ventricle, or **systole.** As the heart relaxes, the natural elastic recoil of the aorta and other arteries provides continuous pressure to maintain blood flow into the periphery until the next surge of blood is received from contraction of the heart. During **diastole,** the relaxation phase of the cardiac cycle, blood pressure in the arterial system decreases to about 70 to 80 mm Hg. In people with arteries "hardened" by deposits of minerals and fatty materials within their walls, or with excessive resistance to blood flow in the periphery resulting from kidney malfunction or nervous strain, systolic pressure may increase from 120 to as high as 300 mm Hg and diastolic pressures may exceed 120 mm Hg.

Young and middle-age blacks at higher risk for subarachnoid hemorrhage. Subarachnoid hemorrhage is a ruptured blood vessel on the brain's surface. This usually fatal category of stroke occurs more frequently in young and middle-aged blacks (12 per 100,000) than comparably aged whites (6 per 100,000). Blacks also suffer higher rates of intracerebral hemorrhage caused by a burst vessel within the interior of the brain. These two categories of stroke account for about one-half of all deaths within 30 days of occurrence. The difference between races could be related to higher rates of hypertension and smoking among blacks.

High blood pressure, or **hypertension,** imposes a chronic and excessive strain on the normal function of the cardiovascular system. Chronic hypertension that is not corrected can eventually lead to **heart failure,** in which the heart muscle weakens and is unable to maintain its pumping ability. In **stroke,** brittle vessels become obstructed or burst to cut off the

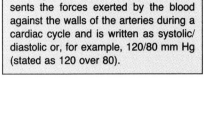

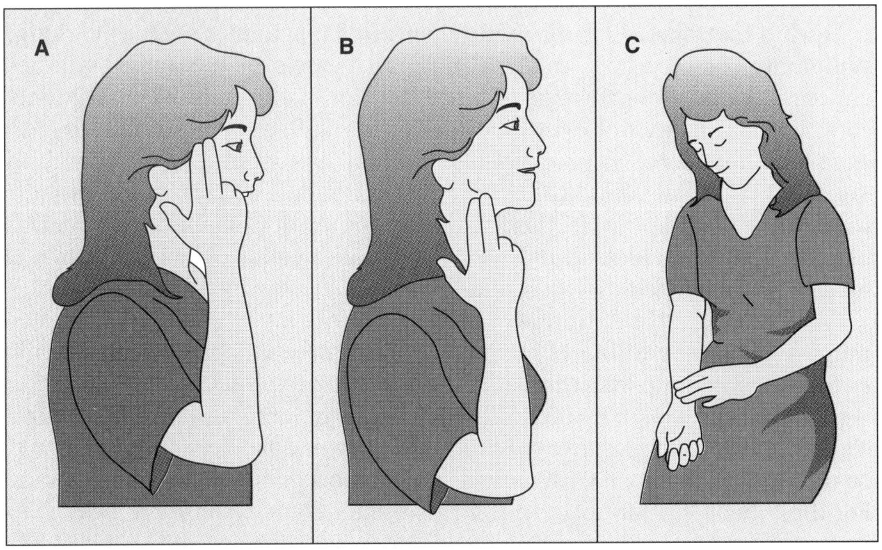

FIG. 12–10. Pulse rate taken at the (A) temporal, (B) carotid, and (C) radial arteries.

Hypertension and race. American blacks overall have twice the incidence of high blood pressure as whites and nearly seven times the rate of severe hypertension. Compounding the issue of race and hypertension is the fact that blacks in the United States have a much greater incidence of elevated blood pressure than blacks in Africa. This has led researchers to focus on the possible causative role of diet, stress, cigarette smoking, and other lifestyle and environmental factors in triggering this chronic blood pressure response in genetically susceptible blacks.

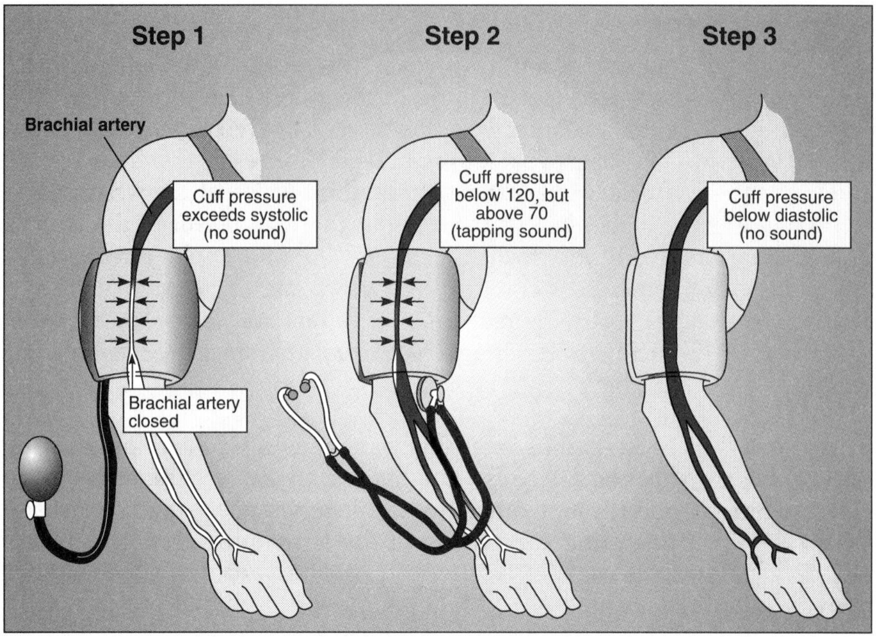

FIG. 12–11. Measurement of blood pressure by auscultation. **Step 1.** A pressure cuff, called a **sphygmomanometer,** is inflated so its pressure exceeds systolic pressure, the highest pressure within the artery. Blood flow is occluded and a brachial pulse (at the elbow fossa) cannot be palpated or heard (auscultated). Note the restriction of blood through the brachial artery. **Step 2.** Pressure within the cuff is reduced by small increments and the examiner listens until a faint sound occurs. This represents blood flowing through the brachial artery. The pressure exerted on the walls of the artery when the first soft tapping sounds occur is called systolic pressure. **Step 3.** As the pressure in the cuff is lowered further, distinct sounds continue to be heard as blood flows through the artery for longer portions of the cardiac cycle. The pressure in the artery when the sounds disappear is diastolic pressure. Blood pressure is expressed as systolic pressure in relation to diastolic pressure (for example, 120 over 80).

blood supply to vital brain tissue. More is said about hypertension in Chapters 19 and 20.

During Exercise. During rhythmic muscular activities such as jogging, swimming, or bicycling, dilation of blood vessels in the active muscles enhances blood flow through a large portion of the body. The alternate contraction and relaxation of the muscles themselves also provides significant pumping force to propel blood through the vessels and return it to the heart. Increased blood flow during moderate exercise causes systolic pressure to rise rapidly in the first few minutes of exercise and level off, usually between 140 and 160 mm Hg, while diastolic pressure remains relatively unchanged.

With straining-type exercises such as the various forms of resistance training (including lifting of barbells), the pressure responses are dramatic as the sustained muscular forces compress the peripheral arteries, causing significant *resistance* to blood flow. This results in rapid and often profound elevation in blood pressure. The additional workload for the heart could be dangerous for those with existing high blood pressure or heart disease. For these people, more rhythmic forms of moderate exercise are desirable.

Body Inversion. Inversion devices that allow a person to hang upside-down have become popular. The belief is that this position can offer relaxation, facilitate a strength-training response, or relieve lower back pain. No one has yet demonstrated with careful research that inverting the body is of any practical medical or physiologic significance, and the maneuver can trigger significant *increases* in blood pressure both at the start and throughout the inversion period. This raises concern about the possible consequences of inversion for people with high blood pressure, or the wisdom of performing exercises in the upside-down position that magnify the normal rise in blood pressure with exercise. Furthermore, a brief period of inversion doubles pressure within the eye (intraocular pressure) in healthy young adults. *Clearly, individuals with eye disorders should refrain from prolonged periods of inverted posture.*

CIRCULATORY FUNCTION IN THE TRAINED AND UNTRAINED

The output of blood from the heart pump, referred to as **cardiac output,** is an important indicator of the functional capacity of the circulation to meet the demands of aerobic activity. Cardiac output is determined by two factors: the rate at which the pump strokes, or **heart rate,** and the quantity of fluid ejected with each stroke, the **stroke volume.** Thus,

Cardiac output = Heart rate × Stroke volume

The blood flow to muscles increases in proportion to the severity of exercise. In relatively sedentary college-aged males, the cardiac output during strenuous exercise increases by about four times the resting level to an average maximum of 20 liters, or 20,000 ml, of blood pumped per minute. Maximal heart rate at this age usually averages 195 beats per minute. Consequently, the "untrained" heart pumps about 103 ml of blood with each beat (20,000 ml ÷ 195) during maximum exercise. This contrasts with world-class endurance athletes whose maximum cardiac output is 35 to 40 liters of blood per minute. For these athletes, maximum heart rate is not appreciably different from that of sedentary people of similar age. Thus, the **stroke volume of the athlete's heart** is about 180 ml of blood per beat.

Cardiac output = Heart rate × Stroke volume

	Cardiac Output	=	Heart Rate	×	Stroke Volume
At rest					
Sedentary	5000 ml	=	70 beats/min	×	71 ml
Trained	5000 ml	=	50 beats/min	×	100 ml
Maximum exercise					
Sedentary	20,000 ml	=	195 beats/min	×	103 ml
Trained	35,000 ml	=	195 beats/min	×	180 ml

Figure 12–12 illustrates the response of cardiac output, stroke volume, and heart rate in relation to oxygen uptake during exercise of increasing severity. The subjects were two groups of men, one group comprising highly trained endurance athletes, while the other consisted of sedentary college

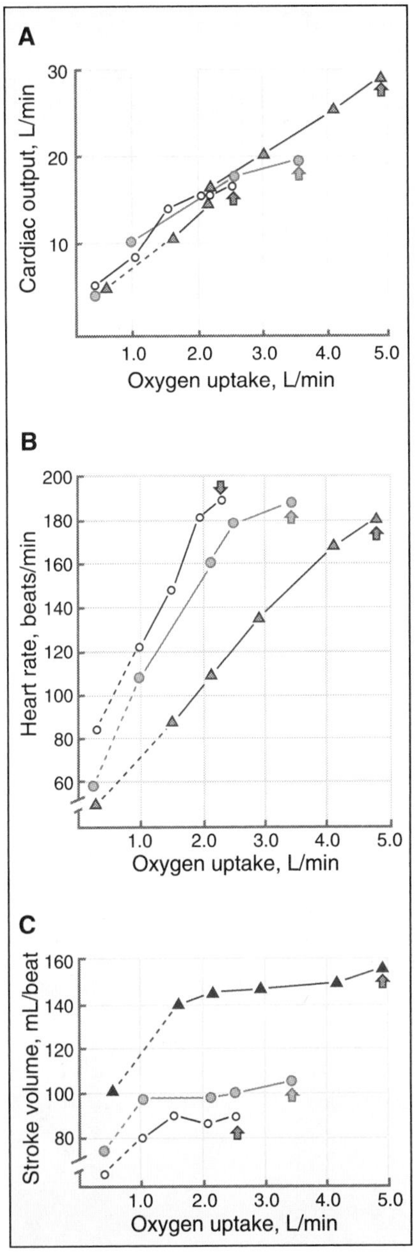

FIG. 12–12. Maximal values for (A) cardiac output, (B) stroke volume, and (C) heart rate in relation to oxygen uptake during upright exercise in endurance athletes (▲) and sedentary college students prior to (○) and following (●) 55 days of aerobic training. Arrows indicate maximal values. (From Saltin, B.: Physiological effects of physical conditioning. *Med. Sci. Sports,* 1:50, 1969.)

students measured before and after a 55-day training program designed to improve aerobic fitness.

Stroke volume makes the difference. A significantly larger stroke volume is the key factor that enables an endurance athlete to pump more blood from the heart each minute than an untrained counterpart.

The researchers observed several important physiologic responses. First, for both trained athletes and students, cardiac output increased in linear fashion in relation to oxygen uptake throughout the major portion of the work range (Figure 12–12A). The distinguishing feature between students and athletes was the athletes' high level of oxygen uptake and corresponding cardiac output capacity. In addition, the 35% improvement in max $\dot{V}O_2$ for the students after training was accompanied by an almost proportionate increase in maximum cardiac output. Second, the stroke volume of the athletes' hearts was considerably larger than that of the untrained students at rest and during exercise (Figure 12–12B). Third, the response pattern for stroke volume during exercise was similar in both groups: the increase was greatest when going from rest to light exercise, and thereafter it was quite small. Fourth, stroke volume increased only slightly from rest to exercise in the untrained men. Thus, their major means to raise cardiac output in response to exercise was by an increase in heart rate. For the trained athletes, on the other hand, *both* heart rate and stroke volume increased to augment blood flow during exercise. Following training, the students' stroke volume (and maximum cardiac output) had increased substantially, but the value was still considerably below that of the athletes. The degree to which both training and genetic factors account for the exceptionally large stroke volumes of successful endurance athletes is still unresolved. Scientists do agree, however, that the ability of the heart trained by exercise to generate a large stroke volume is the result of two factors: an enlarged internal dimension of the left ventricular chamber, and a more forceful contraction that empties the ventricle almost completely with each beat.

Stroke volume improves regardless of age. Numerous studies have documented that an increase in the heart's pumping capacity occurs in healthy men and women of all ages who undertake vigorous physical conditioning programs.

Cardiac output is similar at rest and during submaximal exercise in both sedentary and exercise-trained men and women. Consequently, the large stroke volumes of endurance athletes and the increase in stroke volume of sedentary subjects following aerobic training are accompanied by a proportionate reduction in submaximal exercise heart rate (Figure 12–12C). Although the same value of cardiac output is required during a particular level of exercise after training, this is achieved with a much *lower* heart rate. The reduction in exercise heart rate during a standard bout of submaximal exercise provides a practical means to evaluate physiologic adaptation during training. This is discussed more fully in Chapter 19.

Training lowers heart rate. It is common for the exercise heart rate to be lowered by 12 to 15 beats per minute as a result of an aerobic conditioning program.

Close Association between Cardiac Output Capacity and Max $\dot{V}O_2$. Figure 12–13 displays the relationship between **maximum cardiac output and aerobic capacity.** Included are values for sedentary people as well as elite endurance athletes. The relationship is unmistakable: a low aerobic capacity is closely associated with low maximum cardiac output, whereas the ability to generate a 5- or 6-liter max $\dot{V}O_2$ is always accompanied by a 30- to 40-liter cardiac output.

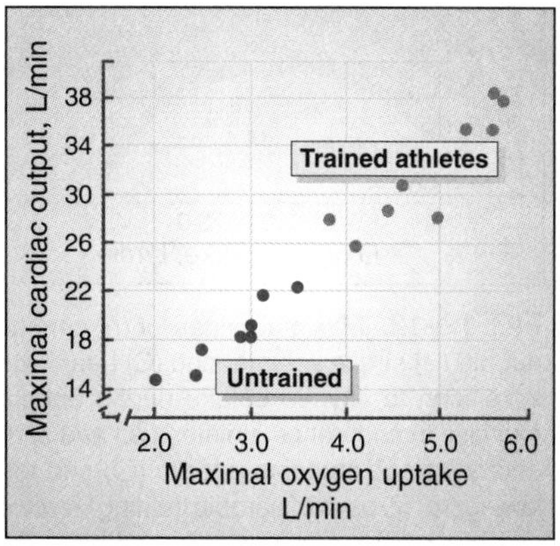

FIG. 12–13. Relationship between maximal cardiac output and max $\dot{V}O_2$.

"Athlete's Heart." *A modest increase in size, or hypertrophy, is a fundamental adjustment of the healthy heart to regular exercise training.* There is greater synthesis of cellular protein as the individual muscle fibers thicken and the contractile elements within each fiber increase in number. This size increase with training is transient, and heart size returns to pretraining levels when training intensity decreases.

*Different **patterns of cardiac enlargement** are associated with various types* *of conditioning*. In endurance athletes, for example, who participate regularly in rhythmic exercise requiring a large cardiac output, the ventricular walls are of normal thickness but the ventricular cavity is enlarged. The greater internal dimensions are certainly in keeping with the development of a large stroke volume that is so beneficial in endurance activities. In contrast, athletes involved in resistance exercise training such as weight lifters, shot putters, and wrestlers, who are regularly subjected to acute episodes of elevated arterial pressure caused by straining-type exercises, have normal ventricular volume but the ventricular wall is thickened. Undoubtedly, this represents compensation for the added workload resistance training imposes on the left ventricle. The consequences of these apparent differences in training response for long-term cardiovascular health are unknown. *There is no scientific evidence, however, that a normal heart can be harmed by exercise training.*

Sonar for the heart. A clearer understanding of the changes in heart size and structure with training has been provided by the ultrasonic technique of echocardiography. With this approach, sound waves are passed through the heart to "map" the dimensions of the muscle itself as well as the volume of its cavities.

SUMMARY

1. The lungs provide a large interface between the body's internal fluid environment and the gaseous external environment. At any one second, there is probably no more than a pint of blood in the pulmonary capillaries.
2. Pulmonary ventilation is geared to maintain favorable concentrations of alveolar oxygen and carbon dioxide to assure adequate aeration of blood flowing through the lungs.
3. Pulmonary airflow depends upon small pressure differences between ambient air and air within the lungs. These differences are brought about by the action of various muscles that work to alter the dimensions of the chest cavity.
4. A forced exhalation against a closed glottis is called a Valsalva maneuver. It can cause a large increase in pressure within the chest and abdominal cavities that compresses the thoracic veins, significantly reducing venous return to the heart.
5. In the lungs and tissues, gas molecules diffuse down their concentration gradients from an area of higher concentration (higher pressure) to one of lower concentration (lower pressure).
6. Gas exchange is so rapid in the healthy lung that equilibrium occurs at about the midpoint of the blood's transit through the pulmonary capillaries. Even with vigorous exercise, the velocity of blood flow through the lungs generally does not restrict the full loading of oxygen and unloading of carbon dioxide.
7. At the tissues, the diffusion gradient favors movement of oxygen from the capillary to the tissues and carbon dioxide from the cells into the blood. In exercise, these gradients are expanded and oxygen and carbon dioxide diffuse rapidly.
8. Hemoglobin, the iron-protein pigment in the red blood cell, increases the oxygen-carrying capacity of whole blood about 65 times above the level of oxygen carried in physical solution dissolved in the plasma.
9. The blood's oxygen transport capacity varies only slightly with normal fluctuations in hemoglobin content. Iron deficiency anemia, however, significantly decreases the blood's oxygen-carrying capacity and consequently reduces aerobic exercise performance.

10. In light to moderate exercise, ventilation increases linearly with oxygen uptake. In vigorous, non-steady-state exercise, ventilation increases disproportionately with oxygen uptake. This sharp upswing in ventilation is related to the onset of blood lactate accumulation.
11. Exercise-induced asthma is an obstructive pulmonary phenomenon that is brought on by evaporative cooling of the airways during exercise. This response is essentially eliminated when humidified air is breathed during exercise. Cigarette smoke also significantly increases airway resistance.
12. Functionally, the heart can be viewed as two separate pumps: one receives blood returning from the body and pumps it to the lungs for aeration, whereas the other receives oxygenated blood from the lungs and pumps it throughout the body.
13. The surge of blood with contraction of the ventricles (and subsequent runoff during relaxation) creates pressure changes within the arterial vessels. Systolic pressure, the highest pressure generated during the cardiac cycle, occurs during ventricular contraction. Diastolic pressure is the lowest pressure reached before the next contraction of the ventricle.
14. Systolic blood pressure increases in proportion to oxygen uptake during rhythmic muscular activities, while diastolic pressure remains relatively unchanged. With straining-type exercises, blood pressures mirror the hypertensive state and may pose a risk to individuals with existing hypertension or heart disease.
15. Cardiac output reflects the functional capacity of the circulatory system. The two factors determining the heart's output capacity are heart rate and stroke volume.
16. Cardiac output increases in proportion to the severity of exercise, from about 5 liters per minute at rest to a maximum of 20 to 25 liters per minute in college-aged men and 35 to 40 liters per minute in elite male endurance athletes. These differences in maximum cardiac output are attributable entirely to the large stroke volumes of the athletes.
17. During exercise, stroke volume rises during the transition from rest to light exercise. Thereafter, cardiac output is augmented primarily by increases in heart rate.
18. Heart rate and oxygen uptake are linearly related throughout the major portion of the exercise range. With aerobic training, this line shifts significantly to the right because of improvements in the heart's stroke volume. Consequently, heart rate becomes significantly reduced at any submaximal exercise level.
19. Cardiac hypertrophy is a fundamental adaptation to the increased workload imposed by exercise training. It results in a stronger heart that can generate a relatively large stroke volume. The pattern of structural and dimensional changes in the left ventricle varies with specific forms of exercise training.

RELATED LITERATURE

Åstrand, P.O., and Rodahl, K.: Textbook of Work Physiology. New York, McGraw-Hill, 1986.

Banner, A.S., et al.: Relation of respiratory water loss to coughing after exercise. *N. Engl. J. Med.*, 311:833, 1984.

Bender, P.R., and Martin, B.J.: Maximal ventilation for exhausting exercise. *Med. Sci. Sports Exerc.*, 17:164, 1985.

Berk, J.L., et al.: Cold-induced bronchoconstriction: role of cutaneous reflexes vs. direct airway effects. *J. Appl. Physiol.*, 63:659, 1987.
Brooks, G.A.: Anaerobic threshold: review of the concept and directions for future research. *Med. Sci. Sports Exerc.*, 17:22, 1985.
Bundgaard, A., et al.: Influence of temperature and relative humidity of inhaled gas on exercise-induced asthma. *Eur. J. Resp. Dis.*, 63:239, 1982.
Carter, R., et al.: Exercise training in patients with chronic obstructive pulmonary disease. Med. Sci. Sports Exerc., 24:281, 1992.
Cordain, L., et al.: Lung volumes of maximal respiratory pressures in collegiate swimmers and runners. *Res. Q. Exerc. Sport*, 61:70, 1990.
Couldry, W.C., et al.: Carotid vs. radial pulse counts. *Phys. Sportsmed.*, 10:67, 1982.
Cox, M.L., et al.: Exercise training–induced alterations of cardiac morphology. *J. Appl. Physiol.*, 61:926, 1986.
Coyle, E.F., et al.: Time course of loss of adaptations after stopping prolonged intense endurance training. *J. Appl. Physiol.*, 57:1857, 1984.
Davis, J.A.: Anaerobic threshold: review of the concept and directions for future research. *Med. Sci. Sports Exerc.*, 17:6, 1985.
Dempsey, J.A.: Is the lung built for exercise? *Med. Sci. Sports Exerc.*, 18:143, 1986.
Donaldson, M.C.: Varicose veins in active people. *Phys. Sportsmed.*, 18:46, 1990.
Effron, M.B.: Effects of resistive training on left ventricular function. *Med. Sci. Sports Exerc.*, 21:694, 1989.
Ehsani, A.A., et al.: Improvement of left ventricular contractile function by exercise training in patients with coronary artery disease. *Circulation*, 74:350, 1986.
Farrell, P.A., et al.: Plasma lactate accumulation and distance running performance. *Med. Sci. Sports Exerc.*, 11:338, 1979.
Fleck, S.J.: Cardiovascular adaptations to resistance training. *Med. Sci. Sports Exerc.*, 20:S146, 1988.
Gaffney, F.A., et al.: Cardiovascular and metabolic responses to static contraction in man. *Acta Physiol. Scand.*, 138:249, 1990.
Haas, F., et al.: Effect of aerobic training on forced expiratory airflow in exercising asthmatic humans. *J. Appl. Physiol.*, 63:1230, 1987.
Hagberg, J.M., et al.: Pulmonary function in young and older athletes and untrained men. *J. Appl. Physiol.*, 65:101, 1988.
Hannum, S.M., and Kasch, F.W.: Acute postexercise blood pressure response of hypertensive and normotensive men. *Scand. J. Sports Med.*, 3:11, 1981.
Harman, E.A., et al.: Intra-abdominal and intra-thoracic pressures during lifting and jumping. *Med. Sci. Sports Exerc.*, 20:195, 1988.
Hickson, R.C., et al.: Reduced training intensities and loss of aerobic power, endurance, and cardiac growth. *J. Appl. Physiol.*, 58:492, 1985.
Holloszy, J.O., and Coyle, E.F.: Adaptations of skeletal muscle to endurance training and their metabolic consequences. *J. Appl. Physiol.*, 56:831, 1984.
Hopkins, S.R., and McKenzie, D.C.: Hypoxic ventilatory response and arterial desaturation during heavy work. *J. Appl. Physiol.*, 67:1119, 1989.
Jones, N.L.: Dyspnea in exercise. *Med. Sci. Sports Exerc.*, 16:14, 1984.
Kaufman, F.L., et al.: Effect of exercise on recovery blood pressure in normotensive and hypertensive subjects. *Med. Sci. Sports Exerc.*, 19:17, 1987.
Keleman, M.H.: Exercise training combined with antihypertensive drug therapy: effects on lipids, blood pressure, and left ventricular mass. *JAMA*, 263:2766, 1990.
LeMarr, J.D., et al.: Cardiorespiratory responses to inversion. *Phys. Sportsmed.*, 11:51, 1983.
Levinson, H., and Cherniack, R.: Ventilatory cost of exercise in chronic obstructive pulmonary disease. *J. Appl. Physiol.*, 25:21, 1968.
Lewis, S.F., et al.: Cardiovascular responses to exercise as a function of absolute and relative workload. *J. Appl. Physiol.*, 54:1314, 1983.
Massic, B.M.: To combat hypertension, increase activity. Phys. Sportsmed., 20:89, 1992.
McArdle, W.D., et al: Exercise Physiology: Energy, Nutrition, and Human Performance, 3rd ed. Philadelphia, Lea & Febiger, 1991.
McFadden, E.R.: Exercise-induced asthma; recent approaches. *Chest*, 93:1282, 1988.
Miles, D.S., et al.: Cardiovascular responses to upper body exercise in normals and cardiac patients. *Med. Sci. Sports Exerc.*, 21:S126, 1989.
Nakamura, M., et al.: Acute effects of cigarette smoke inhalation on peripheral airways in dogs. *J. Appl. Physiol.*, 58:27, 1985.
Pelliccia, A., et al.: The upper limit of physiologic cardiac hypertrophy in highly trained elite athletes. *N. Engl. J. Med.*, 324:295, 1991.

Powers, S.K., et al.: Effects of incomplete pulmonary gas exchange in $\dot{V}O_2$ max. *J. Appl. Physiol.*, 66:2491, 1989.
Reiff, D.B., et al.: The effect of prolonged submaximal warm-up on exercise-induced asthma. *Am. Rev. Respir. Dis.*, 139:479, 1989.
Rode, A., and Shephard, R.J.: The influence of cigarette smoking upon the oxygen cost of breathing in near-maximal exercise. *Med. Sci. Sports*, 3:51, 1971.
Rowell, L.B.: General principles of vascular control. In: Human Circulation: Regulation during Physical Stress. New York, Oxford University Press, 1986.
Rowell, L.B.: Human cardiovascular adjustments to exercise and thermal stress. *Physiol. Rev.*, 4:75, 1974.
Rowland, T.W., et al.: "Athletes heart" in prepubertal children. *Pediatrics*, 79:800, 1987.
Saltin, B.: Physiological effects of physical conditioning. *Med. Sci. Sports Exerc.*, 1:50, 1969.
Saltin, B. and Strange, S.: Maximal oxygen uptake: "old" and "new" arguments for cardiovascular limitation. Med. Sci. Sports Exerc., 24:30, 1992.
Seals, D.R., and Hagberg, J.M.: The effect of exercise training on human hypertension. *Med. Sci. Sports Exerc.*, 16:207, 1984.
Sharp, J.T., et al.: Relative contributions of rib cage and abdomen to breathing in normal subjects. *J. Appl. Physiol.*, 36:608, 1975.
Smith, M.A., et al.: Assessment of beat to beat changes in cardiac output during the Valsalva manoeuvre using bioimpedience cardiology. *Clin. Sci.*, 72:423, 1987.
Voy, R.O.: The U.S. Olympic Committee experience with exercise induced bronchospasm, 1984. *Med. Sci. Sports Exerc.*, 18:328, 1986.
Weltman, A., et al.: The lactate threshold and endurance performance. *Adv. Sports Med. Fitness*, 2:91, 1989.

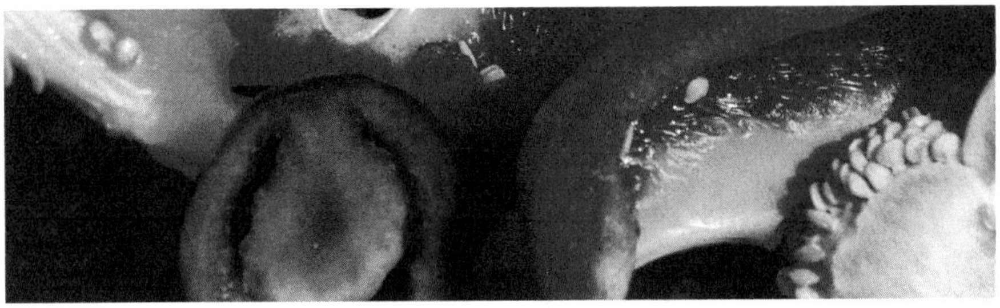

13

ENERGY VALUE OF FOOD AND PHYSICAL ACTIVITY

The energy trapped within the chemical bonds of carbohydrates, lipids, and proteins is extracted during a series of complex chemical reactions and made available to the cells in the form of energy currency: adenosine triphosphate, or ATP. Because the three major food nutrients contain energy, and because all bodily functions require energy, it is possible to classify both food and physical activity in terms of a common denominator, *energy*.

ENERGY CONTAINED IN FOODS: CALORIES

*A **calorie** is a unit of heat used to express the energy value of food.* Although the term appears widely in popular literature, it has a precise scientific meaning. One Calorie (spelled with a capital C) represents the amount of heat necessary to increase the temperature of 1 kg of water, which is slightly more than a quart, by 1° Celsius. A Calorie—or more accurately, a kilocalorie—is abbreviated ***kcal.*** For example, a McDonald's Big Mac hamburger and regular fries contain about 783 kcal and thus the energy to raise the temperature of about 783 quarts (196 gallons) of water by 1° C. This is indeed a relatively large amount of energy. On the other hand, a boiled egg contains only 80 kcal, or the energy required to increase the temperature of about 80 quarts of water by 1° C.

Kilojoule. The accepted international standard for expressing energy is the joule. To convert kcal to **kilojoule** (kJ), multiply the kcal value by 4.2.

MEASUREMENT OF CALORIES

The energy or kcal value of any food can be measured directly by the amount of heat released when it is burned in an apparatus called a ***bomb calorimeter.*** This method of measuring the energy content of foods is known as direct calorimetry.

The bomb calorimeter, illustrated in Figure 13–1, works as follows. A weighed portion of food is placed inside a small chamber filled with oxygen. The food is literally exploded and burned when an electric current ignites a fuse inside the chamber. The heat released as the food burns, termed the ***heat of combustion,*** is absorbed by a surrounding water bath. Because the

Heat of combustion. The heat liberated by the burning or oxidation of food in the bomb calorimeter is referred to as its heat of combustion and represents the total energy value of the food.

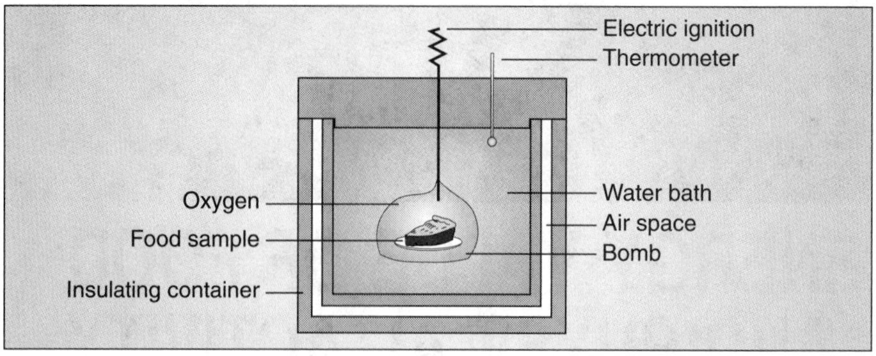

FIG. 13–1. A bomb calorimeter is used to determine the energy value of food.

calorimeter is fully insulated, no heat escapes to the outside. The precise amount of heat absorbed by the water is determined by measuring the increase in water temperature with a sensitive thermometer. For example, when one 4.7 oz, 4-inch sector of apple pie is completely burned in the calorimeter, 350 kcal of heat energy is released. This will raise 3.5 kg, or 7.7 pounds, of ice water to the boiling point.

CALORIC VALUE OF FOODS

Many laboratories have used the bomb calorimeter to determine the energy value of foods.

Heat of Combustion. The burning of 1 g of pure carbohydrate yields a heat of combustion of 4.20 kcal, 1 g of pure protein releases 5.65 kcal, and 1 g of pure lipid yields 9.45 kcal. Because most foods in the diet consist of various proportions of these three nutrients, the caloric value of a given food, such as a hamburger or french fries, is determined by the macronutrient content of an average serving. It is evident from the heats of combustion that the energy content will be greater in a food high in fat than in one that is relatively fat free. For example, the number of calories in 1 cup of whole milk is 160 kcal, whereas the same amount of skimmed milk contains 90 kcal. If someone who normally consumes 1 quart of milk each day switches to skimmed milk, the quantity of calories ingested each year would be reduced by an amount equal to about 11.4 kg (25 lb) of body fat!

When a gram of carbohydrate or lipid is "burned" in the mitochondria (the cell's energy factory), the body liberates the same value of 4.20 kcal for carbohydrate and 9.45 kcal for lipid as did the bomb calorimeter. The energy yield from lipid is more than twice that of carbohydrate because of the difference in structural composition between the two nutrients. As noted in Chapter 1, the chemical formula for a simple carbohydrate always has a ratio of two hydrogen atoms for each atom of oxygen. Lipid molecules, on the other hand, contain significantly more hydrogen than oxygen. The fatty acid palmitic acid, for example, has the structural formula $C_{16}H_{30}O_2$. This means there are more hydrogen atoms that can be cleaved away and oxidized to produce energy during the breakdown of a lipid.

The energy available to the body from protein breakdown is less than that released in the bomb calorimeter. In addition to carbon, hydrogen, and oxygen, proteins contain the element nitrogen. Because the body cannot use nitrogen, it combines with hydrogen to form urea (NH_2CONH_2) that is excreted in the urine. This elimination of hydrogen represents a loss of potential energy. For this reason, the energy yield from 1 g of protein in the body is 4.35 kcal instead of the 5.65 kcal released during its complete oxidation in the bomb calorimeter.

Digestive Efficiency. An important consideration in determining the ultimate caloric yield of ingested macronutrients is the efficiency with which they are made available to the body. Efficiency in this sense refers to completeness of digestion and absorption. Normally, about 97% of carbohydrates, 95% of lipids, and 92% of proteins are digested and absorbed. *When these average* ***digestive efficiencies*** *are considered, the net kcal value for carbohydrate is 4.0, for lipid it is 9.0, and for protein it is 4.0.*

Digestive efficiency. The average percentage for digestive efficiency varies somewhat depending on the particular food. This is especially true for protein, where digestive efficiency ranges from a high of 97% for animal protein to a low of 78% for dried legumes. Furthermore, the available energy from a meal is reduced when it has a high fiber content.

CALORIE VALUE OF A MEAL

By use of net kcal values, the caloric content of a food dish can be determined as long as its composition and weight are known. Suppose, for example, we wished to determine the kcal value for ½ cup of creamed chicken. The weight of this portion is equivalent to 3.5 oz, or about 100 g. Based on laboratory analysis of a standard recipe, the macronutrient composition of the creamed chicken is approximately 20% protein, 12% lipid, 6% carbohydrate, and the remaining 62% is water. Using these compositional values, the kcal in the creamed chicken can be determined as follows: each gram of creamed chicken contains 0.2 g of protein, 0.12 g of fat, and 0.06 g of carbohydrate. Based on net kcal values, 0.2 g of protein contains 0.8 kcal (0.20 × 4.0), 0.12 g of lipid equals 1.08 kcal (0.12 × 9.0), and 0.06 g of carbohydrate yields 0.24 kcal (0.06 × 4.0). The total caloric value of 1 g of creamed chicken would therefore equal 2.12 kcal (0.80 + 1.08 + 0.24). Consequently, a 100 g serving would contain 100 times as much, or 212 kcal. An example of these computations is presented in Table 13–1. Although this table shows the method for calculating the kcal value of ice cream, the same method can be used for a serving of any food. Reducing the portion size by half would of course reduce caloric intake by 50%.

Lipid is the energy-rich nutrient. The variation in energy value of the macronutrients indicates clearly that if extra fat is added in food preparation, or if fat-free substitutes are used, the caloric value of a meal can be affected significantly.

How to Use Appendix A. Fortunately, there is seldom need to compute the kcal value of foods as shown in the example, because the United States

TABLE 13–1. METHOD OF CALCULATING THE CALORIC VALUE OF A FOOD FROM ITS COMPOSITION OF NUTRIENTS

FOOD: ICE CREAM (VANILLA)
WEIGHT: THREE-FOURTHS CUP = 100 GRAMS

	Composition		
	Protein	Fat	Carbohydrate
Percentage	4%	13%	21%
Total grams	4	13	21
In 1 g	0.04 g	0.13 g	0.21 g
Calories per gram	0.16	1.17	0.84
	(0.04 × 4.0 kcal) +	(0.13 × 9.0 kcal) +	(0.21 × 4.0 kcal)

Total calories per g: 0.16 + 1.17 + 0.84 = 2.17 kcal
Total calories per 100 g: 2.17 × 100 = 217 kcal

Department of Agriculture has already made these determinations for almost all foods. What we have done in Appendix A is to present a representative listing of the nutritive and energy value of the more common foods. The nutritive value for each food is expressed per ounce, or 28.4 g, of the food item. The specific values for each food include its calories per ounce as well as its content of protein, fat, carbohydrate, calcium, iron, vitamin B_1, vitamin B_2, fiber, and cholesterol.

Computer Programs Are Helpful. For those with access to a computer-based nutritional analysis system, the task of evaluating nutritional quality is quite easy. When a portion size is specified, the computer taps its memory for that particular food and lists the corresponding nutrient composition. In this way, we can determine the total nutrient intake for any diet and compare it with the Recommended Dietary Allowances specified by the Food and Nutrition Board. This analysis is useful to evaluate nutritional status and to compare individuals and groups in terms of their dietary practices. Major drawbacks with this approach are the considerable time required to enter "coded" food items into the computer and uncertainty regarding portion size. At best, the approximation of "true" nutrient intake by computerized analysis may be off by 10 to 30% even when accurate records are kept.

A CALORIE IS A CALORIE IS A CALORIE

If you examine Appendix A carefully, you will note a rather striking, yet reasonable observation with regard to the energy value of food. Consider, for example, five common foods: raw celery, cooked cabbage, cooked asparagus spears, mayonnaise, and salad oil. To consume 100 kcal of each of these foods, a person must eat 20 stalks of celery, 4 cups of cabbage, 30 asparagus spears, but only 1 tablespoon of mayonnaise or $\frac{4}{5}$ tablespoon of salad oil. The point is that a small serving of some foods contains the equivalent energy value as a large quantity of other foods. Viewed from a different perspective, one would have to consume over 4000 stalks of celery, 800 cups of cabbage, or 30 eggs to supply the daily energy needs of a fairly sedentary individual, while the *same energy* would be supplied by ingesting only $1\frac{1}{2}$ cups of mayonnaise or about 8 oz of salad oil. The major difference is that high-fat foods exist as relatively concentrated sources of energy and contain little water. In contrast, foods low in fat or high in water tend to contain relatively little energy. An important concept, however, is that 100 kcal from mayonnaise and 100 kcal from celery are exactly the same in terms of energy. Simply stated, *a calorie is a calorie is a calorie.* The number of calories contained in foods is additive: the more you eat, the more calories you consume. If the food has a high concentration of calories, as in the case of fatty foods, and you consume even a moderate portion, you will of course consume a large number of calories.

Energy is energy. A calorie is a calorie. There is no difference between calories from an energy standpoint, a calorie being a unit of heat regardless of the food source.

HEAT PRODUCED BY THE BODY

Two techniques, direct and indirect **calorimetry,** are used to determine the energy generated by the body both at rest and during physical activity.

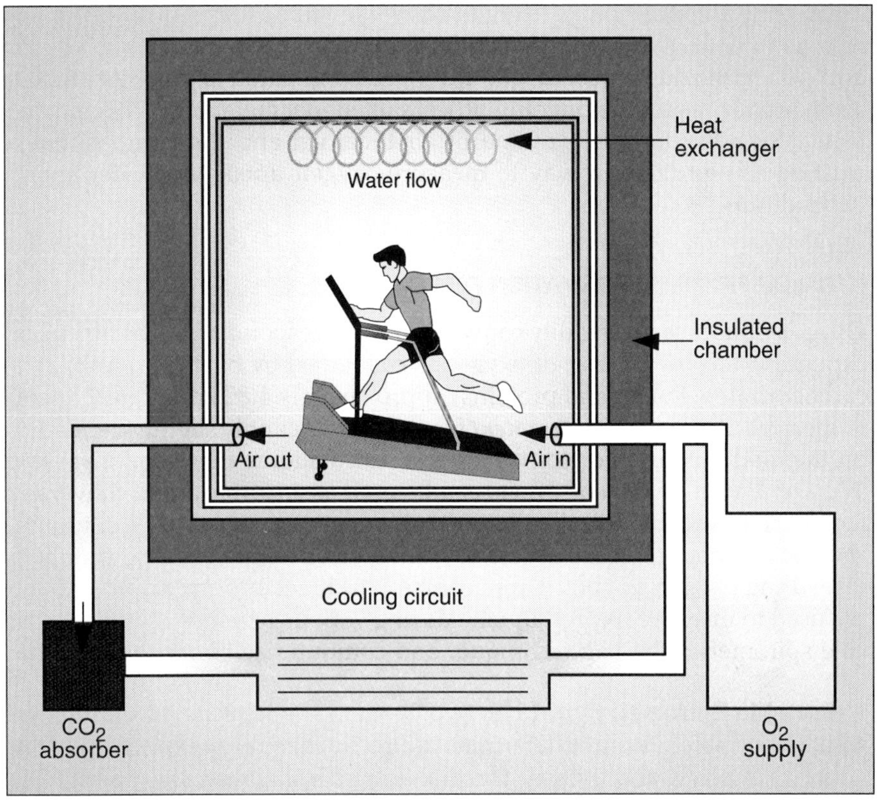

FIG. 13–2. Human calorimeter used to measure heat production.

Direct Calorimetry. The heat produced by the body can be measured in a *calorimeter* similar to the one used to determine the energy content of food. The **human calorimeter** illustrated in Figure 13–2 consists of an airtight chamber with an oxygen supply in which a person can live and work for an extended period. A known volume of water is circulated through a series of coils at the top of the chamber. Because the entire chamber is insulated, the heat produced and radiated by the individual is absorbed by the circulating water. The change in water temperature reflects the energy metabolism for a particular time. To provide adequate ventilation, the subject's exhaled air is drawn from the room and passed through chemicals that remove the moisture and absorb carbon dioxide. Oxygen is then added to the air and recirculated through the chamber.

Human calorimeter. The direct measurement of heat production in humans is of considerable theoretical importance, yet its use and application are rather limited. The calorimeter is relatively small and quite expensive, accurate measurements of heat production are time-consuming, and its use is generally not applicable for energy determinations during common sports, occupational, or recreational activities.

Indirect Calorimetry. *All energy-releasing reactions in the body ultimately depend on the utilization of oxygen.* By measuring a person's oxygen uptake, it is possible to obtain an *indirect* estimate of energy expenditure. Compared to direct calorimetry, **indirect calorimetry** is relatively simple, the equipment is much less expensive, and the technique is highly accurate.

There are two methods of indirect calorimetry: closed-circuit and open-circuit spirometry. The **open-circuit method** is the most widely used to measure oxygen uptake, especially during exercise. In the **closed-circuit method,** the subject breathes and rebreathes from a prefilled container of oxygen. In open-circuit spirometry the subject inhales ambient air that has a constant composition of oxygen (20.9%), carbon dioxide (0.03%), and nitrogen (79.0%) with the remainder inert gases. The changes in oxygen and carbon dioxide percentage in expired air compared to inspired ambient air indirectly reflect the ongoing process of energy metabolism. Thus, analysis of two factors—the volume of air breathed and the composition of exhaled air—provides a way to measure oxygen uptake and infer energy expenditure.

CALORIFIC TRANSFORMATION FOR OXYGEN

Oxygen uptake translates into calories burned. The specific calorific value per liter of oxygen consumed is 4.5 kcal for protein, 4.7 kcal for lipid, and 5.0 kcal for carbohydrate. For convenience, a value of 5 kcal per liter of oxygen consumed is used as an appropriate conversion factor.

Oxygen uptake can be readily converted to a corresponding value for energy expenditure. When 1 liter of oxygen is consumed by burning a mixture of carbohydrates, lipids, and proteins, approximately 4.82 kcal of heat energy is liberated. This ***caloric equivalent for oxygen*** varies only slightly depending on the food mixture. For convenience in calculations, therefore, a value of *5 kcal per liter of oxygen* consumed can be used as an appropriate conversion factor. This amount, 5 kcal, is important because it enables us to determine the body's energy release at rest or during steady-state exercise simply by measuring oxygen uptake. Three common indirect calorimetry procedures are used to measure oxygen uptake during various physical activities: portable spirometry, the bag technique, and computerized instrumentation.

Portable Spirometry. In 1940, two German scientists developed a lightweight, portable system to determine indirectly the energy expended during a variety of physical activities. The box-shaped apparatus, shown in Figure 13–3, weighs approximately 3 kg and is usually carried on the back during the measurement period. The subject breathes through a two-way valve that allows inspiration of ambient air, while exhaled air passes through a meter to measure air volume. Samples of exhaled air are simultaneously collected in small rubber bags attached to the meter. Oxygen uptake is computed by analyzing the expired air for oxygen and carbon dioxide content. Energy expenditure, expressed in kcal, is then computed from the oxygen uptake. An advantage of the **portable spirometer** is that it gives a person considerable freedom to move while being measured. The portable spirometer was used to estimate the energy expenditure for most of the recreational and household activities listed in Appendix A.

Bag Technique. The subject shown in Figure 13–4B is cycling on a stationary ergometer. While exercising, a special headgear is worn to which a two-way breathing valve is attached. The subject breathes in ambient air through one side of the valve and exhales it from the other side into a collection bag. The exhaled air is then analyzed for its oxygen and carbon dioxide composition and volume. Energy expenditure is computed from oxygen uptake just as it is when using the portable spirometer. As can be seen in Figure 13–4A, oxygen uptake is being measured by the **bag technique** during rest.

Computerized Instrumentation. Recent advances in computer and microprocessor technology enable the exercise scientist to efficiently measure metabolic and cardiovascular response to exercise. A computer is interfaced with at least three instruments: a system to continuously sample the airflow from the subject, a meter to record the volume of air breathed, and oxygen

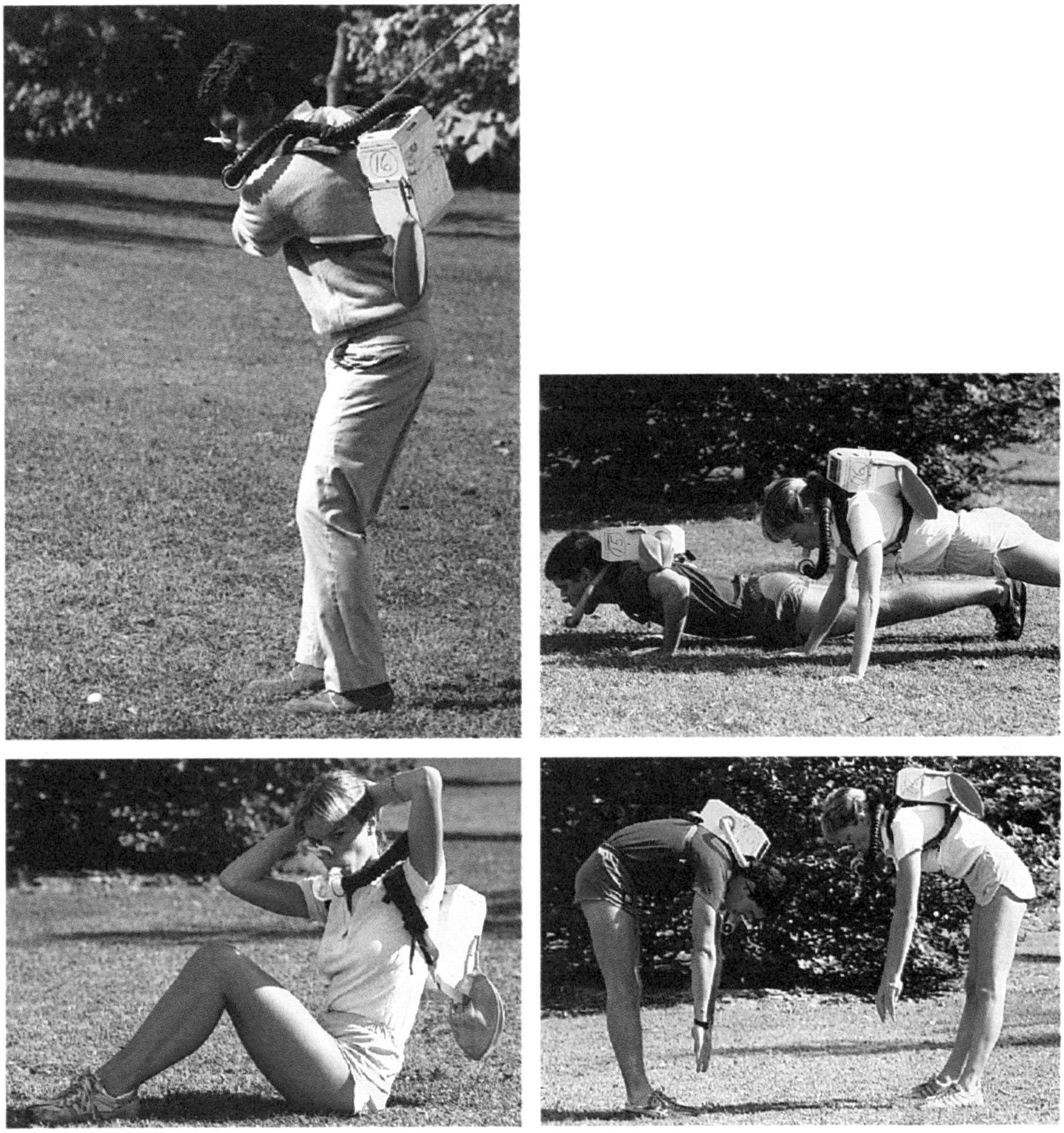

FIG. 13–3. Portable spirometer used to measure oxygen uptake by the open-circuit method during (A) golf, (B) push-up exercise, (C) sit-up exercise, and (D) calisthenic exercise.

and carbon dioxide analyzers to measure the composition of the expired gas mixture. The computer is programmed to perform all the necessary calculations based on electronic signals it receives from the instruments. A printed or graphic display of the data is provided simultaneously during exercise and recovery. More advanced systems include automated blood pressure, heart rate, and temperature monitors, as well as preset instructions to regulate the speed, duration, and workload of treadmills, bicycle ergometers, steppers, rowers, and other exercise devices. Figure 13–5 shows examples of the automated and computerized measurement of metabolic and physiologic responses.

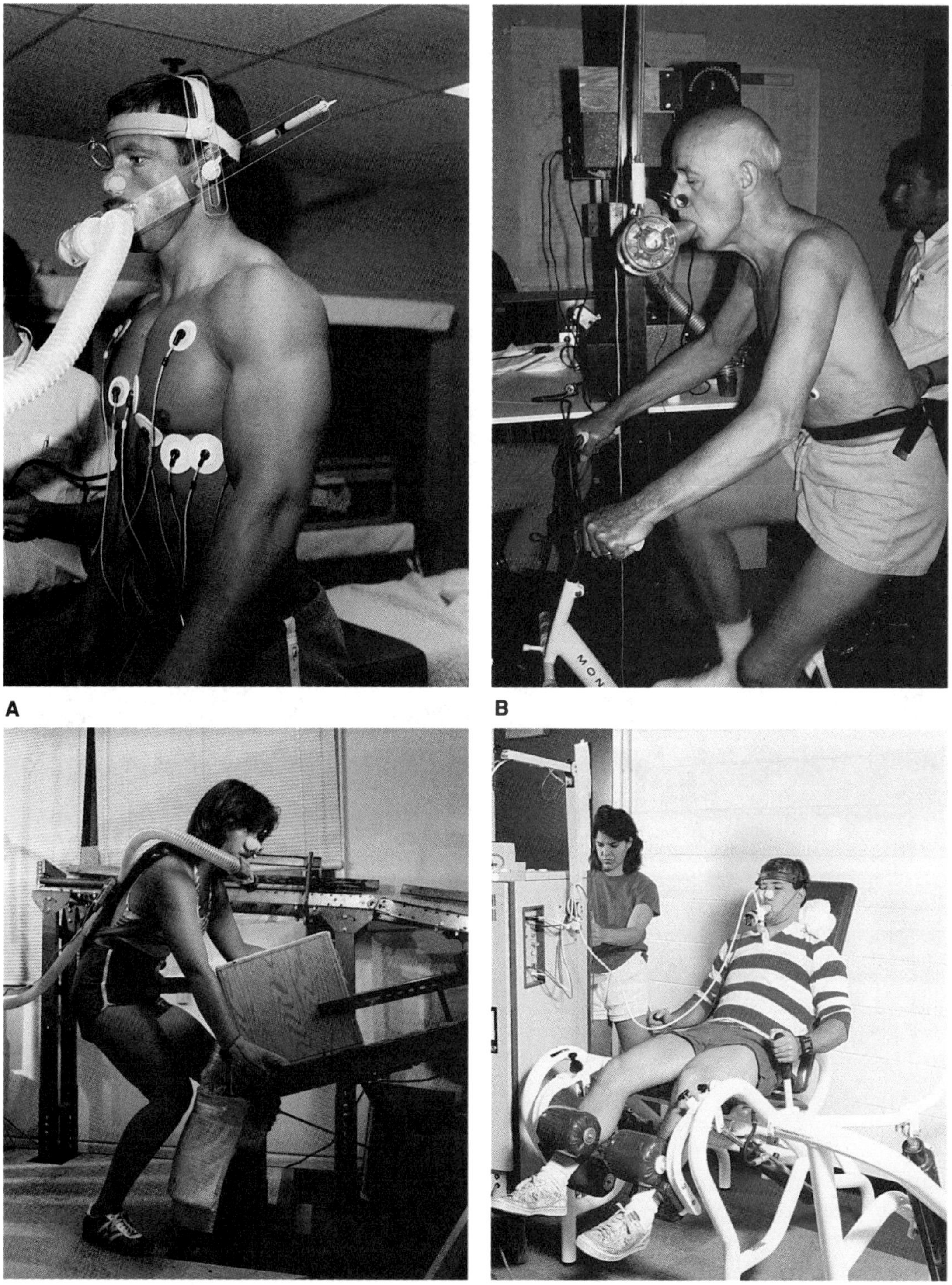

FIG. 13–4. Measurement of oxygen uptake by open-circuit spirometry during (A) rest, (B) cycle ergometry, (C) box lifting, and (D) resistance exercise. (Photos A and C courtesy of Dr. E. Michael.)

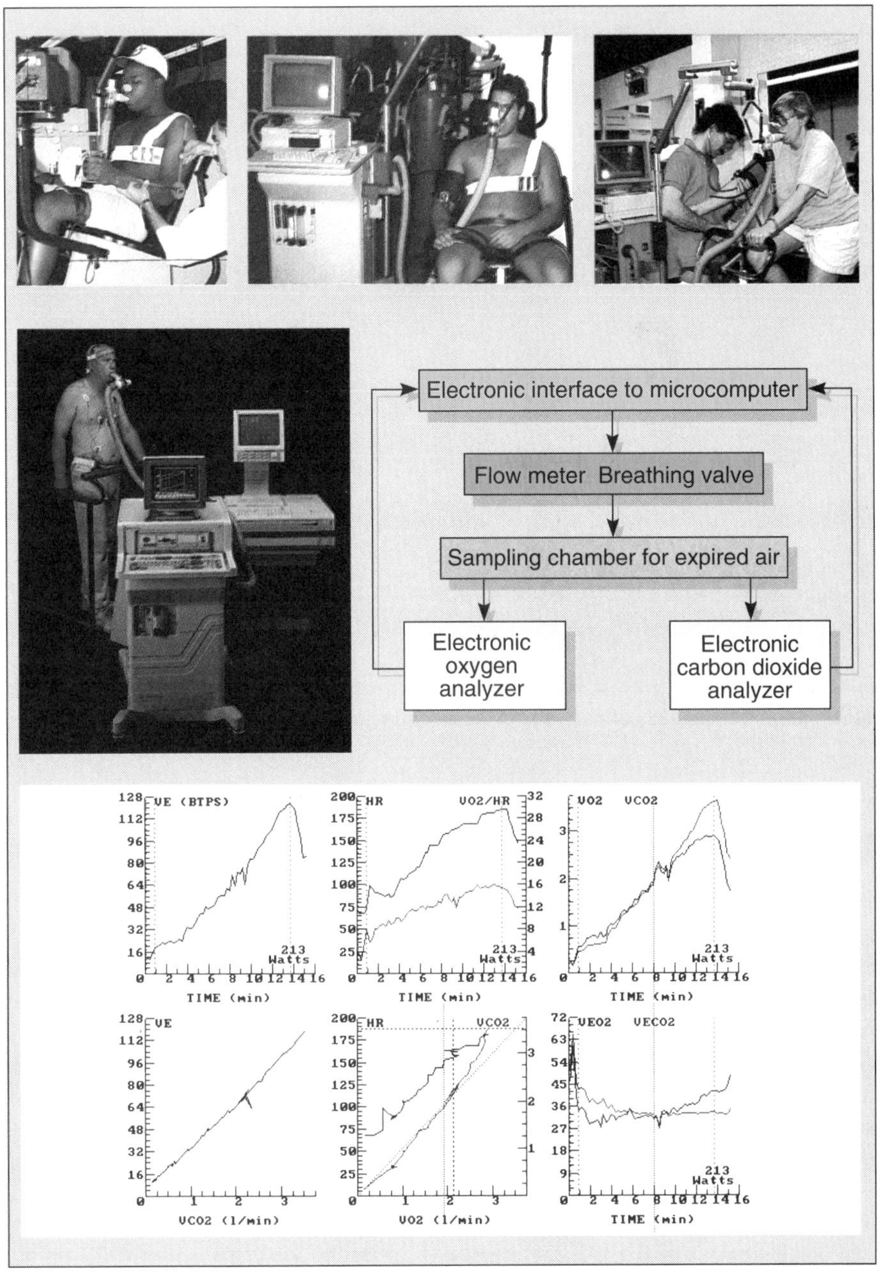

FIG. 13–5. Computerized systems approach for the collection, analysis, and output of physiologic and metabolic data. Photos courtesy of Dr. Dillawar Mistry and Dawn Gillis, Amherst, MA, SensorMedics Corporation, Anaheim, CA, and Hydra Fitness Industries, Belton, TX.)

Computerized instrumentation. Regardless of the sophistication of a particular automated system, the output data are only as good as the accuracy of the measuring devices. In large part, this depends on careful and frequent calibration of the electronic equipment using previously established reference standards.

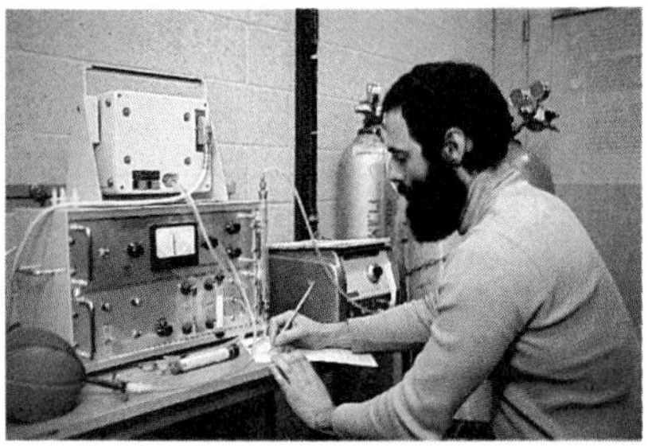

Careful calibration of electronic equipment is crucial for accurate data analysis.

ENERGY EXPENDITURE DURING REST AND PHYSICAL ACTIVITY

Figure 13–6 illustrates that daily energy expenditure is determined by three factors:

- Resting metabolic rate (which includes basal and sleeping conditions plus the added cost of arousal)

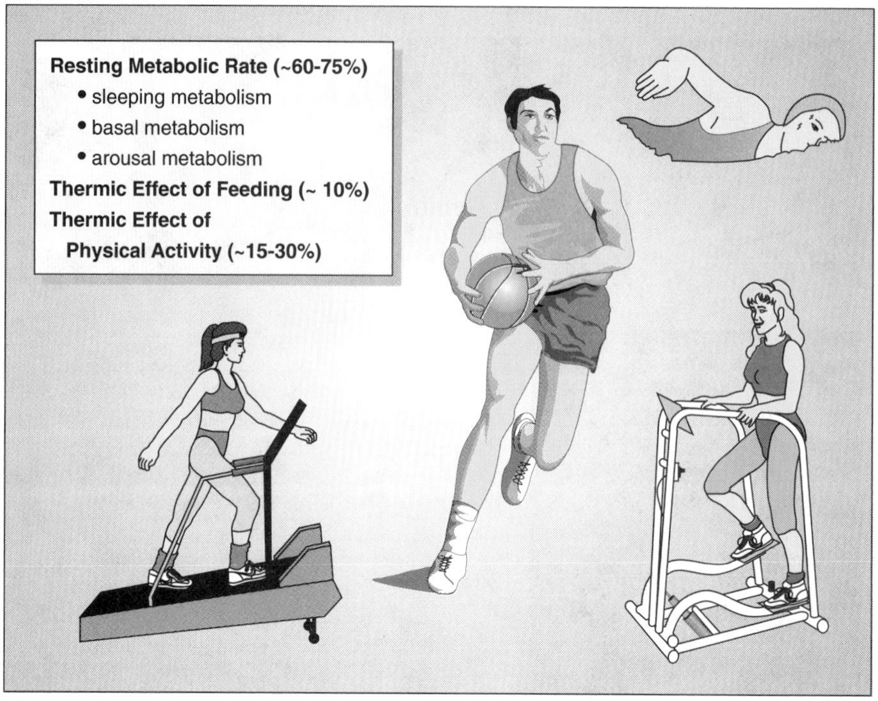

FIG. 13–6. Components of daily energy expenditure for an average 70-kg person.

- Thermogenic influence of food consumed
- Energy expended during and in recovery from physical activity

ENERGY EXPENDITURE AT REST: BASAL METABOLIC RATE

Basal oxygen uptake during rest. Values for oxygen uptake during the BMR test usually range between 160 and 290 ml per minute (0.8 to 1.45 kcal/min), depending upon a variety of factors, especially a person's size.

For each individual, there is a minimum energy requirement to sustain the body's functions in the waking state. This requirement, the ***basal metabolic rate*** (*BMR*), is usually determined by measuring oxygen uptake under standardized laboratory guidelines. No food is eaten for at least 12 hours prior to measurement to eliminate the energy required for digestion and absorption of food. Abstaining from food in this manner is referred to as the ***postabsorptive state.*** In addition, no undue muscular exertion should have occurred for at least 12 hours prior to BMR determination. During the test, the subject lies quietly in a dimly lit, temperature-controlled room. Oxygen uptake is measured after the person has been lying quietly for 30 to 60 minutes.

The measurement of BMR under controlled laboratory conditions provides a convenient method to study the relationship between energy expenditure and body size, gender, and age. The BMR also establishes the important energy baseline for constructing a sound program of weight control by use of diet, exercise, or the effective combination of both.

Influence of Body Size on Resting Metabolism. When individuals of different body size are compared with respect to basal energy metabolism, the value is usually expressed in terms of surface area and not body mass. The results of numerous experiments have provided data on average values of BMR per unit surface area in men and women of different ages.

Figure 13–7 reveals that the BMR is not equal between genders, but

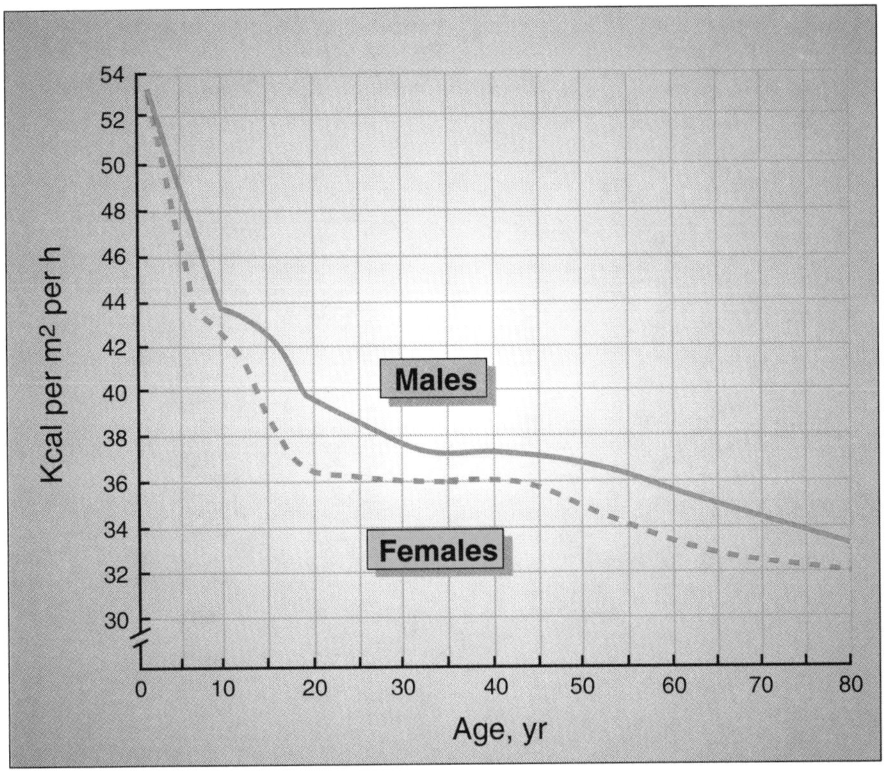

FIG. 13–7. Basal metabolic rate as a function of age and gender. (Data from Altman, P.L., and Dittmer, D.S.: Metabolism. Bethesda, MD, Federation of American Societies for Experimental Biology, 1968.)

Regular exercise blunts a decrease in metabolism with age. Differences in body composition largely explain the 2% decrease in BMR per decade usually observed through adulthood. However, when young and middle-aged endurance athletes were compared, there were no differences in body composition and BMR was similar. Thus, regular exercise can offset the decrease in resting metabolism usually noted with aging.

averages 5 to 10% lower in women at all ages. This lower BMR can be attributed to a woman's larger percentage of body fat and smaller muscle mass. When the BMR is expressed per unit of lean body mass, the observed gender differences become less apparent. While this observation may be of some theoretical importance, the curves shown in Figure 13–7 still describe the BMR in men and women adequately. From ages 20 to 40, average values for BMR are 38 kcal per square meter (m^2) of surface per hour for men, and 36 kcal for women. If one desires a more precise estimate of BMR, the actual average value for a specific age can be read directly from the curves. By using the values for heat production in Figure 13–7, in conjunction with the appropriate value for surface area, it is easy to estimate resting metabolism in kcal per minute and convert this to a total daily requirement. The nomogram in Figure 13–8 provides a simplified method for computing surface area based on stature and mass.

To determine surface area with the nomogram, locate stature on Scale I and mass on Scale II. Connect the two points with a straight edge. The intersection at Scale III gives the surface area in square meters. For example, if stature is 185 cm and mass is 75 kg, surface area according to Scale III on the nomogram is 1.98 m^2.

Estimate of Daily Resting Energy Expenditure. To determine one's approximate energy expenditure or kcal requirement during rest, multiply the appropriate average kcal per unit surface area per hour from Figure 13–7 by the surface area determined from the nomogram. Then multiply this

A close estimate. Estimated values for daily resting energy expenditure based on age, gender, and surface area will usually be within 10% of the kcal value per day had the BMR actually been measured under strict laboratory conditions.

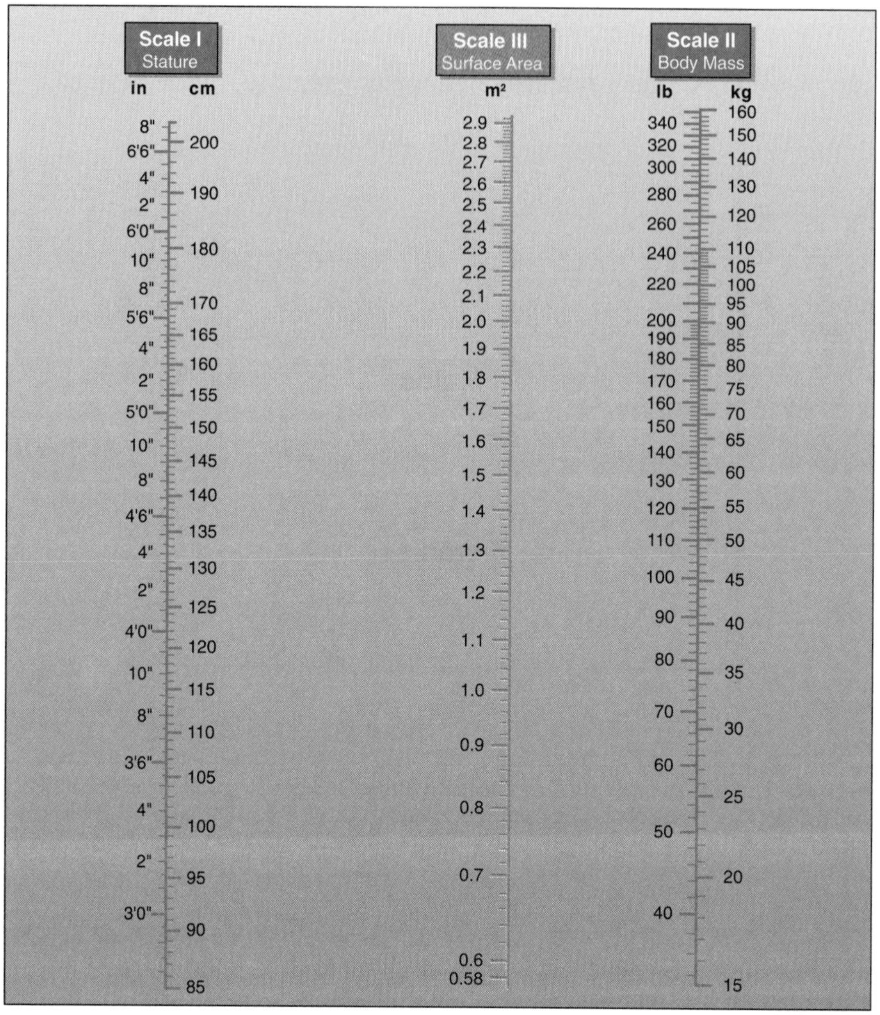

FIG. 13–8. Nomogram to estimate body surface area from stature and mass. (Reproduced from "Clinical Spirometry," as prepared by Boothby and Sandiford of the Mayo Clinic, through the courtesy of Warren E. Collins, Inc., Braintree, MA.)

by 24 to estimate the energy requirement for 24 hours. For a 22-year-old man whose surface area is 2.04 m^2, the minimum daily caloric requirement would be 38 kcal/m^2/h $\times$ 2.04 m^2 $\times$ 24, or 1860 kcal per day. Computing the minimum daily energy requirements based on age and surface area gives a more dependable estimate than simply using the average population value, which for men and women generally ranges between 900 and 1900 kcal a day.

Another method for determining the daily resting energy expenditure would be to compute the caloric equivalent of the total volume of oxygen consumed for basal functions during a 24-hour period. We pointed out in a previous section that approximately 5 kcal of energy is expended for each liter of oxygen consumed during metabolism. Because the value for oxygen uptake during rest generally ranges between 160 and 290 ml/min (average, 235 ml/min), an average value for the energy expended per minute is 1.18 kcal (0.235 $\times$ 5 kcal). Because there are 1440 minutes in a day, the daily resting energy expenditure would theoretically equal 1700 kcal (1440 $\times$ 1.18

Shortcut to estimate daily basal energy expenditure (BEE). Daily BEE (kcal) can be estimated as follows from age (yr), body mass (kg), and stature (cm):

Women: BEE = 655 + (9.6 $\times$ mass) + (1.85 $\times$ stature) − (4.7 $\times$ age)
Men: BEE = 66.0 + (13.7 $\times$ mass) + (5.0 $\times$ stature) − (6.8 $\times$ age)

For example, for a woman with body mass = 62.7 kg, stature = 172.5 cm, and age = 22.4 years, the daily BEE = 65.5 + (9.6 $\times$ 62.7) + 1.85 (172.5) − (4.7 $\times$ 22.4) = 1681.3 kcal.

kcal). This value is only a rough approximation because it does not adjust for differences in body size such as surface area, body mass, or body composition.

DIETARY-INDUCED THERMOGENESIS

For most people, food has a stimulating effect on metabolism attributable mainly to the energy-requiring processes of digesting, absorbing, and assimilating the various nutrients. This **dietary-induced thermogenesis** reaches a maximum within 1 hour after a meal; it can vary between 10 and 25% of the ingested food energy in normal individuals depending on the quantity and type of food eaten.

Thermic effect of food. Protein elicits the greatest thermogenic effect, equal to nearly 25% of the total calories in the protein meal itself.

The calorie-burning effect of protein ingestion has been used by some to argue for a high-protein diet for weight reduction. They maintain that fewer calories are ultimately available to the body with a meal high in protein compared to a lipid or carbohydrate meal of similar caloric value. Although this point may have some validity, other factors must be considered in formulating a prudent weight loss program—not to mention the potentially harmful strain on liver and kidney function brought on by excessive protein intake. For one thing, well-balanced nutrition requires a blend of macronutrients as well as appropriate quantities of vitamins and minerals. In addition, if exercise is combined with food restriction for weight loss, carbohydrate intake is important to power exercise and conserve the lean tissue often lost through dieting.

Research indicates that individuals who have poor control of body mass often have a blunted thermic response to eating. Undoubtedly, this could contribute to considerable accumulation of body fat over a period of years. The important point, however, is that if a person is physically active, the thermogenic effect represents only a small portion of the total daily energy expenditure. It also appears that exercising after eating augments an individual's normal thermic response to food intake. This certainly would support the wisdom of "going for a brisk walk" after eating, especially for those interested in weight control.

Exercise augments thermogenesis. In one study, exercising 30 minutes after eating breakfast nearly doubled the thermogenic effect of the meal compared to the effect of eating without subsequent exercise.

ENERGY EXPENDITURE IN PHYSICAL ACTIVITY

An understanding of resting energy metabolism provides an important frame of reference for the potential to increase daily energy output. According to numerous surveys, about one-third of a person's time is spent in resting activities such as those specified in the test of BMR. The remaining 16 hours are devoted to a wide range of physical activities. Consequently, the total daily energy expenditure can be considerably greater than the basal requirement, depending of course on the intensity, duration, and type of physical activity performed.

Researchers have measured the energy expended during such varied activities as brushing teeth, cleaning house, mowing the lawn, walking the dog, driving a car, playing ping-pong, bowling, dancing, swimming, sawing, and physical activity during space flight. Consider an activity such as rowing continuously at 30 strokes a minute for 30 minutes. If oxygen uptake averaged 2 liters per minute, then in 30 minutes the rower would consume 60 liters of oxygen. Because the utilization of 1 liter of oxygen generates about 5 kcal of energy, the researcher can make a reasonably accurate estimate of the energy expended in exercise. In this instance, the body

Caloric cost of exercise. The portable spirometer shown in Figure 13–3 has been used extensively to determine the energy cost of most daily chores and occupational activities, while the balloon and computer techniques have measured oxygen uptake in activities such as cycling, swimming, skiing, walking, jogging, running, dancing, rowing, and resistance training.

generated 300 kcal (60 liters × 5 kcal) during the exercise period. This value is considered the **gross energy expenditure.** All this energy, however, cannot be attributed solely to the cost of rowing because the 300 kcal value also includes the resting requirement during the 30 minutes. By knowing the exerciser's size (mass = 81.8 kg; stature = 183 cm), surface area can be determined from the nomogram in Figure 13–8. The value for surface area, 2.04 m^2, when multiplied by the average BMR for gender (38 kcal/m^2/h × 2.04 m^2), gives the resting metabolism per hour. This amounts to approximately 78 kcal per hour, or 39 kcal over a 30-minute period. Based on this computation, the **net energy expenditure** required solely for rowing can be determined. It is equal to the total energy expenditure of 300 kcal *minus* the 39 kcal requirement for rest, resulting in a net energy expenditure for rowing of approximately 261 kcal. The net kcal values for other activities would be computed in similar fashion.

Some investigators have measured the daily energy expenditure for men and women in a variety of occupations. This is done by determining the time spent in each activity and the energy expended for the activity. An accurate assessment of the time spent in activities is kept by diary, and energy expenditure is measured with the portable spirometer shown in Figure 13–3. Because it is impractical to carry the spirometer constantly day after day, frequent observations are made for a representative time period. For the miner listed in Table 13–2, who spent 12 hours during the week loading coal, the energy cost of the task ranged from 5.5 to 7.2 kcal per minute. For purposes of computation, an average value of 6.3 kcal per minute was used to represent the energy cost during this time. The total of 26,460 kcal expended during the 1-week period averaged 3780 kcal per day. This value includes the energy expended during the 8-hour work shift,

TABLE 13–2. ENERGY EXPENDITURE OF A COAL MINER IN 1 WEEK*

ACTIVITY	TIME SPENT IN 1 WEEK (H)	(MIN)	RATE OF ENERGY EXPENDED (KCAL/MIN)	ENERGY IN 1 WEEK (KCAL)
Sleep				
In bed	58	30	1.05	3690
Nonoccupational				
Sitting	38	37	1.59	3680
Standing	2	16	1.80	250
Walking	15	0	4.90	4410
Washing and dressing	5	3	3.30	1000
Gardening	2	0	5.00	600
Cycling	2	25	6.60	960
Work				
Sitting	15	9	1.68	1530
Standing	2	6	1.80	230
Walking	6	43	6.70	2700
Cutting	1	14	6.70	500
Timbering	6	51	5.70	2340
Loading	12	6	6.30	4570
Total	168 h			26,460
Average daily energy expenditure				3780

* Data from Garry, R. C., et al.: Expenditure of energy and the consumption of food by miners and clerks. Medical Research Council Report No. 289. Fife, Scotland, Her Majesty's Stationery Office, 1955.

the energy cost of an 8-hour sleeping period, as well as the remaining 8-hour period spent in nonoccupational activities.

ENERGY COST OF RECREATION AND SPORT ACTIVITIES

The energy requirements of various sport and recreational activities are presented in Appendix A. Table 13–3 lists several examples to illustrate the large variation in energy cost that occurs with participation in these types of physical activities. Notice, for example, that volleyball requires about 3.6 kcal per minute, or 216 kcal hourly, for a person weighing 71.4 kg (157 lb). The same person will expend more than twice this amount of energy, or 546 kcal per hour, while swimming the front crawl. Viewed somewhat differently, 25 minutes of swimming requires about the same number of calories as participating in recreational volleyball for 1 hour. If the pace of the swim or volleyball game is increased, the energy expenditure will rise proportionally.

EFFECT OF BODY MASS

Body size often plays an important role with respect to exercise energy requirements, just as it does for BMR. Figure 13–9 illustrates that heavier people generally expend more energy to perform the same activity than people who weigh less. This is because the energy expended during *weight-bearing exercise* increases in proportion to body mass. The relationship is so high that energy expenditure during walking or running can be predicted from body mass with almost as much accuracy as if the actual oxygen uptake were measured. In *non-weight-bearing exercise* such as stationary cycling, on the other hand, there is little relationship between body mass and the energy cost of exercise.

If you weigh more, it costs more. The effect of added mass on energy expenditure occurs whether a person gains weight "naturally" as body fat, or as an acute added load, for example, sports equipment or a weighted vest worn on the torso.

TABLE 13–3. GROSS ENERGY COST FOR SELECTED RECREATIONAL AND SPORTS ACTIVITIES*

ACTIVITY	Kg / Lb	50 / 110	53 / 117	56 / 123	59 / 130	62 / 137	65 / 143	68 / 150	71 / 157	74 / 163	77 / 170	80 / 176	83 / 183
Volleyball		2.5	2.7	2.8	3.0	3.1	3.3	3.4	3.6	3.7	3.9	4.0	4.2
Aerobic dancing		6.7	7.1	7.5	7.9	8.3	8.7	9.2	9.6	10.0	10.4	10.8	11.2
Cycling, leisure		5.0	5.3	5.6	5.9	6.2	6.5	6.8	7.1	7.4	7.7	8.0	8.3
Tennis		5.5	5.8	6.1	6.4	6.8	7.1	7.4	7.7	8.1	8.4	8.7	9.0
Swimming, slow crawl		6.4	6.8	7.2	7.6	7.9	8.3	8.7	9.1	9.5	9.9	10.2	10.6
Touch football		6.6	7.0	7.4	7.8	8.2	8.6	9.0	9.4	9.8	10.2	10.6	11.0
Running, 8 min/mile		10.8	11.3	11.9	12.5	13.1	13.6	14.2	14.8	15.4	16.0	16.5	17.1
Skiing, uphill racing		13.7	14.5	15.3	16.2	17.0	17.8	18.6	19.5	20.3	21.1	21.9	22.7

* Data from Appendix A.

Note: Energy expenditure is computed as the number of minutes of participation multiplied by the kcal value in the appropriate body weight column. For example, the kcal cost of one hour of tennis for a person weighing 150 pounds is 444 kcal (7.4 kcal × 60 min).

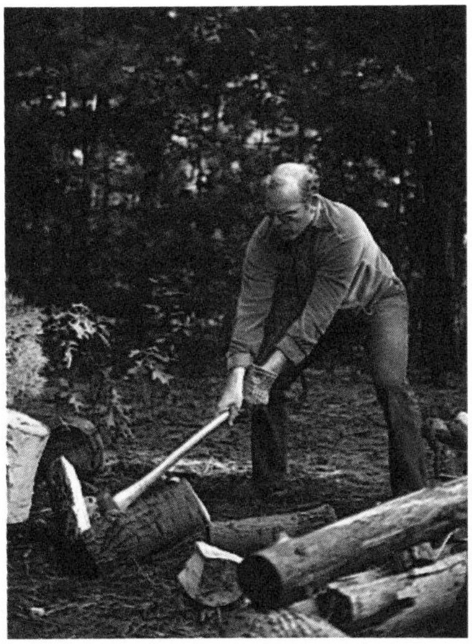

The gross energy expenditure of chopping wood slowly for this 196-pound man is 7.6 kcal/min, or about 450 kcal/hr. (Photo courtesy of Dr. John Edman.)

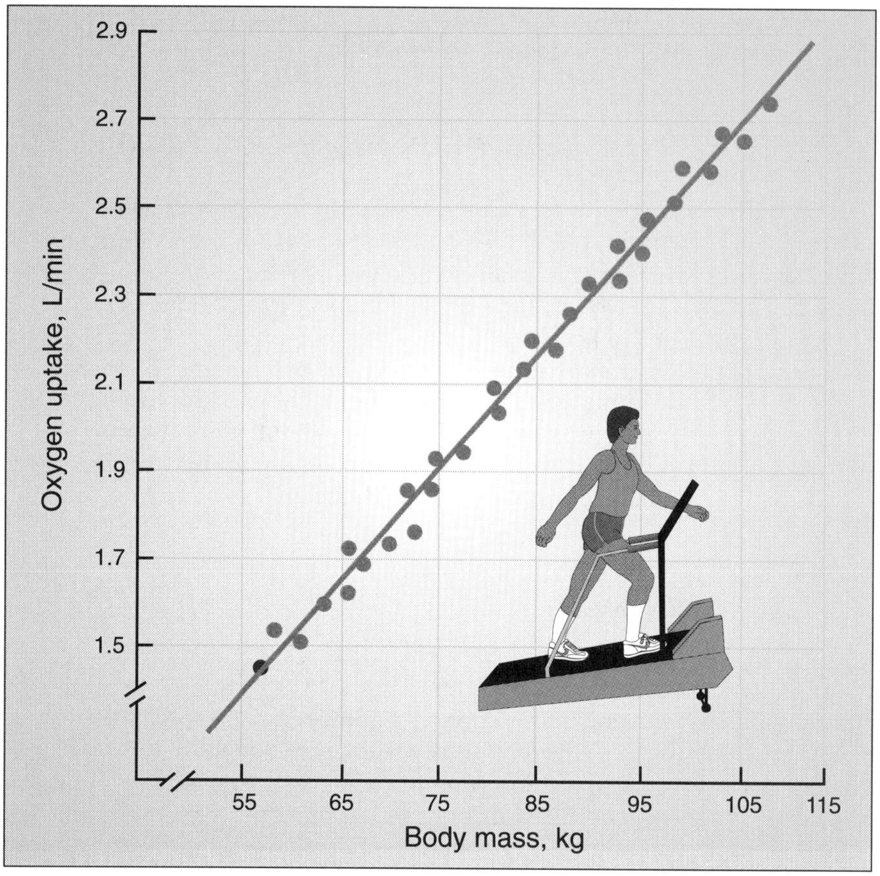

FIG. 13–9. Relationship between body mass and oxygen uptake measured during treadmill walking. (From Laboratory of Applied Physiology, Queens College, Flushing, NY.)

Weight-bearing exercise. In weight-bearing exercise such as walking, running, and cross-country skiing, participants must transport their body mass during the activity. This makes the cost of the exercise closely linked to body mass.

A practical application of these findings is that walking and other forms of weight-bearing exercise provide a substantial caloric expenditure for heavier people. Notice in Table 13–3 that the energy expended in playing tennis or volleyball for a person weighing about 83 kg is considerably greater than for a person 20 kg lighter. When the caloric cost is expressed in terms of body mass, that is, as kcal per minute per kilogram of body mass (kcal/min/kg), the difference in caloric cost is reduced considerably between men and women of different size. Keep in mind, however, that although the average energy expended playing tennis may be 0.109 kcal/min/kg regardless of race, gender, or body mass, the *total* energy expended by the heavier player is considerable, simply because the body mass must be transported—and this requires proportionately more total energy. Appendix A presents a comprehensive list of the gross energy expended in relation to body mass during household, recreational and sport, and occupational and industrial activities. These figures represent average values that can vary considerably depending on skill and pace of performance.

How to Use Appendix A. Refer to the column that comes closest to your present body mass. Multiply the number in this column by the number of minutes you spend in an activity. Suppose an individual weighs 62.3 kg (137 lb) and spends 30 minutes playing a casual game of billiards. To determine the energy cost of participation, multiply the caloric value per minute (2.6 kcal) by 30 to obtain the 30-minute gross expenditure of 78 kcal. If the same individual does aerobic dance for 45 minutes, the gross energy expended would be calculated as 6.4 kcal × 45 minutes, or 288 kcal.

AVERAGE DAILY RATES OF ENERGY EXPENDITURE

A committee of the United States Food and Nutrition Board proposed various norms to represent average rates of energy expenditure for men and women in the United States. These standards apply to people whose occupations could be considered between sedentary and active, and who participate in some recreational activities such as weekend swimming, golf, and tennis. As shown in Table 13–4, the average daily energy expenditure is 2700 kcal for men and 2000 kcal for women between the ages of 23 and 50. As seen in the bottom part of the table, about 75% of the average person's day is spent in fairly sedentary activity. This predominance of physical *inactivity* has prompted some sociologists to refer to the modern-day American as *Homo sedentarius,* a term that is probably all too appropriate.

Walking is the most popular activity. A survey by the President's Council on Physical Fitness and Sports revealed that for 36% of American men and 51% of American women, walking was the most prevalent form of exercise, regardless of occupation or race. It is probably a fair estimate that only about 50% of adult Americans engage in physical activities requiring an energy expenditure much above the resting level!

Table 13–5 summarizes data on the daily energy expenditure for people with different occupations from Scotland; data are also included for Swiss peasants and English army cadets. The number in each group varied from 10 to 30, and the subjects were studied for 1 week. Although the average daily energy expenditure increased for each occupational group, as presented from top to bottom in the table, there was considerable variation within a particular group. This was attributed to differences in the time

TABLE 13–4. AVERAGE DAILY RATES OF ENERGY EXPENDITURE FOR MEN AND WOMEN LIVING IN THE UNITED STATES*

	Age (yr)	(kg)	(lb)	(cm)	(in)	Energy Expenditure (kcal)
Men	15–18	66	145	176	69	2800
	19–22	70	154	177	70	2900
	23–50	70	154	178	70	2700
	51+	70	154	178	70	2400
Women	15–18	55	120	163	64	2100
	19–22	55	120	163	64	2100
	23–50	55	120	163	64	2000
	51+	55	120	163	64	1800

AVERAGE TIME SPENT DURING THE DAY FOR MEN AND WOMEN

Activity	Time (h)
Sleeping and lying	8
Sitting	6
Standing	6
Walking	2
Recreational: sports or exercises	2

* Data from Food and Nutrition Board, National Research Council, Recommended Dietary Allowances, 8th rev. ed., National Academy of Sciences, Washington, DC, 1980. From McArdle, W. D. Katch, F. I., Katch, V. L.: Exercise Physiology. Philadelphia, Lea & Febiger, 1991.

TABLE 13–5. DAILY RATES OF ENERGY EXPENDITURE FOR VARIOUS OCCUPATIONS*				
		Energy Expenditure, kcal per day		
	Occupation	Average	Minimum	Maximum
Men	Elderly retired	2330	1750	2810
	Office workers	2520	1820	3270
	Coal mine clerks	2800	2330	3290
	Laboratory technicians	2840	2240	3820
	Older industrial workers	2840	2180	3710
	University students	2930	2270	4410
	Building workers	3000	2440	3730
	Steel workers	3280	2600	3960
	Army cadets	3490	2990	4100
	Older peasants (Swiss)	3530	2210	5000
	Farmers	3550	2450	4670
	Coal miners	3660	2970	4560
	Forestry workers	3670	2860	4600
Women	Older housewives	1990	1490	2410
	Middle-aged housewives	2090	1760	2320
	Laboratory assistants	2130	1340	2540
	Assistants in department store	2250	1820	2850
	University students	2290	2090	2500
	Factory workers	2320	1970	2980
	Bakery workers	2510	1980	3390
	Older peasants (Swiss)	2890	2200	3860

Data from Durnin, J.V.G.A., and Passmore, R.: Energy, Work and Leisure. London, Heinemann Educational Books, 1967. From McArdle, W. D., Katch, F. I., Katch, V. L.: Exercise Physiology. Philadelphia, Lea & Febiger, 1991.

devoted to recreational pursuits. Also important were differences in the type of work done within each specific profession. Because of recreational activities, one elderly retired man was almost as active as the least energetic of the coal miners and forestry workers. His daily energy expenditure was therefore much higher than the average for his group.

CLASSIFICATION OF WORK

All of us at one time or another have done some type of physical work that we would classify as exceedingly "difficult." This might be walking up a long flight of stairs, shoveling a snow-filled driveway, running to catch a bus, loading and unloading furniture on a truck, digging a deep trench, skiing through a snow storm, or running in soft beach sand. There are two factors to consider in rating the difficulty of a particular task: the amount of *time* it takes and the *intensity* of the effort. Both factors may vary considerably. For example, two people of the same body size could expend an equal amount of energy completing the same task. One might exert extreme effort over a short period, while the other could exert less effort over a longer period. This can be illustrated for running a 26-mile marathon at various speeds. One runner might run at maximum pace and complete the race in a little more than 2 hours. Another runner of equal fitness might select a slower more leisurely pace and complete the run in 3 hours. In this

TABLE 13–6. FIVE-LEVEL CLASSIFICATION OF PHYSICAL ACTIVITY IN TERMS OF INTENSITY OF EFFORT*

LEVEL	ENERGY EXPENDITURE			
	Men kcal · min	l · min	ml · kg · min	METs
Light	2.0–4.9	0.40–0.99	6.1–15.2	1.6–3.9
Moderate	5.0–7.4	1.00–1.49	15.3–22.9	4.0–5.9
Heavy	7.5–9.9	1.50–1.99	23.0–30.6	6.0–7.9
Very heavy	10.0–12.4	2.00–2.49	30.7–38.3	8.0–9.9
Unduly heavy	12.5–	2.50–	38.4–	10.0–
	Women kcal · min	l · min	ml · kg · min	METs
Light	1.5–3.4	0.30–0.69	5.4–12.5	1.2–2.7
Moderate	3.5–5.4	0.70–1.09	12.6–19.8	2.8–4.3
Heavy	5.5–7.4	1.10–1.49	19.9–27.1	4.4–5.9
Very heavy	7.5–9.4	1.50–1.89	27.2–34.4	6.0–7.5
Unduly heavy	9.5–	1.90–	34.5–	7.6–

* l · min based on 5 kcal per liter of oxygen; ml · kg · min based on 65-kg man and 55-kg woman; one MET is equivalent to the average resting oxygen uptake. Modified from McArdle, W. D., Katch, F. I., Katch, V. L.: Exercise Physiology. Philadelphia, Lea & Febiger, 1991.

example, the intensity of exercise is the factor distinguishing how the work is completed. In another situation, two people may run at the same speed, but one may run twice as long as the other. Here, exercise duration becomes the important consideration.

Several classification systems have been proposed for rating the difficulty of work in terms of its intensity. The five-level classification system presented in Table 13–6 rates the difficulty of work based on energy expended by average men and women performing physical effort throughout a workday. The energy intensity that corresponds to a particular rating is expressed in kcal per minute and **METs**, a MET being defined as a multiple of the resting metabolism. *One MET is equivalent to the average for resting metabolism or oxygen uptake.* Physical work performed at 2 METs requires twice the resting metabolism, 3 METs is three times the resting energy expenditure, and so on.

Most tasks require only a moderate energy expenditure. As a frame of reference for evaluating the intensity of effort, most industrial jobs and household tasks require an energy expenditure that is less than 3 times resting level, or the equivalent of 3 METs.

SUMMARY

1. A calorie or kilocalorie (kcal) is a measure of heat used to express the energy value of food. This food energy is directly measured in a bomb calorimeter.

2. The heat of combustion represents heat liberated by the complete oxidation of food. For fats, carbohydrates, and proteins, these gross energy values are 9.45, 4.2 and 5.65 kcal per gram, respectively.
3. Digestive efficiency refers to the proportion of ingested food that is actually digested and absorbed for use by the body. This represents about 97% for carbohydrates, 95% for fats, and 92% for proteins. Thus, the net energy values are 4, 9, and 4 kcal per gram for carbohydrate, fat, and protein, respectively.
4. The calorific values for the various macronutrients can be used to compute the caloric content of any meal as long as the carbohydrate, fat, and protein composition is known.
5. From an energy standpoint, a calorie is a unit of heat energy regardless of the food source. Thus, it is incorrect to consider 300 kcal of chocolate ice cream any more fattening than 300 kcal of watermelon, 300 kcal of pepperoni pizza, or 300 kcal of bagels and sour cream.
6. Direct and indirect calorimetry are the two methods for determining the body's rate of energy expenditure. With direct calorimetry, actual heat production is measured in an appropriately insulated calorimeter. Indirect calorimetry infers energy expenditure from measurements of oxygen uptake and carbon dioxide production, using either closed- or open-circuit spirometry.
7. The open-circuit method of indirect calorimetry is the most practical means for indirectly quantifying energy expenditure during a variety of physical activities. The most common indirect procedures involve the use of either a portable spirometer, meterologic balloons (the bag technique), or computerized instrumentation.
8. A person's total daily energy expenditure is the sum total of the energy required in basal and resting metabolism, thermogenic influences (especially the thermic effect of food), and the energy generated in physical activity.
9. The BMR is the minimum energy required to maintain vital functions in the waking state. The BMR is proportional to the surface area of the body. It is also related to age and generally is higher for men than for women; these influences are largely attributable to variation in lean body mass.
10. Different classification systems exist for rating the strenuousness of physical activities. These include ratings based on (1) the ratio of energy cost to resting energy requirement, (2) the oxygen requirement in ml/kg/min, or (3) multiples of the resting metabolic rate, or METs.
11. The average daily energy expenditure is estimated to be 2700 to 2900 kcal for men and 2000 to 2100 for women between the ages of 15 and 50 years. Great variability in daily energy expenditure exists, however, largely determined by an individual's physical activity level.
12. It is possible to classify different occupations as well as athletic groups by daily rates of energy expenditure. Within any classification, however, there is great variability due to energy expended in recreational pursuits. In addition, heavier individuals expend more energy in physical activity than their lighter counterparts.

RELATED LITERATURE

Belko, A., et al.: Effect of energy and protein intake and exercise intensity on the thermic effect of food. *Am. J. Clin. Nutr.*, 43:863, 1986.

Bray, G.: The acute effect of food intake on energy expenditure during cycle ergometry. *Am. J. Clin. Nutr.*, 27:254, 1974.

Calloway, D.H., and Zanni, E.: Energy requirements and energy expenditure of elderly men. *Am. J. Clin. Nutr.*, 33:2088, 1980.

Cohen, J.L., et al.: Cardiorespiratory responses to ballet exercise and the $\dot{V}O_2$ max of elite ballet dancers. *Med. Sci. Sports Exerc.*, 14:212, 1982.

Durnin, J.V.G.A., and Passmore, R.: Energy, Work and Leisure. London, Heinemann, 1967.

Garry, R.C., et al.: Expenditure of energy and the consumption of food by miners and clerks. Medical Research Council, Report No. 289. Fife, Scotland, Her Majesty's Stationery Office, 1955.

Guthrie, H.A.: Introductory Nutrition, 7th ed. St. Louis, C.V. Mosby, 1988.

Hickson, J.F., Jr., and Wolinsky, I. (Eds.): Nutrition in Exercise and Sport. Boca Raton, FL, CRC Press, 1989.

Kannagi, T., et al.: An evaluation of the Beckman Metabolic Cart for measuring ventilation and aerobic requirements during exercise. *J. Cardiac Rehab.*, 3:38, 1983.

Kashiwazaki, H., et al.: Correlations of pedometer readings with energy expenditure in workers during free-living daily activities. *Eur. J. Appl. Physiol.*, 54:585, 1986.

Katch, V., et al.: Basal metabolism of obese adolescents: age, gender and body composition effects. *Int. J. Obes.*, 9:69, 1985.

Keys, A., et al.: Basal metabolism and age of adult men. *Metabolism*, 22:579, 1973.

Kleiber, M.: The Fire of Life: An Introduction to Animal Energetics. Huntington, NY, Krieger, 1975.

LeBlanc, J., et al.: Hormonal factors in reduced post prandial heat production of exercise trained subjects. *J. Appl. Physiol.*, 56:772, 1984.

Livesey, G., and Elia, M.: Estimation of energy expenditure, net carbohydrate utilization and net fat oxidation and synthesis by indirect calorimetry: evaluation of errors with special reference to detailed composition of fuels. *Am. J. Clin. Nutr.*, 47:608, 1988.

McArdle, W.D., et al.: Metabolic and cardiovascular adjustment to work in air and water at 18, 25, and 33°. *J. Appl. Physiol.*, 40:85, 1976.

McArdle, W.D., et al.: Aerobic capacity, heart rate, and estimated energy cost during women's competitive basketball. *Res. Q.*, 42:178, 1981.

McArdle, W.D., et al.: Exercise Physiology: Energy, Nutrition, and Human Performance, 3rd ed. Philadelphia, Lea & Febiger, 1991.

Meredith, C.N., et al.: Body composition and aerobic capacity in young and middle-aged endurance-trained men. *Med. Sci. Sports Exerc.*, 19:557, 1987.

Miles, D.S., et al.: Effect of dietary fiber on the metabolizable energy of human diets. *J. Nutr.* 118:1075, 1988.

Montoye, H.J., and Taylor, H.L.: Measurement of physical activity in population studies. *Hum. Biol.*, 56:195, 1984.

Norton, A.C.: Portable equipment for gas exchange. In: Assessment of Energy Metabolism in Health and Disease. Columbus, OH, Ross Laboratories, 1980.

Parham, E.S., et al.: Weight control content of women's magazines: bias and accuracy. *Int. J. Obes.*, 10:19, 1987.

Poehlman, E.T., et al.: Resting metabolic rate and post prandial thermogenesis in highly trained and untrained males. *Am. J. Clin. Nutr.*, 47:793, 1988.

Rothwell, N.J., and Stock, J.: Luxuskonsumption, diet-induced thermogenesis and brown fat: the case in favor. *Clin. Sci.*, 64:64, 1983.

Schutz, Y., et al.: Diet-induced thermogenesis measured over a whole day in obese and non-obese women. *Am. J. Clin. Nutr.*, 40:542, 1984.

Segal, K.R., et al.: Thermic effects of food and exercise on lean and obese men of similar lean body mass. *Am. J. Physiol.*, 252:E110, 1987.

Snellen, J.W.: Studies in human calorimetry. In: Assessment of Energy in Health and Disease. Columbus, OH, Ross Laboratories, 1980.

Trembly, A., et al.: Diminished dietary thermogenesis in exercise-trained human subjects. *Eur. J. Appl. Physiol.*, 52:1, 1983.

BODY COMPOSITION AND WEIGHT CONTROL

II

An excess accumulation of body fat is undesirable for a variety of reasons. From a health standpoint, medical problems exist for which obesity or "overfatness" is considered a risk factor and for which a reduction in excess fat is desirable. Also, being too fat is often accompanied by changes in personality and behavior patterns frequently manifested as depression, withdrawal, self-pity, and aggression.

The first step in formulating an effective program for weight control is to appraise body size objectively. It is possible to be heavy and even overweight according to established charts, yet possess only a moderate amount of body fat. Many athletes, for example, are quite muscular but are otherwise lean in terms of their overall body composition. For such people, a program of dietary modification or exercise for purposes of weight control may be unnecessary. Such an approach would be prudent, however, for others who may be 5 to 10 kg "overfat." Of even greater importance is the need for effective weight control among the increasingly large segment of the population afflicted with "creeping obesity." During the adult years, body mass and body fat can increase insidiously to the point that the amount of body fat exceeds even the most liberal limits for normalcy. It is at this point that the health-related aspects of obesity become a serious concern. Unfortunately, correction of adult-acquired obesity through dietary intervention or exercise is much more difficult than its early prevention.

The chapters that follow deal with topics relevant to body composition, obesity, and weight control. Chapter 14 discusses the underlying rationale for evaluating body composition in terms of body fat and lean body mass. In Chapter 15, we define "overweight" in terms of acceptable limits of body fat for a particular age range for men and women. We discuss the interrelated factors often associated with obesity as well as the efficacy of diet and exercise as a treatment for the overfat condition. Chapter 16 deals with weight control. We discuss the question of weight loss and weight gain within the framework of the "energy balance equation." In addition, a strategy is presented for quantifying food intake, and incorporating exercise and caloric restriction to achieve a desired rate of weight loss. Chapter 17 is concerned with applying the principles of behavior modification, with emphasis on weight reduction by means of dietary modification and increased energy expenditure through moderate physical activity.

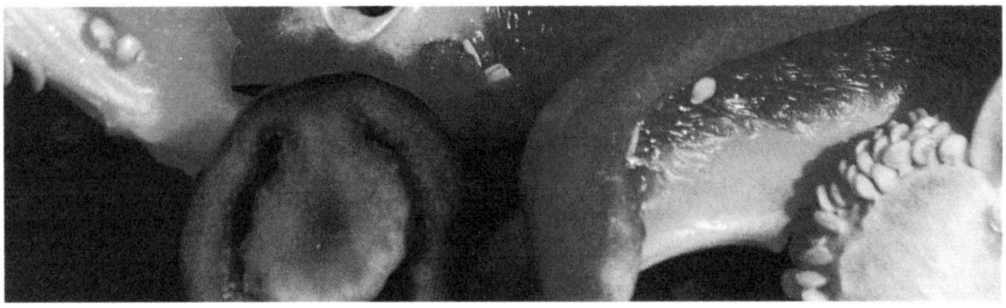

14

EVALUATION OF BODY COMPOSITION

In the early 1940s, **Dr. Albert Behnke,** a U.S. Navy physician and foremost authority on body composition, made detailed measurements of the size, shape, and structure of 25 professional football players, many of whom had achieved All-American status while in college. According to military standards at that time, a person whose body mass was 15% above the average "weight-for-height," as determined from insurance company statistics, was designated as overweight and rejected by the military. When these standards were applied to the football players, whose body mass ranged from 72.3 to 118.2 kg, 17 of them were classified as too fat and unfit for military service. However, a more careful evaluation of each player's body composition revealed that 11 of the 17 overweight players actually had a relatively low percentage of body fat—the excess mass resulted primarily from their large muscular development.

These data were among the first to illustrate clearly that the popular height-weight tables provide little information about the quality or composition of an individual's body mass. A football player may indeed weigh much more than some "average," "ideal," or "desirable" body mass based on the height-weight tables, but more than likely this athlete is not exces-

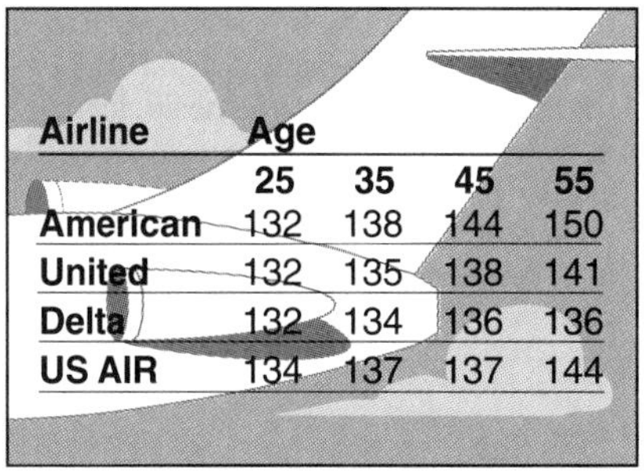

Airline	Age 25	35	45	55
American	132	138	144	150
United	132	135	138	141
Delta	132	134	136	136
US AIR	134	137	137	144

Weight limits eased. The upper limit for body weight for female flight attendants is now based on age. Below are the limits, by airline, for a woman whose stature averages 162.6 cm, or 64 in.

Height-weight tables. The height-weight tables are statistical landmarks based on average ranges of body mass for which the mortality rate was lowest, without regard to specific causes of death or the quality of health (morbidity) prior to death.

sively fat or in need of reducing body mass. The extra weight consists of a considerable muscle mass. *Thus, "**overweight**" refers only to body mass in excess of some standard, usually the average mass for a specific stature.* The use of **height-weight tables** can be misleading for a person who actually wants to know: How "fat" or "overfat" am I?

Not all excess weight is bad weight. If football players followed the height-weight guidelines, it's a good bet that they would cease playing football and might even jeopardize their overall health by undertaking a crash or bizarre diet regimen.

During the past 50 years, many laboratory procedures have been developed to analyze the body in relation to its structural components. Some techniques are time-consuming and require sophisticated laboratory equipment, whereas others are fairly simple and inexpensive. In this chapter, we analyze the gross composition of the human body and present the rationale underlying various indirect methods for partitioning the body into two basic compartments, *body fat* and *lean body mass.* In addition, simple methods are presented for determining body composition in terms of percent body fat, pounds of fat, and lean body mass.

GROSS COMPOSITION OF THE HUMAN BODY

*Three **major structural components of the human body** include muscle, fat, and bone.* Because there are marked gender differences in body composition, a convenient basis for comparison is to employ the concept proposed by Dr. Behnke of a **Reference man** and **Reference woman** as depicted in Figure 14–1.

Reference Man and Reference Woman. Compared with the Reference female, the Reference male is taller by 10.2 cm and heavier by 13.3 kg, his skeleton weighs more (10.4 vs. 6.8 kg), and he has a larger muscle mass (31.3 vs. 20.4 kg) and lower total fat content (10.5 vs 15.3 kg). These gender differences exist even when the amount of fat, muscle, and bone are expressed as a percentage of body mass. This is particularly true for body fat, which represents 15% of total body mass for Reference man and 27% for his female counterpart. The concept of reference standards does not mean that men and women should strive to achieve this body composition, nor that the Reference man and woman are in fact "average" or desirable. The models do, however, provide a useful frame of reference to compare individuals in terms of body composition.

Reference man and woman. The Reference man and Reference woman are theoretical models based on average physical dimensions from detailed measurements of thousands of individuals who were subjects in large-scale anthropometric and nutrition-assessment surveys. The reference models provide a useful frame of comparision when making inter-individual and intra-individual assessments of body composition.

ESSENTIAL AND STORAGE FAT

According to the Reference model, total body fat exists in two depots or storage sites.

Essential Fat. The first depot, termed **essential fat,** is the fat stored in the marrow of bones as well as in the heart, lungs, liver, spleen, kidneys, intestines, muscles, and lipid-rich tissues of the central nervous system. This fat is required for normal physiologic functioning. In the female, essential fat includes the additional **gender-specific fat.** It is not at all clear whether this fat is expendable or serves as reserve storage. The mammary glands and pelvic region are probably primary sites for the component of essential fat, although the precise quantitative amounts are unknown.

Gender-specific essential fat. The contribution of breast fat has been estimated to be no higher than 4% of body mass for women whose total body fat content varied from 14 to 35%. This means that sites other than the breasts contribute a large proportion of gender-specific essential fat (perhaps the lower body region that includes the pelvis and thighs).

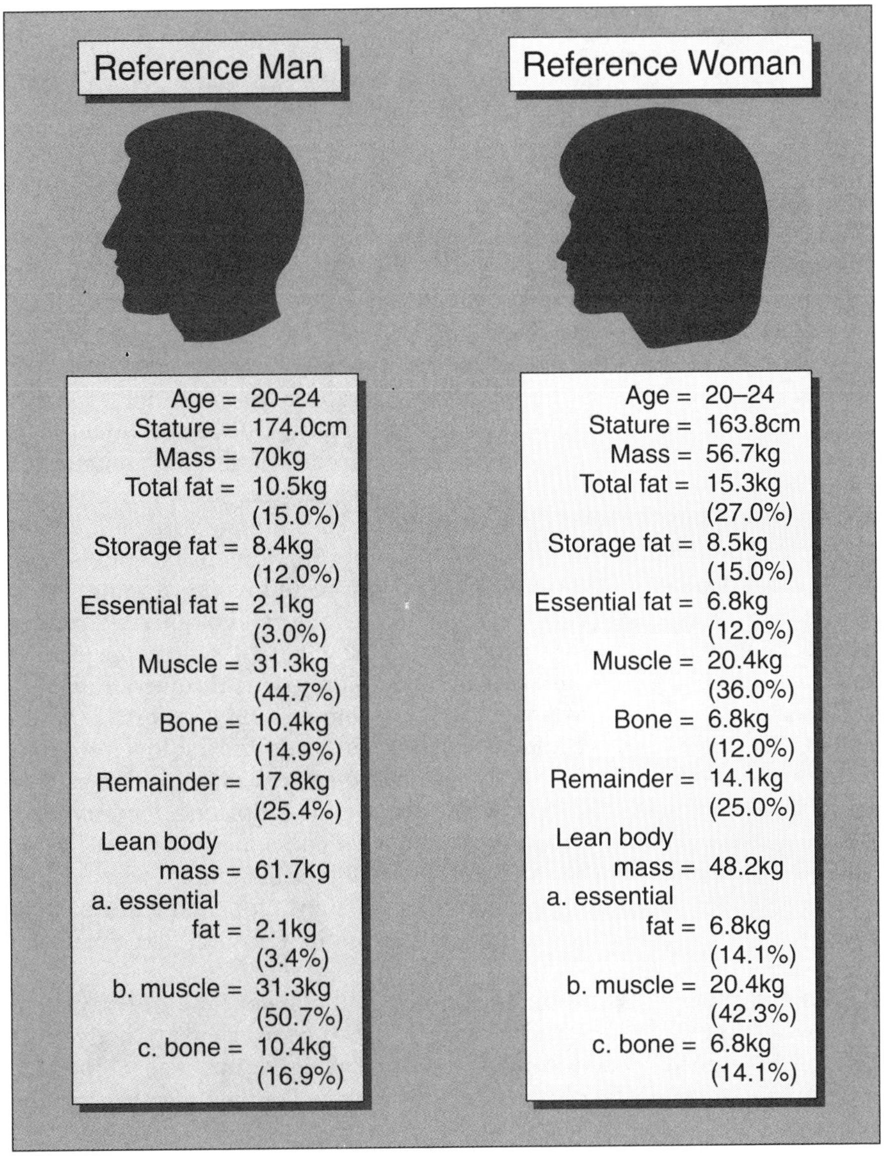

FIG. 14–1. Body composition of Reference man and Reference woman.

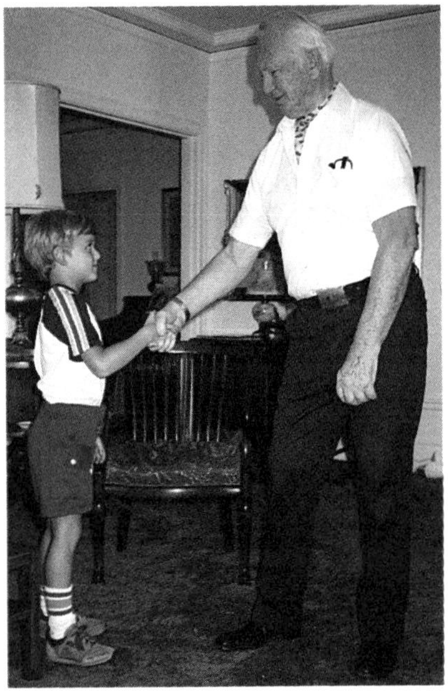

Albert Behnke, MD, developed the concept of the Reference man and Reference woman.

Storage Fat. The other major depot, the **storage fat,** consists of fat that accumulates in adipose tissue. This nutritional reserve includes the fatty tissues that protect the various internal organs as well as the larger subcutaneous fat volume beneath the skin surface. Although the proportional distribution of storage fat in males and females is similar (12% of body mass in males, 15% in females), the total quantity of essential fat in females, which includes the gender-specific fat, is three times higher than in males. More than likely, this additional fat is biologically important for childbearing and other hormone-related functions.

MINIMAL STANDARDS FOR LEANNESS

There appears to be a biologic lower limit beyond which a person's body mass cannot be reduced without impairing health status.

Lean body mass. In normally hydrated healthy adult males, the only difference between lean body mass and fat-free body mass is that lean body mass includes the "essential" lipid-rich stores in bone marrow, brain, spinal cord, and internal organs.

Lean Body Mass (Men). In men, this lower limit is referred to as **lean body mass** and is calculated as body mass minus the mass of storage fat. For Reference man, lean body mass is equivalent to 61.6 kg, which includes approximately 3% or 1.9 kg of essential fat. This amount of fat presumably is a lower limit, and any encroachment into this reserve may impair normal body function and capacity for exercise. Body fat values approaching this 3% "lower limit" have been obtained for champion male athletes in various sports. The fat content of world-class marathon runners, for example, ranges from about 4 to 8%. This is only slightly above the quantity of essential fat that apparently cannot be reduced. The low fat content and body mass for these athletes reflects, to some degree, positive adaptation to the severe energy requirements of distance training. Also, a low percentage of body fat facilitates heat loss during high-intensity exercise and reduces the load of excess weight to be transported while running.

Considerable variation is found in the lean body mass of different groups of male athletes, with values ranging from a low of 48.1 kg in some jockeys to a high of 116.1 kg for an Olympic champion discus thrower. Table 14–1 presents data on the physique and body composition of selected professional male athletes who could be classified as "underfat" or "overweight." There are striking differences between these groups in body size as well as in body fat, lean body mass, the lean-to-fat ratio, and various girth measures. The defensive backs and offensive backs are "underfat" in relation to Reference man (or any other nonathletic standard), whereas the linemen and shot putters are clearly "overweight" for their stature (their mass per unit stature exceeds the 90th percentile for nonathletic males).

Minimal weight. The concept of minimal weight in females, which incorporates about 12% essential fat, is equivalent to lean body mass in males that includes 3% essential fat.

Minimal Weight (Women). In contrast to the lower limit of body mass for males that includes about 3% essential fat, the lower limit of body mass for the Reference female, termed **minimal weight,** includes 12 to 14% essential fat (essential fat plus gender-specific fat). For the Reference female,

TABLE 14–1. PHYSIQUE AND BODY COMPOSITION OF "UNDERFAT" PROFESSIONAL FOOTBALL PLAYERS AND "OVERWEIGHT" OFFENSIVE AND DEFENSIVE PROFESSIONAL FOOTBALL LINEMEN AND SHOT-PUTTERS

	DEFENSIVE BACKS (ALL-PRO)				OFFENSIVE BACK (ALL-PRO, N = 1)	OFFENSIVE LINEMEN (DALLAS, 1977, N = 10)	DEFENSIVE LINEMEN (DALLAS, 1977, N = 5)	SHOT PUTTERS (OLYMPIC, N = 13)
VARIABLE	1	2	3	4				
Age, y	27.1	30.2	29.4	24.0	32	—	—	24.0
Stature, cm	184.7	181.9	187.2	181.5	184.7	193.8	197.6	187.0
Mass, kg	87.9	87.1	88.4	88.9	90.6	116.0	116.5	112.3
Relative fat, %	3.9	3.8	3.8	2.5	1.4	18.6	13.2	14.8
Absolute fat, kg	3.4	3.3	3.4	2.2	1.3	21.6	15.4	16.6
Lean body mass, kg	84.5	83.8	85.0	86.7	89.3	94.4	101.1	95.7
Lean/fat ratio	24.8	25.3	25.0	39.4	68.6	4.3	6.57	5.77

(From Katch, V. I., and Katch, V. L.: The body composition profile: Techniques of measurement applications. Clin. Sports Med., *3*:31, 1984.)

minimal weight is equivalent to 48.2 kg. In general, body fat levels in the leanest women in the population do not fall below about 12% of body mass. This probably represents the lower limit of fatness for most women in good health.

It should be emphasized that the concept of female minimal weight is based on theoretical considerations, with little actual data. In carefully conducted experiments, however, values lower than 10% body fat are rarely reported. Data from female distance runners constitute an exception: a value of 5.9% body fat was reported for one runner who weighed 52.6 kg. Corroboration of such findings with a larger sample will probably result in modification of the lower limits of minimal body mass.

Underweight and Thin. The terms underweight and thin are not necessarily synonymous. In some cases they describe physical characteristics that differ considerably. In one study, for example, structural characteristics were compared between thin or "skinny" females and women who were normal in body fat or obese. The objective of the research was to determine if body frame size (as measured by bone widths at four sites on the trunk and four on the extremities) differed among these three groups who varied markedly in body fat.

Light is not necessarily lean. Appearing thin or skinny does not necessarily mean that skeletal frame size is diminutive or that the body's total fat content is excessively low.

The results were unexpected. While the thin females were indeed relatively low in body fat—18.2% compared with 25% body fat for the normal-size women and 32% for the obese group—there were *no differences* in average structural dimensions among the three groups! What this means is that for women of approximately the same stature, the level of body fat was not predictive of a small, medium, or large frame size as assessed from bone widths.

LEANNESS, EXERCISE, AND MENSTRUAL IRREGULARITY

Researchers have suggested that physically active females in general, as well as females in specific sports associated with excessive leanness, increase their chances of either a delayed onset of menstruation, an irregular menstrual cycle **(oligomenorrhea),** or complete cessation of menses **(amenorrhea).** For example, female ballet dancers as a group are quite lean and report a greater incidence of **menstrual irregularity,** eating disorders, and higher mean age at menarche compared to age-matched females who are not dancers. The speculation is that the body in some way "senses" when energy reserves are inadequate to sustain pregnancy, and thus ceases ovulation to prevent conception. Maintenance of at least 17% body fat is often cited as the "critical level" for the onset of menstruation and 22% fat as the level required to maintain a normal cycle. Some have argued that hormonal and metabolic disturbances which affect the menses are triggered if body fat falls below these levels.

Menstrual irregularity is prevalent among athletic women. One-third to one-half of female athletes in certain sports have some menstrual irregularity.

Altered menstruation means bone loss. When menstrual function is irregular or absent in premenopausal women, they face an increased risk of musculoskeletal injury during exercise.

Leanness Is Not the Only Factor. Although the lean-to-fat ratio does appear to be important for normal menstrual function (perhaps through the role of peripheral fat in converting androgens to estrogens), other factors must be considered. Many active females are significantly below the proposed critical level of 17% body fat, yet have normal menstrual cycles and maintain a high level of physiologic capacity. On the other hand, there are women athletes with average levels of body fat who are amenorrheic. In addition, when the menstrual cycle returns to normal, it is not always associated with an increase in body mass or body fat. These observations have led researchers to focus on the role of physiologic and psychologic stress, including that provided by exercise training, in influencing normal menstrual function. More recently, nutritional inadequacy and energy imbalance among athletes with irregular menstrual function have also been identified as possible predisposing factors.

There are currently many outstanding female distance runners, gymnasts, and body builders engaged in highly structured and vigorous training programs who have normal menses and who compete at a body fat level below 17%. In a study from one of our laboratories, 30 female athletes and 30 nonathletes with body fat below 20% were compared for menstrual cycle regularity. For women who ranged between 11 and 15% body fat, 4 athletes and 3 nonathletes had regular cycles, whereas 7 athletes and 2 nonathletes had irregular cycles or were amenorrheic. For the total sample, 14 athletes and 21 nonathletes had regular cycles. These data corroborate other findings and cast doubt on the hypothesis of a critical fat level of 17 to 22%.

Consideration must also be given to the complex interplay of physical, nutritional, genetic, hormonal, psychologic, and environmental factors as well as regional fat distribution as they affect menstrual function. Research shows that for active women, an intense bout of exercise triggers the release of an array of hormones some of which have antireproductive properties. It remains to be determined whether regular bouts of heavy exercise have a cumulative effect sufficient to alter normal menses. When young amenorrheic ballet dancers sustained injuries that prevented them from exercising, normal menstruation resumed although body mass remained unchanged. For most women, exercise-associated disturbances in menstrual function can be reversed with changes in lifestyle without serious consequences. If a critical fat level does exist, it is probably specific for each woman and may change throughout life.

In light of current knowledge on this topic, approximately 13 to 17% body fat should be regarded as the lower range of body fatness associated with regularity of menstrual function. The risks of sustained amenorrhea on the reproductive system are undetermined; the well-documented danger to bone mass is presented in Chapter 7. Failure to menstruate or cessation of the normal cycle should be evaluated by a gynecologist or endocrinologist because it may reflect a significant medical condition such as pituitary or thyroid gland malfunction or premature menopause. Additional studies are needed to define the lower limits of body fatness compatible with regular menstruation, and to determine if low body fat per se modifies hormonal regulation of ovulatory patterns.

Delayed Onset of Menstruation and Cancer Risk. Researchers now suggest that the delayed onset of menarche generally observed in chronically active young females provides a positive health benefit. Female college athletes who started training in high school or earlier show a lower lifetime occurrence of cancer of the breast and reproductive organs, as well as cancers not involving the reproductive system, compared to their nonathletic counterparts. This **lower cancer risk** with delayed onset of menstruation may be linked to the production of less total estrogen or a less potent form of estrogen over a lifetime. Lower body fat levels may also be involved, because fatty tissues convert androgens to estrogen.

COMMON LABORATORY METHODS TO ASSESS BODY COMPOSITION

The fat and lean components of the human body have been determined by two general procedures. One measures body composition *directly* by chemical analysis. The second approach assesses body composition *indirectly* with hydrostatic weighing or with simple circumferences, fatfold measurements, or other procedures. While direct methods form the basis for indirect techniques and are useful in animal research and for human cadaver analysis, indirect procedures permit the accurate assessment of body composition in living people.

Direct Assessment. Although there is considerable research on the direct measurement of body composition in various species of animals, few studies have chemically determined human fat content. Such analyses are time-consuming and tedious, require specialized laboratory equipment, and involve many ethical and legal problems in obtaining cadavers for research purposes.

While body fatness varies considerably, the composition of the skeletal mass and lean tissues remains relatively stable. The constancy of these tissues has enabled researchers to develop mathematical equations to determine the body's fat and lean percentages. This is indeed fortunate, as the direct method for assessing the fat content of cadavers, while of considerable theoretical importance, obviously cannot be used with live subjects.

Indirect Assessment. Three indirect procedures are commonly used to assess body composition. The first involves **Archimedes' principle** as applied to hydrostatic weighing. With this method, percent body fat is computed from body density (the ratio of body mass to body volume). The second approach assesses body composition through the measurement of fatfolds to estimate subcutaneous body fat. The third procedure involves the prediction of body fat from circumference (girth) measurements. Both circumference and fatfold measurements are of practical significance because body fat can be predicted simply and accurately.

Assess the composition of the body. It is the indirect, noninvasive procedures that enable us to assess the fat and nonfat components of living persons.

HYDROSTATIC WEIGHING

ARCHIMEDES' PRINCIPLE

About 2000 years ago, the Greek mathematician Archimedes discovered a basic principle that is currently applied in the evaluation of body composition. An itinerant scholar of that time described the interesting circumstances surrounding the event:

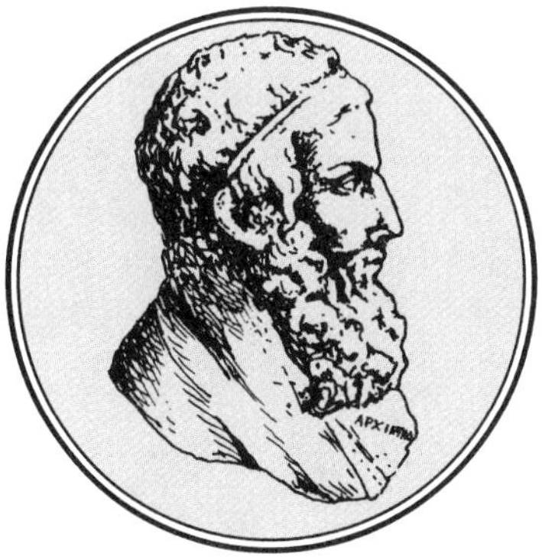

> King Hieron of Syracuse suspected that his pure gold crown had been altered by substitution of silver for gold. The King directed Archimedes to devise a method for testing the crown for its gold content without dismantling it. Archimedes pondered over this problem for many weeks without succeeding, until one day, he stepped into a bath filled to the top with water and observed the overflow. He thought about this for a moment, and then, wild with joy, jumped from the bath and ran naked through the streets of Syracuse shouting "Eureka! Eureka! I have discovered a way to solve the mystery of the King's crown."

Archimedes reasoned that a substance such as gold must have a volume proportionate to its mass, and the way to measure the volume of an irregular object such as the crown was to submerge it in water and collect the overflow. Archimedes took a lump of gold and silver, each having the same mass as the crown, and submerged each in a container full of water. To his delight, he discovered that the crown displaced more water than the lump of gold and less than the lump of silver. What this meant was that the crown was indeed composed of both silver and gold, as the King had suspected.

Essentially, what Archimedes evaluated was the **specific gravity** of the crown (ratio of the mass of the crown to the mass of an equal volume of water) compared to the specific gravities for gold and silver. Archimedes probably also reasoned that an object submerged in water is buoyed up by a counterforce that equals the mass of the water it displaces. This buoyancy force supports an object in water against the downward pull of gravity, causing the object to lose weight in water. *Because the object's loss of weight in water equals the weight of the volume of water it displaces, we can redefine specific gravity as the ratio of the weight of an object in air divided by its loss of weight in water*. Thus,

$$\text{Specific gravity} = \text{Weight in air} \div \text{Loss of weight in water}$$

where

$$\text{Loss of weight in water} = (\text{Weight in air} - \text{Weight in water})$$

In practical terms, suppose the crown weighed 2.27 kg in air and 0.13 kg less, or 2.14 kg, when weighed underwater (Figure 14–2). The specific gravity of the crown would then be computed by dividing the weight of the crown (2.27 kg) by its loss of weight in water (0.13 kg), which results in a specific gravity of 17.7. Because this ratio is considerably different than the specific gravity of gold (19.3), we too can conclude: "Eureka! Eureka! the crown is a fraud!"

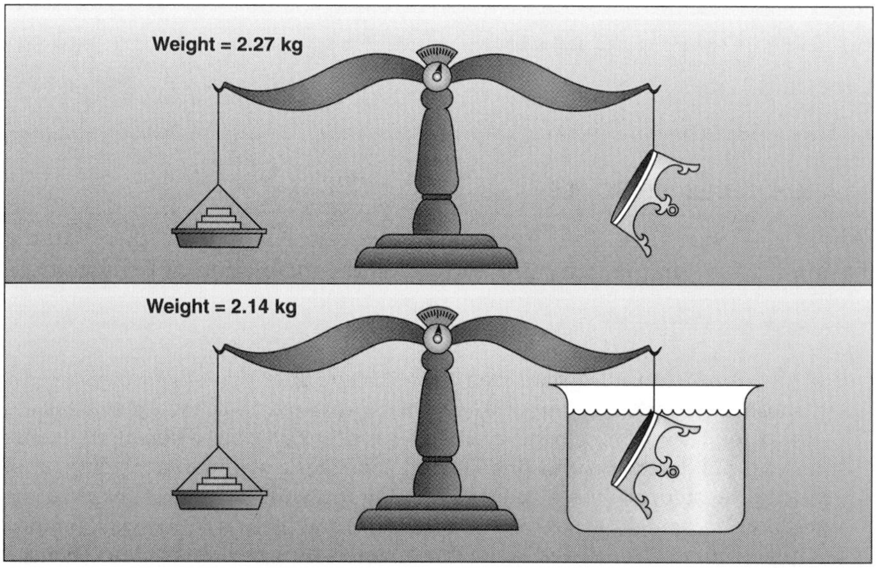

FIG. 14–2. Archimedes' solution for determining the gold content of the king's crown.

The physical principle Archimedes discovered can be applied directly to the assessment of body composition in humans. This is achieved by determining the body's volume by water submersion in relation to the total body mass. Because density is mass per unit volume (that is, body mass ÷ body volume), we can compute the density of the body once the mass and volume are known.

DETERMINING BODY DENSITY

For illustrative purposes, suppose a 50 kg person weighs 2 kg when submerged completely underwater. According to Archimedes' principle, the buoyancy or counterforce of the water equals 48 kg. The 48 kg loss of body weight in water equals the weight of the displaced water. Because the density of water at any temperature is known, we can compute the volume of water displaced. In this example, 48 kg (48,000 g) of water is equal to a volume of 48 liters or 48,000 cc (1 g water = 1 cm^3 by volume, or 1 g/cc, at 39.2° F). If the person were measured at the cold-water temperature of 39.2° F, no density correction would be necessary. In practice, researchers use warmer water and apply the appropriate density value for water at the particular temperature. The density of the subject, computed as mass ÷ volume, would be 50,000 g (50 kg) ÷ 48,000 g/cc, or 1.0417 g/cc. This particular value for body density is about midway between the density value of 0.90 g/cc for fat extracted from adipose tissue and 1.10 g/cc for fat-free tissue. Once body density has been established, the next step is to determine the corresponding percentage of body fat.

Fat-free tissue. The assumed densities for the components of the fat-free mass at body temperature of 37° C are: water, 0.993 g/cc; mineral, 3.000 g/cc; protein, 1.340 g/cc.

COMPUTING PERCENT BODY FAT AND MASS OF FAT AND LEAN TISSUE

The relative percentage of fat in the human body can be estimated with a simple equation that incorporates body density. This equation was derived from the theoretical premise that the **densities of fat and fat-free tissues** remain relatively constant (fat = 0.90 g/cc; fat-free tissue = 1.10 g/cc), even with large variations in both total body fat and the lean tissue components of bone and muscle. Thus, the relative contributions of fat and lean components to total body mass can be determined from an algebraic expression that relates these proportions to the density of the whole body. The following equation, derived by Berkeley scientist Dr. William Siri, is used to compute percent body fat by incorporating the determined value of body density:

Siri equation: Percent body fat = 495 ÷ Body density − 450

The body density value of 1.0417 g/cc determined for the subject in the previous example can now be substituted in the Siri equation for percent body fat as follows:

Percent body fat = 495 ÷ 1.0417 − 450 = 25.2% fat

The mass of fat can then be calculated by multiplying body mass by percent fat:

Fat mass (kg) = Body mass (kg) × [Percent fat ÷ 100]
= 50 kg × 0.252 = 12.6 kg

Resting and total daily energy expenditure predicted from lean body mass. Use the following equations to estimate your resting energy expenditure (REE) and total daily energy expenditure (TDEE) from lean body mass (LBM*) using the following equations:

(1) REE (kcal/d) = 21.6 (LBM, kg) + 370

If, for example, LBM = 70 kg, then:

REE = 21.6(70) + 370 = 1882 kcal/d

(2) TDEE (kcal/d) = 26.0 (LBM, kg) + 682

If, for example, LBM = 70 kg, then:

TDEE = 26.0(70) + 682 = 2502 kcal/d

* Compute LBM as outlined on pp. 241–242, this Chapter. *Source:* Cunningham, J.J.: Body composition as a determinant of energy expenditure: a synthetic review and a proposed general prediction equation. *Am. J. Clin. Nutr.* 54:963, 1991.

Lean body mass is calculated by subtracting the mass of fat from body mass:

Lean body mass (kg) = Body mass (kg) − Fat mass (kg)
= 50 kg − 12.6 kg = 37.4 kg

In this example, then, 25.2%, or 12.6 kg, of the 50 kg body mass is fat. The remaining 37.4 kg is the lean body mass. For simplicity we will use the term lean body mass, although we realize that by subtracting out the total body fat yields a remainder that is "fat-free." The true calculation of lean body mass in males includes the essential fat; in females, the lean body mass (termed minimal weight) also includes the gender-specific essential fat.

Possible Limitations. The generalized density values of 1.10 and 0.90 g/cc for lean and fat tissues, respectively, are average values for young and middle-aged adults. Although these values are assumed to be constants, this may not be the case. For example, the density of the lean body mass is estimated to be significantly *greater* for blacks than for whites (1.113 vs. 1.100 g/cc). The existing equations to calculate body composition from body density in whites, therefore, would tend to *overestimate* the lean body mass (and *underestimate* percent body fat) when applied to blacks.

In addition to racial differences, applying constant density values for the various tissues to growing children or aging adults could also add uncertainty in predicting body composition. For example, the density of the skeleton is probably in continual change during growth as well as during the well-documented demineralization of osteoporosis with aging. This would make the actual density of the fat-free tissue of young children and the elderly *lower* than the assumed constant of 1.10 g/cc and result in *overestimation* of percent body fat. With highly trained and select groups of athletes such as professional football players, champion long-distance runners, and champion body builders, the density of the fat-free component could theoretically exceed 1.10 g/cc. This would cause an *underestimation* of relative fat.

MEASUREMENT OF BODY VOLUME

Determining body mass and calculating body density, percent body fat, and lean body mass are quite simple. The more difficult task is the accurate assessment of body volume, which is usually measured by the procedure of ***hydrostatic weighing.***

Hydrostatic weighing (also referred to as underwater weighing) computes body volume as the difference between body weight measured in air and body weight measured during water submersion. In other words, body volume equals the loss of weight in water with the appropriate temperature correction for water density. Figure 14–3 illustrates the procedure for measuring body volume by hydrostatic weighing.

A diver's belt is usually secured around the waist so the subject does not float toward the surface during submersion. While seated with the head out of the water, the subject makes a forced maximal exhalation as the head is lowered beneath the water. The breath is held for several seconds while

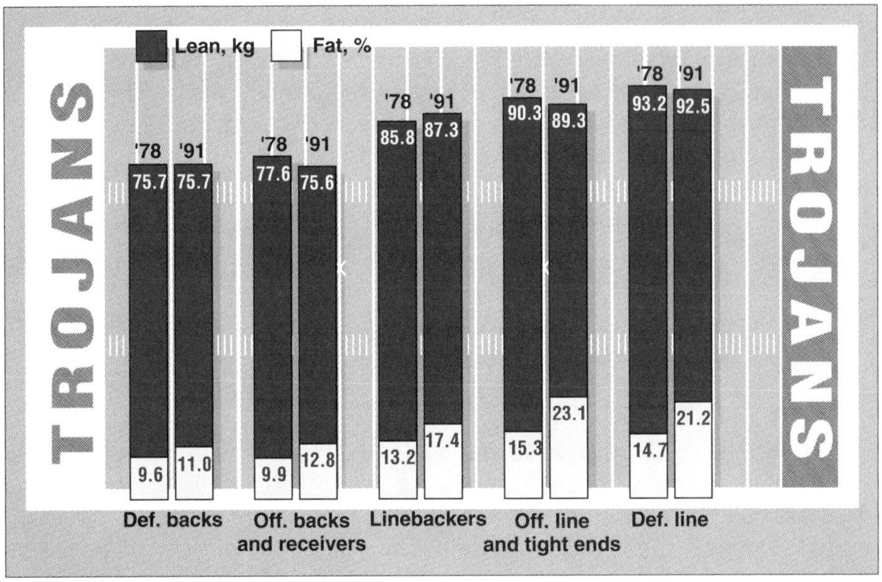

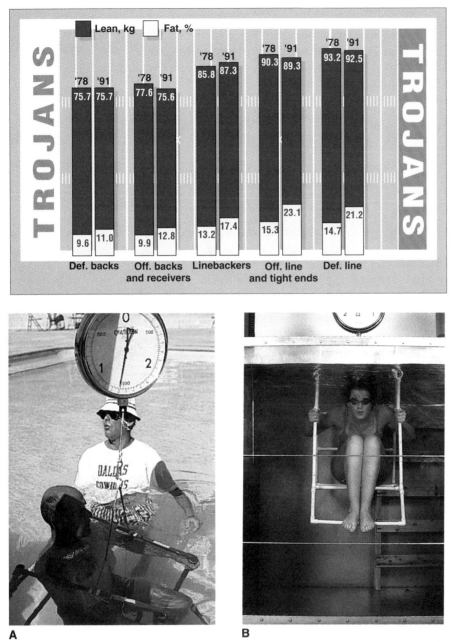

Percent body fat and lean body mass of collegiate football players over a 13-year period. A perennial powerhouse, the Trojans of the University of Southern California, are compared for body fat and lean body mass in 1978 and 1991. For the team as a whole, the average body mass remained the same at 96.6 kg, yet body fat for all positions was larger in 1991. Data Courtesy of Dr. Robert Girandola, Department of Exercise Science, University of Southern California, Los Angeles, CA, 1991.

A B

FIG. 14–3. Different methods of measuring body volume by the underwater weighing method.

the underwater weight is recorded. Eight to twelve repeated weighings are made to obtain a dependable underwater weight score. This amount of practice is given because there is a predictable "learning curve" in making a forced exhalation during submersion. Even when achieving a full exhalation, a small volume of air, the ***residual lung volume,*** remains in the lungs. This air volume, however, is measured for each subject just before, during, or following the underwater weighing and its buoyant effect is subtracted in the calculation of body volume. Water temperature is also recorded to correct for the density of water at the time of weighing.

EXAMPLES OF CALCULATIONS

Let us put theory into practice again in the sequence of steps to compute body density, percent fat, mass of fat, and lean body mass. The subjects are two professional football players: an offensive guard and a quarterback. The following measurements were made:

	OFFENSIVE GUARD	QUARTERBACK
Body weight	110 kg	85 kg
Underwater weight	3.5 kg	5.0 kg
Residual lung volume	1.2 L	1.0 L
Water temperature correction factor	0.996	0.996

Because the loss of weight in water is equal to volume, the body volume of the offensive guard is 110 kg − 3.5 kg = 106.5 kg or 106.5 liters; for the quarterback, body volume is 85 kg − 5.0 kg = 80.0 kg or 80 liters. Dividing body volume by the water temperature correction factor of 0.996 increases body volume slightly for both players (106.9 liters for the guard and 80.3 liters for the quarterback). Because residual lung volume also contributes to buoyancy, this volume is subtracted. The body volume of the offensive guard then becomes 105.7 liters (106.9 liters − 1.2 liters); for the quarterback, 79.3 liters (80.3 liters − 1.0 liters).

Body density is then computed as mass ÷ volume. For the offensive guard, body density is 110 kg ÷ 105.7 liters = 1.0407 kg/liter or 1.0407 g/cc. For the quarterback, body density is 85.0 kg/79.3 liters = 1.0719 g/cc.

The percentage of fat is computed from the Siri equation:

$$\text{Percent body fat} = 495 \div \text{Body density} - 450$$

Offensive guard	Quarterback
495 ÷ 1.0407 − 450 = 25.6%	495 ÷ 1.0719 − 450 = 11.8%

The total mass of the body fat is calculated as follows:

$$\text{Fat mass} = \text{Body mass} \times (\text{Percent fat} \div 100)$$

Offensive guard	Quarterback
110 kg × 0.25 = 28.2 kg	85 kg × 0.118 = 10.0 kg

Lean body mass is calculated as follows:

$$\text{Lean body mass} = \text{Body mass} - \text{Fat mass}$$

Offensive guard	Quarterback
110 kg − 28.2 kg = 81.8 kg	85 kg − 10.0 kg = 75.0 kg

This analysis of body composition illustrates that the offensive guard possesses more than twice the percentage body fat as the quarterback (25.6% vs. 11.8%) and almost three times as much total fat (28.2 kg vs. 10.0 kg). On the other hand, lean body mass, which provides a good indication of muscle mass, is also much larger for the guard than for the quarterback. Although the guard is 25 kg heavier than the quarterback, similar differences in body composition occur for people of the same body mass, especially between physically active and sedentary people. These results point up the crucial role of body composition analysis in determining the fat and lean components of the body. We believe it is inadequate to rely solely on body mass as the index of "acceptability" for assessing body size and shape.

FATFOLD MEASUREMENTS

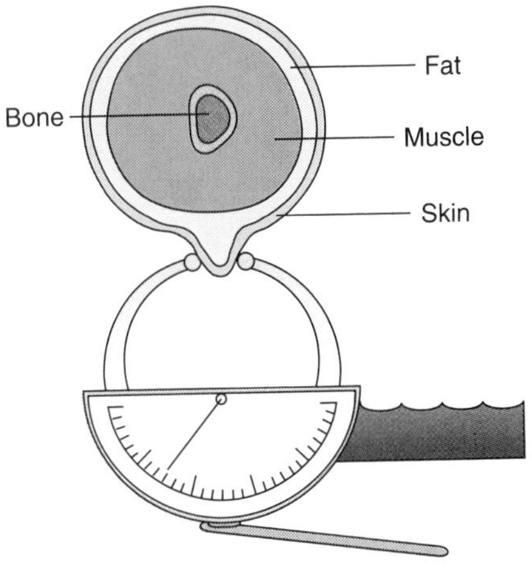

Hydrostatic weighing is a widely used indirect method for assessing body composition. When laboratory facilities are unavailable, simpler alternative procedures can be used to predict body fatness. Two of these procedures, the measurement of subcutaneous fatfolds and girths or circumferences, require relatively inexpensive equipment. The rationale for **fatfold measurements** to estimate total body fat is that a relationship exists between the fat located directly beneath the skin and internal fat, and that both of these measures are related to body density.

By 1930, a special pincer-type caliper was used to measure subcutaneous fat at selected sites on the body with relative accuracy. The caliper works on the same principle as the micrometer used to measure distance between two points. The procedure for measuring fatfold thickness is to grasp a fold of skin and subcutaneous fat firmly with the thumb and forefingers, pulling it away from the underlying muscle tissue following the natural contour of the fatfold. The caliper is applied with its jaws exerting constant tension of 10 g/mm^2 at their point of contact with the skin. The thickness of the double layer of skin and subcutaneous tissue is then read directly from the caliper dial and recorded, in millimeters, within several seconds after applying the full force of the caliper. This is done to avoid undue compression of the fatfold when taking the measurements.

The most common areas for measuring fatfolds are at triceps, subscapular, suprailiac, abdominal, and upper thigh sites. All measures are taken on the right side of the body with the subject standing. A minimum of two or three measurements are made at each site, and the average value is used as the fatfold score. When fatfolds are measured for research purposes, the investigator has had considerable experience and is consistent in duplicating values for the same subject on the same day, consecutive days, or even weeks apart. Figure 14–4 shows the anatomic location of the five most **frequently measured fatfold sites:**

- **Triceps:** Vertical fold measured at the midline of the upper arm halfway between the tip of the shoulder and tip of the elbow
- **Subscapular:** Oblique fold measured just below the bottom tip of the scapula
- **Suprailiac:** Slightly oblique fold measured just above the hip bone; the fold is lifted to follow the natural diagonal line at this point
- **Abdominal:** Vertical fold measured 1 inch to the right of the umbilicus
- **Thigh:** Vertical fold measured at the midline of the thigh, two-thirds of the distance from the kneecap to the hip

Fatfolds are sometimes taken on the medial, lateral, and posterior calf and on the anterior chest wall at the level of the armpit. However, depending on the individual's degree of fatness, these measurements are often difficult.

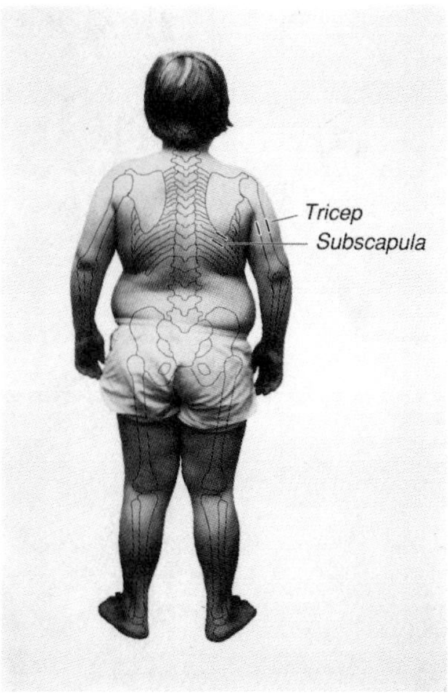

Tracking excessive fatness in childhood. Triceps and subscapular fatfolds are useful indices for tracking changes in subcutaneous fat in the trunk and extremity regions. (Photo courtesy of V. Katch.)

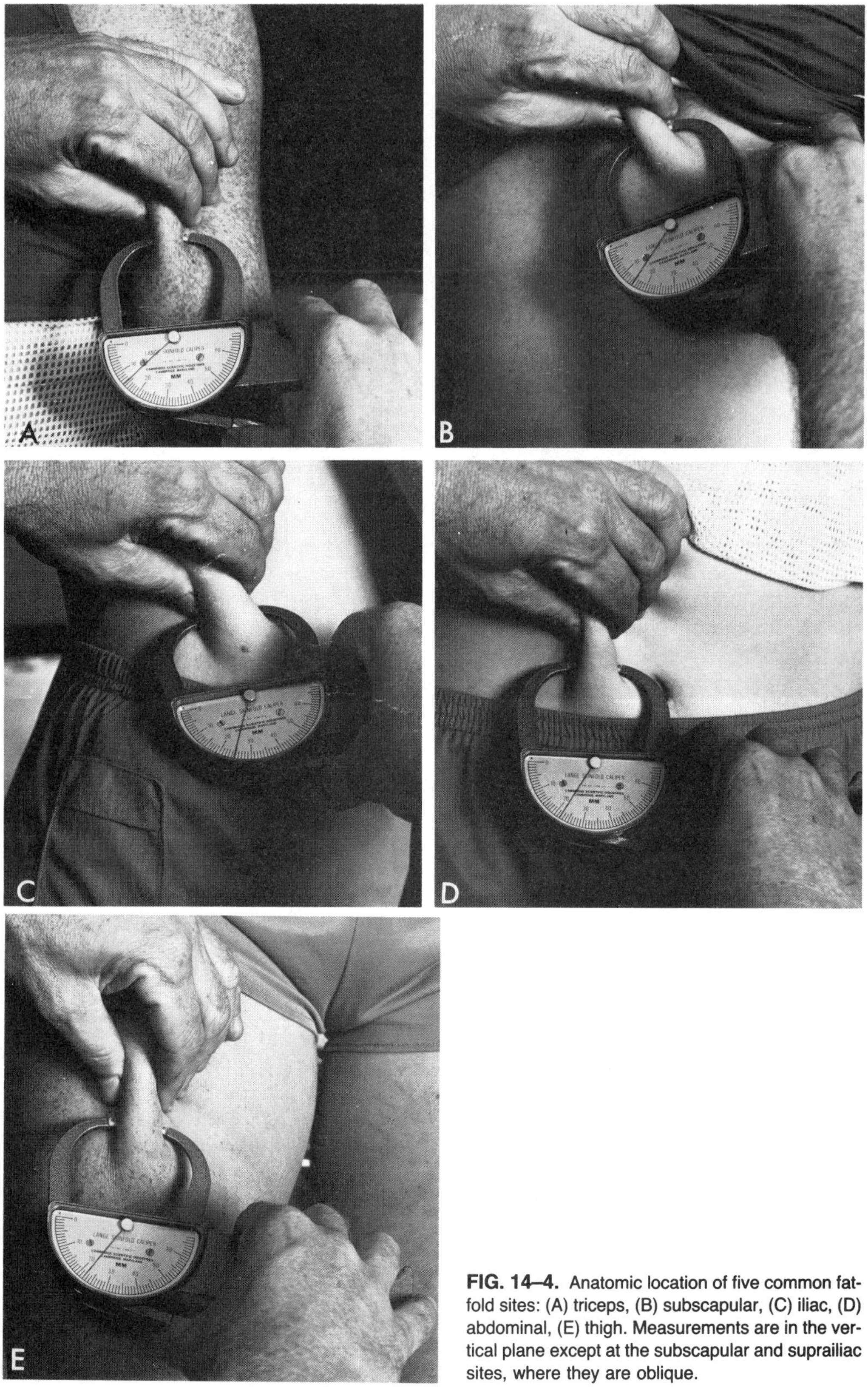

FIG. 14–4. Anatomic location of five common fatfold sites: (A) triceps, (B) subscapular, (C) iliac, (D) abdominal, (E) thigh. Measurements are in the vertical plane except at the subscapular and suprailiac sites, where they are oblique.

USEFULNESS OF FATFOLD SCORES

Fatfold measurements provide meaningful information concerning body fat and its distribution. There are basically two ways to use fatfolds. The first is to sum the scores as an indication of relative fatness among individuals. This "sum of fatfolds" can also be used to reflect changes in fatness before and after a physical conditioning regimen. Changes in individual fatfold values as well as the total fatfold score can then be evaluated on either an absolute or percentage basis.

From the fatfold data shown in Table 14–2, obtained from a 22-year-old female college student before and after a 16-week exercise program, the following observations can be made:

1. The largest changes in fatfold thickness occurred at the suprailiac and abdominal sites.
2. The triceps showed the largest decrease and the subscapular the smallest decrease when changes were expressed as percentages.
3. The total reduction in subcutaneous fatfolds at the five sites was 16.6 mm, or 12.6% below the starting condition.

A second way to use fatfolds is in conjunction with mathematical equations designed to predict body density or percent body fat. These equations are **"population specific,"** and predict fatness fairly accurately for subjects similar in age, gender, state of training, fatness, and race to those on whom the equations were derived. When these criteria are met, the predicted value of fatness for an individual is usually within 3 to 5% of the body fat assessed by hydrostatic weighing.

Equations have been developed in our laboratories to predict body fat from triceps and subscapular fatfolds. The equations most useful for predicting total body fat in young women and men are:

Young women, ages 17 to 26 years

$$\% \text{ Body fat} = 0.55(A) + 0.31(B) + 6.13$$

Young men, ages 17 to 26 years

$$\% \text{ Body fat} = 0.43(A) + 0.58(B) + 1.47$$

where A = triceps fatfold (mm) and B = subscapular fatfold (mm)

Using the fatfold data for the woman who participated in the 16-week conditioning program, percent body fat can be computed before and after

TABLE 14–2. CHANGES IN SELECTED FATFOLDS FOR A YOUNG WOMAN DURING A 16-WEEK EXERCISE PROGRAM

FATFOLDS, MM	BEFORE	AFTER	ABSOLUTE CHANGE	PERCENT CHANGE
Triceps	22.5	19.4	−3.1	−13.8
Subscapular	19.0	17.0	−2.0	−10.5
Suprailiac	34.5	30.2	−4.3	−12.8
Abdomen	33.7	29.4	−4.3	−12.8
Thigh	21.6	18.7	−2.9	−13.4
Sum	131.3	114.7	−16.6	−12.6

training using the equation for young women. Substituting the pretraining fatfold values for triceps (22.5 mm) and subscapular (19.0 mm), percent body fat is computed as:

$$\begin{aligned}\%\text{ Body fat} &= 0.55(A) + 0.31(B) + 6.13\\ &= 0.55(22.5) + 0.31(19.0) + 6.13\\ &= 12.38 + 5.89 + 6.13\\ &= 24.4\%\end{aligned}$$

Substituting the post-training values for triceps (19.4 mm) and subscapular (17.0 mm) fatfolds, percent body fat is computed as:

$$\begin{aligned}\%\text{ Body fat} &= 0.55(19.4) + 0.31(17.0) + 6.13\\ &= 10.67 + 5.27 + 6.13\\ &= 22.1\%\end{aligned}$$

Determining percent body fat before and after a conditioning or weight control program provides a convenient means to evaluate alterations in body composition that often are not reflected by changes in body mass.

Fatfolds and Age. For young adults, approximately one-half of the body's total fat is subcutaneous and the remainder is internal fat. With advancing age, a proportionately greater quantity of fat is deposited internally in comparison to subcutaneous fat. Thus, the same fatfold score reflects a greater total percentage of body fat as one gets older. For this reason, age-adjusted or ***generalized equations*** that account for age should be used when predicting body fat from fatfolds or girths (see next section) for older men and women.

Not for All People. Although fatfolds have been widely used in the allied health professions to predict percent body fat, a major drawback is that the person taking the measurements must have considerable experience with the proper techniques to obtain consistent values. With extremely obese people, the thickness of the fatfold often exceeds the width of the caliper's jaws! The particular caliper used may also contribute to measurement error. Because there are no standards to compare results between different investigators, it is difficult to determine which sets of fatfold data are "best" to use. Thus, prediction equations developed by a particular researcher (which may be highly valid for the sample measured) may result in large errors in prediction when another person takes the measurements.

GIRTH MEASUREMENTS

The measurement of **circumferences** (or girths) provides a valid assessment of body fat that is free from some of the limitations imposed by the fatfold technique. A linen or plastic measuring tape is applied lightly to the skin surface so that the tape is taut but not tight. This procedure avoids skin compression that produces artificially low scores. Duplicate measurements are taken at each site and the average is used. Figure 14–5 displays the anatomic landmarks for the various girths used to assess body fatness:

- **Abdomen:** One inch above the umbilicus
- **Buttocks:** Maximum protrusion with the heels together
- **Right thigh:** Upper thigh just below the buttocks
- **Right upper arm:** Arm straight, palm up and extended in front of the body, measured at the midpoint between the shoulder and the elbow

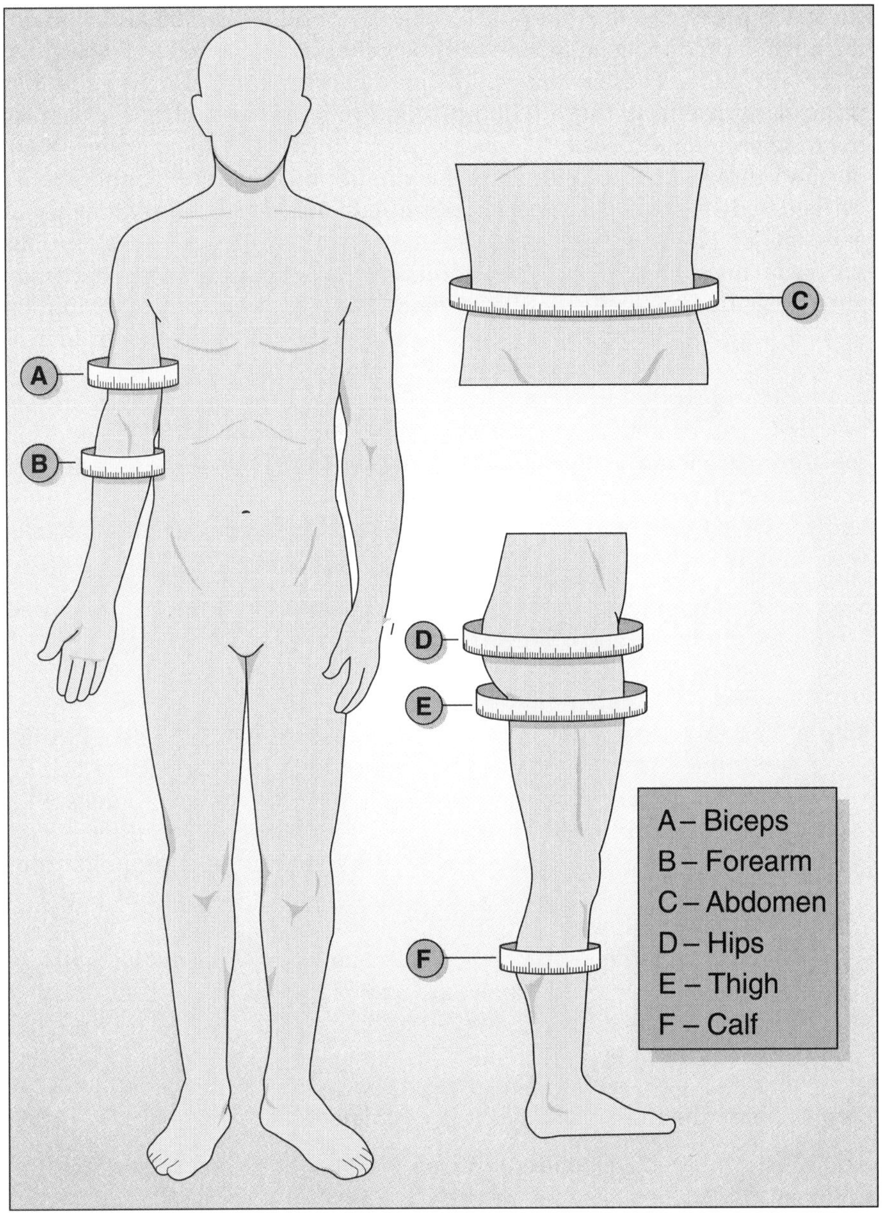

FIG. 14–5. Anatomic landmarks for the various girths.

- **Right forearm:** Maximum girth with the arm extended in front of the body with palm up
- **Right calf:** Widest girth midway between the ankle and knee

Different prediction equations have been developed based on gender and age. The equations for these groups have been cross-validated on different samples with good results.

USEFULNESS OF GIRTH MEASUREMENTS

The girth-based predictions are most useful in ranking individuals within a group according to their relative fatness. If one uses the equations and

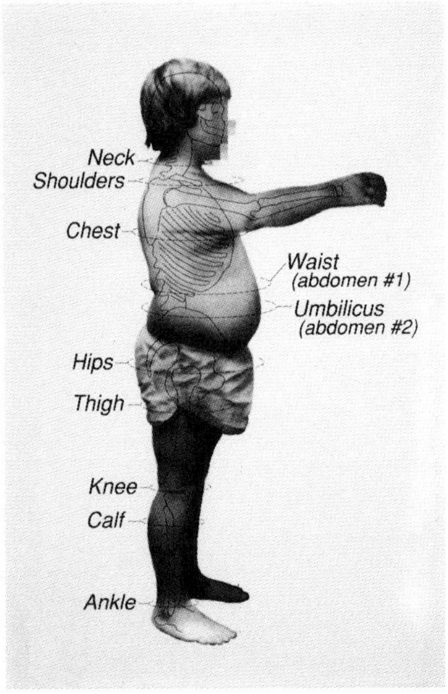

Tracking changes in girths can evaluate changes in growth. Measurement of girths during childhood and adolescence provides useful information about body composition. Body fat can be predicted from girths in children using tables appropriate for age and gender. (Photo courtesy of V. Katch.)

constants presented in Appendix C for young and older men and women, the error in predicting an individual's percent body fat is generally between ± 2.5 and 4.0%. These relatively low prediction errors make the equations particularly useful to those without access to laboratory facilities, because the measurements are easy to take and a tape measure is inexpensive. Keep in mind, however, that the equations are population specific and should *not* be used to predict fatness in individuals who (1) appear very thin or very fat, or (2) have been involved for a number of years in strenuous sports or resistance training. In addition to predicting percent body fat, girth measures are well suited for determining patterns of fat distribution on the body as well as changes in fat patterning following weight loss.

Predicting Body Fat from Girths. From the appropriate tables in Appendix C, we can substitute the corresponding constants A, B, and C in the formula shown at the bottom of each table. One addition and two subtraction steps are required. The following five-step example shows how to compute percent fat, fat mass, and lean body mass for a 21-year-old man who weighs 79.1 kg:

Step 1. The upper arm, abdomen, and right forearm girths are measured with a cloth tape and recorded to the nearest ¼ inch: upper arm = 11.5 in. (29.21 cm); abdomen = 31.0 in. (78.74 cm); right forearm = 10.75 in. (27.30 cm)

Step 2. The three constants A, B, and C corresponding to the three girths are determined from the Appendix: Constant A, corresponding to 11.5 in. = 42.56; Constant B, corresponding to 31.0 in. = 40.68; Constant C, corresponding to 10.75 in. = 58.37

Step 3. Percent body fat is computed by substituting the appropriate constants in the formula for young men shown at the bottom of Chart 1 in Appendix C as follows:

$$\begin{aligned}\text{Percent fat} &= \text{Constant A} + \text{Constant B} - \text{Constant C} - 10.2\\ &= 42.56 + 40.68 - 58.37 - 10.2\\ &= 83.24 - 58.37 - 10.2\\ &= 24.87 - 10.2\\ &= 14.7\%\end{aligned}$$

Step 4. Next, the mass of body fat is calculated:

$$\begin{aligned}\text{Fat mass} &= \%\text{ fat} \div 100 \times \text{Body mass}\\ &= 14.7 \div 100 \times 79.1\text{ kg}\\ &= 0.147 \times 79.1\text{ kg}\\ &= 11.63\text{ kg}\end{aligned}$$

Step 5. Finally, lean body mass is determined:

$$\begin{aligned}\text{LBM} &= \text{Body mass} - \text{Fat mass}\\ &= 79.1\text{ kg} - 11.63\text{ kg}\\ &= 67.5\text{ kg}\end{aligned}$$

OTHER INDIRECT PROCEDURES TO ASSESS BODY COMPOSITION

There are **alternative indirect procedures** that enable the researcher to gain valuable information about body composition.

Ultrasound. A lightweight, portable **ultrasound** meter is used to measure the distance between the skin and the fat-muscle layer, and between that layer and bone. The ultrasound meter operates by emitting high-frequency sound waves that penetrate the skin surface. The sound waves pass through adipose tissue until they reach the muscle layer, where they are reflected from the fat-muscle interface to produce an echo that returns to the ultrasound unit. The time for sound waves to be transmitted through the tissues and back to the receiver is converted to a distance score that is displayed on an easy to see readout.

With the ultrasound technique, we have evaluated the pattern of fat gain and loss on the trunk and extremities in athletes and in obese and normal-weight nonathletes before and after sports and exercise training. Figure 14–6 shows the ultrasound meter for recording fat and muscle thickness. The use of ultrasound for "mapping" muscle and fat thickness at various body sites and estimating total body fat is a useful and valid technique in body composition assessment.

World-record measurements. The following are astounding facts about body size and composition listed in the 1990 *Guinness Book of World Records.* Heaviest weight for a male: 1400 lb, 634.9 kg; and female: 880 lb or 399.1 kg; lightest human: 4.7 lb emaciated female dwarf at age 17 (26.5 in. in stature). Her final weight was 13 lb at age 20. At birth, she weighed 2.5 lb; most fat removed during surgery: 140 lb of adipose tissue from the abdomen of a 798 lb man; largest biceps: 26⅛ in. in a male who weighed 362 lb; smallest biceps: 4 in.; largest chest girth: 124 in. (315 cm).

Bioelectric Impedance Analysis (BIA). The principle underlying this technique is based on the fact that flow of electricity is facilitated through hydrated fat-free tissue and extracellular water compared to fat tissue. This occurs because of the greater electrolyte content (and thus lower electrical resistance) of the fat-free component. Consequently, impedance to the flow of electric current is directly related to the level of body fat. With the **BIA technique,** electrodes are placed on the hands and feet, a painless localized electric signal is introduced, and the impedance or resistance to current flow is determined. The value for impedance is then converted to body density, which in turn is converted to percent body fat by use of the Siri equation explained earlier in this chapter.

A factor that affects the accuracy of BIA is the need for the subject to maintain a normal hydration level, because either dehydration or overhydration affects the body's electrolyte concentration. This will alter current flow *independent* of real changes in body fat. More specifically, loss of body water decreases the impedance measure to yield a lower percent fat, whereas overhydration produces the opposite effect. Even under conditions of normal hydration, the prediction of body fat may be questionable in relation to values obtained from hydrostatic weighing. In fact, the technique may be less accurate than the anthropometric methods that use girths and

BIA technique: proceed with caution. A recent study has questioned the validity of using BIA to evaluate change in body composition. Researchers studied the individual data from seven experiments with adults who incurred a change in body mass and lean body mass resulting from a diet or diet and exercise program. The results were quite clear; the mathematical equations that form the foundation of the BIA technique were unable to successfully predict change in body composition even when there was a 20% change in body mass or lean body mass!

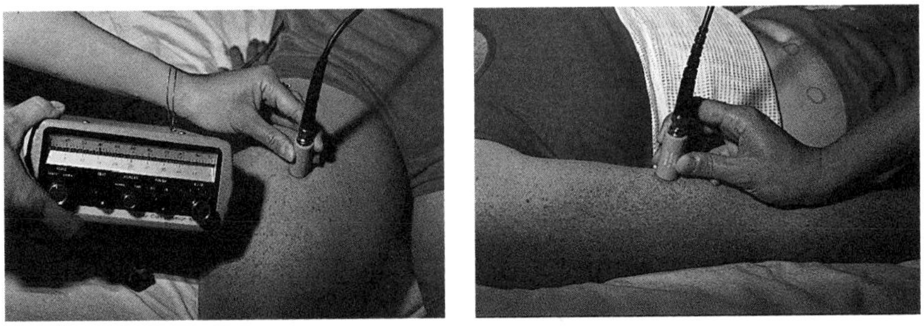

FIG. 14–6. Ultrasound measurement. (A) Portable body composition meter that includes a display scale to provide a direct readout of distance between skin-to-fat, fat-to-muscle, and muscle-to-bone. (B) Measurement of upper arm fat and muscle thickness.

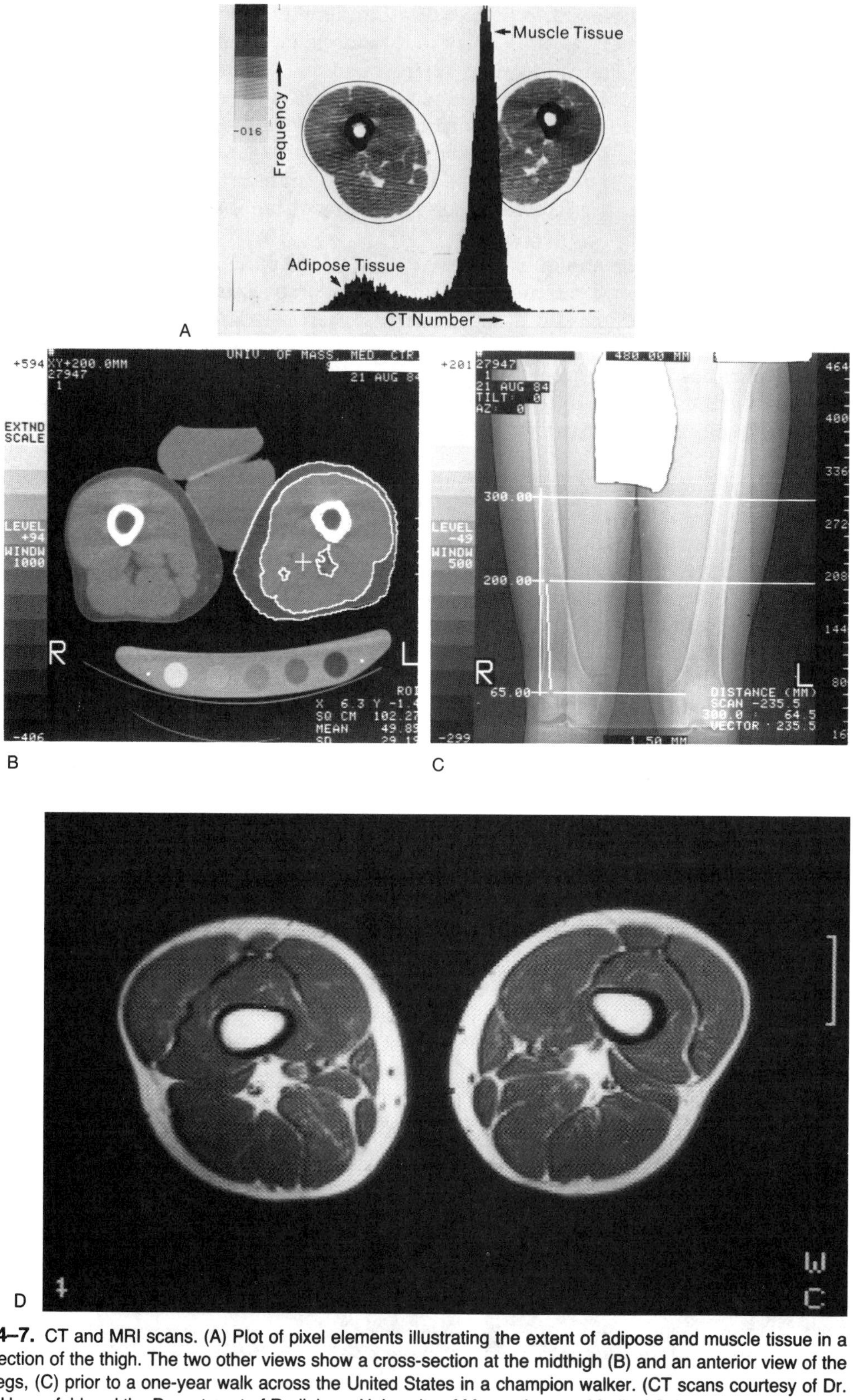

FIG. 14–7. CT and MRI scans. (A) Plot of pixel elements illustrating the extent of adipose and muscle tissue in a cross-section of the thigh. The two other views show a cross-section at the midthigh (B) and an anterior view of the upper legs, (C) prior to a one-year walk across the United States in a champion walker. (CT scans courtesy of Dr. Steven Heymsfeld and the Department of Radiology, University of Massachusetts Medical School, Worcester, MA.) (D) MRI scan of the midthigh of the younger author (F.K.) before a 13-week resistance training program. (MRI scan courtesy of the Radiology Department, Bay State Medical Center, Springfield, MA.)

fatfolds to predict body fat. Skin temperature, which is influenced by ambient conditions, also affects whole-body resistance. Thus, the predicted body fat value is significantly lower in a warm compared to a cold environment. There is conflicting evidence on whether BIA can detect small changes in body composition during weight loss. At best, BIA is another noninvasive, indirect means to assess body composition provided that measurements are made under conditions strictly standardized for both ambient temperature and level of hydration.

Computed Tomography (CT) and Magnetic Resonance Imaging (MRI). The **CT and MRI** scanning procedures produce radiographic images of sections of the body. In the first studies that used CT to evaluate body composition, researchers were able to differentiate fat accumulation accurately in the abdominal area. By use of appropriate computer software, the scan provides pictorial and quantitative information for total tissue area, total fat area, and intra-abdominal fat area. The top panels of Figure 14–7 shows CT scans of both upper legs and a cross section at the midthigh in a professional walker who completed an 11,200 mile walk through the 50 United States in 50 weeks. A comparison of CT scans prior to and after the walk showed a significant increase in the total cross section of muscle area and corresponding decrease in subcutaneous fat in the midthigh region. In recent studies using CT scans, scientists have been able to determine the relationship between the outer thickness of fat at the abdomen and visceral fat within the abdominal cavity. Surprisingly, there is little relation in both males and females between these "external" and "internal" depots of fat.

The newer technology of MRI, shown in Figure 14–7D, provides valuable information about the body's tissue compartments. In MRI, electromagnetic radiation in the presence of a strong magnetic field is used to excite the hydrogen nuclei of water and lipid molecules. This causes the nuclei to give off a detectable signal that can then be rearranged under computer control to provide a visual representation of body tissues. The MRI procedure can be used effectively to evaluate changes in a tissue's lean-to-fat components. This has been done to evaluate changes in the cross-sectional area of muscle following resistance exercise training and during growth and aging.

Dual-Energy X-ray Absorptiometry **(DEXA)** is another high-technology procedure that permits quantification of fat and muscle not only around the bony areas of the body, but also in areas where there is no bone present. The DEXA procedure is an accepted clinical tool for assessment of spinal osteoporosis and related bone disorders. The underlying principle of DEXA is that the bone and soft tissue areas of the body can be penetrated to a depth of about 30 cm by two distinct x-ray energies. Specialized computer software then reconstructs an image of the underlying tissues. Examples of DEXA are illustrated in Figure 14–8 A, B, C and D. A whole scan of the body takes approximately 12 minutes, and the computer-generated report quantifies bone mineral, total fat mass, lean mass, and lean mass and bone mineral, and the percentage of fat mass for the entire skeleton and subregions of the body. Selected regions of the body can also be pinpointed for more in-depth analysis.

Another technique known as **dual-photon absorptiometry** also plays a key role in evaluating the bone mineral content of the spine and femur, two areas that characteristically become demineralized in osteoporosis.

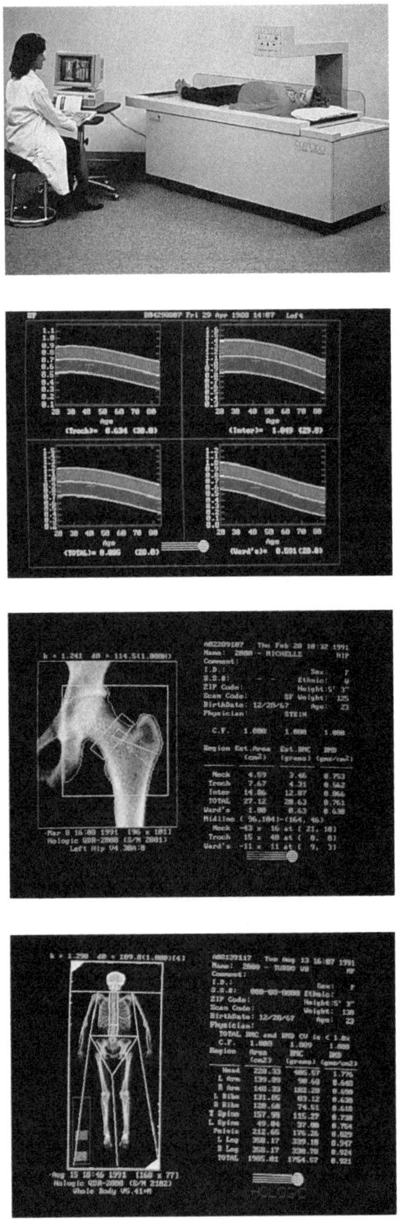

FIG. 14–8. A. Example of a patient undergoing a whole body scan using the DEXA procedure. Scans of the spine and hip can be performed in 2 to 3 minutes, and whole body scans take 11 to 14 minutes. B. Four areas of the body are compared to reference values in light and darker blue. C. Close-up view of the proximal femur. D. Whole body scan with related body composition report. (Photos courtesy of Hologic, Inc., 590 Lincoln Street. Waltham, MA 02154.)

AVERAGE VALUES FOR BODY COMPOSITION

Average values for body fat in samples of men and women throughout the United States are presented in Table 14–3. Also included are values representing plus and minus one standard deviation to give some indication of the amount of variation or spread from the average: the column headed "68% Variation Limits" indicates the range of values for percent body fat that includes one standard deviation, or about 68 of every 100 persons measured. As an example, the average percent body fat of young men from the New York sample is 15.0%, and the 68% variation limits are from 8.9 to 21.1% body fat. Interpreting this statistically, it could be expected that for 68 of every 100 young men measured, values for percent fat would range between 8.9 and 21.1%. Of the remaining 32 young men, 16 would possess more than 21.1% body fat, while for the other 16 men, body fat would be less than 8.9%. Certainly a body fat value within the 68% variation limits could be considered normal. In the next chapter we discuss what is considered abnormal or excessive fatness.

TABLE 14–3. AVERAGE VALUES OF PERCENT BODY FAT FOR YOUNGER AND OLDER WOMEN AND MEN FROM SELECTED STUDIES

STUDY	AGE RANGE	STATURE CM	MASS KG	% FAT	68% VARIATION LIMITS
Younger Women					
North Carolina, 1962	17–25	165.0	55.5	22.9	17.5–28.5
New York, 1962	16–30	167.5	59.0	28.7	24.6–32.9
California, 1968	19–23	165.9	58.4	21.9	17.0–26.9
California, 1970	17–29	164.9	58.6	25.5	21.0–30.1
Air Force, 1972	17–22	164.1	55.8	28.7	22.3–35.3
New York, 1973	17–26	160.4	59.0	26.2	23.4–33.3
North Carolina, 1975		166.1	57.5	24.6	—
Massachusetts, 1993	17–30	165.3	57.7	21.8	16.7–27.2
Older Women					
Minnesota, 1953	31–45	163.3	60.7	28.9	25.1–32.8
	43–68	160.0	60.9	34.2	28.0–40.5
New York, 1963	30–40	164.9	59.6	28.6	22.1–35.3
	40–50	163.1	56.4	34.4	29.5–39.5
North Carolina, 1975	33–50	—	—	29.7	23.1–36.5
Massachusetts, 1993	31–50	165.2	58.9	25.2	19.2–31.2
Younger Men					
Minnesota, 1951	17–26	177.8	69.1	11.8	5.9–11.8
Colorado, 1956	17–25	172.4	68.3	13.5	8.3–18.8
Indiana, 1966	18–23	180.1	75.5	12.6	8.7–16.5
California, 1968	16–31	175.7	74.1	15.2	6.3–24.2
New York, 1973	17–26	176.4	71.4	15.0	8.9–21.1
Texas, 1977	18–24	179.9	74.6	13.4	7.4–19.4
Massachusetts, 1993	17–30	178.2	76.3	12.9	7.8–18.1
Older Men					
Indiana, 1966	24–38	179.0	76.6	17.8	11.3–24.3
	40–48	177.0	80.5	22.3	16.3–28.3
North Carolina, 1976	27–50	—	—	23.7	17.9–30.1
Texas, 1977	27–59	180.0	85.3	27.1	23.7–30.5
Massachusetts, 1993	31–50	177.1	77.5	19.9	13.2–26.5

Modified from McArdle, W.D., Katch, F.I., and Katch, V.L.: Exercise Physiology. 3rd ed. Philadelphia, Lea & Febiger, 1991.

Representative Samples Are Lacking. Although considerable data are available concerning average body composition for many groups of men and women of different ages and fitness levels, there has been no systematic evaluation of the body composition of representative samples from the general population that would warrant setting up precise norms or desirable values of body composition. At this time, the best we can do is to present the average values from various studies of different age groups.

A general conclusion based on these data is that, with increasing age, the percentage of body fat tends to rise in both men and women. This average change does not necessarily mean the trend should be interpreted as desirable or "normal." Changes in body composition with age could occur because the aging skeleton becomes demineralized and porous; such a process reduces body density because of the decrease in bone density. Another reason for the relative increase in body fat with age is reduction in the level of daily physical activity. Adaptation to a more sedentary lifestyle could increase the deposition of storage fat and reduce the quantity of muscle mass. This would occur even if the daily caloric consumption remained unchanged.

Keep active and keep lean. Research indicates that participation in vigorous physical activities after age 35 can retard the "average" increase in body fatness so common in middle age. Even at ages 70 and older, if former athletes keep physically active, their bone mass also will be superior, compared to average individuals of the same age.

Desirable Body Mass. Although an excess of body fat is undesirable for good health and fitness, an optimum level of body fat or body mass for a particular individual cannot be precisely stated. More than likely, this optimum varies from person to person and is greatly influenced by genetic factors. *Based on data from physically active young adults and competitive athletes, it would be desirable in our opinion to strive for a body fat content of 15% for men (certainly less than 20%) and about 25% for women (certainly less than 30%).* An "optimal" or "desirable" body mass can be computed using a desired level of body fat as follows:

Desirable body mass = Lean body mass ÷ (1.00 − % fat desired)

Suppose a 91 kg (200 lb) man, who has 20% body fat, wishes to know the weight he should attain so that this new lower body weight would contain 10% body fat. The computations would be as follows:

$$\text{Fat mass} = 91\text{ kg} \times .20 = 18.2\text{ kg}$$

$$\text{Lean body mass} = 91\text{ kg} - 18.2\text{ kg} = 72.8\text{ kg}$$

$$\begin{aligned}\text{Desirable body mass} &= 72.8\text{ kg} \div (1.00 - 0.10)\\ &= 72.8\text{ kg} \div 0.90\\ &= 80.9\text{ kg (178 lb)}\end{aligned}$$

$$\begin{aligned}\text{Desirable fat loss} &= \text{Present body mass} - \text{Desirable body mass}\\ &= 91\text{ kg} - 80.9\text{ kg} = 10.1\text{ kg (22.2 lb)}\end{aligned}$$

A lot of talk but not much change. The federal Centers for Disease Control reveals that about 27% of women and 24% of men are "significantly overweight"—values that are virtually unchanged from the early 1960s. The problem is even worse among minorities and the poor.

If this man lost 10.1 kg of body fat, his new body mass of 80.9 kg would have a fat content equal to 10% of body mass.

We believe that the notion of an upper and lower limit around the desired weight, rather than a precise value, is the best recommendation when prescribing optimal levels of body composition. Furthermore, weight loss should always be accompanied by a planned, systematic program of increased physical activity. This will reduce reliance on drastic dieting and

A desirable range for goal weight. For practical purposes, a desirable weight range is recommended rather than one specific goal weight. In most instances, this range should lie within 1 or 2 kg of the computed "desirable body mass." For example, if the desirable body mass is 135 lb, one should strive for a body mass that ranges from 133 to 137 lb.

increase the likelihood that the lost weight will be mostly fat and not lean tissue.

SUMMARY

1. Standard "height-weight" tables reveal little about an individual's body composition, which can vary considerably at any given body mass and stature. A person can be overweight without being overfat.
2. Total body fat consists of essential fat and storage fat. Essential fat is that present in bone marrow, nerve tissue, and the various organs; it is generally required for normal physiologic function. Storage fat is the energy reserve that accumulates mainly as adipose tissue beneath the skin.
3. True gender differences appear to exist for quantities of essential fat. Although storage fat values for men and women average 12% and 15% of body mass, respectively, the essential fat differences are large and amount to 3% for men and 12% for women. This difference is probably related to childbearing and hormonal functions.
4. It appears that a person cannot reduce below the essential fat level and still maintain good health.
5. Menstrual irregularities and cessation of menstruation occur among some groups of female athletes, especially among women who train hard and maintain low levels of body fat. The precise interaction between the physiologic and psychologic stress of intense, regular training, hormonal balance, energy and nutrient intake, and body fat requires further study.
6. A positive aspect may exist between the delayed onset of menarche observed in chronically active young females and health, because such individuals show a lower lifetime occurrence of cancer of the reproductive organs and other types of cancer.
7. The two most popular indirect methods for assessing body composition are hydrostatic weighing and prediction methods from fatfolds and circumferences (anthropometry). Hydrostatic weighing involves the determination of body density and subsequent estimation of percent body fat; this assumes a constant density for human fat and fat-free tissues. Lean body mass is calculated by subtracting fat mass from body mass.
8. Part of the error inherent in predicting body fat from whole body density lies in the assumptions concerning the density of the body's fat and nonfat components. Actual values for the density of each component probably vary from assumed constants in relation to race, age, and athletic experience. At this point in time, firm data are lacking for improving the theoretically based constants.
9. The prediction methods to assess body composition employ equations developed from relationships between selected fatfolds and girths with body density and percent fat. These equations are "population specific" because they are most accurate with subjects similar to those from which the equations were derived.
10. The techniques of ultrasound, computerized tomography, magnetic resonance imaging, and absorptiometry show promise for assessing

body composition, regional and internal fat distribution, and changes in body fat patterns with exercise and weight loss.

RELATED READINGS

Aloia, J.F., et al.: Relationship of menopause to skeletal and muscle mass. *Am. J. Clin. Nutr.*, 53:1378, 1991.

Baumgartner, R.N. et al.: Bioelectric impedance for body composition. In: Exercise and Sport Sciences Reviews, Vol. 18. Edited by K.B. Pandolf and J.O. Holloszy. Baltimore, Williams & Wilkins, 1990.

Baumgartner, R.N., et al.: Body composition in elderly people: effect of criterion estimates on predictive equations. *Am. J. Clin. Nutr.*, 53:1345, 1991.

Behnke, A.R., and Wilmore, J.H.: Evaluation and Regulation of Body Build and Composition. Englewood Cliffs, NJ, Prentice-Hall, 1974.

Body Composition in Animals and Man. Washington, DC, National Academy of Sciences, Publication 1598, 1968.

Brooks-Gunn, J., et al.: The relation of eating problems and amenorrhea in ballet dancers. *Med. Sci. Sports Exerc.*, 19:41, 1987.

Brozek, J., et al.: Densitometric analysis of body composition: revision of some quantitative assumptions. *Ann. N.Y. Acad. Sci.*, 110:113, 1963.

Bullen, B.A., et al.: Endurance training effects on plasma hormonal responsiveness and sex hormone excretion. *J. Appl. Physiol.*, 56:1453, 1984.

Claessens, A.L., et al.: Growth and menarcheal status of elite female gymnasts. *Med. Sci. Sports Exerc.*, 24:755, 1992.

Davies, P.S.W., et al.: The distribution of subcutaneous and internal fat in man. *Ann. Human Biol.*, 13:189, 1986.

Durenberg, P., et al.: Changes in fat-free mass during weight loss measured by bioelectrical impedance and by densitometry. *Am. J. Clin. Nutr.*, 49:33, 1989.

Forbes, G.B., et al.: Is bioimpedance a good predictor of body composition change? *Am. J. Clin. Nutr.*, 56:4, 1992.

Fowler, P.A., et al.: Total and subcutaneous adipose tissue in women: the measurement of distribution and accurate prediction of quantity by using magnetic resonance imaging. *Am. J. Clin. Nutr.*, 54:18, 1991.

Freedson, P.S., et al.: Physique, body composition, and psychological characteristics of competitive female body builders. *Phys. Sportsmed.*, 11:85, 1983.

Frisch, R.E., et al.: Delayed menarche and amenorrhea in ballet dancers. *N. Engl. J. Med.*, 303:17, 1980.

Frisch, R.E., et al.: Lower lifetime occurrence of breast cancer and cancers of the reproductive system among former college athletes. *Am. J. Clin. Nutr.*, 45:328, 1987.

Frisch, R.E., et al.: Lower prevalence of non-reproductive cancers among female former college athletes. *Med. Sci. Sports Exerc.*, 21:250, 1989.

Heyward, V.H.: Predictive accuracy of three field methods for estimating relative body fatness of nonobese and obese women. *Int. J. Sport Nutr.*, 2:75, 1992.

Hortobagyi, T., et al.: Comparison of four methods to assess body composition in black and white athletes. *Int. J. Sport Nutr.*, 2:60, 1992.

Hortobagyi, T., et al.: Relationships of body size, segmented dimensions, and ponderal equivalents to muscular strength in high-strength and low-strength subjects. *Int. J. Sports Med.*, 11:349, 1990.

Johnston, F.E.: Body fat deposition in adult obese women. I. Patterns of fat distribution. *Am. J. Clin. Nutr.*, 47:225, 1988.

Kaiserauer, S., et al.: Nutritional, physiological, and menstrual status of distance runners. *Med. Sci. Sports Exerc.*, 21:120, 1989.

Katch, F.I., and Hortobagyi, T.: Validity of surface anthropometry to estimate upper arm muscularity, including changes with body mass loss. *Am. J. Clin. Nutr.*, 52:591, 1990.

Katch, F.I., and Katch, V.L.: Measurement and prediction errors in body composition assessment and the search for the perfect prediction equation. *Res. Q. Exerc. Sport*, 51:249, 1980.

Katch, F.I., and Katch, V.L.: The body composition profile: techniques of measurement and applications. *Clin. Sports Med.*, 3:31, 1984.

Katch, F.I., and McArdle, W.D.: Validity of body composition prediction equations for college men and women. *Am. J. Clin. Nutr.*, 28:105, 1975.
Katch, F.I.: Cross validation of body composition prediction equations in obese, male adults. *Am. J. Hum. Biol.*, (in press, 1993).
Katch, V.L., et al.: Gender dimorphism in size, shape, and body composition of child-onset obese and nonobese adolescents. *Int. J. Obesity*, 15:267, 1991.
Kohrt, W.M., et al.: Body composition of healthy sedentary and trained, young and older men and women. *Med. Sci. Sports Exerc.*, 24:832, 1992.
Lohman, T.G., et al. (eds.): Anthropometric Standardization Reference Manual. Champaign, IL., Human Kinetics Books, 1988.
Loucks, A.B.: Effects of exercise training on the menstrual cycle: existence and mechanisms. *Med. Sci. Sports Exerc.*, 22:275, 1990.
McArdle, W.D., et al.: Exercise Physiology: Energy, Nutrition, and Human Performance, 3rd ed. Philadelphia, Lea & Febiger, 1991.
Rubeffe-Scrive, M.L., et al.: Fat cell metabolism in different regions in women: effect on menstrual cycle, pregnancy, and lactation. *J. Clin. Invest.*, 75:1973, 1985.
Schutte, J.E., et al.: Density of lean body mass is greater in Blacks than Whites. *J. Appl. Physiol.*, 56:1647, 1984.
Shangold, M.M., et al.: Evaluation and management of menstrual dysfunction in athletes. *JAMA*, 262:1665, 1990.
Tran, Z.V., and Weltman, A.: Generalized equation for predicting body density of women from girth measurements. *Med. Sci. Sports Exerc.*, 21:101, 1989.
Vogel, J.A., and Kasper, M.J.: Body fat assessment in women: special considerations. *Sportsmed.*, 13:245, 1992.
Wadden, T.A., et al.: Body fat deposition in adult obese women. Changes in fat distribution accompanying weight reduction. *Am. J. Clin. Nutr.*, 47:229, 1988.
Weltman, A., et al.: Accurate assessment of body composition in obese females. *Am. J. Clin. Nutr.*, 48:1179, 1988.
Yang, M.V.: Body composition and resting metabolic rate in obesity. In: Obesity and Weight Control. Edited by R.T. Frankle and M.V. Yang. Rockville, MD, Aspen Press, 1988.

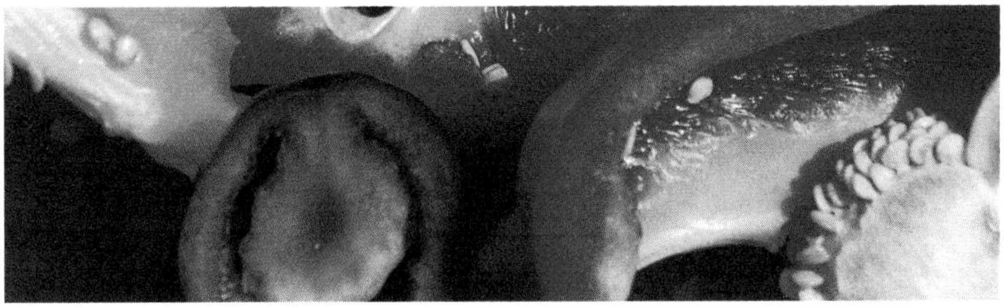

15

OBESITY

Americans consume more fat per capita than any nation in the world. We also consume more than 90% of the foods high in saturated fats and processed sugars. The end result of this national preoccupation with food and effortless living is that an estimated 50 million men and 60 million women between the ages of 18 and 79 (and 10 to 12 million teenagers) are "too fat" and need to reduce. If these overfat men and women consumed 600 fewer calories each day to reduce to a "normal" body fat value (achievable in 68 days for men and 101 days for women), the reduced caloric intake would equal 5.7 trillion calories. This energy could supply the yearly residential electricity demands of Boston, Chicago, San Francisco, and Washington, DC, or 1.3 billion gallons of gasoline to fuel about 1 million autos for a year!

OBESITY: OFTEN A LONG-TERM PROCESS

Obesity often begins in childhood. When this occurs, the chances for adult obesity are three times greater compared to children of normal body mass. Simply stated, a child generally does not "grow out of" an obesity problem.

Often a gradual process. In the Western world, the average 35-year-old male gains between 0.2 and 0.8 kg of fat each year until the sixth decade of life despite a progressive decrease in food intake.

Excessive fatness also develops slowly during adulthood with ages 25 to 44 being the years of greatest fat accretion. Middle-aged men and women invariably weigh more than their college-aged counterparts of the same stature.

In one longitudinal study, the fat content of 27 adult men increased an average of 6.5 kg over a 12-year period from ages 32 to 44. This was equal to the group's total gain in body mass over the duration of the study. Women are the biggest weight gainers with about 14% putting on more than 13.6 kg between the ages of 25 and 34. The extent to which this "creeping obesity" during adulthood reflects a normal biologic pattern is unknown.

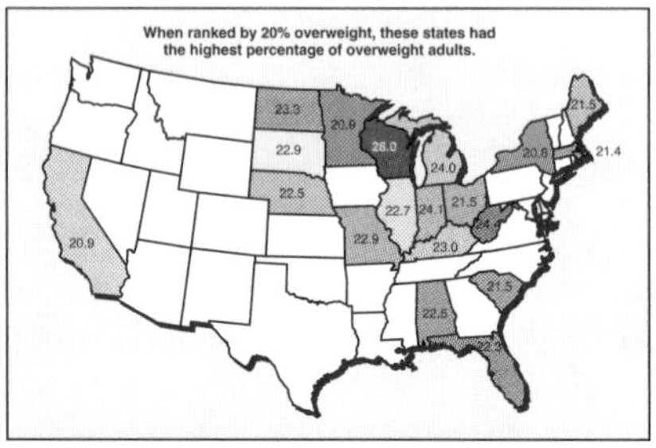

Wisconsin wins! States in the upper Midwest have the highest percentage of overweight adults in the United States. Wisconsin's top ranking is linked to the state's high intake of fat-rich foods such as cheese, butter, ice cream, bacon, and sausage.

Not Necessarily Overeating. Until recently, the major cause of obesity was believed to be overeating. If obesity were truly a unitary disorder, and gluttony and overindulgence were the only factors associated with an increase in body fat, the easiest way to reduce permanently would surely be to cut back on food. Of course, if it were that simple, obesity would soon be eliminated as a major health problem. Obviously, other influences are operating such as genetic, environmental, social, and perhaps racial. Research also suggests that differences in specific factors may predispose a person to excessive weight gain. These include: eating patterns, eating environment, food packaging, and body image; biochemical differences related to resting metabolic rate, dietary-induced thermogenesis, level of spontaneous activity or "fidgeting," and basal body temperature; levels of cellular adenosine triphosphatase, lipoprotein lipase, and other enzymes; and the metabolically active brown adipose tissue.

It is difficult to partition the cause or causes of obesity into distinct categories because they probably overlap. It seems fairly certain that the treatment procedures devised so far—whether diets, surgery, drugs, psychological methods, or exercise, either alone or in combination—have not been particularly successful in solving the problem on a long-term basis. There is optimism, nonetheless, that as researchers continue to investigate the many facets of obesity, as well as to test and quantify various treatment modalities, significant progress will be made to conquer this major health problem.

Physical Activity: An Important Component. Observations of older men and women who maintain an active lifestyle suggest that the pattern of fat gain in adulthood can be significantly attenuated. *In fact, increases in body fat may be more a function of activity level than of age.* For both young and middle-aged men who exercised regularly, the time spent in activity was inversely related to their body fat level. Surprisingly, no relationship emerged between body fat and caloric intake. This suggested that the greater body fat among the active middle-aged men compared to their younger counterparts was the consequence of less-vigorous training and *not* greater food intake. Such findings indicate that the trend for increases in body fat with aging can be somewhat blunted with increases in daily physical activity.

Evidence has been presented recently that **reduced energy expenditure is a crucial factor** in the magnitude of weight gain in infants born to overweight mothers compared to infants born to lean mothers. Up to 3 months of age, the infants in the two groups could not be distinguished in terms of anthropometry (fatfolds and body mass index), resting metabolic rate, or energy intake. From age 3 months to 1 year, however, the total energy expenditure of the infants who later became overweight was significantly lower, by 21%, compared to the infants who maintained a normal weight gain. In another study, the 24-hour energy expenditure was measured in young adult Native Americans and correlated with the rate of change in body mass over a two-year period. The estimated risk of gaining more than 7.5 kg in body mass was four times higher in people with a low compared to a high 24-hour energy expenditure.

Exercise can counter age trends for fat. Research indicates that the trend toward greater body fat with aging can be blunted with increases in daily physical activity.

HEALTH RISKS OF OBESITY

Nearly 37 million Americans weigh 20% or more above their desirable body mass. More than 12 million of these men and women are severely obese and at high risk of developing a variety of diseases related to their obesity. Although it has been argued that a moderate excess in body fat is not in itself harmful, a 1985 report of a 14-member panel convened at the National Institutes of Health concluded that **obesity should be viewed as a disease.** This is because there are multiple biologic hazards at surprisingly low levels of excess fat, representing only about 2 to 5 kg above desirable body mass. In fact, it is now argued rather convincingly that obesity is a powerful heart disease risk that may be equal to that of smoking, elevated blood lipids, and hypertension.

It is well established that chronic disease is more prevalent among obese people than in individuals with normal body fat. While it is not clear to what degree obesity causes a specific medical problem, the increased **risk of medical and health complications** includes the following: hypertension and stroke, renal disease, gallbladder disease, diabetes mellitus, pulmonary diseases, problems with anesthesia during surgery, osteoarthritis and gout, breast and endometrial cancer, abnormal plasma lipids and lipoproteins, impaired cardiac function, menstrual irregularities and toxemia in pregnancy, psychological trauma, flat feet and intertriginous dermatitis (infection in fatfolds), organ compression by adipose tissue, and impaired heat tolerance.

Excess fat is the health risk. When rigorous standards for determining body fat levels are applied, excess body fat, and not body mass per se, is the important factor that links being overweight to an increased risk for cardiovascular disease.

Heart disease risk. An eight-year study of nearly 116,000 female nurses concluded that all but the thinnest women were at increased risk for heart attack and chest pains. Women of average body mass had 30% more heart attacks than the women of low body mass, while the risk for the moderately overweight was 80% higher than for the lightest women. That means that women who gained just 9 kg from their late teens to middle age doubled their heart attack risk.

Weight loss improves the lipid profile. Obesity is a common cause of lipid disorders—weight loss is one of the most effective treatments.

Functional trauma. From a psychological perspective, overweight individuals score lower in the usual defenses for maintaining self-esteem, show lower feelings of value as family members, and feel less self-acceptance and self-satisfaction.

CRITERIA FOR OBESITY: HOW FAT IS TOO FAT?

A variety of criteria have been used to establish a person's level of body fatness.

PERCENT BODY FAT AS A CRITERION.

The line of demarcation between normal body fat levels and obesity is somewhat arbitrary. In the previous chapter we suggest that the **normal range of body fat** in adult men and women encompasses at least plus and minus one unit of variation from the average population value. That variation unit is approximately 5% body fat for men and women between the ages of 17 and 50 years. Within this statistical boundary, overfatness would correspond to any value for percent body fat that exceeds the average value for age and gender, plus 5%. For young men, whose fat mass averages 15%, the borderline for obesity is 20% body fat. For older men, average percent fat is approximately 25%. Consequently, overfatness for this group

Where it's at is what counts! Body fat distribution predicts the health hazards of obesity: diabetes, hyperlipidemia, hypertension, and coronary heart disease.

Waist-to-hip-ratio. Measure your **waist-to-hip-ratio** to determine if your abdominal girth is too large:

- Measure your waist at your navel while standing relaxed, not pulling in your stomach
- Measure around your hips, over the buttocks where the girth is largest
- Divide the waist measure by the hip measure

would be a body fat content in excess of 30%. For young women, obesity corresponds to a body fat content above 30%, while for older women, borderline obesity would be about 37% body fat. It should be emphasized, however, that although the average population value for percent body fat increases with age, this does not necessarily mean that men and women should be expected to get fatter as they grow older. *To the contrary, the **criterion for overfatness** should probably be that established for younger men and women: above 20% for men and above 30% for women.*

There is also a gradation of obesity that progresses from the upper limit of normal—20% for men and 30% for women—to as high as 50 to 70% of body mass in the excessively obese. Common terms for the gradations in obesity include "pleasantly plump" for those just above the cutoff, to moderately obese, excessively obese, and massively obese. The last category includes people who weigh in the range of 170 to 275 kg and whose fat content is above 55% of body mass, often 60 to 65% or higher! In this situation, body fat exceeds lean body mass and obesity may be a life-threatening condition.

Standards for Overfatness

Men—above 20%
Women—above 30%

REGIONAL FAT DISTRIBUTION AS A CRITERION

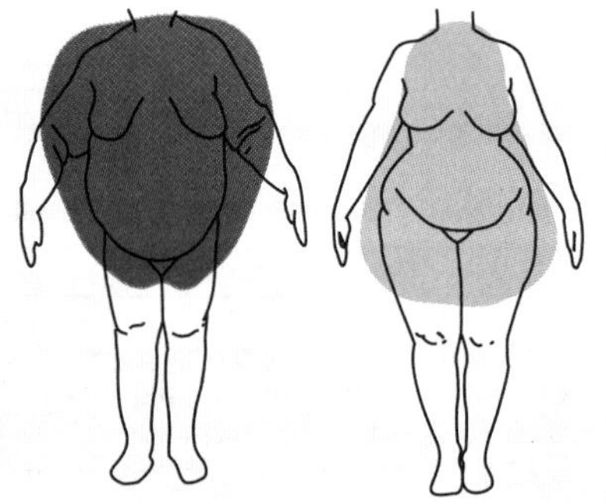

Apples and pears—it's the shape that counts. The pattern of fat deposition plays a key role in disease. Men and women shaped like apples, in whom excess weight is carried above the waist (also referred to as android), have higher blood levels of glucose, greater blood triglyceride levels, and more hypertension. Such individuals are at greater risk for diabetes and death from heart disease, and women also have an increased risk for developing cancers of the breast and uterus.

Adipose cells display remarkable diversity depending upon where they are concentrated. Some cells are highly efficient at taking up excess calories from the bloodstream, while others readily release their stored energy for use by other tissues. This helps to explain why certain fat deposits are so difficult to reduce. It is also apparent that the ***patterning of adipose tissue distribution,*** independent of total body fat, alters the health risk of obesity. For example, waist-to-hip ratios that exceed 0.80 for women and 0.95 for men are associated with an increased risk of death from coronary artery disease as well as a variety of illnesses, most notably diabetes, elevated triglycerides, hypertension, and general overall mortality. This may be because excess fat in the abdominal area (central or **android-type obesity,** most prevalent in males) is more active metabolically—and thus more active in processes related to heart disease—than fat located in the hips and thighs (peripheral or **gynoid-type obesity,** most prevalent in females).

To some extent, a person's pattern of fat distribution is inherited and is probably governed by the regional activity of **lipoprotein lipase,** or *LPL,* the rate-limiting enzyme for triglyceride uptake by the fat cell. LPL is the important enzyme that facilitates the processing and storage of fat molecules by the adipocytes (fat cells). Variations in the activity level of this enzyme probably account for the differences in fat distribution among people, or the changes in a person's fat distribution that occur in pregnancy and middle age.

FAT CELL SIZE AND NUMBER

The size and number of fat cells have also been proposed as a means to identify and study what is normal and abnormal with regard to body fatness. The body increases its quantity of adipose tissue in two ways. The first is by enlarging or filling existing fat cells with more fat; this is referred to as **fat cell hypertrophy.** The second way is by increasing the total number of fat cells, or **fat cell hyperplasia.**

Abdominal obesity in females. Abdominal obesity increases a woman's risk for developing cancers of the breast and uterine lining. Women with a large waist-to-hip ratio are 15 times more likely to develop endometrial cancer compared to women of similar weight who carry their excess pounds below the waist.

Methods for Determining Fat Cell Size and Number. Researchers have used a variety of techniques to study adipose cellularity. The most accurate method was developed in the 1960s in the laboratory of **Dr. Jules Hirsch** at Rockfeller University in New York City. The technique involves sucking small fragments of subcutaneous tissue, usually from the upper back, buttocks, abdomen, and back of the upper arm, into a syringe through a needle inserted directly into a fat depot. The adipose tissue is then treated chemically so that the fat cells can be separated and counted.

Once the number of cells is determined for a known mass of fat tissue, the average quantity of fat per cell is determined by dividing the amount of fat in the sample by the total number of cells it contains. If the body's fat mass is known, a reasonable estimate can be made of the total number of fat cells in the body. Let us assume that a person weighs 70 kg and is 18% fat as determined by underwater weighing. The mass of fat for this person is computed as body mass multiplied by body fat and equals 12.6 kg. Dividing this value by the average content of fat per cell gives the total number of fat cells in the body.

Enzymes determine where fat is deposited. The larger amount of the fat-storing enzyme lipoprotein lipase or LPL possessed by females may explain their relatively larger fat content compared to males. Differences in fat distribution patterns between genders may also be enzymatically related because the fat cells of the hip, thigh, and breast region produce considerable LPL in the female, while for males the abdominal fat cells are active with the enzyme.

$$\text{Total number of fat cells} = \text{Mass of body fat} \div \text{Fat content per cell}$$

In this example, if the average fat cell holds 0.53 micrograms (μg) of lipid, then the 12.6 kg of body fat contains 23.8 billion fat cells.

In one of our laboratories, the **needle biopsy procedure** coupled with photomicrographic techniques was used to extract and measure the average size of fat cells in the buttocks, abdomen, and upper back area. Figure 15–1 shows the biopsy procedure from the buttocks region and a photomicrograph of the fat cells, which are counted and measured for diameter and volume. For the middle-aged professor whose total fat content prior to a successful marathon run was 14.4 kg (83.4 kg body mass, 17.2% body fat) with 0.68 μg of lipid per cell, the total number of fat cells was estimated at 21.2 billion.

VARIETY OF HUMAN OBESITIES

It is simple enough to establish standards for obesity, but it is not easy to distinguish between the gradations of obesity. Attempts have been made to describe obesity types based on the amount, distribution, and texture of fat tissue. The idea of a classification scheme is appealing because it permits quantification of the phenotype and evaluation of a variety of hormonal and biochemical correlates of obesity. In Figure 15–2 the top panel presents six **phenotypic patterns** that have been observed in female obesity (comparable data are unavailable for males). The photographs in the lower panel complement several of the outline patterns and show examples of severe, intractable obesity. The four photographs at the right show the effects of a 35-kg weight loss over 15 months in a 49-year-old woman. Most of the weight lost was from the large abdominal panniculus, which was partially removed surgically. Note that even with a relatively large decrease in overall body mass, the pattern of the phenotype remains relatively invariant. Considerably more research in the area of obesity clas-

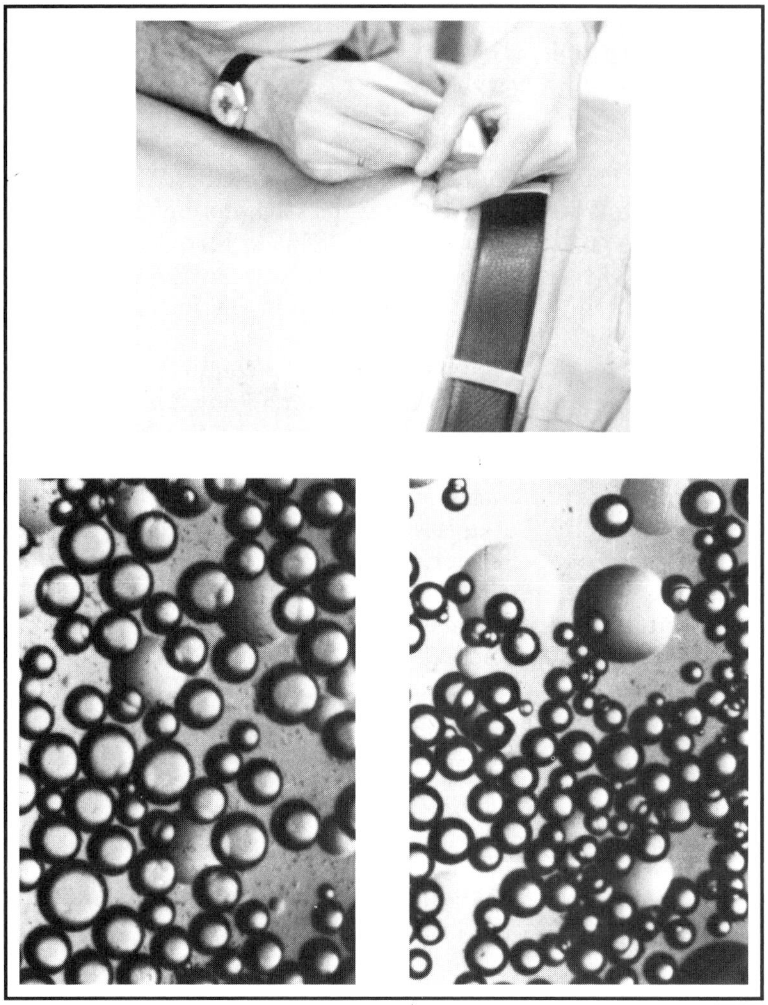

FIG. 15–1. (Upper panel) Needle biopsy procedure to extract fat cells in the upper buttocks region. The biopsy needle is placed beneath the skin surface after the area is anesthetized. Small tissue fragments are literally sucked from the site of the incision into a syringe. (Bottom panels) Photomicrographs of fat cells biopsied from the buttocks of the middled-aged, physically active professor. The large spherical structures in the background are lipid droplets. During a period of relative inactivity prior to six months of marathon training (5 days a week, 10 to 16 miles per day), the average fat cell diameter was 8.6% larger than following training. On average, the volume of fat in each cell decreased by 18.2% compared to pretraining values.

sification is needed in males and females of all ages, particularly in conjunction with anthropometric, metabolic, and biochemical studies.

FAT CELL SIZE AND NUMBER IN NORMAL AND OBESE ADULTS

Number of cells is an important factor. The major structural difference in adipose tissue mass between obese and nonobese people is the number of fat cells.

Comparative studies of **adipose cellularity in obese and nonobese humans** show conclusively that fat accumulation is brought about either by storage of fat in existing adipocytes (hypertrophy), by actual formation of new fat cells (hyperplasia), or by a combination of both hypertrophy and hyperplasia.

Figure 15–3 graphically compares the body mass, total fat mass, and cell

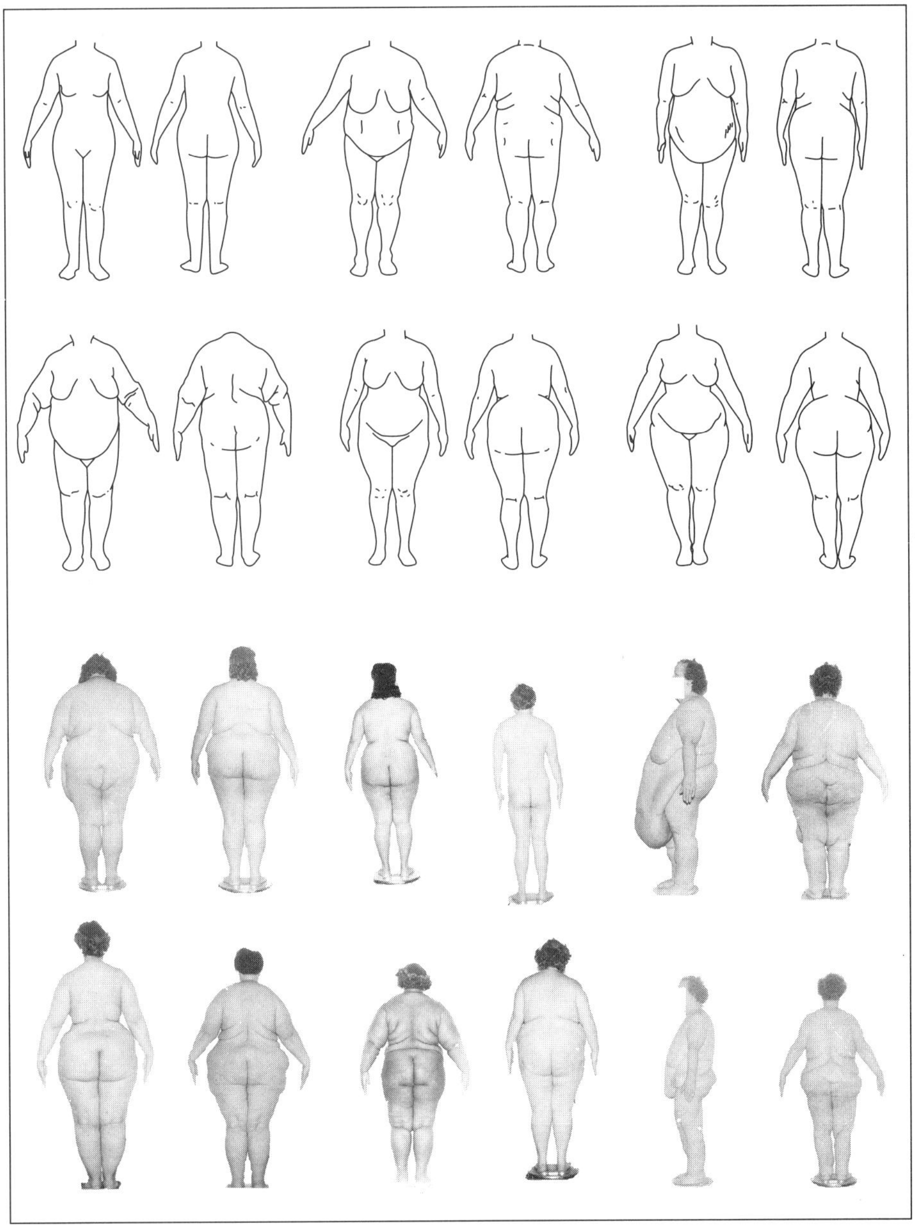

FIG. 15–2. (Upper panel) Patterns of female body form illustrating the varieties of human obesity. (Lower panel) Photographs showing several of the body patterns as well as an example of intractable obesity where the abdominal paniculus was estimated to weigh over 35 kg prior to weight loss. (Photos and outline patterns courtesy of the late Dr. L.S. Craig.)

Types of Obesity

TYPE	LOCATION OF EXCESS FAT
1	Total body (most common)
2	Subcutaneous fat on the trunk (android)
3	Subcutaneous fat in the lower body (gynoid)
4	Visceral fat in abdomen (intra-abdominal fat)

Classification proposed by Dr. Claude Bouchard, Physical Activity Sciences Laboratory. Laval University. Quebec, Canada.

Genetics may set the stage. Our genetic makeup does not necessarily cause obesity, but it does influence susceptibility. In the right disease-producing environment (sedentary and stressful, with easy access to food), the susceptible individual will gain weight—and possibly lots of it.

size and number in a group of 20 subjects clinically classified as obese and in 5 nonobese subjects. The body mass of the obese subjects averaged more than twice that of the nonobese, while their total fat content was nearly three times as large. The mass of body fat in the obese ranged from 42 to 103 kg; the average for the nonobese was about 18 kg. Further analysis of body fat indicated that the quantity of fat per cell averaged about 35% higher in the obese subjects. In addition, the total number of fat cells in the obese was nearly three times greater than in the nonobese: 75 billion fat cells versus 27 billion.

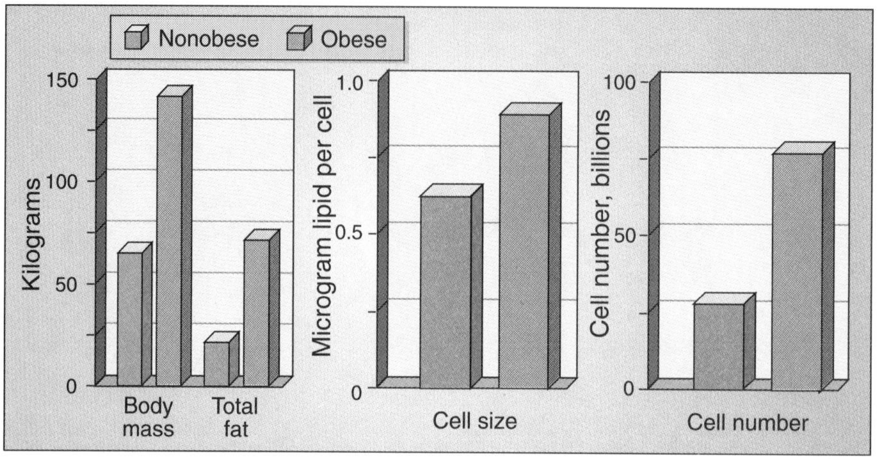

FIG. 15–3. Comparison of body mass, total body fat, cell size, and cell number in obese and nonobese subjects. (Modified from Hirsch, J., and Knittle, J.: Cellularity of obese and nonobese human adipose tissue. *Fed. Proc.*, 29:1518, 1970.)

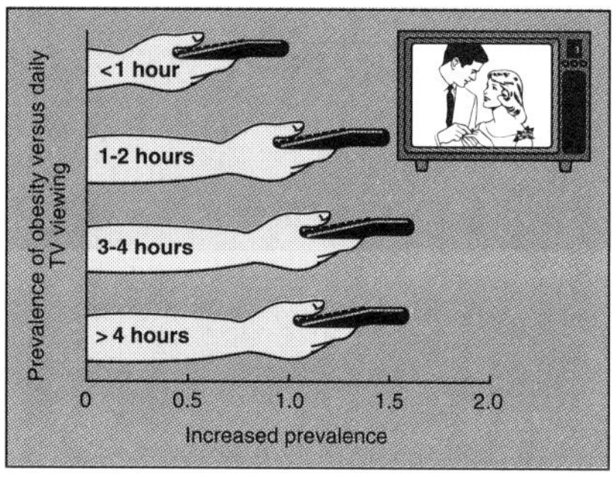

TV viewing affects the risk of obesity. In a study relating TV watching and obesity in 4,771 adult females, those who watched 3 to 4 hours or more of TV daily had twice the prevalence of obesity as women who watched less than 1 hour. One should not infer cause and effect based on this study. Excessive TV viewing may contribute to obesity, but conversely, obesity may contribute to more TV watching. It seems reasonable to propose that increased TV watching leaves less time for exercise, while at the same time allowing more time to consume excess calories.

In an international study to determine factors at home that could affect children's education, excessive TV viewing once again played a large role. While the study was unrelated to health factors, the findings support the notion that children devote a large part of their nonschool day to an activity that ranks low in energy expenditure!

We can further examine the importance of fat cell number in obesity by relating total body fat to both cell size and cell number. The data in the left side of Figure 15–4 demonstrate the strong positive relationship between total fat mass in the obese and the number of fat cells. The person with the lowest fat content had the fewest number of fat cells, while the fattest subject had considerably more cells. On the other hand, the data displayed in the right panel of Figure 15–4 show that there was little relationship between total body fat in the obese and the average size of fat cells. This suggests that there may be some biologic upper limit to how large fat cells can become. After this size is reached, cell number probably becomes the key factor determining the extent of obesity. Even if the size of normal fat cells could double, this would not account for the tremendous difference in the fat content of obese and nonobese people. The excessive mass of

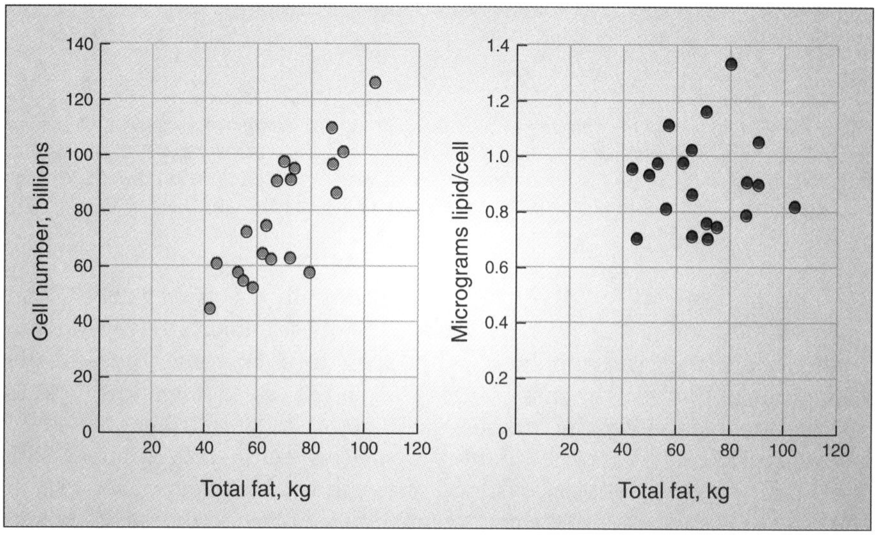

FIG. 15–4. Adipose cell number (left) and size (right) related to the body's total mass of fat.

adipose tissue in obesity, therefore, must occur by fat cell hyperplasia. As a frame of reference, an average nonobese person has about 25 to 30 billion fat cells. For the moderately obese this number is between 60 and 100 billion, while for the massively obese the fat cell number may be as high as 300 billion or more!

FAT CELL SIZE AND NUMBER AFTER WEIGHT REDUCTION

If a **weight reduction** program achieves normal body mass and fatness, then the individual fat cells will shrink and actually become smaller than those of people who have never been obese. These findings for weight reduction in obese adults are depicted in Figure 15–5. In this study, 19 obese subjects who initially weighed 149 kg reduced body mass by 45.8 kg, weighing 103 kg at the end of the first part of the experiment. Prior to weight reduction the number of fat cells averaged 75 billion. This number remained essentially unchanged with weight reduction. The average size of the fat cells, on the other hand, was reduced 33% from 0.9 to a normal value of 0.6 μg of fat per cell. When they lost 28 kg more, the subjects attained a normal body mass. Cell number again remained unchanged, while cell size continued to shrink to about one-third the size of the fat cells in normal, nonobese subjects. Other experiments have confirmed these findings in both adults and young children.

You can shrink them but you can't lose them. Weight reduction in obese adults is accompanied by a decrease in the size of fat cells but no change in fat cell number. This is a somewhat pessimistic outlook for the obese person who hopes to stay permanently reduced.

The formerly obese person who reduces body mass and body fat to near average values still is not "cured" of obesity, at least in terms of the number of fat cells. Clinical evidence reveals that such formerly obese individuals have extreme difficulty maintaining their new body size. It is tempting to suggest that the large number of relatively small fat cells in the reduced obese is somehow related to appetite control, causing the person to crave

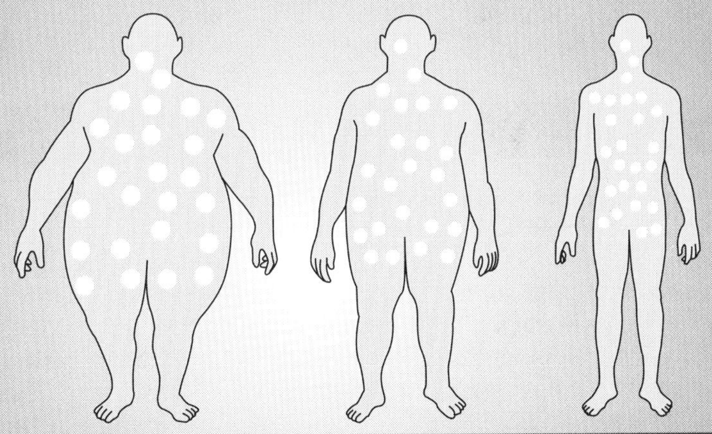

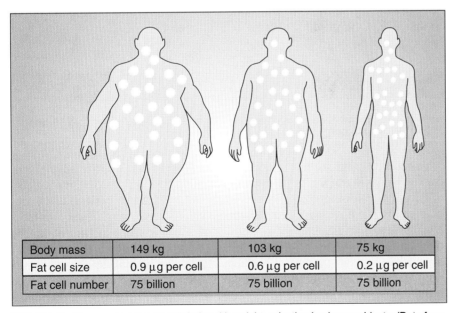

Body mass	149 kg	103 kg	75 kg
Fat cell size	0.9 μg per cell	0.6 μg per cell	0.2 μg per cell
Fat cell number	75 billion	75 billion	75 billion

FIG. 15–5. Changes in adipose cellularity with weight reduction in obese subjects. (Data from Hirsch, J.: Adipose cellularity in relation to human obesity. In: Advances in Internal Medicine, Vol. 17. Edited by G.H. Stollerman. Chicago, Year Book, 1971.)

food, overeat, and regain the lost weight. Some nutritionists have linked the repetitive yo-yo-like cycle of weight loss and weight gain often noted among the obese to the "plight of the starving fat cells."

FAT CELL SIZE AND NUMBER AFTER WEIGHT GAIN

An interesting series of studies on the development of human obesity was conducted at the University of Vermont. Over a 40-week period, adult male volunteers with an initial average body fat content of 15% deliberately tripled their normal daily caloric intake to about 7000 kcal. For a typical subject, body mass increased by 25% and body fat nearly doubled, to 28.2% of body mass. Consequently, of the 12.7 kg gained by overeating, 10.5 kg were caused by increased deposition of body fat.

In a similar experiment with a group of nonobese subjects who had no previous personal or family history of obesity, body mass increased an average of 16.4 kg from voluntary overeating. When the size and number of fat cells were compared before and after the four-month period of **weight gain**, the average size of the fat cells had increased substantially with *no change* in cell number. When the subjects reduced to their normal weight through caloric restriction, body fat was decreased and the adipocytes returned to their original size. These results indicate that the acquisition of fat by overeating in adults occurs primarily by filling existing adipocytes with more lipid rather than by increasing the number of new fat cells.

Although you can't lose them, you can make more of them. In mature-onset severe obesity, hypercellularity may accompany the greatly increasing size of the existing fat cells.

New Fat Cells May Also Develop.

There is also evidence that in adult-onset moderate to massive obesity, in which an already fat adult becomes even fatter, new adipocytes may develop in addition to the hypertrophy of existing cells. This is because fat cells have an upper size limit of about 1.0 μg of lipid per cell. In the massively obese (60% body fat; about 170% of normal weight), almost all fat cells have attained their hypertrophic limit and more cells may be recruited from the preadipocyte pool to increase cell number.

DEVELOPMENT OF ADIPOSE CELLULARITY

The **development and growth of adipose tissue** can be broadly categorized based on animal and human research.

Animal Studies. Studies of fat cell development in different animal species reveal two ways that fat depots develop. The most extensive studies of fat cell development have been conducted with rats because these mammals appear to develop fat in a manner similar to humans. They also have a relatively short life span, so various diets and exercise regimens can be readily studied during the growth cycle. Figure 15–6 illustrates the generally upward trending curves for body mass, fat mass, and fat cell size and number in the rat during the first six months of life. Note that both cell number and size increase during weeks 6 through 15. Then, as the animals become heavier, the additional increase in body fat occurs because existing cells became filled with fat, not because new fat cells develop.

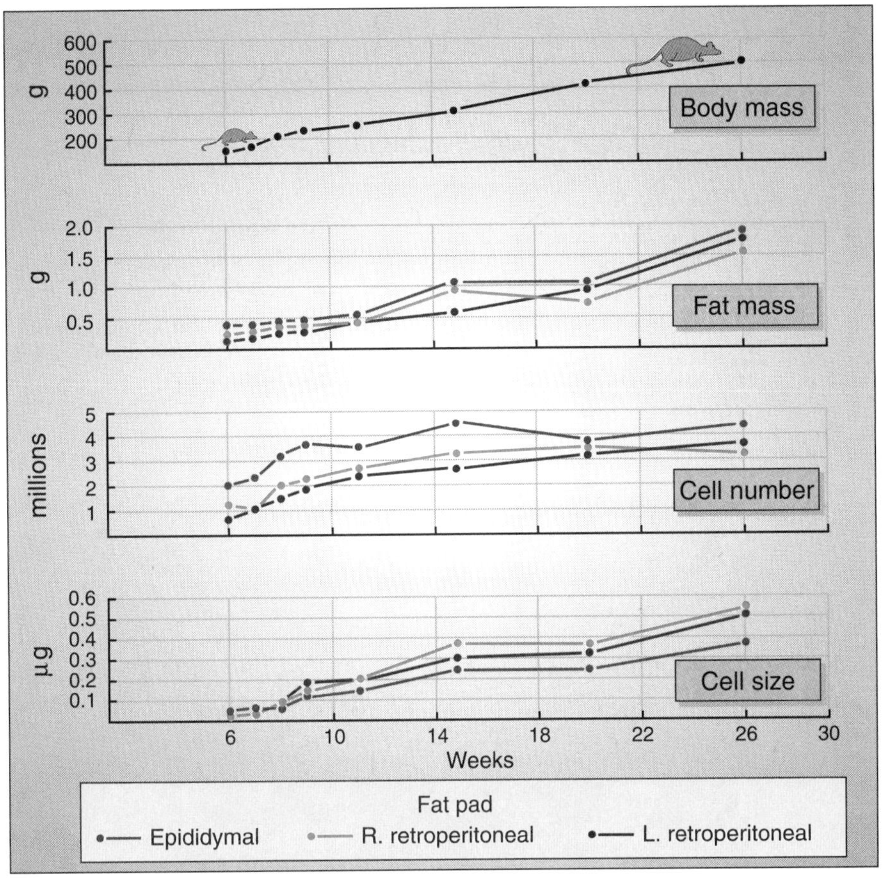

FIG. 15–6. Changes in body mass, fat mass, cell number, and cell size in rats during the first six months of growth. (From Hirsch, J., and Han, P.W.: Cellularity of rat adipose tissue: effects of growth, starvation, and obesity. *J. Lipid Res.*, 10:77, 1969.)

Human Studies. In contrast to the many longitudinal studies of animals during growth, the data in humans are not based on long-term studies of the same individuals, but rather of different individuals at different ages. With this cross-sectional approach, fat cell size and number were determined for 34 infants and children who ranged in age from a few days to 13 years old. The top panel of Figure 15–7 illustrates the relationship between fat cell size and number and age. The value for average cell size in normal adults is shown at the right of the figure.

These data suggest that the size of adipocytes in newborn infants and children up to age 1 year is about one-fourth that of the adult. It is also evident that fat cells triple in size during the first six years of life with little further increase to age 13. Data on the size of adipose cells during adolescence are scarce. We can assume, however, that cell size increases further during this growth period because in adulthood adipocytes are significantly larger than at age 13.

The bottom panel of Figure 15–7 illustrates data on fat cell number from birth to age 13. Cell number increases fairly rapidly during the first year of life, being about three times greater at 1 year than at birth. Scientists

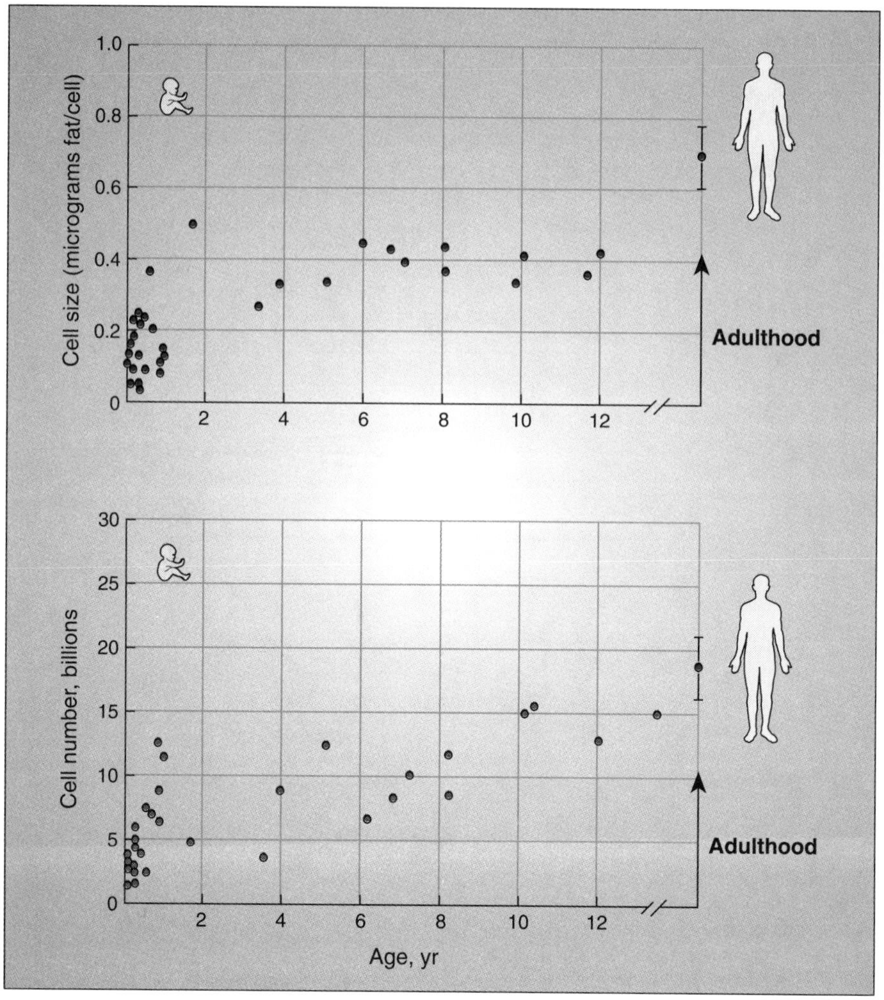

FIG. 15–7. Changes in fat cell size (top) and number (bottom) from birth to adulthood.

believe that most of the fat cells existing prior to birth are formed during the last three months of pregnancy. After the first year of life, cell number increases more gradually up to about age 10. As is the case with cell size, the number of cells formed after age 13 continues to increase during the adolescent growth spurt until adulthood; thereafter, there is little further increase in cell number.

Thus, there appear to be three general periods when the number of fat cells increases significantly: the last trimester of pregnancy, the first year of life, and the adolescent growth spurt. It is during adulthood that the total number of fat cells probably cannot be altered to any significant degree; an exception is in extreme adult obesity, when further cell proliferation can occur. However, there are still no data to indicate clearly if the final number of adult fat cells in humans can be modified through some form of intervention early in life. A fundamental question remains, "Can fat cell number be altered before adulthood, or is overfatness predetermined primarily by the genetic code?"

Is cell number predetermined? It is impossible to state with certainty whether the rate of fat cell development in humans can be reversed, or at least slowed down.

MODIFICATION OF ADIPOSE CELLULARITY

Although the precise causes for fat cell development are poorly understood, it does appear that certain practices could modify the process. In humans, for example, a mother's nutritional practices during pregnancy may modify the body composition of the developing fetus. Babies born to women whose weight gain exceeded 18 kg during gestation had significantly larger fatfold thickness than the offspring of women who followed the recommended weight gain during pregnancy. Bottle feeding and early introduction of solid food may also be associated with development of obesity. Conversely, breast feeding, allowing the infant to set the limits to food consumption, and delayed introduction to solid food may prevent overfeeding and development of poor eating habits with subsequent obesity.

Research with animals suggests that alterations in fat cell size and number can be achieved in two ways: modification of early nutrition, and exercise.

NUTRITIONAL INFLUENCES

Prevention is better than cure. Early prevention of obesity through exercise and diet, rather than correction of obesity once it is present, may be the most effective method to curb the "overfat" condition so common in children and adults.

Early **nutritional intervention** can influence the development of body fatness and adipose cellularity at a later period in an animal's life. In one study, large numbers of rats were redistributed at birth, giving some mothers large litters of 22 animals and others small litters of 4 animals. After weaning at 21 days, both groups had unlimited access to food. At weaning and at each subsequent five-week period to 20 weeks of age, the body mass of animals from the large (calorically deprived) litters was significantly lower than for the other group. This suggests that early food restriction caused a permanent effect on body mass even though both groups of animals had free access to food after weaning.

Figure 15–8 shows that the underfed group reached a definite plateau in the number of fat cells by 15 weeks of age. In contrast, cell number continued to increase in the overfed animals from small litters. In both groups, cell size increased progressively during the 20-week experiment. *These data certainly suggest there may be a critical time during the early growth period when permanent modifications in adipose tissue occur.*

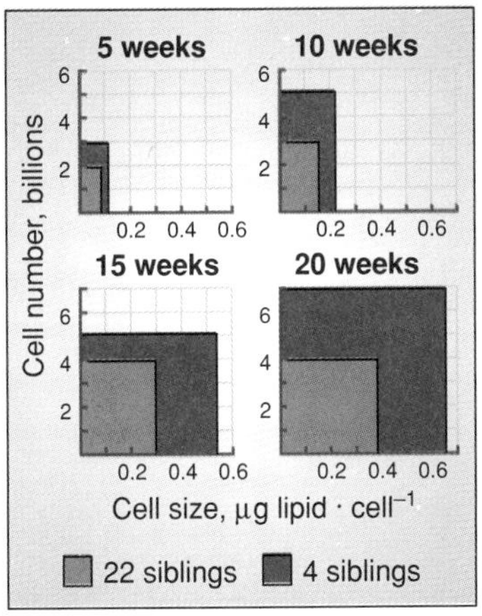

FIG. 15–8. Changes in cell size and number in animals raised in small and large litters. (Adapted from Knittle, J., and Hirsch, J.: Effect of early nutrition on the development of rat epididymal fat pads: cellularity and metabolism. *J. Clin. Invest.*, 47:2091, 1968.)

Clearly, there are difficulties in extrapolating experimental results from rats to humans. However, some striking similarities in adipose tissue development are apparent in humans and rats. The excessive quantity of body fat in obese humans is associated primarily with the large number of fat cells and, to a lesser extent, with increased size of individual cells. When obese adults lose considerable weight, the number of fat cells remains unchanged and total body fat is reduced almost exclusively through decreasing fat cell size. Similar findings for fat cell number occur with adult rats. When these animals are calorically deprived either by acute starvation or more prolonged semistarvation, the decrease in body mass is only temporary and is rapidly reinstated upon refeeding. The weight loss is due to decrease in fat cell size with no corresponding change in cell number. When the starved animals again have normal access to food, their fat cells refill to normal size. Except in already obese animals, overfeeding of adults produces an increase in total fat, but—as with humans—this increase is brought about by "stuffing" of existing cells rather than by increases in cell number. Thus, in both adult humans and rats, dietary manipulation generally does not affect adipose cell number; changes in the total quantity of body fat are brought about primarily by cellular enlargement. Furthermore, when the fat content is reduced, cell size shrinks accordingly, only to expand again when the body's content of fat is restored.

If the influence of early nutrition in rats is paralleled by similar effects in humans, then overfeeding during childhood may increase the tendency toward adult obesity. Based on limited evidence, it certainly seems prudent to encourage the parents of young children to avoid overfeeding their youngsters because this may temper their proclivity towards obesity as adults.

EXERCISE INFLUENCES

Only a few experiments have evaluated the contribution of exercise to modifying cell size and number in adipose tissue. Figure 15–9 summarizes the results of one such experiment on the growth of rats. In this study, an exercise group with free access to food was subjected to a 14- to 16-week program of swimming early in life. The animals swam in plastic barrels 6 days a week. Initially the exercise sessions lasted 15 minutes; they were gradually lengthened until the animals were swimming for 6 hours a day at the end of 4 weeks. They continued to swim for this duration until the end of the experimental period, when they were sacrificed and analyzed for fat content and adipose cellularity. During the experiment, two adult groups of rats remained sedentary; one group had free access to food and water, while the other group was calorically restricted to maintain their body mass at the same level as the exercising group.

The results were convincing: animals given unlimited food but forced to exercise for 15 weeks gained weight more slowly and had a lower final body mass than the sedentary, freely eating rats. Because both groups

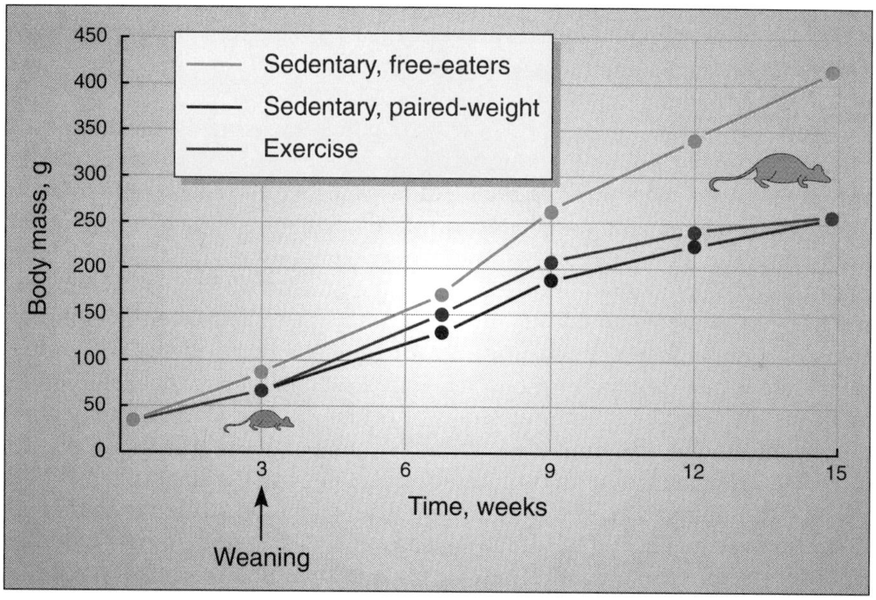

FIG. 15–9. Effects of exercise and food restriction on body mass of rats. (From Oscai, L., et al.: Effects of exercise and of food restriction on adipose tissue cellularity. *J. Lipid Res.*, 13:588, 1972.)

consumed the same number of calories each day, the lower rate of weight gain in the exercisers was attributed to the increased caloric requirements of exercise. It was also shown that the total fat content was about four times higher in the nonexercising group than in the freely eating exercise group. The **exercise intervention** during growth caused a significantly lower level of body fat resulting from smaller cell size *and* cell number.

The total fat content of the sedentary, food-restricted group was also lower than that of the sedentary animals who could eat freely. Reducing food intake resulted in a decrease in cell size and cell number. When the body fat of the food-restricted and exercised animals was compared, the exercisers had fewer fat cells and less fat per cell even though the final body mass of both groups was approximately equal. The results demonstrate that exercise performed *early* during the growth period depresses the development of fat cells.

In a follow-up experiment, the fat-retarding effects of exercise or diet early in an animal's life were studied to determine whether either would reduce fat accumulation in adulthood. Three groups of animals were used: an exercise group, a sedentary group with free access to food and water, and a sedentary group with restricted food intake. Exercise and food restriction were terminated after 28 weeks. Several animals from each group were then sacrificed and compared for growth, body fat, and adipose cell size and number. The remaining animals were subjected to 34 weeks of sedentary living without exercise and were allowed unlimited food and water. The animals were then sacrificed and the groups compared for body mass, cell size, and cell number. The data in Figure 15–10 show that the exercised and food-restricted animals weighed less at 28 weeks of age than the sedentary, free-eaters.

During the 34 weeks of inactivity, the previously exercised animals con-

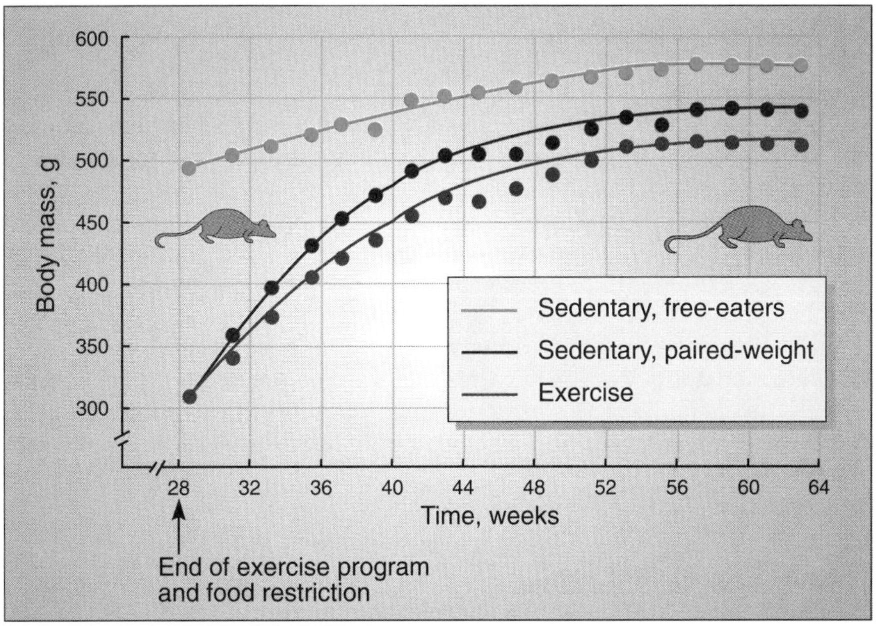

FIG. 15–10. Effects of exercise and food restriction on body mass in rats followed by no exercise with unlimited access to food. (Data from Oscai, L., et al.: Exercise or food restriction: effect on adipose tissue cellularity. *Am. J. Physiol.*, 277:901, 1974.)

tinued to maintain a lower body mass than the sedentary animals. Thus, the exercise program performed earlier in life caused a reduction in body mass that was still evident at the end of the experiment. Comparing cell size and number at the end of the training period revealed that the exercise group had fewer and smaller fat cells than either sedentary group of animals. These results agreed with the previous experiment. After 34 weeks of inactivity, the exercise group still had a lower final body mass and reduced total body fat content than sedentary counterparts, as well as significantly fewer fat cells. Fourteen to 16 weeks of exercise begun early in life and then terminated retarded the expansion and proliferation of fat cells during the growth period to adulthood. This occurred even though the exercise period was followed by 34 weeks of inactivity.

If these findings can be applied to humans, it is possible that a modification of diet, physical activity, or both, when begun early in life, may aid in controlling the proliferation of new fat cells and filling up of existing ones. Programs of exercise and weight control begun later in life and maintained thereafter can be effective in lowering the body's total quantity of fat. As far as we know, only cell size can be reduced, not cell number. If exercise or dietary intervention is discontinued, then the existing adipose tissue mass is likely to increase again by expansion of the cellular volume.

SPOT REDUCTION: DOES IT WORK?

The underlying basis for the notion of **spot reduction** is that an increase in a muscle's activity facilitates relatively greater fat mobilization from the fat storage areas in proximity to the muscle. Therefore, by localized exercise of a specific body area, more fat will be selectively reduced from that area than if exercise of the same caloric intensity is performed by a different muscle group. For example, advocates of spot reduction would recommend large numbers of sit-ups or side bends for a person with excessive abdominal fat. Whereas the promise of spot reduction with exercise is attractive from an aesthetic standpoint, a critical evaluation of the research does not support this notion.

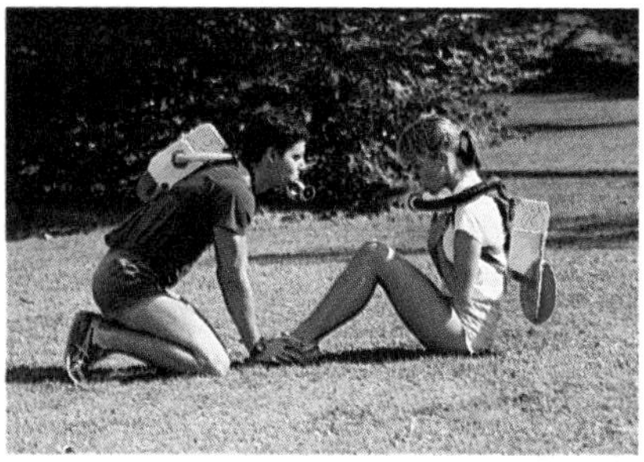

Spot reduction doesn't work. Current knowledge of energy supply indicates that exercise stimulates the mobilization of fat through hormones that act on fat depots throughout the body. The areas of greatest fat concentration or enzyme activity probably supply the greatest amount of this energy. There is no evidence that fatty acids are released to a greater degree from fat pads directly over the exercising muscle.

To examine the claims for spot reduction critically, comparisons were made of the girths and subcutaneous fat stores of the right and left forearms of high-caliber tennis players. As expected, the dominant or playing arm was significantly larger than the nondominant arm because of the modest muscular hypertrophy associated with the exercise overload provided by tennis. Measurements of fatfold thickness, however, showed *no difference* in the quantity of subcutaneous fat in the two forearms. Clearly, prolonged exercise was not accompanied by reduced fat deposits in the playing arm.

There is no doubt that the negative caloric balance created through regular exercise can significantly contribute to a reduction in total body fat. This fat, however, is not reduced selectively from the exercised areas but rather from total body fat reserves, and usually from the areas of greatest fat concentration.

WHERE ON THE BODY DOES FAT REDUCTION OCCUR?

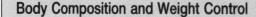

An often asked question concerning fat loss is, "Where on the body do changes occur when weight is lost?" To help answer this question, alterations in body composition were evaluated in 26 initially obese females at successive 2.3 kg (5 lb) decrements of weight loss. Weight loss was induced by caloric restriction and an exercise program consisting of 45-minute sessions 3 days a week for 14 weeks. Body composition assessment included 5 fatfolds, 9 girths, and densitometry to determine absolute and relative body fat and lean body mass. Figure 15–11 displays the changes in body composition, fatfolds, and girths for three subgroups that reduced body mass by 2.3, 4.5, and 9.1 kg. A 4.5 kg loss in body mass produced approximately twice the amount of change in overall body composition compared to changes observed at 2.3 kg. When weight loss doubled from 4.5 to 9.1 kg, the corresponding alteration in body composition was almost

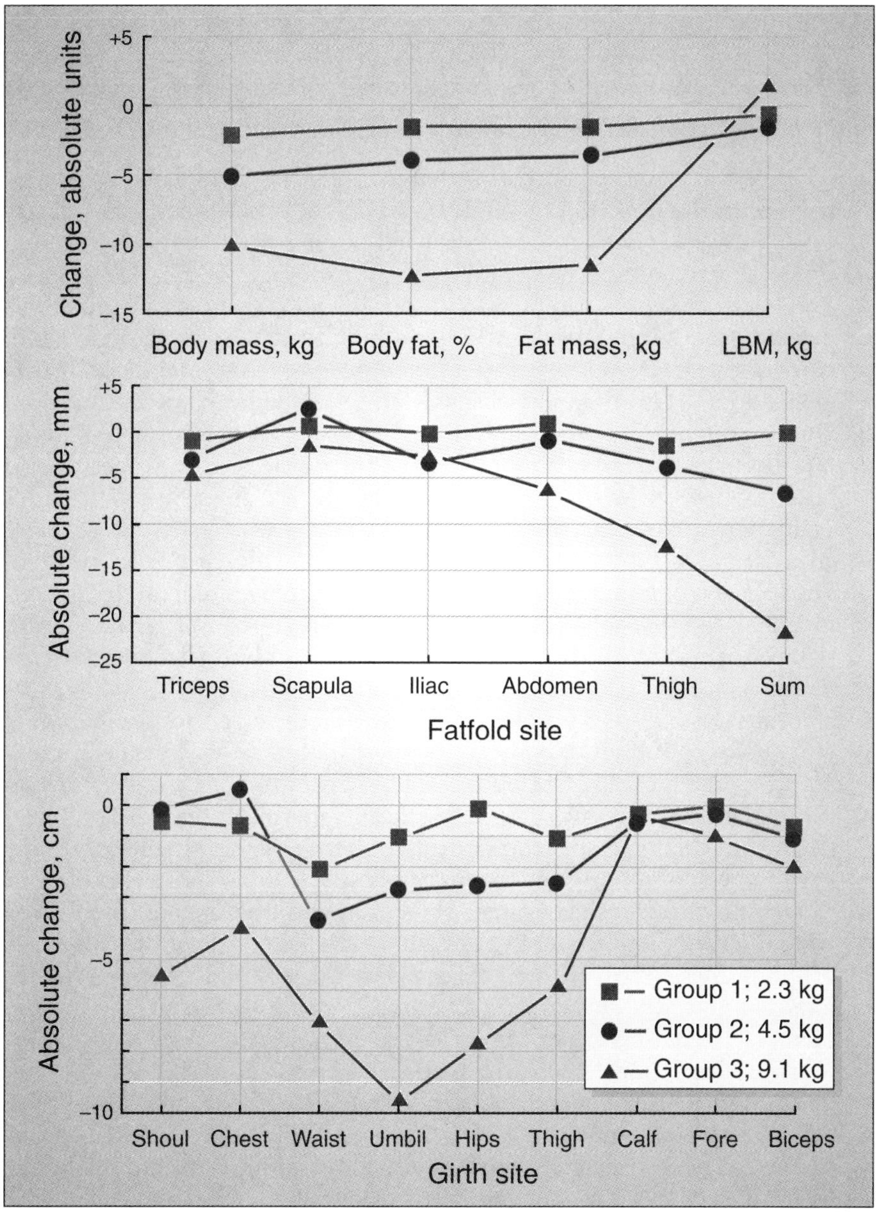

FIG. 15–11. Changes in body composition with specified amounts of loss in body mass. (Top) Body mass, body fat, fat mass, and lean body mass (LBM). (Middle) Fatfolds. (Bottom) Girths.

three times as great. This occurred for changes in fat mass, sum of 5 fatfolds, and sum of 11 girths. It is noteworthy that there was an approximately two-fold greater change in fatfolds and girths in the trunk region compared to the extremities. In addition, the proportional changes in body composition and anthropometry apparently mirror changes in loss of body mass up to 4.5 kg. Thereafter, the relative alteration in body composition becomes more pronounced and is apparently not related to the amount of additional weight loss up to 9.1 kg. Additional studies are needed to quantify the magnitude of change in overall body composition with additional losses in body mass.

SUMMARY

1. Obesity is a complex disorder related to numerous factors that tip energy balance in the direction of weight gain. What is becoming increasingly clear, however, is that a reduced level of energy expenditure through physical inactivity plays a significant contributory role.
2. There are numerous health risks associated with surprisingly low levels of excess body fat. These include an increased risk for hypertension, coronary heart disease, diabetes, renal disease, abnormal blood lipids, gallbladder and pulmonary disease, and various forms of cancer.
3. Obesity is usually defined in terms of excessive quantities of total body fat. There is probably no biologic reason for men and women to get fatter as they grow older. Therefore, the standards for overfatness for adult men and women should probably be those established for younger adults, namely, above 20% body fat for men and above 30% for women.
4. The location of adipose tissue should also be considered; fat distributed in the abdominal region (android-type obesity) poses a greater health risk compared to fat deposited at the thigh and buttocks (gynoid-type obesity).
5. Another classification for obesity is based on the size and number of fat cells. Before adulthood, body fat increases in two ways: by enlargement of individual fat cells, termed fat cell hypertrophy, or by an increase in the total number of fat cells, termed fat cell hyperplasia. Fat cells probably reach some biologic upper limit in size, so that cell number becomes the key factor determining the extent of obesity.
6. The number of fat cells becomes stable sometime before adulthood; any weight gain or loss thereafter is usually related to a change in the size of the individual cells. In extreme cases, fat cell number may increase in adults once the hypertrophic limit is reached for cell size.
7. Increases in the number of fat cells appear to involve three critical periods: the last trimester of pregnancy, the first year of life, and the adolescent growth spurt prior to adulthood.
8. Fat cell development in animals is influenced by dietary restriction and exercise. These effects are most prominent during early growth when the rate of fat cell division can be retarded.
9. Selective reduction of fat at specific body areas by "spot exercise" does not work.

RELATED READINGS

Berry, E.M., et al.: The role of dietary fat in human obesity. *Int. J. Obes.*, 10:123, 1986.
Björntorp, P.: Adipose tissue in obesity. In: Recent Advances in Obesity Research, Vol. 4. Edited by J. Hirsch and T.B. Van Itallie. London, Libby, 1985.
Björntorp, P.: Classification of obese patients and complications related to the distribution of surplus fat. *Am. J. Clin. Nutr.*, 45:1120, 1987.
Björntorp, P.: Adipose tissue distribution and function. *Int. J. Obes.*, 15:67, 1991.
Bogardus, C., et al.: Familial dependence on resting metabolic rate. *N. Engl. J. Med.*, 315:96, 1986.
Bortz, W.M.: Disease and aging. *JAMA*, 248:1203, 1982.
Bouchard, C., and Perusse, L.: Heredity of body fat. *Annu. Rev. Nutr.*, 8:259, 1988.
Bouchard, C., et al.: Inheritance of the amount and distribution of human body fat. *Int. J. Obes.*, 72:205, 1988.
Bouchard, C. et al.: The genes in the constellation of determinants of regional fat distribution. *Int. J. Sports Nutr.*, 15:9, 1991.
Bray, G.A.: The energetics of obesity. *Med. Sci. Sports Exerc.*, 15:32, 1983.
Bray, G.A.: Effects of obesity on health and happiness. In: Handbook of Eating Disorders. Edited by K.D. Brownell and J.B. Foreyt. New York, Basic Books, 1986.
Campaigne, B.N.: Body fat distribution: metabolic consequences and implications for weight loss. *Med. Sci. Sports Exerc.*, 22:291, 1990.
Chumlea, W.C., et al.: Adipocytes and adiposity in adults. *Am. J. Clin. Nutr.*, 34:1798, 1981.
Davies, P.S.W., et al.: The distribution of subcutaneous and internal fat in man. *Ann. Human Biol.*, 13:189, 1986.
Drenick, E.J.: Risk of obesity and surgical indications. *Int. J. Obes.* 5:387, 1980.
Duston, H.P.: Obesity and hypertension. *Ann. Intern. Med.*, 103:1047, 1985.
Forbes, G.G., et al.: Genetic factors in abdominal obesity, a risk factor for stroke. *N. Engl. J. Med.*, 318:1070, 1988.
Garn, S.M.: Continuities and changes in fatness from infancy through adulthood. *Curr. Probl. Pediatr.*, 15:1, 1985.
Gartmaker, S.L., et al.: Increasing pediatric obesity in the United States. *Am. J. Dis. Child.*, 141:535, 1987.
Greenwood, M.R.C.: Adipose tissue: cellular morphology and adipose tissue development. *Ann. Intern. Med.*, 103:996, 1985.
Greenwood, M.R.C., and Pitmann-Waller, V.: Weight control: a complex, varied, and controversial problem. In: Obesity and Weight Control. Edited by R.I. Frankle and M.-V. Yang, Gaithersburg, MD, Aspen, 1988.
Gwinup, G., et al.: Thickness of subcutaneous fat and activity of underlying muscles. *Ann. Intern. Med.*, 74:408, 1971.
Hagar, A., et al.: Adipose tissue cellularity in obese school girls before and after dietary treatment. *Am. J. Clin. Nutr.*, 31:68, 1978.
Hannon, B.M., and Lohman, T.G.: The energy cost of overweight in the United States. *Am. J. Publ. Health*, 68:765, 1978.
Health implications of obesity. National Institutes of Health Consensus Development Conference Statement, Vol. 5, No. 9. Washington, DC, U.S. Government Printing Office, 1985.
Hirsch, J., and Han, P.W.: Cellularity of rat adipose tissue: effects of growth, starvation and obesity. *J. Lipid Res.*, 10:77, 1969.
Hirsch, J., and Knittle, J.: Cellularity of obese and nonobese human adipose tissue. *Fed. Proc.*, 28:1516, 1970.
Hubert, H.B., et al.: Obesity as an independent risk factor for cardiovascular disease: a 26-year follow-up of participants in the Framingham Heart Study. *Circulation*, 67:968, 1983.
Iverius, P.H. and Brunzell, J.D.: Obesity and common genetic metabolic disorders. *Ann. Intern. Med.*, 103:1050, 1985.
Jeffrey, R., et al.: Weight cycling and cardiovascular risk factors in obese men and women. *Am. J. Clin. Nutr.*, 55:641, 1992.
Johnson, F.E.: Health implications of childhood obesity. *Ann. Intern. Med.*, 103:1068, 1985.
Katch, F.I., et al.: Effects of situp exercise training on adipose cell size and adiposity. *Res. Q. Exerc. Sport*, 55:242, 1984.
Knittle, J., and Hirsch, J.: Effect of early nutrition on the development of rat epididymal fat pads: Cellularity and metabolism. *J. Clin. Invest.*, 47:2091, 1968.

Kramer, M.S.: Do breast feeding and delayed introduction of solid food protect against subsequent obesity? *J. Pediatr.* 98:883, 1981.
Krotkiewski, M., et al.: Impact of obesity on metabolism in men and women—importance of regional adipocyte size in man. *J. Clin. Endocrinol. Metabol.*, 72:1150, 1983.
Larsson, B., et al.: The health consequences of moderate obesity. *Int. J. Obes.*, 5:97, 1981.
Lauer, M.S., et al.: The impact of obesity on left ventricular mass and geometry. *JAMA*, 266:231, 1991.
Leibel, R., and Hirsch, J.: Metabolic characterization of obesity. *Ann. Intern. Med.*, 103:1000, 1985.
Manson, J.E., et al.: A prospective study of obesity and risk of coronary heart disease in women. *N. Engl. J. Med.*, 322:822, 1990.
McArdle, W.D., et al.: Exercise Physiology: Energy, Nutrition, and Human Performance, 3rd Ed. Philadelphia, Lea & Febiger, 1991.
Meredith, C.N., et al.: Body composition and aerobic capacity in young and middle aged endurance-trained men. *Med. Sci. Sports Exerc.*, 19:557, 1987.
Noland, M., and Kearney, J.T.: Anthropometric and densitometric responses of women to specific and general exercise. *Res. Q.*, 49:322, 1978.
Oscai, L., et al.: Effects of exercise and of food restriction on adipose tissue cellularity. *J. Lipid Res., 13:588, 1972.*
Ostlund, R.E., et al.: The ratio of waist-to-hip circumference, plasma insulin level, and glucose intolerance as independent predictors of the HDL_2 cholesterol level in older adults. *N. Engl. J. Med.*, 332:229, 1990.
Ravussin, E., et al.: Reduced rate of energy expenditure as a risk factor for body-weight gain. *N. Engl. J. Med.*, 318:467, 1988.
Rebuffe-Scrive, M., et al.: Regulation of human adipose tissue metabolism during the menstrual cycle, pregnancy, and lactation. *J. Clin. Invest.*, 75:1973, 1985.
Roberts, S.B., et al.: Energy expenditure and intake in infants born to lean and overweight mothers. *N. Engl. J. Med.*, 318:461, 1988.
Roche, A.F.: The adipocyte-number hypothesis. *Child. Dev.* 52:31, 1981.
Ross, J.G., and Pate, R.R.: The National Children and Youth Fitness Study. II: A summary of findings. *JOHPERD*, 58:51, 1987.
Salans, L.B., et al.: Experimental obesity in man: cellular character of the adipose tissue. *J. Clin. Invest.*, 50:1005, 1971.
Salans, L.B., et al.: Studies of human adipose tissue: adipose cell size and number in nonobese and obese patients. *J. Clin. Invest.*, 52:929, 1973.
Schlundt, D.G., et al.: The role of breakfast in the treatment of obesity: a randomized clinical trial. *Am. J. Clin. Nutr.*, 55:645, 1992.
Schutz, Y., et al.: Diet-induced thermogenesis measured over a whole day in obese and nonobese women. *Am. J. Clin. Nutr.*, 40:542, 1984.
Segal, K.R., et al.: Body composition, not body weight, is related to cardiovascular disease risk factors and sex hormone levels in man. *J. Clin. Invest.*, 80:1050, 1987.
Segal, K.R., et al.: Thermic effects of food and exercise in lean and obese men of similar lean body mass. *Am. J. Physiol.*, 252:E110, 1987.
Sims, E.A.H., and Horton, E.S.: Endocrine and metabolic adaptation to obesity and starvation. *Am. J. Clin. Nutr.*, 21:1455, 1968.
Stunkard, A.J.: An adoption study of human obesity. *N. Engl. J. Med.*, 314:193, 1986.
Van Itallie, T.B.: Health implications of overweight and obesity in the United States. *Ann. Intern. Med.*, 103:983, 1985.
Willett, W.C., et al.: New weight guidelines for Americans: justified or injudicious? (editorial). *Am. J. Clin. Nutr.*, 53:1102, 1991.

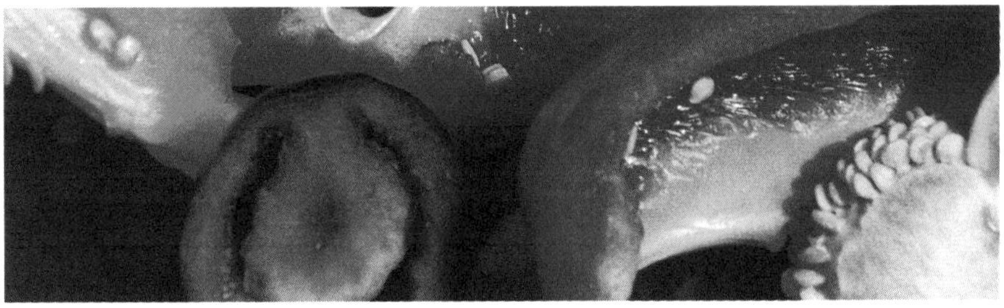

16

WEIGHT CONTROL

It is truly remarkable that the body mass of most adults fluctuates only slightly during the year. In the United States, the annual intake of food averages nearly 900 kg and includes 280 eggs, 7 kg of breakfast cereal, 84 kg of meat, 91 kg of fruit, 114 kg of vegetables, 31 kg of bread, and 429 soft drinks, 8 liters of wine, 96 liters of beer, and 8 liters of liquor! This is rather impressive considering that only a slight but prolonged excess can cause substantial weight gain. Eating just an extra handful of peanuts each day, for example, causes a weight gain of about 10 kg over a year. The fact that the body mass of most adults remains fairly stable illustrates the body's exquisite regulatory control in balancing caloric intake with daily energy expenditure. *It is only when the number of calories ingested as food exceeds the daily energy requirements that excess calories are stored as fat in adipose tissue.* To prevent an increase in body mass and body fat because of caloric imbalance, an effective weight control program must establish a balance between energy input and energy output.

The literally hundreds of consumer health type books that advocate exotic diets or exercise plans for weight loss have one thing in common: they all claim their plans are so easy to follow that results can be guaranteed! If

Americans are desperately trying to lose weight. Of 29 million serious dieters in the United States in 1991, 20.6 million were female. For this group, 630 million pounds were lost and 489 million regained. The difference in calories "burned up" converts to a whopping 1 billion 89 million caloric deficit for fat loss—enough energy to walk 10,890,000 miles (at 100 calories per mile) or the one-person equivalent of 12.9 years of continuous walking without rest at a 15 minute per mile pace!

Weight loss as big business. Studies by the diet industry indicate that at any given time, up to 50 million Americans are dieting. Small wonder that the weight loss business is a source of large financial profit—often at the expense of consumers who are looking for a fast and easy way to shed excess pounds from products that rarely do what their claims state.

Diet's composition does make a difference. The composition of the diet influences the efficiency of how the body converts a caloric excess to stored fat. Excess fat calories are almost effortlessly converted into storage fat by the body. Only about 3% of the energy in ingested fat is required to convert these excess calories to body fat, whereas 25% of the calories in excess carbohydrates are "burned" in the conversion process.

Athletes are often the worst offender. Fad and bizarre diets are particularly troublesome to those who work in sports medicine and athletics, where reports consistently document the use of potentially dangerous weight control behaviors among athletes.

this were true, and a simple procedure could maintain the "perfect" body size permanently, then the large number of overfat Americans could be cured easily. Even when a particular diet plan becomes popular through an advertising blitz "documenting" dramatic weight loss, these schemes often jeoparidize the dieter's health.

DIETING IS NOT WITHOUT RISK

Many professional organizations have voiced strong opposition to extreme dietary practices for rapid weight loss, in particular the low-carbohydrate, high-fat, and high-protein diets. In the following sections we review those approaches to weight loss.

KETOGENIC DIETS

Advocates of **ketogenic diets** emphasize *carbohydrate restriction* while often ignoring the total caloric intake. Their rationale is that with minimal carbohydrate for energy, the body must metabolize its fat stores. This supposedly generates sufficient ketone bodies (by-products of incomplete fat breakdown) to suppress appetite and cause urinary loss of these "unburned" calories to account for weight loss. It is argued that this caloric excretion will be so great that the dieter need not be concerned with caloric intake, as long as carbohydrates are restricted. At best, the calories lost through urinary excretion of ketones equal only 100 to 150 a day. This would account for a small weight loss of approximately 0.45 kg (1 lb) a month—not very appealing when the major portion of the diet amounts to a lipid intake as high as 60 to 70% of total calories. Also, any initial weight loss on this diet may be largely the result of dehydration brought about by an extra solute load on the kidneys that increases the urinary loss of water. Such water loss is of no lasting significance in a program designed to reduce body fat.

Compared to a standard well-balanced, low-calorie diet, ketogenic diets show no advantage in facilitating loss of body fat. In fact, such low-carbohydrate diets have potential to cause significant loss of lean tissue. This is because the body will use lean tissue protein to synthesize the important fuel glucose that becomes depleted through dietary restriction. This is certainly an undesirable side effect for a diet designed to bring about fat loss. High-fat low-carbohydrate diets are also potentially hazardous in a number of ways. For one thing, the diet can raise serum uric acid levels and lower potassium levels; this facilitates undesirable cardiac arrhythmias, causes acidosis, aggravates kidney problems from the extra solute burden placed on the renal system, elevates blood lipids to increase heart disease risk, depletes glycogen reserves and contributes to a state of fatigue, and causes relative dehydration. This diet is definitely contraindicated during pregnancy because adequate carbohydrate availability is essential for proper fetal development.

The focus on weight begins in youth. Of about 3,000 middle school children studied, by the eighth grade 55% of girls believe they are fat (13% actually are) and 50% have dieted. For the boys, 28% consider themselves fat (13% are) and 25% have dieted. According to experts in nutrition and body image, this inordinate preoccupation with body weight can be blunted if parents will help children accept their bodies and discourage them from crash dieting.

STARVATION DIETS

A **starvation diet** or therapeutic fast may be recommended in severe obesity in which body fat exceeds 40% of body mass. Such diets are usually prescribed for up to 3 months, but usually as a "last resort" prior to undertaking more extreme medical approaches that include various surgical treatments. This **very-low-calorie diet** or VLCD approach to weight loss is predicated on the hope that abstinence from food will break established dietary habits, which in turn may improve the long-term prospects for success. Such diets may also depress appetite, which could help the patient comply with the diet plan.

It is difficult to maintain an active lifestyle while on a very low calorie diet. If a person fasts even for several days and then attempts to exercise, deterioration in performance and fatigue are likely to occur. Because adequate carbohydrates are not consumed, glycogen stores in the liver and muscles are rapidly depleted, and this will impair most tasks requiring sustained muscular effort.

Daily medications are usually prescribed and include calcium carbonate or antihistamines for nausea; bicarbonate of soda and potassium chloride to maintain consistency of body fluids; mouthwash and sugar-free chewing gum for bad breath (owing to high levels of fat metabolism) that persists as long as fasting continues; and various bath oils for dry skin. Clearly, for most individuals, starvation is not an "ultimate diet" or proper approach to weight control. Furthermore, the success rate of prolonged fasting is poor. And because the lean tissue lost through such extreme dieting may not all be regained as weight is put back, the "new" body mass may now possess an ever greater percentage of body fat!

Renewed interest in VLCD regimens. The approach of VLCD was first published in the medical literature in 1929. In the late 1970s, there was renewed interest in VLCDs as a viable method to help treat obesity. First and foremost was the question of whether or not VLCD was truly effective as a treatment modality. While there are still no firm answers to this and other questions about VLCDs, scientists from around the world are continuing to study the VLCD approach in hopes of obtaining more theoretical and practical information about this method of obesity treatment. What is known is that VLCDs cause rapid weight loss **and** weight regain once the VLCD is discontinued. What seems to be universally agreed is that dramatic changes in lifestyle (that include both exercise and behavior modification) probably offer the most effective chance for longer-term success.

HIGH-PROTEIN DIETS

The **high-protein diet** has been extolled as the "last chance diet" for the obese as well as people who are less overweight. The argument is that a protein diet causes appetite suppression through the body's excessive reliance on fat mobilization. This effect has yet to be supported with careful research. An accompanying claim is that the elevated calorie-burning thermic effect of dietary protein, as well as its relatively lower coefficient of digestibility, ultimately reduce the net calories available from proteins compared to a well-balanced meal of equal caloric value. Although this point may have some validity, many other factors must be considered in formulating a sound weight loss program—not to mention the potentially harmful strain on kidney and liver function and the accompanying dehydration, electrolyte imbalance, and lean tissue loss resulting from excess protein intake.

When the protein is in fluid form, the "miracle liquid" is made palatable with artificial flavoring and often includes a blend of ground-up animal hooves and horns, skin, and connective tissue mixed in a broth with enzymes and tenderizers to "predigest" it. In 1979, according to the Food and Drug Administration, this particular kind of protein elixir and others like it were associated with 58 deaths. Sixteen of the victims were obese women who lost an average of 38 kg within 2 to 8 months. None had a previous history of heart disease; they all died suddenly while on the diet or shortly thereafter. Table 16–1 summarizes the principles and the main advantages and disadvantages of some of the popular dietary approaches to weight loss.

The heart may also suffer. With extremes of dieting, there is the distinct possibility that lean tissue loss may occur disproportionately from critical organs such as the heart.

Potentially bad source of protein. Liquid protein is often not of the highest quality in terms of the amino acid mixture, and is generally lacking in required vitamins and minerals.

What's your choice—good nutrition, money, fitness, or sex? A survey in *American Health* magazine posed the question, "What would you choose if offered the choice of losing 10 pounds, winning $2500, completing a 5-mile race, or having great sex four times in a weekend?" The clear winner for both genders was the money. The second choice was the sex weekend for the men, while the women chose losing 10 pounds. For both men and women, completing the 5-mile run was last. Of interest was that 86% of respondents would give up sex for money, and that it would require $4 to 5 million dollars for a lifetime of celibacy.

MAINTENANCE OF GOAL WEIGHT IS A DIFFICULT TASK

While most diets produce weight loss during the first several weeks, the weight lost is largely body water. In addition, loss of lean tissue is usually

TABLE 16–1. PRINCIPLES, ADVANTAGES, AND DISADVANTAGES OF SOME POPULAR DIETARY APPROACHES TO WEIGHT LOSS

METHOD	PRINCIPLE	ADVANTAGES	DISADVANTAGES	COMMENTS
Surgical procedures	Alteration of the gastrointestinal tract changes capacity or amount of absorptive surface	Caloric restriction is less necessary	Risks of surgery and post-surgical complications include death	Radical procedures include stapling of the stomach and removal of a section of the small intestine (a jejunoileal bypass)
Fasting	No energy input assures negative energy balance	Weight loss is rapid (which may be a disadvantage) Exposure to temptation is reduced	Ketogenic A large portion of weight lost is from lean body mass Nutrients are lacking	Medical supervision is mandatory and hospitalization is recommended
Protein-sparing modified fast	Same as fasting except protein or protein with carbohydrate intake presumably helps preserve lean body mass	Same as in fasting	Ketogenic Nutrients are lacking Some unconfirmed deaths have been reported, possibly from potassium depletion	Medical supervision is mandatory Popular presentation was made in Linn's *The Last Chance Diet*
One-food-centered diets	Low caloric intak favors negative energy balance	Being easy to follow has initial psychological appeal	Being too restrictive means nutrients are probably lacking Repetitious nature may cause boredom	No food or food combination is known to "burn off" fat Examples include the grapefruit diet and the egg diet
Low-carbohydrate/high-fat diets	Increased ketone excretion removes energy-containing substances from the body Fat intake is often voluntarily decreased; a low caloric diet results	Inclusion of rich foods may have psychological appeal Initial rapid loss of water may be an incentive	Ketogenic High-fat intake is contraindicated for heart and diabetes patients Nutrients are often lacking	Popular versions have been offered by Taller and Atkins; some have been called the "Mayo," "Drinking Man's," and "Air Force" diets
Low-carbohydrate/high-protein diets	Low caloric intake favors negative energy balance		Expense and repetitious nature may make it difficult to sustain	If meat is emphasized, the diet becomes one that is high in fat The Pennington diet is an example
High-carbohydrate/low-fat diets	Low caloric intake favors negative energy balance	Wise food selections can make the diet nutritionally sound	Initial water retention may be discouraging	The Pritikin diet is an example

Source: Modified and reprinted by permission from Reed, P.B.: Nutrition: An Applied Science. Copyright © 1980 by West Publishing Co. All Rights Reserved.

significant with extremes of dieting, especially in the early phase of very low calorie dieting. Unless a person maintains reduced caloric intake for a considerable time, the weight is eventually regained. The net result is a return to original body size, often at the expense of feelings of hunger and other psychological stress during the diet plan. Anyone who has seriously tried to maintain a diet knows the difficulty encountered. While it is certainly possible to lose significant weight through dieting, few people have the self-control to stick with a diet plan long enough to achieve permanent success.

A review of the scientific literature dealing with weight loss reveals that people who have initial success are usually *unsuccessful* in permanently maintaining their desired body size. This has been pointed out in numerous follow-up studies of patients who participated in weight loss programs in which caloric intake was carefully regulated. In an early survey of the effectiveness of obesity clinics during a 10-year period, the dropout rate varied between 20 and 80%. Of those who remained in a program, no more than 25% lost as much as 9 kg, and only 5% lost 18 kg or more.

In a follow-up study of 121 patients, illustrated in Figure 16–1, much of the reduced weight was maintained for the first 12 to 18 months. The tendency to regain weight was independent of the length of the fast, extent of weight lost, or age at onset of obesity. Return to original weight occurred in one-half of the subjects within 2 or 3 years, and only 7 patients remained at their reduced weight after 7 years.

Not very successful. Five-year results from Denmark indicate the ineffectiveness of rapid weight loss with either very low calorie diets (VLCD) or obesity surgery (gastroplasty) on long-term weight reduction. Those on the VLCD lost a maximum average of 22 kg while the group receiving surgery lost 26 kg. Success was defined as maintaining a weight loss of at least 10 kg. After 5 years the success rate was a disappointing 3% for the diet group and 16% for the surgery group. Such statistics are rather discouraging and indicate that the long-term maintenance of a particular low-calorie diet is extremely difficult; it is especially difficult in the relaxed atmosphere of home, where access to food is relatively easy.

THE ENERGY BALANCE EQUATION

Before a person develops a plan for favorably modifying both body mass and body composition, the rationale underlying the **energy balance equation** must be considered. *The equation states that body mass will remain constant when caloric intake equals caloric expenditure.* The top of Figure 16–2 shows the ideal situation in which energy input (calories in food) *exactly balances* energy output (calories expended in daily physical activities). As long as this equilibrium is maintained within narrow limits, there will be relatively little fluctuation in body mass. The middle part of the figure depicts what happens all too frequently when energy input *exceeds* energy output. Under such conditions, the number of calories consumed in excess of daily requirements is stored as fat in adipose tissue. As we will discuss shortly, *3500 "extra" kcal through either increased intake or decreased output will equal approximately 1 pound (0.45 kg) of stored body fat.* The bottom of the figure illustrates what occurs when energy intake is ***less than*** energy output. In this case, the body obtains the required calories from its energy stores and body mass and fat become reduced.

Excess Intake = Fat Gain. Accumulating fat is the body's way of keeping track of the extra calories consumed above the required level. The body simply does not forget about the extra slice of cheese, bagel with cream cheese, additional helping of pepperoni pizza, or three super scoops of chocolate chip cookie mix ice cream with hot fudge!

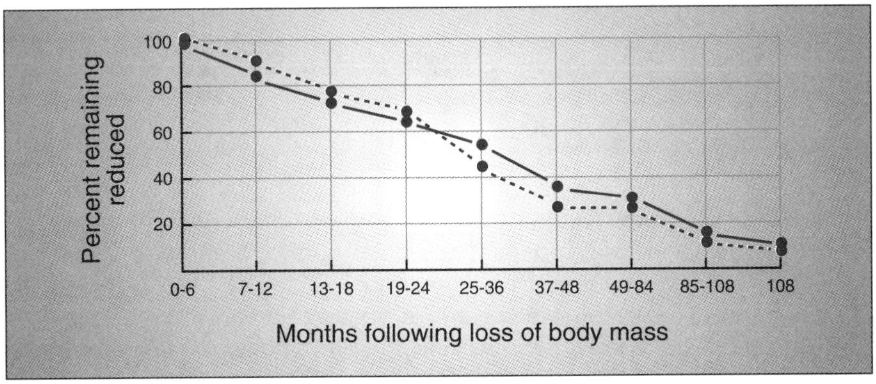

FIG. 16–1. Percent of patients remaining at reduced weights at various time intervals following accomplished weight loss. The solid line represents 60 subjects with obesity onset before age 21. (From Johnson, D., and Drenick, E.J.: Therapeutic fasting in morbid obesity. *Arch. Intern. Med.*, 137:1381, 1977.)

Just a little extra goes a long way. Over a 40-year period between ages 25 and 65, the average woman consumes more than 18 metric tons of food. During this time, she would gain about 11 kg (24 lb) from a daily excess of only 350 mg (0.012 oz) in food intake.

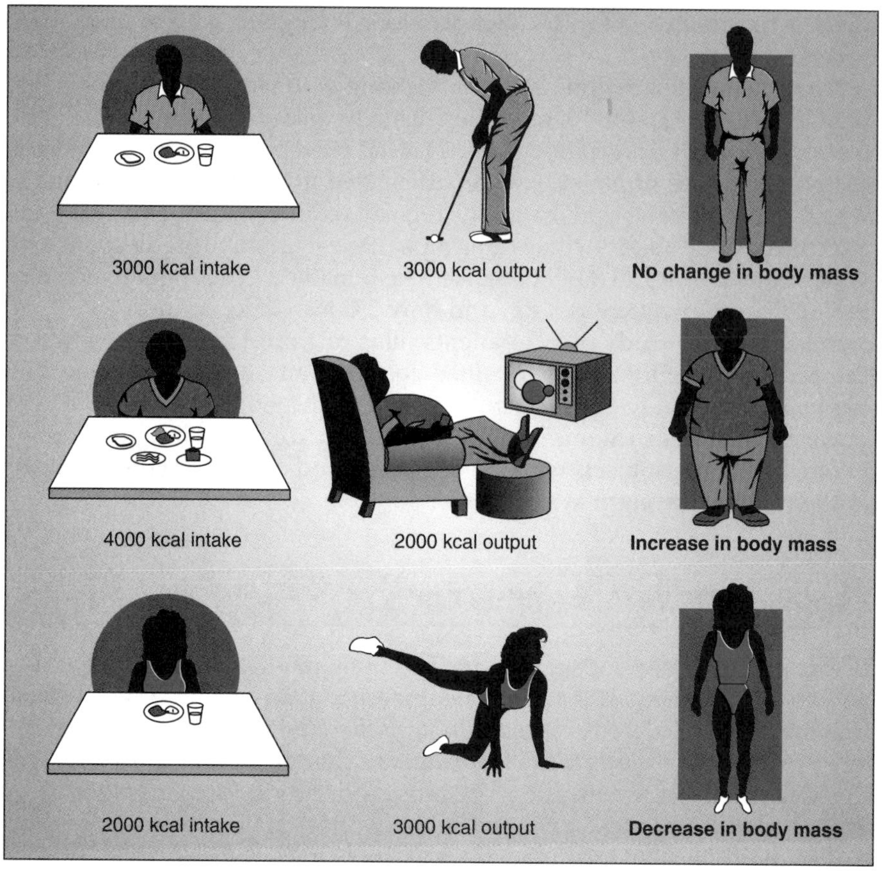

FIG. 16–2. The energy balance equation.

There are three **ways to "unbalance" the energy balance equation** to cause weight loss:

> **Tipping the scale.** Unbalancing the energy balance equation is the most important step to weight loss. Energy input must be reduced below energy output, or energy output must be increased above energy input. In each situation, weight loss will occur.

1. Maintain energy input and *decrease* caloric intake below daily energy requirements
2. Maintain caloric intake and *increase* caloric output through additional physical activity
3. Combine methods 1 and 2 by decreasing daily food intake and increasing daily energy expenditure

Energy input = Energy output → Stable body mass	
Energy input > Energy output → Increase in body mass	
Energy input < Energy output → Decrease in body mass	

To understand the sensitivity of the energy balance equation in weight control, consider what happens when daily calorie intake exceeds output by only 100 kcal. This could occur by eating just one extra banana each day. Annually, the surplus number of ingested calories would be 365 days × 100 kcal or 36,500 kcal. Because 0.45 kg (1 lb) of body fat contains about 3500 kcal, the small daily increase in caloric intake would cause a gain of 10.4 kg, or 4.7 lb, of fat in one year. If the same energy imbalance was maintained, then theoretically there would be a gain in fat mass of 23.6 kg (52 lb) in 5 years! On the other hand, reducing daily food intake by only

100 kcal and increasing energy expenditure a similar amount by jogging a mile each day would reduce total body fat by 9.5 kg (21 lb) in a year.

We believe that one of the major reasons weight control is often unsuccessful is because most Americans have great difficulty curbing their appetite and getting their body moving. We are all impressed by modern technologies that provide convenience rather than relying on the body's own power for movement and exercise. In the next chapter, we discuss practical ways to help twentieth century man and woman fight the battle of energy balance and avoid defeat by twenty-first century technologies.

Excess calories accumulate fat. Each 0.45 kg (1 lb) of adipose tissue is about 87% fat, or 395 g × 9 kcal/g = 3555 kcal. There is simply no getting around the fact that when total extra calories consumed add up to about 3500, approximately 0.45 kg of extra fat is gained. This cannot be undone by magic potions, trick diets, or special formula foods.

PERSONAL ASSESSMENT OF ENERGY INTAKE AND ENERGY OUTPUT

An objective assessment of food intake and energy expenditure provides the frame of reference for unbalancing the energy balance equation to favorably modify both body mass and body composition.

Energy Intake. Section II B of the *Study Guide* illustrates the step-by-step procedure to assess both nutrient and energy intake by means of a 3-day dietary survey. Studies have shown that people who calculate caloric intake from daily records of food consumption are usually within approximately 10% of the number of calories actually consumed. For example, suppose the caloric value of your daily food intake were directly measured in the bomb calorimeter and averaged 2130 kcal. If you kept a careful 3-day dietary history to estimate caloric intake, the daily value would fall between about 1920 and 2350 kcal. As long as you maintain a careful record, the accuracy of caloric determinations will be within acceptable limits.

Careful record keeping of food intake accomplishes two things: (1) it provides the dieter with an objective list of the foods actually consumed (rather than a "guesstimate" of what has been eaten), and (2) it triggers an important aspect of the weight control process that must occur before success can be achieved: self-realization and awareness of current food habits and preferences. Most people who keep meticulous records are often "shocked" not only at how much they actually eat, but the wide range of foods they consume. For many people, eating becomes an unconscious act—so much so that they have difficulty remembering what was eaten, let alone the quantity consumed, the frequency of eating, or the situations that trigger the urge to eat.

Energy Output. In addition to caloric restriction through dieting, we believe that a physically active lifestyle is crucial to long-term success. This does not mean playing a token game of tennis twice a year, going for a swim on weekends during the summer, or walking to the store when the car is being repaired. Modifying personal exercise habits entails a serious commitment to changing the daily routine to include regular periods of moderate to vigorous physical activity. A first step in that direction is to obtain a detailed picture of your current pattern of physical activity as outlined in Secton II C of the *Study Guide*.

Serious commitment to a new lifestyle. Increasing energy expenditure through physical activity, while not unpleasant in itself, does require changes in time allocation and lifestyle that many people are unwilling to make. Reducing body size through diet and exercise is only half the battle; staying reduced requires a serious commitment to a new lifestyle.

UNBALANCING THE ENERGY BALANCE EQUATION

Estimating energy intake and energy output provides useful information with regard to the energy balance equation. Monitoring changes in body mass helps to complete the picture. If body mass remains stable from week to week, this means that caloric intake is matched to the caloric requirements of daily living. On the other hand, if body mass increases, then the intake of calories exceeds those expended for rest plus other daily energy needs. *It is simply not possible to consume more calories than are expended without increasing body mass.* There is no way of avoiding this! If weight loss is occuring, the equilibrium has been disturbed in favor of less input (food) and more output (activity).

DIETING TO TIP THE ENERGY BALANCE EQUATION

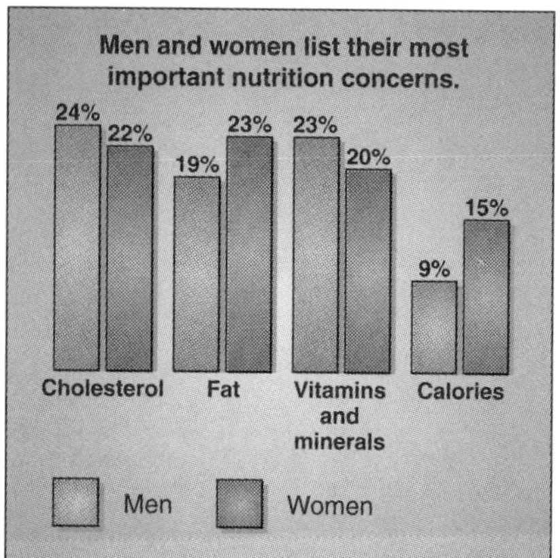

Source: American Dietetic Association

A prudent dietary approach to weight loss unbalances the energy balance equation by reducing energy intake, usually by about 500 to 1000 kcal a day below the daily expenditure. Caloric restriction of more than 1000 kcal per day is poorly tolerated over a long time, plus this form of semi-starvation increases the chances for poor nourishment. Suppose an obese woman who consumes 2800 kcal daily and maintains body mass at 80 kg wishes to reduce by 5 kg. She decides to maintain her activity level but decreases daily food intake to create a caloric deficit of 1000 kcal. Thus, instead of consuming 2800 kcal, she takes in only 1800 daily. In 7 days, the caloric deficit would equal 7000 kcal (1000 kcal/day × 7 days). This would be accompanied by a corresponding loss of approximately 0.9 kg (2 lb) of body fat. Actually, more than 0.9 kg would be lost during the first week because the carbohydrate stores, which contain fewer calories per kg than fat and considerably more water, would be metabolized to the greatest extent. To reduce fat content by an additional 1.4 kg, the reduced daily caloric intake of 1800 kcal would have to be maintained for another 10.5 days. By adhering to the 1800 kcal diet, she would reduce body fat at the rate of 0.45 kg of fat every 3.5 days provided the daily energy output remained unchanged.

While the mathematics of weight loss through caloric restriction are rather straightforward, two basic assumptions could, if violated, greatly reduce the effectiveness of the diet. The *first assumption* is that energy expenditure remains relatively unchanged throughout the period of dieting. This is somewhat difficult to control, however, as there can be large variation in a person's daily and weekly energy expenditure. For some people, caloric restriction and its tendency to deplete the body's carbohydrate stores can cause lethargy. This will actually decrease the level of daily energy expenditure. In addition, as body mass is reduced, the energy cost of physical activity decreases proportionately. This also causes the energy output side of the equation to become smaller. The *second assumption* is that a dieter will persevere with a reduced caloric intake until the desired body size is achieved. These two assumptions could probably be met quite adequately if humans functioned without variation. If weight loss were indeed proportional to caloric restriction, progressive decrease in body mass would depend solely on the extent of caloric deprivation. However, changes take place during caloric restriction that affect the rate of weight loss. One such change is in the resting metabolic rate.

It takes a while to lose fat. Short periods of caloric restriction are often encouraging to the dieter, but result in a large percentage of water and carbohydrate loss per unit of body weight loss with only a minimal decrease in body fat. As weight loss continues, however, a larger proportion of body fat is used for energy to make up the caloric deficit created by food restriction.

SET-POINT THEORY: A CASE AGAINST DIETING

When reviewing the scientific literature on the success of weight loss through dieting, we must conclude that dieting usually does not work over the long term. Surely, a person can crash off weight in a short time by simply not eating. This success is short-lived, however, and eventually the urge to eat wins out and weight is regained. By the **set-point theory,** the reason for this failure lies in a "set-point" for body mass that differs from what the dieter would like to have. Proponents of the theory argue that each person has an internal control mechanism, a set-point, probably located deep within the brain's *hypothalamus,* that drives the body to maintain a particular level of body fat. In a practical sense, this would be your body mass when you are not counting calories. The problem is that we all have a different set-point, and various factors such as the drugs fenfluramine, amphetamine, and nicotine, as well as exercise, lower the particular setting—while dieting has *no effect.* Each time we manage to reduce our fat level below our "natural" set-point by dieting, the body makes internal adjustments to resist this change and conserve body fat.

Resting Metabolism Is Lowered. One well-documented occurrence is the dramatic reduction in resting metabolic rate with weight loss. In fact, this decrease in metabolism is often greater than the decrease attributable to the weight lost. For example, severe caloric restriction depresses resting metabolism by as much as 45%! *This calorie-sparing defense may even become more apparent with repeated bouts of dieting so that depression of resting metabolism is enhanced with each subsequent attempt to reduce caloric intake.* This greatly conserves energy and causes dieting to become progressively less effective. As a result, a plateau in weight loss is reached and further decreases in body mass are considerably less than predicted simply from the energy deficit caused by caloric restriction. When the rewards of one's efforts are no longer apparent, the dieter usually quits and reverts to previous eating behaviors.

Metabolism, the body's defense against weight change. Caloric restriction brings about significant depression of resting metabolism as the body defends against weight loss. Even when a person attempts to gain weight above normal level by means of overeating, the body resists this change through an increase in resting metabolism.

Figure 16–3 displays the results from a study of 6 obese men in whom body mass, resting oxygen uptake (minimal energy requirement), and caloric intake were carefully monitored for 31 consecutive days. The subjects consumed 3500 kcal per day for the first 7 days of the experiment. For the remaining 24 days the daily caloric intake was markedly reduced to 450 kcal. During the pre-diet period, body mass and resting oxygen uptake remained stable. For this group, 3500 kcal a day was just adequate to balance the daily energy expenditure. However, when the subjects began dieting, both body mass and resting metabolism declined but the percentage decline in metabolism was greater than the decrease in body mass. The dashed line represents expected weight loss for this 450-kcal diet. The decline in resting metabolism actually conserved energy, causing the diet to become progressively less effective. More than half the total weight loss occurred within the first 8 days of the diet, and the remainder during the final 16 days. This slowing of the theoretical weight loss curve often leaves the dieter frustrated and discouraged.

WEIGHT CYCLING: GOING NOPLACE FAST

The futility of repeated cycles of weight loss and weight gain, the so-called **yo-yo effect,** is shown in studies in which food efficiency is evaluated by the ratio of body mass change to ingested calories. *In general, weight gain occurs more readily with repeated cycles of weight loss.* In one study, animals required twice the time to lose the same weight during a second period of caloric restriction and only one-third the time to regain it! Furthermore, if

Disconcerting news. Although being overweight clearly raises the chances for heart trouble, the failure to keep weight off might be even worse. Repeated bouts of weight loss and weight gain further increase the risk of dying from a heart attack. In fact, the risk is almost 70% higher in those who take weight off and put it on again, compared to people whose weight stays reasonably steady.

A lifetime of weight cycling can be a killer. Researchers are now divided about the need to continually try to shed excess weight. Men and women between 30 and 44 years old who repetitively diet, losing and regaining hundreds of pounds during this time, are at greater risk of death overall and death from heart disease than people whose weight remains relatively stable. Most researchers agree that there is still need to reduce excess weight for health reasons, yet the opinion is not unanimous. Dr. David Garner, director of the Eating Disorders Research Program at Michigan State University, questions the appropriateness of treating obesity at all: "There's little scientific justification for continuing to treat obesity, given what we already know." Dr. Garner was referring to the 90 to 95% failure rate of dieters to maintain their weight loss. Undoubtedly, there will be research to explore the interrelationships between weight cycling, body composition, patterns of food intake, illness, and increased mortality.

In the meantime, what should people do? It is our position that people who need to reduce excess weight must face the reality that keeping weight off requires a full-time effort, especially when using dieting only. People who eat little or nothing for a week or two and then gain it all back may be putting themselves in double jeopardy in terms of health. Going on a diet without significantly increasing energy expenditure will probably result in relapse, thus setting the person up for another attempt at weight loss and eventual regain of the lost weight—and increased risk for illness.

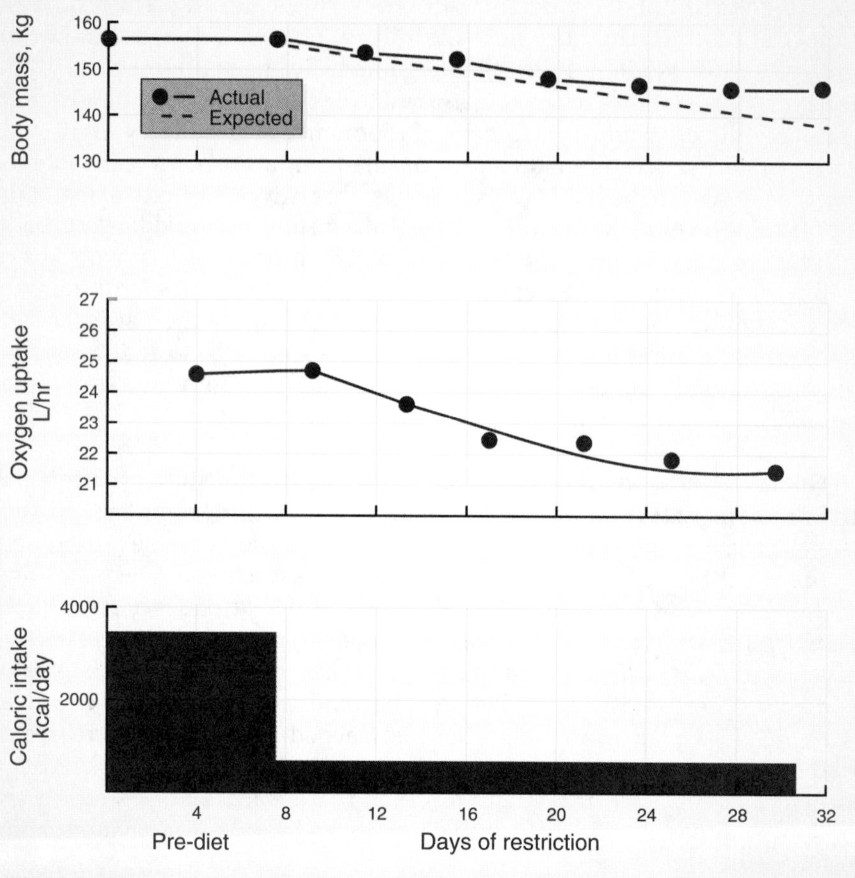

FIG. 16–3. Effects of two levels of caloric intake on changes in body mass and resting oxygen uptake. (Adapted from Bray, G.: Effect of caloric restriction on energy expenditure in obese subjects. *Lancet*, 2:397, 1969.)

the body is unable to regain its lean tissue at the rate it was lost through dieting, then fat may be replaced instead.

Recent research provides further disconcerting news for those desiring permanent fat loss. It now appears that when obese people lose body mass, the adipocytes increase their level of lipoprotein lipase, the enzyme that facilitates fat synthesis and storage. The effect of these high enzyme levels is to make it easier for the formerly obese to regain fat—and the fatter people are before their weight loss, the more lipoprotein lipase they produce when they reduce. This suggests that the fatter people are originally, the more vigorously their bodies attempt to regain lost weight. Such findings provide an additional biologic mechanism to explain the great difficulty the obese encounter in maintaining weight loss.

Although the set-point theory may be unwelcome news for those who possess a set-point that is tuned "too high," the good news is that regular exercise may lower the set-point toward a more desirable level. Concurrently, regular exercise conserves and even increases lean body mass, raises resting metabolism, and brings about enzymatic changes that facilitate fat breakdown in the tissues, all of which would make dieting more effective.

For overweight men and women who exercise regularly, food intake tends to drop initially despite the increase in energy output, and body fat decreases. Eventually, as an active lifestyle is maintained, caloric intake balances the daily energy requirement so body mass is stabilized at a new, lower level.

Good news for exercisers. When exercise is part of a weight loss program, either alone or in combination with dieting, a smaller reduction in resting metabolism occurs than when weight loss relies solely on dieting. This makes it easier for people who exercise to take weight off and keep it off.

HOW TO SELECT A DIET PLAN

The most difficult aspect of dieting is deciding exactly what foods to include in the daily menu. There are literally hundreds of diet plans to choose from—water diets, drinker's diets, fruit or vegetable diets, egg diets, meat diets, fast-food diets, ice cream diets, "eat to win" diets, and name of city diets such as the New York City or Beverly Hills diet, not to mention the potentially dangerous varieties of high-fat, low-carbohydrate, and high-protein diets. Some authors have even preached that it is not total calories that contribute to weight loss, but the order in which foods are eaten! One popular diet book claims that eating a grapefruit every morning counteracts the effects of high-calorie foods; another suggests that drinking extra water dilutes the calories in the food ingested. Of course, such claims are ludicrous, but for those desperate to shed excess weight, such misinformation reinforces negative eating behaviors. As a result, it is easy to repeat a vicious cycle of failures. Someone who wants to reduce by a given amount tries a particular diet plan that, for whatever reason, is ineffective. The dieter, who may have lost a few pounds, is easily discouraged and quickly regains weight. After a pep talk or some counseling by friends, another attempt is made, this time with a diet "guaranteed" to work! The cycle continues, usually with the same results—the dieter has not changed appreciably in appearance and is still overfat.

Eat healthful foods but in smaller amounts. For weight loss, it is generally unwise to follow some packaged exotic diet plan in a popular book or magazine. Instead, dieters should eat well-balanced meals but in smaller quantities.

WELL BALANCED BUT LESS OF IT

A calorie-counting approach to weight loss should provide a well-balanced diet containing all of the essential nutrients. The general recommendation is that reducing diets should contain the RDA for the micronutrients and protein with reduced amounts of cholesterol and saturated fats and the remainder consisting predominantly of unrefined, fiber-rich, complex carbohydrates. *Calories do count*; the trick is to keep within the daily limit specified by the rate of fat loss desired. Recall from the previous section that our daily energy expenditure is largely determined by two factors: the resting energy requirement, and the energy expended in daily physical activities. As long as a diet is nutritionally sound, it really is not important what we eat, but rather how many calories are consumed. If a true caloric deficit exists and input is less than output, weight loss will occur independent of the diet's composition of carbohydrate, lipid, or protein. When obese patients consumed either a high-fat or high-carbohydrate 800 kcal diet, weight loss for both groups was nearly identical, as was the percentage of fat lost during a 10-day period. During weight loss, the initial decrease in body mass occurs primarily from water loss and some depletion of carbohydrate reserves. As the diet progresses, a larger amount of body fat is metabolized to make up the energy deficit created by dieting.

There are no magic potions. There is simply no compelling evidence that popular "fad" diets have any advantage over a calorically restricted, well-balanced diet. No magic metabolic mixture will assure more effective weight loss than can be achieved with a well-balanced, low-calorie diet.

Consult a knowledgeable professional for assistance. A professional with expertise in nutrition, exercise, and the energetics of weight control should be consulted if planning a diet that deviates from the recommended low-calorie but well-balanced meal plan. Check out credentials carefully. Remember, some fancy-looking diplomas of "weight counselors" can be purchased through mail order!

USING THE COMPUTERIZED MEAL PLAN AND EXERCISE APPROACH

The computerized meal and exercise plan discussed in Chapter 10 and illustrated in Appendix D is an alternative weight loss method for combining diet with exercise. The projected weight loss curve provides a picture of the progress likely to be made if a person follows the nutrition and exercise recommendations. As we point out in Chapter 17, it is crucial to modify both eating and exercise behaviors if positive and permanent changes are to occur in body size and composition. The weight loss curve on the computer printout is not a straight line, but rather is curvilinear to account for changes that generally occur in metabolism and body composition as the individual progresses through the program.

There are three major advantages to using a computer in the diet and exercise prescription.

1. Because meal plans are based on the dietary exchange method, a person's preferred foods can easily be substituted within a given meal to offer tremendous variety in planning daily menus. This flexibility maintains nutritional adequacy of meals and assures constancy to the recommended caloric intake.
2. The difference between the computer meal plan for dieting and the myriad of "typical diets" is that the computer plan allows direct participation in creating well-balanced meals. It is unnecessary to follow a preset selection of foods, often drawn up by some self-appointed "expert." People who actively participate in their meal planning are much more likely to remain with the program. A person who choses to eat a particular food probably will; having to eat disliked foods as part of a diet regimen is negative reinforcement and usually leads to failure. The same is true for exercise. If a plan calls for jogging and the person passionately dislikes it, what are the chances of keeping active? Slim of course. We all know men and women who refuse to exercise regularly because they have been led to believe that prolonged running is the only beneficial exercise. With a choice of activities and an appropriate starting level, the chances are excellent for rapid progress. To this end, the computer stands ready with its variety of choices.
3. The computerized exercise prescription allows a person to change activities and still use about the same recommended number of calories. For example, if it rains and jogging is impractical, the computer printout offers alternatives such as swimming, circuit-training, cycling, or racquetball. The example in the Appendix shows the caloric equivalence between walking, swimming, cycling, and nine sports activities. Without a computer, such calculations would require hundreds of hours, particularly because the exercise output is matched to the diet plan and both are individualized to the participant's weight loss goals.

EXERCISING TO TIP THE ENERGY BALANCE EQUATION

The precise contributions of sedentary living and excessive caloric intake to obesity are not clearly understood. What is clear is that an increased level of daily physical activity can impact significantly on energy balance.

NOT SIMPLY A PROBLEM OF GLUTTONY

In the past, it was generally accepted that obesity was the result of excessive food intake. Clearly, then, the proper approach to weight loss would be some form of caloric restriction by dieting. This view of obesity is overly simplistic, as available evidence indicates that excess weight gain often parallels reduced physical activity rather than an increase in energy intake. In fact, among active young and middle-aged endurance-trained men, body fat was inversely related to energy expenditure; no relationship existed between body fat and food consumption. Among the physically active, those who eat the most often weigh the least and are the most fit! In the United States, per capita caloric intake has steadily decreased over the past 80 years, yet body mass and body fat have slowly increased. Americans now eat 5 to 10% fewer calories than they did 20 years ago, yet they weigh an average of 2.3 kg more. Certainly, if food consumption were the culprit, this reduction in caloric intake should bring the national body mass to a lower, not higher level!

> **Gluttony is not the culprit.** One is hard pressed for evidence that groups of overweight men and women actually eat more, on average, than people of normal weight.

This pattern holds for children too. Obese infants do not characteristically consume more calories than the recommended dietary standards. Infant offspring of obese parents often have lower resting metabolism and less spontaneous movements than infants of normal-weight parents. This suggests that subdued movement patterns are abnormal and may reflect an inherited characteristic. Time-in-motion photography to document activity patterns of elementary school students clearly showed that overweight children were considerably less active than their normal-weight peers, and their excess weight was not related to food intake. The caloric intake of obese high school girls and boys was actually below that of their nonobese peers. This observation that fat people often eat the same or even less than thinner ones is also true for adults over a broad age range as they become less active and slowly begin to add weight. Consequently, reducing caloric intake is inappropriate as the only method to combat the overfat condition.

> **TV watching the #1 activity.** Sports participation declines steadily throughout the teen years. In one survey, "watching TV" was the highest scoring activity among all teenage groups, rating 87% among 18-year olds.

INCREASED ENERGY OUTPUT IS WORTH CONSIDERING

It is increasingly clear that men and women of all ages who maintain a physically active lifestyle or become involved in aerobic exercise programs maintain a desirable level of body composition. Increased caloric output with exercise provides a significant option for unbalancing the energy balance equation. Only recently, however, has this approach to bring about desirable weight loss and body composition changes come into prominence. Two arguments have generally been raised against the exercise option. One is the belief that exercise inevitably increases the appetite so that any caloric deficit is rapidly made up by proportionately greater food intake. The second argument is that the calorie-burning effects of exercise are so small that a reasonable use of exercise would only "dent" the body's fat reserves compared to using starvation or semistarvation. Let's take a closer look at these two misconceptions.

> **Exercise does not always stimulate appetite.** Short-term increases in physical activity do not always increase caloric intake in proportion to the calories expended during exercise. In fact, some individuals show no increase in food intake with moderate daily exercise.

Effects of Exercise on Food Intake.

Sedentary people do not always maintain a fine balance between energy expenditure and food intake. For them, the daily caloric intake generally exceeds their low energy requirement. This lack of precision in regulating food intake at the low end of the physical activity spectrum may account

> **Balance between energy intake and energy expenditure.** Regular physical activity contributes to the normal functioning of the brain's feeding control mechanisms to bring about a balance between energy intake and energy expenditure.

for the "creeping obesity" common in highly mechanized and technically advanced societies. On the other hand, for individuals who regularly exercise, appetite control is in a "reactive zone" where it is simpler to match food intake with daily energy expenditure.

In considering the **effects of exercise on appetite and food intake,** a distinction must be made between the type and duration of exercise. There is no question that lumberjacks, farm laborers, and certain athletes who regularly perform hard physical labor often consume about twice the daily calories (4000 to 6000 kcal) as more sedentary people (2000 to 3000 kcal). Endurance athletes such as marathon runners, cross-country skiiers, and cyclists consume about 4000 to 5000 kcal daily, yet these men and women are among the leanest in the world. Obviously, this extreme food intake is required just to meet the energy demands of training!

Effects of Exercise on Energy Expenditure. The second misconception concerns the number of calories expended through regular exercise—the idea that a person must perform an inordinate amount of exercise to lose body fat. We have all heard the statistics that a person has to chop wood for 10 hours, golf for 20 hours, perform mild calisthenics for 22 hours, play ping-pong for 28 hours or volleyball for 32 hours, or run 35 miles just to reduce body fat by 0.45 kg. Understandably, such a commitment is overwhelming to the overweight person who plans to reduce by 10 or 15 kg or more. Looking at it from a different perspective, however, if a person played golf only 2 hours (about 350 kcal per day) for 2 days a week (700 kcal), it would take about 5 weeks, or 10 golfing days, to lose 0.45 kg of fat (3500 kcal). Assuming golf was played year-round, golfing 2 days a week would result in a 4.5 kg loss of fat during the year provided food intake remained fairly constant. While most of us would probably not play golf this frequently (nor are we likely to play golf for 20 consecutive hours), the point is that *the calorie-expending effects of exercise are cumulative:* a caloric deficit of 3500 kcal is equivalent to a 0.45 kg fat loss whether it occurs rapidly or systematically over time.

The caloric expenditure values for the physical activities presented in Appendix A should not be considered absolute. These are "average" values, applicable under "average" conditions when applied to the "average" person of a given body mass. However, these values do provide a good approximation of energy expenditure and are useful in establishing the caloric cost of an exercise program.

Just a small but regular excess can add up to quite a bit. For a person who originally weighs 120 kg (263 lb), an intake of only 218 extra calories daily for 22 years could result in a body mass of 340 kg, or 748 lb!

Energy expenditure values are "averages." Understandably, a wide range of values for energy expenditure in a specific activity is possible because of individual differences in performance style and technique as well as the intensity of participation, and because of environmental factors such as terrain, temperature, and wind resistance.

It's what's burned during exercise that counts. With moderate exercise as performed by most people for weight control, the contribution of recovery metabolism—the so-called afterglow—to total energy expenditure is probably quite small because recovery from such exercise is rapid.

The fatter you are, the more you'll lose. The effectiveness of exercise for weight loss is linked to the degree of obesity at the start.

EXERCISE IS EFFECTIVE

Regular aerobic exercise, with or without dietary restriction, brings about favorable changes in body mass and body composition. Even conventional resistance training combined with caloric restriction results in maintenance of lean body mass compared to a weight loss program that relies exclusively on dieting. As a general rule, persons who are obese lose weight and fat more readily through exercising than do their normal-weight counterparts. In addition, exercise provides significant positive "spin-off" because it alters body composition (reduced fat with maintenance or even small increase in lean tissue) in such a way that the resting metabolism is maintained or even increased. This reduces the body's tendency to store calories.

A person planning to exercise for weight control should consider factors such as frequency, intensity, and duration as well as the specific form of exercise. Ideal activities are continuous, big muscle aerobic activities that have a moderate to high caloric cost, such as walking, running, rope skipping, cycling, and swimming. Many recreational sports and games are also effective in reducing body mass, although precise quantification of energy expenditure is difficult during such activities. These aerobic exercises burn considerable calories, stimulate lipid metabolism, reduce body fat, establish favorable blood pressure responses, and generally promote cardiovascular fitness. An extra 300 kcal expended with moderate jogging daily for 30 minutes causes a 0.45 kg fat loss in about 12 days. Over a year's time, this theoretically represents a total caloric deficit equivalent to about 13.6 kg (30 lb) of body fat!

There's no one "best" aerobic exercise. There is generally no selective effect of running, walking, or bicycling; each is equally effective in altering body composition, provided the duration, frequency, and intensity of exercise are similar.

A Dose-Response Relationship. A direct **dose-response relationship** has been demonstrated between weight loss and time spent exercising. In fact, the total energy expended is probably the most important factor that influences the effectiveness of an exercise program for weight loss. Thus, an overfat person who begins exercising lightly with slow walking, for example, can accrue a considerable caloric expenditure simply by extending the *duration* of the exercise. This effect of duration offsets the inability (and inadvisability) of a previously sedentary, obese person beginning an exercise program at high intensity. Furthermore, because the energy cost of weight-bearing exercise such as walking is proportional to body mass, the overweight person expends considerably more calories to perform these tasks as someone of normal weight.

The importance of exercise duration for weight loss was illustrated in a study of three groups of men who exercised for 20 weeks by walking and running for either 15, 30, or 45 minutes per session. Compared to a sedentary control group, the three exercise groups significantly decreased their total body fat, fatfolds, and waist girth. When comparisons were made between the three groups, the 45-minute training group lost more body fat than either the 30- or 15-minute group. This was directly attributed to the greater caloric expenditure of the longer exercise period.

Start Slowly. A person beginning an exercise program for weight loss should adopt long-term goals, exert personal discipline, and restructure both eating and exercise behaviors. It is often counterproductive to include unduly rapid training progressions because many obese men and women initially are psychologically resistant to physical training. During the first few weeks, slow walking is replaced by intervals of walking and jogging that eventually lead to continuous jogging. Allow at least 6 to 8 weeks for observable changes to occur. Behavioral approaches should also be applied to cause meaningful lifestyle changes that will increase physical activity (see Chapter 17). For example, walking or bicycling can replace use of the auto, stair climbing can replace the elevator, and manual tools can replace power tools.

Begin slowly and progress steadily. The initial stage of an exercise program for a previously sedentary, overfat person should be developmental in nature and should aim toward achieving a high total energy expenditure during workouts.

Table 16–2 shows the effectiveness of regular exercise for weight loss. In this study, 6 sedentary, obese young men exercised 5 days a week for 16 weeks by walking for 90 minutes at each session. The men lost nearly 6 kg of body fat; this represented a decrease in body fat from 23.5 to 18.6%. In addition, physical fitness and work capacity improved, as did the level of high-density lipoprotein (15.6%) and the high- to low-density lipoprotein ratio (25.9%).

TABLE 16–2. CHANGES IN BODY COMPOSITION AND BLOOD LIPIDS IN 6 OBESE YOUNG ADULT MEN DURING A 16-WEEK WALKING PROGRAM

VARIABLE	PRE-TRAINING*	POST-TRAINING	DIFFERENCE
Body mass, kg	99.1	93.4	−5.7†
Body density, g/ml	1.044	1.056	+0.012†
Body fat, %	23.5	18.6	−4.9†
Fat mass, kg	23.3	17.4	−5.9†
Lean body mass, kg	75.8	76.0	+0.2
Sum of fatfolds, mm	142.9	104.8	−38.1†
HDL cholesterol, mg/100 ml	32.0	37.0	+5.0†
HDL/LDL cholesterol	0.27	0.34	+0.07†

* Values are means.
† Statistically significant.
Source: From Leon, A.S., et al.: Effects of a vigorous walking program on body composition, and carbohydrate and lipid metabolism of obese young men. *Am. J. Clin. Nutr.*, 33:1776, 1979.

The more you become active, the more calories you'll burn. Exercise frequency is important when considering exercise for weight loss.

Regularity Is the Key. Based on available research, it appears that at least 3 days of training per week is required to bring about favorable body weight changes through exercise. More frequent exercise is even more effective. This frequency effect is most likely the direct result of the added calories burned by the extra exercise. *Although it is difficult to precisely determine a threshold energy expenditure for weight and fat loss, the calorie-burning effect of each exercise session should be at least 300 kcal.* This can be achieved with 30 minutes of moderate to vigorous running, swimming, or bicycling, or less intense walking for at least 60 minutes.

DIET PLUS EXERCISE

Combine diet and exercise for best results. Regular aerobic exercise plus reduced food intake increases fat loss, improves distribution of body fat, and conserves lean body mass. An additional bonus is that regular exercise is associated with a decrease in blood pressure, a more favorable lipoprotein profile, and improved carbohydrate metabolism.

A negative caloric balance produced by either food restriction or exercise can cause desirable modifications in both body mass and percent body fat. Certainly, combinations of exercise and diet offer considerably more flexibility for achieving a negative caloric balance than either exercise alone or diet alone. Adding regular exercise to the program of weight control facilitates a more permanent fat loss than does total reliance on caloric restriction.

If weight reduction is attempted only by reducing food intake, then one must consider how many calories to consume. While there are no hard and fast rules, considerable experimental and clinical data show that adverse psychological changes can occur if caloric intake is reduced too severely over an extended period. In addition, prolonged dieting increases the chances of developing a variety of nutritional deficiencies. A prudent alternative is to blend diet with exercise. Certainly it is easier to create a daily caloric deficit of 1000 kcal by combining diet and exercise than using either one alone.

Most nutrition experts agree that a loss in body fat of up to 0.9 kg (2 lb) *each week* is within acceptable limits, although a steady 0.5 to 1.0 lb a week loss may be even more desirable. This guideline for an **acceptable limit of weight loss** is partially based on the observation that people who have been successful losing weight lost no more than about 0.9 kg a week during the period of caloric deficit.

Setting a Target Time. Suppose the target time selected to achieve a 9 kg (20 lb) fat loss is 20 weeks. The average weekly deficit must therefore be 3500 kcal; the daily caloric deficit is then 500 kcal (3500 ÷ 7). To achieve this deficit by dieting, daily caloric intake must be reduced by 500 kcal. Remember, this level of caloric restriction needs to be maintained for 5 months to achieve the desired fat loss of 0.45 kg per week or 9 kg total. However, if the dieter performed a half hour of moderate exercise equivalent to 350 "extra" kcal 3 days a week, then the weekly caloric output would increase by 1050 kcal (3 days per week × 350 kcal per exercise session). With this additional exercise, the caloric restriction necessary to lose 0.45 kg of fat each week would now only have to reach 2450 kcal instead of 3500. The additional 1050 kcal is "burned" during the weekly exercise. Instead of excluding 500 kcal from the daily diet, the caloric intake need only be reduced by 350 kcal, because the daily contribution of exercise averages 150 kcal (1050 kcal per week ÷ 7). If the same exercise were undertaken 5 days a week, the daily food intake could be increased an additional 100 calories and the 0.45 kg per week fat loss would still be attained. If the duration of the 5 day per week workouts was extended from 30 minutes to 1 hour, then *no reduction* in food intake would be necessary to lose weight, because the required 3500 kcal deficit would be created entirely through extra physical activity.

If the intensity of the 1-hour exercise performed 5 days a week was then increased by only 10% (cycling at 22 instead of 20 miles per hour, running a mile in 9 instead of 10 minutes, swimming each 50 yards in 54 seconds instead of 60 seconds), the number of exercise calories burned each week would increase an additional 350 kcal (3500 kcal/wk × 10%). This new weekly deficit of 3850 kcal, or 550 kcal per day, would actually permit the dieter to increase daily food intake by 50 calories and still lose a pound of fat each week!

Exercise keeps muscle and burns fat. Exercise provides a protein-sparing effect that causes a greater portion of the caloric deficit to be made up from the breakdown of body fat.

Clearly, physical activity can be used effectively by itself or in combination with mild dietary restriction to trigger weight loss. Perhaps equally important, the feelings of intense hunger and other psychological stress may be minimal compared with a similar weight loss program that relies exclusively on food restriction. Furthermore, exercise protects against the usual lean tissue loss when weight reduction is achieved by diet alone. **Lean tissue is preserved** because regular exercise enhances the breakdown of fat from the body's adipose depots. In addition, exercise increases protein buildup in skeletal muscle, while at the same time retarding its rate of breakdown.

OPTIMAL DURATION OF AN EXERCISE PLUS DIET PROGRAM

Figure 16–4 shows the composition of the average daily weight loss for water, protein, and fat that occurred during 24 days of a low-calorie diet consisting of 1000 kcal of carbohydrates per day. In addition to caloric restriction, all subjects exercised daily for 2.5 hours in a prescribed activity program. During the first 3 days, water loss represented 70% of the weight loss. The contribution of water to weight loss became progressively less as the program continued, and during days 11 to 13, water loss represented only 19% of the weight lost. In addition, the proportion of fat loss increased from 25 to 69% during this period. From days 21 to 24, 85% of the weight loss occurred by a reduction in body fat with no corresponding increase

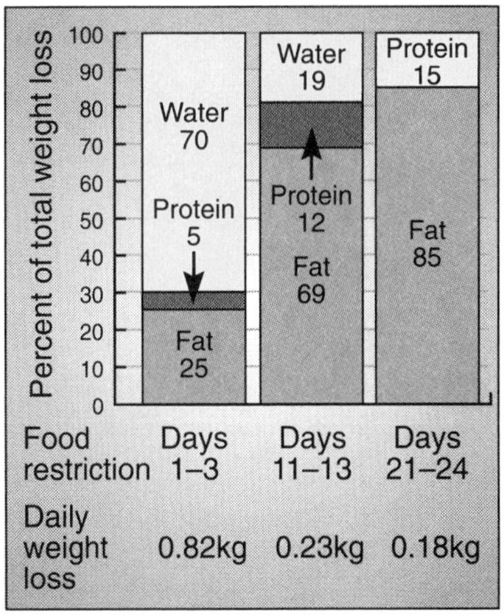

FIG. 16–4. Percentage composition of weight loss at the start, middle, and end of 24 days of food restriction (1000 kcal per day) plus enforced exercise of 2.5 hours per day. (From Grande, F.: Nutrition and energy balance in body composition studies. In Techniques for Measuring Body Composition. Washington, DC, National Academy of Sciences–National Research Council, 1961.)

Drink plenty of fluids. It is important to consume adequate fluid while dieting. The total amount of fat lost during weight reduction, however, is the same regardless of the quantity of fluid ingested.

in water loss. The percentage of weight loss from protein increased from 5% initially to 12% during days 11 to 13, and to 15% by the end of the period of caloric restriction.

Figure 16–5 illustrates the important concept that the caloric equivalent of weight loss increases with the duration of caloric restriction. *This is why it is so important to maintain a caloric deficit for an extended period; dieting for short duration results in a larger percentage of water and carbohydrate loss per unit of weight reduction with only a minimal decrease in body fat.*

SUMMARY OF RESULTS ON CALORIC IMBALANCE

The results of the prior studies that have evaluated various approaches to establish a caloric imbalance can be summarized as follows:

- Exercise combined with dietary restriction is a more effective approach for achieving a long-term negative caloric balance as compared with exercise or diet alone.

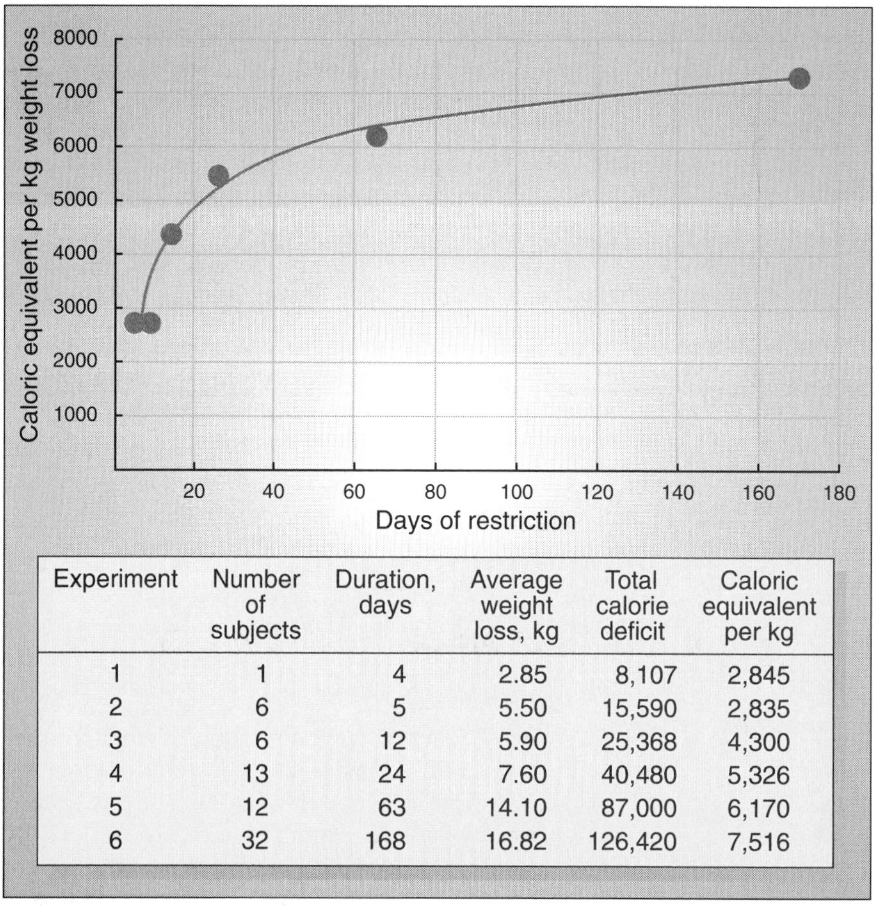

Experiment	Number of subjects	Duration, days	Average weight loss, kg	Total calorie deficit	Caloric equivalent per kg
1	1	4	2.85	8,107	2,845
2	6	5	5.50	15,590	2,835
3	6	12	5.90	25,368	4,300
4	13	24	7.60	40,480	5,326
5	12	63	14.10	87,000	6,170
6	32	168	16.82	126,420	7,516

FIG. 16–5. Caloric equivalent of weight loss in relation to the duration of caloric restriction. Each data point represents an experiment as summarized in the accompanying box. (Adapted from Grande, F.: Nutrition and energy balance in body composition studies. In Techniques for Measuring Body Composition. Washington, DC, National Academy of Sciences–National Research Council, 1961.)

- During the first few days of weight reduction, the rapid weight loss is due primarily to loss in body water and carbohydrate; longer periods of weight reduction are associated with a substantially greater loss of fat per unit of weight loss.
- Water intake should not be restricted when beginning weight reduction because this can precipitate dehydration with no additional fat loss.
- Undesirable psychological and medically related problems may occur with prolonged caloric restriction maintained below minimal energy requirements.
- Weight loss by diet alone causes significant loss of muscle mass. Exercise protects against lean tissue losses; thus, more of the weight lost is fat.

A RADICAL APPROACH: A CHALLENGE TO EXERCISE AND HEALTH PROFESSIONALS

If exercise is to play a key role in weight control, it seems logical that dramatically more exercise must be prescribed if there is to be a real chance at permanent weight loss. We believe strongly that such an approach should be tried. We propose that 7 days a week of aerobic exercise of at least 1 hour duration be performed as the **ultimate "exercise prescription" for weight control.** We think this has a chance to work without even adhering to a reduced caloric intake! An analogy akin to a medical prescription is germane. If a physician prescribes medication three times daily for 6 weeks, then that is what one should do if treatment is to succeed. The same reasoning should hold for a weight control prescription. Three days a week of 30 minutes per session, even if performed strenuously, may be too low a "dose." The challenge to the exercise and health professional who deals intimately with various aspects of weight control is to prescribe large doses of exercise and see to it that the prescription is followed. Naturally, such large doses should be led up to gradually, proceeding from sensible and obtainable goals at the start of a program until the body can tolerate more exercise. At present, there is no research that can lend validity to our assertions concerning such an "aggressive" approach compared to conventional methods. However, the conventional methods have thus far not been too successful. Carefully controlled studies with long-term follow-up would ultimately prove or disprove the effectiveness of this radical approach to weight control.

SUMMARY

1. Long-term weight control through dietary restriction generally is unsuccessful for the major number of participants in such programs.
2. There are three ways to unbalance the energy balance equation and bring about weight loss: reduce caloric intake below daily energy expenditure, maintain regular food intake and increase energy output, and combine both methods by decreasing food intake and increasing energy expenditure.
3. A caloric deficit of 3500 kcal created through either diet or exercise is the equivalent to the calories in 1 lb (0.45 kg) of adipose tissue.

4. Dieting for weight loss can be effective if done properly. The disadvantages of semistarvation, however, are significant and include loss of lean body tissue, lethargy, possible malnutrition and metabolic disorders, and decrease in the basal energy expenditure. Some of these factors actually conserve energy and cause the diet to be less effective.
5. Repeated cycles of weight loss and weight gain cause the body to increase its ability to conserve energy. This ultimately leads to greater difficulty in achieving weight loss with subsequent dieting, and makes regaining the lost weight easier.
6. The calorie-expending effects of exercise are cumulative, so that a little exercise performed routinely has a dramatic effect over time. The role of exercise in appetite suppression or stimulation is unclear. Over time, most athletes eventually consume enough calories to counterbalance caloric expenditure—but many of these athletes are the leanest in the world.
7. Combinations of exercise and diet offer a flexible and effective approach to weight control. Exercise enhances the mobilization and utilization of fat, thus increasing loss of fat mass, and at the same time retards lean tissue loss.
8. The rapid weight loss during the first few days of caloric deficit is due primarily to loss in body water and carbohydrate. Continued weight reduction is associated with a greater loss of fat per unit of weight loss.

RELATED READINGS

Alban, H.J., et al.: Metabolic response to low- and very-low-calorie diets. *Am. J. Clin. Nutr.*, 49:745, 1989.

American College of Sports Medicine: Position statement on proper and improper weight loss programs. *Med. Sci. Sports Exerc.*, 15(1):1X, 1983.

American Medical Association: A critique of low-carbohydrate ketogenic weight reduction regimens (a review of Dr. Atkins' Diet Revolution). *JAMA*, 224:1418, 1978.

Atkinson, R.L., and Pi-Sunyer, F.X.: Very-low-calorie diets. *Am. J. Clin. Nutr.*, S56, 175S, 1992.

Ballor, D.L., et al.: Resistance weight training during caloric restriction enhances lean body weight maintenance. *Am. J. Clin. Nutr.*, 47:19, 1988.

Baron, J.A., et al.: A randomized controlled trial of low carbohydrate and low fat/high fiber diets for weight loss. *Am. J. Publ. Health*, 76:1293, 1986.

Blackburn, G.L., et al.: The very-low-calorie diet: a weight reduction technique. In: Handbook of Eating Disorders. Edited by K.D. Brownell and J.P. Foreyt. New York, Basic Books, 1986.

Blackburn, G.L., et al.: Weight cycling: the experience of human dieters. *Am. J. Clin. Nutr.*, 49:1105, 1989.

Bouchard, C., et al.: Long-term exercise training with constant energy intake. In: Effect on body composition and selected metabolic variables. *Int. J. Obesity*, 14:57, 1990.

Brownell, K.D., et al.: The effects of repeated cycles of weight loss and regain in rats. *Physiol. Behav.*, 38:459, 1986.

Brownell, K.D., et al.: Weight regulation practices in athletes: analysis of metabolic and health effects. *Med. Sci. Sports Exerc.*, 19:546, 1987.

Bullen, B.A., et al.: Physical activity of obese and non-obese adolescent girls appraised by motion picture sampling. *Am. J. Clin. Nutr.*, 14:211, 1964.

Buono, M.J., et al.: Effects of a diet and exercise program on blood lipids, cardiorespiratory function, and body composition in obese women. *Med. Sci. Sports Exerc.*, 17:189, 1985.

Cyborski, C.K.: Deaths associated with the protein-sparing fast. *JAMA*, 239:971, 1978.

Donohoe, C.T., Jr., et al.: Metabolic consequences of dieting and exercise in the treatment of obesity. *J. Consult. Clin. Psychol.*, 52:829, 1984.

Drenick, E.J., and Johnson, D.: Therapeutic fasting in morbid obesity—long term follow-up. *Arch. Intern. Med.*, 137:1381, 1977.

Dullo, A.G., and Girardier, L.: Adaptive changes in energy expenditure during refeeding following low-calorie intake: evidence for a specific metabolic component favoring fat storage. *Am. J. Clin. Nutr.*, 52:415, 1990.

Elliot, D.L., et al.: Sustained depression of the resting metabolic rate after massive weight loss. *Am. J. Clin. Nutr.*, 49:93, 1989.

Epstein, L.H., and Wing, R.R.: Aerobic exercise and weight. *Addictive Behaviors*, 5:371, 1980.

Frank, A., et al.: Fatalities on the liquid-protein diet: an analysis of possible causes. *Int. J. Obesity*, 5:243, 1981.

Grande, F.: Nutrition and energy balance in body composition studies. In: Techniques for Measuring Body Composition. Washington, DC, National Academy of Sciences–National Research Council, 1961.

Herring, J.L., et al.: Effect of suspending exercise training on resting metabolic rate in women. *Med. Sci. Sport Exerc.*, 24:59, 1992.

Hill, J.O., et al.: Effects of exercise and food restriction on body composition and metabolic rates in obese women. *Am. J. Clin. Nutr.*, 46:622, 1987.

Innes, J.A., et al.: Long term follow-up of therapeutic starvation. *Br. Med. J.*, 2:356, 1974.

Isner, J.M., et al.: Sudden unexpected death in avid dieters using the liquid-protein-modified fast. *Circulation*, 60:1401, 1979.

Johnson, M.L., et al.: Relative importance of inactivity and overeating in energy balance in obese high school girls. *Am. J. Clin. Nutr.*, 44:779, 1986.

Karvonen, M.J., et al.: Consumption and selection of food in competitive lumber work. *J. Appl. Physiol.*, 6:603, 1954.

Katch, F.I., et al.: Effects of physical training on the body composition and diet of females. *Res. Q.*, 40:99, 1969.

Kern, P.A., et al.: The effects of weight loss on the activity and expression of adipose-tissue lipoprotein lipase in very obese humans. *N. Engl. J. Med.*, 322:1053, 1990.

Kessey, R.E.: A set-point theory of obesity. In: Handbook of Eating Disorders. Edited by K.D. Brownell and J.P. Foreyt. New York, Basic Books, 1986.

Keys, A., et al.: The Biology of Human Starvation. Minneapolis, University of Minnesota Press, 1970.

King, M.A., and Katch, F.I.: Changes in body density, fatfolds, and girths at 2.3 kg increments of weight loss. *Hum. Biol.*, 58:709, 1986.

Kissileff, H.R., et al.: Acute effects of exercise on food intake in obese and nonobese women. *Am. J. Clin. Nutr.*, 52:240, 1990.

Krotkiewski, M., et al.: Increased muscle dynamic endurance associated with weight reduction on a very-low-calorie diet. *Am. J. Clin. Nutr.*, 51:321, 1990.

Lambert, O., and Hansen, E.S.: Effects of excessive caloric intake and caloric restriction on body weight and energy expenditure at rest and light exercise. *Acta Physiol. Scand.*, 114:135, 1982.

Leon, A.S., et al.: Effects of a vigorous walking program on body composition, and carbohydrate and lipid metabolism of obese young men. *Am. J. Clin. Nutr.*, 32:1776, 1979.

Lissner, L., et al.: Variability of body weight and health outcomes in the Framingham population. *N. Engl. J. Med.*, 324:1839, 1991.

Manore, M.M., et al.: Energy expenditure at rest and during exercise in nonobese female cyclical dieters and in nondieting control subjects. *Am. J. Clin. Nutr.*, 54:41, 1991.

McArdle, W.D., and Magel, J.R.: Weight management: diet and exercise. In: The Medical Aspects of Clinical Nutrition. Edited by J. Bland and N. Shealy. New Canaan, CT, Keats, 1983.

McArdle, W.D., and Toner, M.M.: Application of exercise for weight control: the exercise prescription. In: Eating Disorders Handbook: Complete Guide to Understanding and Treatment, edited by R. Frankle and M.-U. Yang. Rockville, MD, Aspen Publishers, 1988.

Meredith, C.N., et al.: Body composition and aerobic capacity in young and middle-aged endurance-trained men. *Med. Sci. Sports Exerc.*, 19:557, 1987.

Miller, W.C., et al.: Diet composition, energy intake, and exercise in relation to body fat in men and women. *Am. J. Clin. Nutr.*, 52:426, 1990.

Mirkin, G.B., and Shore, R.N.: The Beverly Hills diet: dangers of the newest weight loss fad. *JAMA*, 246:2235, 1981.

Molé, P.A., et al.: Exercise versus depressed metabolic rate produced by severe caloric restriction. *Med. Sci. Sports Exerc.*, 21:29, 1989.

Moyer, C.L., et al.: Body composition changes in obese women on a very low calorie diet with and without exercise. *Med. Sci. Sports Exerc.*, 17:292, 1985.

Newmark, S.R., and Williamson, B.: Survey of very-low-calorie weight reduction diets: I. Novelty diets. *Arch. Intern. Med.*, 143:1195, 1983.
Newmark, S.R., and Williamson, B.: Survey of very-low-calorie weight reduction diets: II. Total fasting, protein-sparing modified fasts, chemically defined diets. *Arch. Intern. Med.*, 143:1423, 1983.
Pavlov, K.N., et al.: Exercise as an adjunct to weight loss and maintenance in moderately obese subjects. *Am. J. Clin. Nutr.*, 49:1115, 1989.
Pi-Sunyer, F.X.: Exercise in the treatment of obesity. In: Obesity and Weight Control. Edited by R.T. Frankle and M.-V. Yang. Rockville, MD, Aspen Publishers, 1988.
Pollock, M.L., et al.: Effects of mode of training on cardiovascular function and body composition of adult men. *Med. Sci. Sports*, 7:139, 1975.
Rodin, J., et al.: Weight cycling and fat distribution. *Int. J. Obesity*, 14:303, 1990.
Rolland-Cachera, M.F., and Bellisle, F.: No correlation between adiposity and food intake: why are working class children fatter? *Am. J. Clin. Nutr.*, 44:779, 1986.
Rosen, L.W., and Hough, D.O.: Pathogenic weight-control behaviors of female college gymnasts. *Phys. Sportsmed.*, 16:141, 1988.
Sims, E.A.H., and Danforth, E., Jr.: Expenditure and storage of energy in man (perspective). *J. Clin. Invest.*, 79:1019, 1987.
Slattery, M.L., and Jacobs, D.R., Jr.: The interrelationships of physical activity, physical fitness, and body measurements. *Med. Sci. Sports Exerc.*, 19:564, 1987.
Sours, H.E., et al.: Sudden death associated with very low caloric weight reduction regimens. *Am. J. Clin. Nutr.*, 34:453, 1981.
Staten, M.A.: The effect of exercise on food intake in men and women. *Am. J. Clin. Nutr.*, 53:27, 1991.
Thompson, D.A., et al.: Acute effects of exercise intensity on appetite in young men. *Med. Sci. Sports Exerc.*, 20:227, 1988.
Thornton, J.S.: Feast or famine: eating disorders in athletes. *Phys. Sportsmed.*, 18:116, 1990.
Trembly, A., et al.: The effect of exercise training on resting metabolic rate in lean and moderately obese individuals. *Int. J. Obesity*, 10:511, 1986.
Trembly, A., et al.: Exercise training with constant energy intake. 2: Effect on glucose metabolism and resting energy expenditure. *Int. J. Obesity*, 14:75, 1990.
Troisi, R.J., et al.: Cigarette smoking, dietary intake, and physical activity: effects on body fat distribution—the Normative Aging Study. *Am. J. Clin. Nutr.*, 53:1104, 1991.
Van Dale, D., and Saris, W.H.M.: Repetitive weight loss and weight regain: effects on weight reduction, resting metabolic rate, and lipolytic activity before and after exercise and/or diet treatment. *Am. J. Clin. Nutr.*, 49:409, 1989.
Van Dale, D., et al.: Weight maintenance and resting metabolic rate 18–40 months after a diet/exercise treatment. *Int. J. Obesity*, 14:347, 1990.
Wadden, T.A.: Very low calorie diets: their efficacy, safety, and future. *Ann. Intern. Med.*, 99:675, 1983.
Wadden, T.A., et al.: Long-term effects of dieting on resting metabolic rate in obese outpatients. *JAMA*, 264:707, 1990.
Weissman, C., et al.: Semistarvation and exercise. *J. Appl. Physiol.*, 60:2035, 1986.
Welle, S.L.: Some metabolic effects of overeating in man. *Am. J. Clin. Nutr.*, 44:718, 1986.
Williamson, D.F., et al.: Smoking cessation and severity of weight gain in a national cohort. *N. Engl. J. Med.*, 324:739, 1991.
Wilmore, J.H.: Appetite and body composition consequent to physical activity. *Res. Q. Exerc. Sport.*, 54:415, 1983.
Woo, R., et al.: Voluntary food intake during prolonged exercise in obese women. *Am. J. Clin. Nutr.*, 36:478, 1982.
Young, J.C., et al.: Prior exercise potentiates the thermic effect of a carbohydrate load. *Metabolism*, 35:1048, 1986.
Zuti, W.B., and Golding, L.A.: Comparing diet and exercise as weight reduction tools. *Phys. Sportsmed.*, 4:49, 1976.

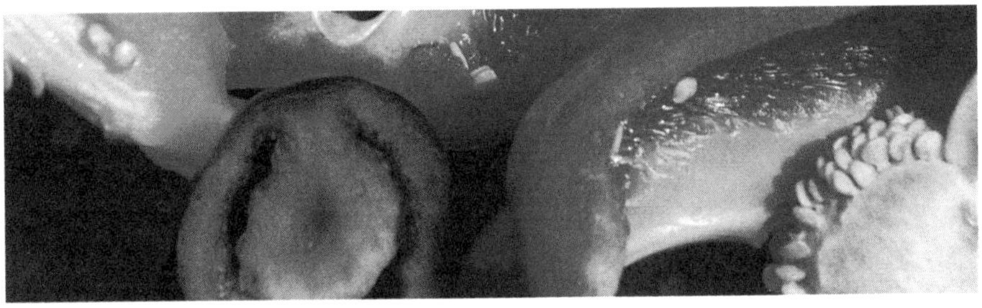

17

MODIFICATION OF EATING AND EXERCISE BEHAVIORS

The human organism is remarkably adaptable. People can modify existing food and exercise behavior patterns as long as they establish a clear-cut need for change and see a good possibility for success. One of the techniques to alter behavior is referred to by psychologists as behavior therapy or **behavior modification.** This approach helps the person to identify, control, and modify undesirable behaviors so they become desirable.

An example of the application of behavior modification is the treatment of **anorexia nervosa** and **bulimia nervosa.** These disordered eating behaviors occur mostly in young women and are associated with severe psychological problems.

In one study, women hospitalized for treatment of anorexia nervosa were found to walk an average of 11 km (7 miles) around the hospital compared to a distance of 8 km (5 miles) walked by women of normal body weight living at home. This hyperactivity was used as the behavioral modifier to induce patients to eat and subsequently gain weight. For example, patients were permitted to walk only if they made a daily weight gain. Any time the patient's body mass was at least 0.22 kg above that of the previous day, she was allowed 6 hours of unrestricted activity outside the hospital.

Within 1 week, significant improvement was noted. On average, body mass increased 1.8 kg per week during the 6 weeks of hospitalization.

Warning signs of disordered eating behaviors*

Anorexia nervosa

- Preoccupation with being too fat
- Ritualistic concern with dieting and counting calories
- Excessive concern about body weight, size, and shape
- Severe shifts in mood
- Compulsive need for continuous, vigorous physical activity
- Maintenance of a skinny look (body weight less than 85% of expected weight)
- Refusal to eat to gain weight, and wearing of baggy clothes to disguise thin-looking appearance

Bulimia nervosa

- Excessive concern about body weight, size, and shape
- Frequent gains and losses in body weight
- Visits to the bathroom following meals
- Compulsive dieting after binge-eating episodes
- Severe shifts in mood (depression, loneliness)
- Secretive eating

How high school students rate their body image–underweight, overweight, or just right.

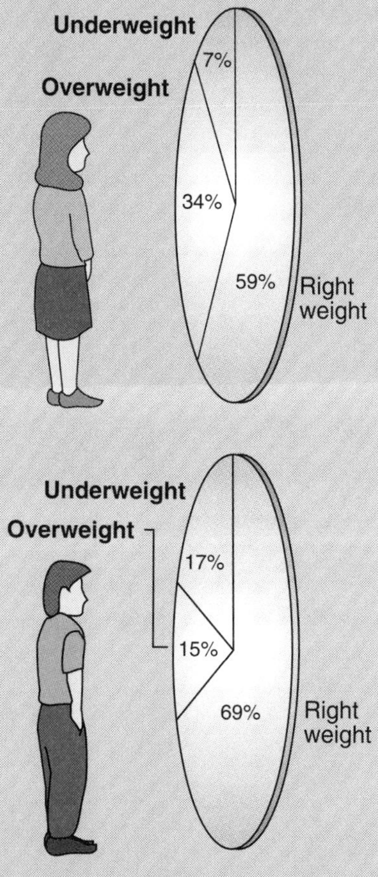

Source: 1990 Centers for Disease Control survey of 11,631 high school students

Characteristics of disordered eating behaviors

In anorexia nervosa (relentless pursuit of thinness), the person:

- Maintains body weight less than 85% of that expected for weight, stature, and bone structure
- Has intense fear of gaining weight or becoming fat, despite being clearly underweight or thin appearing
- Has altered perception of body weight, size, or shape, feeling the body is "too fat" (when in fact the person is skinny or underweight)
- In females, misses a minimum of three consecutive menstrual cycles

In bulimia nervosa (binging and purging to remain thin), the person:

- Has recurrent episodes of consuming large amounts of food (binging)
- Feels a lack of control during binging
- Tries to undo a binge by regular periods of self-induced vomiting, abuses laxatives and diuretics (water pills), restricts eating (fasts), or undertakes inordinate amounts of exercise
- Binges a minimum of twice a week for at least 3 months
- Is overly concerned with physical attributes (weight, size, shape)

* Based in part on the American Psychiatric Association's Diagnostic Criteria for Anorexia Nervosa and Bulimia Nervosa. In Diagnostic and Statistical Manual of Mental Disorders, revised 3rd ed. (*DSM-III-R*). Washington, DC, American Psychiatric Association, 1987.

Physical consequences of disordered eating behaviors (Anorexia nervosa)

- Cold intolerance (hands and feet)
- Loss of monthly menstrual periods
- Loss of sexual desire

- Loss of muscle mass and body fat
- Thin, dull, and brittle hair
- Dry, scaly, and itchy skin
- Digestive irregularities
- Lunago (hair) growth over the body
- Dental problems
- Constipation
- Dehydration
- Brittle bones (from mineral depletion)
- Cardiac arrhythmias

When a model is not the ideal. In 1967, professional models weighed only 8% less than the average American woman. Today, their average weight is 23% lower than the national average for women. Thus, it should occasion little surprise that eating disorders and unrealistic weight goals are so rampant among females of all ages in our culture.

Physical consequences of disordered eating behaviors (Bulimia nervosa)

- Digestive irregularities (gas, bloating, cramps)
- Constipation
- Loss of tooth enamel
- Swollen glands in the neck region
- Bags under the eyes
- Broken facial blood vessels
- Dehydration (causes fluid/mineral imbalance)
- Cardiac arrhythmias (from acid/base imbalance)
- Problems with vision
- Fainting
- Internal bleeding

Another application of behavior modification for an eating disorder involved the treatment of a 17-year-old woman who weighed 23 kg. The search for a positive reinforcer was unsuccessful until she began to complain about the sedative effects of a particular drug that was administered as part of her treatment. The doctors used this aspect of her behavior (complaint) as the reinforcer. Following each day when there was a further loss or no change in body weight, the sedative drug was administered. On the other hand, a 0.11 kg weight gain resulted in a smaller drug dose; for a 0.23 kg weight gain, an even smaller dose was given; and if 0.45 kg was gained, no drug was administered. With the decrease in drug dosage serving as the positive reinforcer, the young woman eventually gained an average of 2.7 kg each week. Ultimately, normal dietary patterns were established and systematic weight gain occurred.

In the following sections we present some **basic principles of behavior modification** with special application to weight reduction by means of dietary modification and increased physical activity. We use four basic steps in applying these principles:

1. Describing the behavior to be modified
2. Replacing established patterns of behavior with more desirable behaviors
3. Developing techniques to control behaviors
4. Providing positive reinforcement or reward for controlling, altering, or modifying undesirable behaviors

EATING BEHAVIOR

We usually eat for two reasons. First, we consume food because we are truly hungry. This hunger enables us to maintain a food intake to supply the energy to power the body's vital processes and sustain life. Second, we eat to satisfy our appetite, which in America is usually "programmed" to be stimulated three times daily. It appears that human eating behavior is intimately tied to both external or environmental cues as well as to internal physiologic cues that signal a real need for caloric intake. The external **"food cues"** include the sight of food; its packaging, display, and advertising; the time and physical environment in which the food is eaten; and the taste, smell, and size of portions.

Behaviors are important. Compared to the obese condition, the lean state is characterized by healthier eating behaviors and an increased level of daily physical activity.

External Cues. Several experiments have demonstrated how **external factors influence eating behavior.** In one study, normal and obese subjects were deceived into believing they were participating in an elaborate psychological experiment. In actuality, the experimenters wished to determine whether or not the visual presence of food affected eating behavior. After missing lunch, the subjects were tested for their response to meaningless psychophysical stimuli. They were then left in a room to complete a questionnaire supposedly concerned with the experiment. In the room, subjects found either 1 or 3 roast beef sandwiches and soda. They were told to eat as much as they wanted and to help themselves to more food from the refrigerator. When 3 sandwiches were left in view, the obese subjects consumed an average of 2.3 sandwiches compared with 1.9 eaten by the normal-sized subjects; when only 1 sandwich was in view, the obese subjects ate fewer sandwiches (1.5) than the nonobese subjects (2.0).

Behavioral links. Even after finishing the most delicious and satisfying meal, most of us could be coaxed into eating "just a bit more" of a delicious piece of pie or homemade cheesecake even if we felt full. Such overeating, although quite common, occurs more in obese than in lean people.

Another experiment concerned the effects of taste on eating behavior. Before the experiment, obese subjects normally consumed 3500 kcal daily while nonobese subjects consumed 2200 kcal. Then, for 3 weeks, subjects in both groups were offered a bland liquid diet; the normal-weight subjects continued to consume 2200 kcal of this liquid meal daily, whereas the obese subjects decreased caloric intake to only 500 kcal. This demonstrated that obese subjects were influenced considerably more by the taste of food then by its caloric content. Such results illustrate how external cues can significantly affect eating behavior, especially in the obese.

PSYCHOLOGICAL FACTORS INFLUENCE EATING BEHAVIOR

Mood state affects eating behavior. Daily events quite unrelated to food itself can trigger the urge to eat. For many with a weight problem, overeating increases with feelings of stress, anger, or boredom.

Depression, frustration, boredom, "uptight" or anxious feelings, guilt, sadness, or anger are often linked to periods of excessive food intake. The prospective dieter must learn to make an accurate appraisal of his or her eating behavior not only in terms of the quantity and frequency of eating but also of the specific circumstances linked to food intake. A first step in such a self-analysis is to become keenly aware of daily caloric intake (refer to the *Study Guide*, Section II B). Once this is accomplished, "undesirable" food cues can be eliminated and a new set of desirable eating responses substituted for previously learned behaviors.

MODIFICATION OF EATING BEHAVIOR

A cure for the blues. Twice as many women (52%) eat when they're depressed compared to men (27%). Chocolate rates first for 43% of women and ice cream ranks as the best bet for 34% of men. Women (38%) also are more likely than men (19%) to binge eat when they're depressed.

While numerous treatment approaches have been used for weight control, none has been particularly successful in achieving long-term success. In fact, one doctor well known for his work in the treatment of obesity has stated: "Most obese patients won't even come for treatment. Those who do come often drop out, and the ones that don't drop out don't lose much weight. Finally, those who do lose weight usually regain it." Unfortunately, research provides ample support for this statement, especially with regard to long-term weight loss. The success record is less than encouraging and underscores the difficulties encountered with most traditional weight control programs.

An apparent breakthrough was made in the treatment of obesity in 1967 when a behavioral psychologist reported the results of a 1-year program using behavior modification techniques. Treatment sessions were conducted for 30 minutes three times a week over a 4- to 5-week period. Subsequent sessions were conducted at 2-week intervals for 12 weeks; thereafter, sessions were held only once a month or as needed. The total number of sessions attended by each person varied from 16 to 41 during the year. Of the 8 obese women in the program, 3 lost more than 18 kg and 5 lost more than 12 kg. The magnitude of this weight loss was the highest ever reported for a group not confined to a hospital or clinic. Figure 17–1 shows the results for 3 of the 8 women in the study. The results are impressive because normally only about 1 of 4 obese subjects who seek treatment loses more than 10 kg, and only 1 in 20 loses more than 18 kg. Numerous studies that applied similar behavior modification techniques have verified these findings.

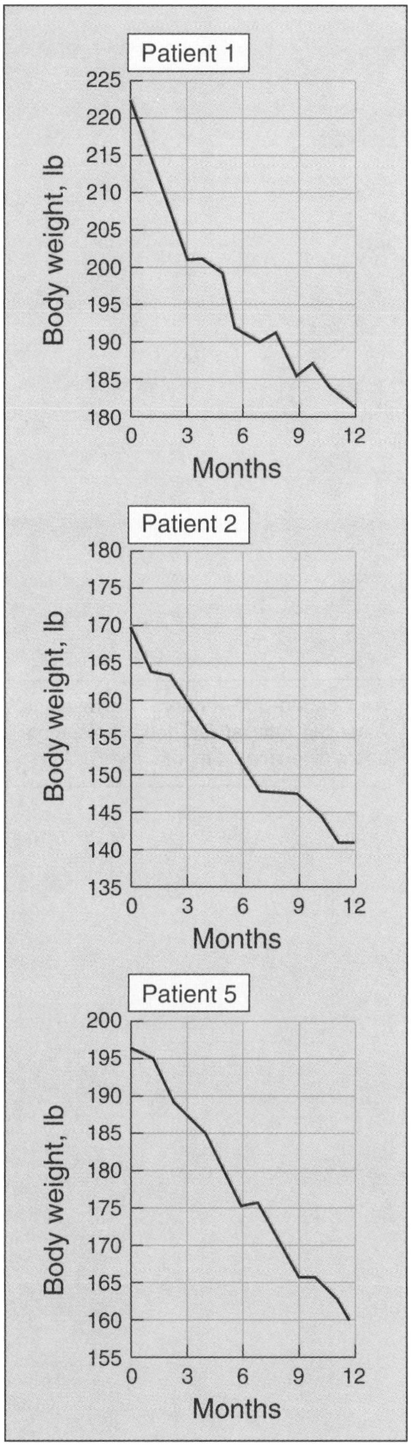

FIG. 17–1. Weight profile of 3 women undergoing behavior therapy for overeating. (From Stuart, R.B.: Behavioral control of overeating. *Behav. Res. Ther.*, 5:364, 1967.)

DESCRIBING THE BEHAVIOR TO BE MODIFIED

The first step in **eating behavior modification** is to **describe the various eating behaviors** of the overweight person, not to change the diet immediately. The person is asked to keep meticulous records and to answer the following questions:

- Where were meals eaten?
- When were meals eaten?
- What was the mood, feeling, or psychological state during the meal?
- How much time was spent at the meal?
- What activities were engaged in during the meal (watching TV, driving a car, sewing)?
- Who was present during the meal?
- What and how much food was eaten?

This time-consuming and often annoying record keeping provides the dieter with objective information concerning personal eating behaviors. *A careful examination of such records will reveal certain recurring patterns of behavior associated with eating*. For example, the dieter may discover that feelings of depression are usually followed by eating candy; that he or she eats snacks while watching television, gets hungry at a particular time of day, goes on an ice-cream binge after an argument, or never eats breakfast or lunch at the kitchen table. Once an analysis is made of eating behaviors, the next step is to substitute alternative behaviors to replace those for which a clear pattern has been established.

SUBSTITUTING ALTERNATIVE BEHAVIORS

Many acceptable behaviors can replace a particular established set of undesirable behavior patterns. Below are several examples of existing behaviors associated with eating, as well as possible **substitute behaviors:**

Established behavior patterns	Replacement behavior
• Eating candy while driving	• Singing along with the radio while driving
• Eating snacks while watching television	• Sewing, painting, or writing letters while watching television
• Feeling hungry at 4:00 P.M.	• Going for a walk at 4:00 P.M.
• Eating ice cream after an argument	• Doing 10 repetitions of an exercise after an argument
• Never eating breakfast or lunch at the kitchen table	• Eating breakfast and lunch only at the kitchen table
• Visiting the kitchen during TV commercials	• Jogging in place; doing sit-ups

While numerous other examples can be given, the major aim of this approach is clear: *to create new associations to replace the old established patterns of behavior.*

DEVELOPING TECHNIQUES TO CONTROL EATING

There are many useful **techniques for gaining control over eating behaviors** once undesirable environmental cues and associated behaviors have been identified and replaced or modified. Examples include the following:

An "eating-out" nation. The average American eats at fast food restaurants about nine times a month.

- **Make the act of eating foods a ritual.** Limit eating to one place in the house and, no matter what foods you eat, follow a set routine. For example, use a placemat, set the table with silverware, and use the same dishes at each meal. Do this for main meals as well as for snacks. One dieter who continually snacked between meals curbed this habit by dressing up in a tuxedo and eating by candlelight for each meal and snack—snacking between meals soon stopped. To discourage bread eating, take only one slice of bread at a time and toast it before eating. For each slice, get up from the table, unwrap the loaf and take out a slice, rewrap the loaf and replace it in the cupboard, toast the slice, and return to the table to eat it. Following an inconvenient routine to obtain some "special" food item often suppresses desire for the food.
- **Use smaller dishes.** The impetus to finish a meal may not be the food per se, but the desire to view an empty plate or glass.
- **Eat slowly.** Fight the urge to eat quickly by taking more time at meals. You can do this by cutting food into smaller pieces and chewing each piece 10 to 15 times before swallowing. Another technique is to place the knife, spoon, or fork back on the table after each two or three bites, and allow for a 1- or 2-minute rest pause between mouthfuls.

Other Useful Techniques. Delaying, substituting, and avoiding are three behavioral strategies for interrupting poor eating behaviors recommended by the YMCA in their weight management program. Try these examples:

- **Delaying.** Add time or steps between the links in the behavior chain:
  Slow down the eating pace
  Take a roundabout way to the kitchen
  Purchase individual-size packages of snacks
  Put off unplanned eating as long as possible—mail a letter, read a book, mow the lawn

- **Substituting.** Break the behavior chain with activities incompatible with eating:
  Pleasant activities—read, go for a walk, listen to music, do hobbies
  Required activities—plan the budget, pay bills, do errands, clean house
- **Avoiding.** Keep yourself out of situations where food is visible or accessible:
  Stay out of the kitchen or other areas associated with eating
  Do not combine eating with other activities such as reading, TV watching, or driving
  When finished eating, remove dishes and food from the table
  Scrape excess food directly into the garbage

PROVIDE POSITIVE REINFORCEMENT OR REWARDS

The long-term rewards of achieving goal weight through a prudent, yet effective weight control program are three-fold: improvement in personal appearance, subtle but meaningful changes in psychological behavior, and better overall health and fitness.

Aside from these inherent long-term benefits, other more immediate reinforcers can facilitate the weight loss program. After achieving and maintaining a given amount of weight loss (e.g., 2 kg) for several months, buy yourself a new article of clothing; after the next substantial weight loss (4 kg), go on a trip. Continue to give rewards until you attain your eventual goal. Another useful technique is to maintain a chart to plot weight changes. Keep separate charts to record daily caloric intake from food (*Study Guide*, Section II B) and caloric expenditure in exercise (*Study Guide*, Section II C), as well as recording changes in various body dimensions such as the abdomen, buttocks, thighs, and arms.

Reward success. Dieters should set up short-term goals and provide interim rewards as they progress toward a realistic goal weight.

The reinforcing power of money can also be used as incentive, especially in a group situation. For example, group members turn over a given amount of money to the group leader at the start of the program. A portion of the deposit is returned to the members as they lose specified amounts of weight (e.g., $10 per pound). If a member quits the program or fails to maintain the weight loss for at least 1 week, the deposit is forfeited and divided equally among the remaining participants at the end of a specified time.

Many variations of schemes like these are possible. Remember that merely providing information about techniques for modifying eating behavior will not in itself assure their continued use. *Encouragement and positive reinforcement in addition to self-discipline must be built-in features of a weight control program.* They provide support until the participant learns to master eating behaviors and achieve the proper balance between energy intake and expenditure.

Weight loss in the '90s. Nutrition experts are encouraged about a gradual shift away from crash diets and rigid weight loss programs and a movement toward more sensible eating and regular exercising. Good advice for the '90s:
- Be realistic in your weight loss goals
- Consume more fruits and vegetables
- Exercise regularly
- Reduce intake of dietary fat

EXERCISE BEHAVIOR

In the past, it was generally accepted that obesity was the result of excessive food intake. Clearly, the effective approach to weight control would be some form of caloric restriction through dieting. However, research on eating patterns and exercise behaviors of the obese shows consistently that a low caloric output due to physical inactivity, rather than an inordinately high caloric intake, is often the prime factor associated with weight gain.

Do the obese overeat? One is hard pressed for evidence that groups of overweight individuals actually eat more on average than people of normal weight.

In the early 1940s, psychologists pointed out that only a small percentage of obese people participated in physical activities within the range usually observed for nonobese people of the same age and gender. This characteristic sedentary behavior pattern of the obese has been consistently demonstrated in subsequent research. *The finding is that the food intake of the obese is generally no greater than for people of normal body size.*

Research conducted at Tufts University and Harvard Medical School indicated that for teenagers and younger children, the more hours a child watched TV, the greater the likelihood that the child was obese. More specifically, the prevalence of adolescent obesity increases 2% for each hour of television viewed daily. Also, the earlier in life TV watching begins, the greater the obesity and the more profound the problem becomes in teenage years. For most of us, the excess weight gained throughout life closely parallels a reduction in daily energy expenditure rather than an increase in caloric intake.

Table 17–1 compares the extent of participation in weekly physical activities as well as average daily caloric intake of 28 obese and 28 normal-weight high school girls. While **time-in-motion analysis** revealed *little difference* between the two groups in the amount of time spent sitting, standing, grooming, baby-sitting, driving in a car, or doing housework, a considerable difference was noted for the extent of participation in active sports and other strenuous activities. "Extra" physical activity was engaged in for 4 hours a week on average by the obese, compared to 11 hours for their nonobese counterparts. In addition, the obese girls consumed 27% *fewer* calories each day than the nonobese girls; only 3 of 28 obese girls consumed more than 2500 kcal.

In a similar study conducted several years later with young boys, the findings were almost identical: obese boys consumed fewer calories each day than a nonobese group. Daily food intake averaged 3011 kcal for the obese and 3476 kcal for the nonobese boys during the school year, and 3430 and 4628 kcal for the obese and lean boys, respectively, during 8 weeks of summer camp. Researchers observed little difference between groups in time spent in light and moderate exercise; however, participation in strenuous activities was less for the obese than for the nonobese boys.

The observation that **obese children are generally less active** than leaner children is also true for adults as they become sedentary and begin to add

TABLE 17–1. PHYSICAL ACTIVITY AND CALORIE INTAKE OF OBESE AND NONOBESE ADOLESCENT GIRLS

	WEEKLY PHYSICAL ACTIVITY (HOURS)							
GROUP	SLEEP, LYING STILL, AWAKE	SITTING	STANDING	GROOMING	BABY-SITTING	PLAYING PIANO, DRIVING CAR	HOUSE-WORK	ACTIVE SPORTS AND OTHER VIGOROUS ACTIVITY
Obese	61	81	1	7	1	1.4	3.6	4
Nonobese	63	75	3	10	1	1.2	3.3	11

DAILY CALORIE INTAKE (KCAL/DAY) GROUP	2500	2500–2000	2000	AVERAGE
Obese	3	6	19	1,965
Nonobese	15	10	3	2,706

Source: Johnson, M.L., et al.: Relative importance of inactivity and overeating in the energy balance of obese high school girls. *Am. J. Clin. Nutr.*, 4:37, 1956.

weight. In one experiment, physical activity levels were compared for groups of obese and nonobese men and women who were matched for age, occupation, and socioeconomic background. Physical activity expressed in miles walked each day was assessed by means of pedometers. Total mileage walked was recorded daily for 1 week by the women and for 2 weeks by the men. The results for the women were unequivocal: the average distance walked by the obese women was about 41% less than for women of normal weight. Total distance walked each day averaged 3.2 km for the obese and 7.9 km for the nonobese. For the men, the comparison was similar: the obese men walked on average 39% less than nonobese counterparts.

All these data clearly illustrate that *inactivity* is a major behavioral characteristic of the obese. Consequently, for effective weight loss, the obese must not only relearn or modify existing eating behaviors, but also reverse a sedentary lifestyle.

Pedometers access physical activity. Pedometers are small instruments usually hooked from a belt worn around the waist. The pedometer is calibrated to the person's stride length and is operated by an internal pendulum that registers each stride. Another popular form of motion device measures vertical movement by means of an accelerometer and uses this information to measure calories burned.

MODIFICATION OF EXERCISE BEHAVIOR

Learning to replace daily periods of inactivity with activity requiring a greater energy expenditure may seem a difficult task. *Experiencing enjoyment and success in physical activity is the most important aspect of this relearning process.* Only a few people will continue to participate in exercise if it is so taxing that little or no enjoyment is possible. A good example is running. It is not much fun to run for a minute or two when the end result is shortness of breath, wobbly legs, and a "stitch" in the side. All the personal motivation one can muster cannot overcome the feelings of genuine discomfort when pursuing unrealistic goals. Even jogging for 5 minutes at a relatively slow pace is not easy, especially for people who have previously been sedentary. However, walking and walking/jogging as well as other physical activities can be enjoyable if the chance for *success* is maximized. This necessitates a carefully planned, systematic approach with long-term rather than short-term goals. If the long-term goal is to jog continuously for 30 minutes each day, then the beginner should plan to achieve this goal over a period of weeks or months, rather than trying to run this distance on the first or second day.

How to maintain a desirable body composition. Individuals who maintain physically active lifestyles or who become involved in appropriate exercise programs generally maintain a desirable level of body composition.

Exercise compliance. Factors such as cigarette smoking, a previously sedentary lifestyle, lack of family support, and disruptive events such as illness all negatively influence an individual's compliance in an exercise program for weight loss. Compliance is greatly enhanced, however, if the person enrolls in a program of *supervised* exercise.

DESCRIBING THE BEHAVIOR TO BE MODIFIED

The first step is to determine the daily pattern of physical activity, including such minimal requirements as sleeping, eating, going to the bathroom, and bathing. An activity profile can be constructed by keeping a daily record of the actual time spent in the various activities for 3 consecutive days as illustrated in the *Study Guide,* Section II C. The activity profile for a physically active college professor during a typical day of summer vacation is also presented in the *Study Guide,* Section II C. This record includes a description of the activity, its duration, and its energy requirements. The actual caloric values for the physical activities are included in Appendix A.

Any hope of changing the profile of daily physical activity is predicated on an accurate appraisal of the activities that make up the day. Once this is done, the next step in **exercise behavior modification** is to substitute more strenuous activities for those that rate low in energy expenditure.

Keep it fun. If there is little chance for enjoyment and success when exercising, then most people will become discouraged and discontinue participation. In psychological behavior terms, they have received negative reinforcement from the activity.

SUBSTITUTING ALTERNATIVE BEHAVIORS

Moderate to strenuous physical activity can easily replace sedentary activities only when the dieter is willing to become more physically active. There are many ways to increase energy expenditure within the time allotted to daily routines. *The important consideration is to determine when and how to make changes.* For example:

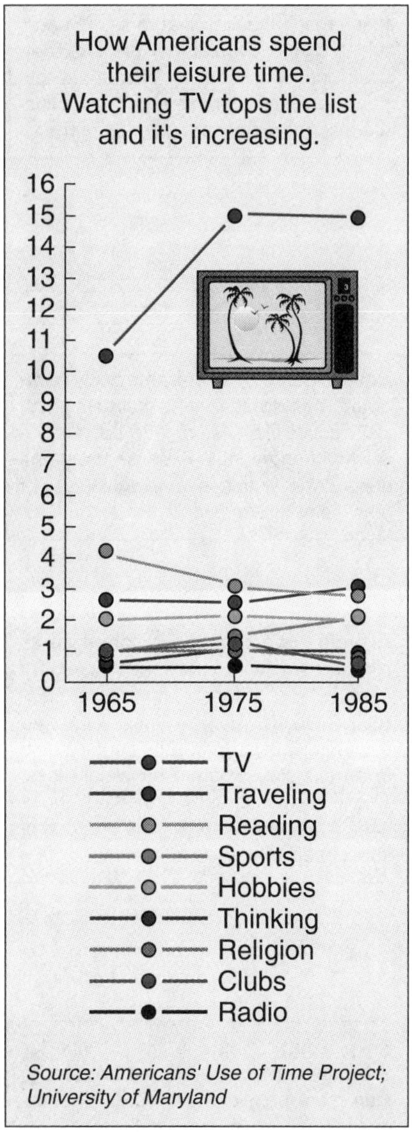

TV watching and the prevalence of obesity. Compared with women who watched TV less than 1 hour a day, women who spent 4 hours a day in front of the TV had more than double the prevalence of obesity.

- When driving to work, park a half mile away and walk the remaining distance; brisk walking to and from the car each day, 5 days a week, will burn up the caloric equivalent of about 3.2 kg of fat in 1 year
- When taking public transportation, get off 8 to 10 stops early and walk the remaining distance
- When traveling relatively short distances, walk instead of taking a cab or bus
- Don't go to a restaurant for lunch; instead, participate in some form of physical activity, such as walking, that you can continue for 30 to 45 minutes
- Wake up an hour early and take a brisk walk, cycle, row, or swim before breakfast
- Replace the cocktail hour with 20 minutes of exercise
- Replace coffee breaks with exercise breaks
- Walk up and down several flights of stairs after each hour at work
- Sweep the sidewalks in front of your house or apartment

  One of our dear older colleagues, a world-renowned scientist, used to sweep the perimeter of a four-square-block park in San Francisco for 2 hours a day, 6 days a week! He did this not only as a public service, but to augment his generally sedentary lifestyle with physically demanding tasks to maintain his arm and leg strength. At 84 years of age and no longer able to work in the park, he substituted what he termed "arm aerobics" as his exercise—he carried two 3 pound dumbbells around his apartment several times a day.
- When going on a family outing, allow time for exercise.
  - Get out of the car before reaching your destination; let your family drive the rest of the way while you walk or jog
  - Instead of eating at half-time or intermission at sports events, walk around the stadium or arena; climb up and down stairs instead of using elevators or escalators
- Replace the hired help and undertake some of these tasks yourself:
  - Gardening
  - Mowing the lawn
  - Painting
  - Washing and waxing the car
  - Walking the dog
  - Plowing the driveway
- During television commercials, run in place, jump rope, jog up and down stairs, or perform vigorous calisthenics
- Replace power tools and appliances with manually operated devices:
  - Lawn care equipment
  - Automatic household appliances such as vacuum cleaners, eggbeaters, ice cream maker, juicers
  - Saws
  - Drills

Snow shovelers
Garage doors
- Play golf without a golf cart or caddy
- Walk or jog up and down the beach in addition to sunbathing

Identifying possible areas for activity modification is easy because today's men and women are accustomed to an automated, labor-saving society. Humans are slaves to machines; we have learned to live the "easy life." Learned behaviors, however, can be changed or at least modified; the major requirement is willingness to commit to a new lifestyle that incorporates more vigorous activities within the fabric of the daily routine. Unfortunately, most of us are too locked into daily routines to even try to modify present behavior. There may be a few things we are willing to do, such as yard work now and then or going for a brisk walk at lunchtime. However, it takes a real commitment to sweep the streets, jog around the block, bicycle to and from work, or walk up and down stairs without feeling embarrassed or self-conscious. People must overcome social pressures and constraints to attain permanent changes in lifestyle.

Substitute the active for the inactive. From the perspective of physical activity, the most difficult task in rearranging a daily routine is to replace conveniences with tasks that require more effort.

Nordic skiing and stair-climbing are tops for first time exercisers

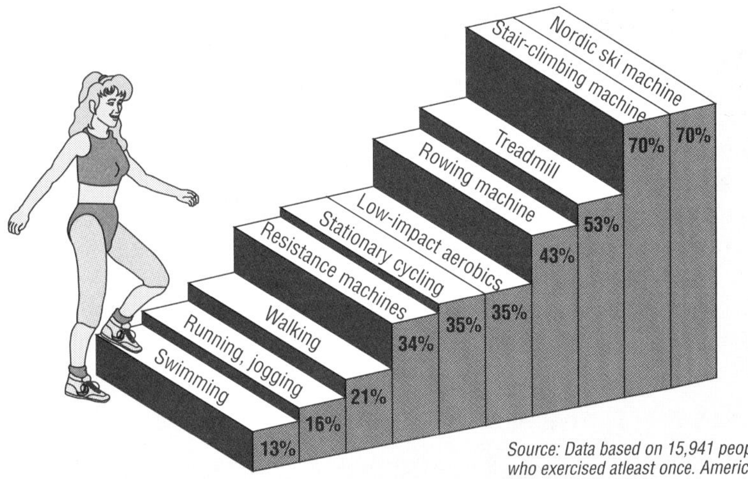

Source: Data based on 15,941 people who exercised atleast once. American Sports Data, Inc. 1990

How Americans started their exercise program.

DEVELOPING TECHNIQUES TO MAXIMIZE EXERCISE SUCCESS

Several techniques can be used to **maximize exercise success** in a program of weight control. These techniques may not apply to team or individual sports in which skill or competition are the key elements (tennis, badminton, basketball, golf, racquetball, squash), but to activities such as jogging, bicycling, swimming, and calisthenic exercises.

- **Progress slowly.** People who have been sedentary should not try to accomplish too much in the first few weeks. Instead of running 1 mile initially, briskly walk 1 block; instead of trying to cycle 15 km, cycle 5; instead of trying to do 100 sit-ups, do 10. Over time, the amount of exercise can be progressively increased.
- **Include variety.** Rather than perform the same exercise over and over again in a given time, vary the exercise as well as the number of repe-

Become goal oriented. Mastery of preset goals provides immediate positive reinforcement and minimizes the chance for failure. At the same time, the fun aspect of the activity is maximized because of the feeling of personal achievement.

titions. For example, instead of jogging continuously around the track, intersperse other forms of exercise: jog for 2 minutes, skip for 1 minute, hop on the right foot 20 times, hop on the left foot 20 times, jump up and down 20 times, skip 1 minute, jog 3 minutes—and so on, until you reach the desired end point.

- **Become goal oriented.** There are three ways to exercise using goal-oriented behavior:

  Exercise for a certain amount of time

  Continue to exercise until you reach a predetermined number of repetitions or distance

  Combine both of the preceding approaches

  Select one of these approaches depending on your personal preference. If a track is available, the total distance run becomes a convenient guide. One limitation with this approach, however, is the tedium of repetitively running the same route with little change in scenery. An alternative is to mark off a given distance (your house to the store, the store to the playground, the playground to the house), and then run this route. If exercise for a specific time is the goal, then walk or run a predetermined route such as around a track or through the neighborhood. The latter alternative has the advantage of changing sceneries. For the novice jogger who may only run continuously for a minute or two between rest intervals, the goal should be to cover a given distance, such as running from a big tree to the fence post, the fence post to the red car, and the red car to the stop sign.
- **Be systematic.** Set aside certain times during the day to exercise. Don't permit outside factors such as watching television, shopping, and doing housework to interfere with daily physical activity.
- **Be comfortable.** Wear clothes conducive to exercising. You need not be concerned with what clothes to wear while swimming or skiing, as the choices are limited and obvious. Many activities have no established patterns of dress, so follow your personal preferences. On hot and humid days, wear light clothing to permit rapid heat loss.

Changing exercise habits is not easy. Federal statistics confirm that changing exercise habits is not something that can be easily accomplished. For example, 42% of individuals living in Kentucky and 52% of people in the District of Columbia reported they were completely sedentary with no leisure-time physical activity during a one-month period. These are the highest values reported in the U.S. The statistics were more encouraging for people residing in Montana and Colorado where approximately 80% of individuals said they did engage in physically active, leisure-time pursuits.

PROVIDE POSITIVE REINFORCEMENT OR REWARDS

Positive reinforcement should be intimately linked to exercise, especially for the beginner.

- **Keep charts to record progress.** Fill in the chart as soon as you achieve the preset goal. Such charts provide immediate feedback and serve to maintain motivation and interest.
- **Exercise with a buddy or in small groups.** A workout is often more enjoyable when performed in small groups of two or three people. Having to make commitments to others can be a subtle form of motivation to help ensure exercise on a regular schedule.
- **Provide rewards.** Self-made competition can be effective for achieving preset goals. This is especially true for beginners, who usually need some incentive. We have found that a simple game helps people maintain a high degree of self-motivation. The game can be played by as many persons as desired. The object is to perform a given amount of exercise, and a painted button is awarded when the exercise goal is achieved. A predetermined reward is given for accumulating 10 buttons.

  To start, obtain 16 white shirt buttons and paint 10 of them a favorite color. Each of the remaining white buttons is equal to a given number of minutes of exercise. We make a 5-minute exercise period equal to 1 white button. When 6 white buttons have been accumulated (equal to 30 minutes of exercise), they are traded in for a painted button. A person who secures 10 painted buttons wins the game and receives a reward. The reward is chosen in advance, and can be anything the participant wants. We suggest that the painted buttons be stored in a prominent place in the house, where family members can keep track of progress and provide encouragement and support. For people just beginning to exercise, the goal is to achieve 5 painted buttons each week. The exercise equivalent for each button can be increased as exercise capacity improves.

For purposes of illustration, suppose 30 minutes of exercise is made to equal 1 painted button. For the person who weighs 90 kg and accumulates 5 painted buttons each week by walking briskly, the "extra" caloric expenditure due to walking would be equal to approximately 1200 kcal per week, 4800 kcal per month, or the equivalent of 7.5 kg of fat per year. Obviously, if this person maintained a corresponding decrease in calorie intake, the rate and quantity of fat loss would double!

Reward success with rewards. Simple games and rewards can offer the positive feedback and reinforcement so important to successful weight loss. As long as the player places value on the reward, the process of striving to achieve it takes on new meaning and offers at least a fighting chance for success. Also, rewards can take the form of positive reinforcement. Something as simple as "you look great" is an intrinsic reward that can mean a great deal. All of us need "rewards" for the things we do—sometimes it's the little ones that mean the most.

SUMMARY

1. Behavior modification techniques enable an individual to identify, control, and modify undesirable eating and exercise behaviors so that they become desirable in terms of weight control and good health.
2. Eating behaviors appear to be linked to a variety of external environmental cues as well as internal physiologic cues related to a need to eat. The external cues may influence eating behavior in the obese to a greater extent than for normal-weight counterparts.
3. Behavior modification attempts to identify undesirable established food cues and behaviors, and substitute them with a new set of desirable eating responses. Positive reinforcement is a key to successful behavior replacement.
4. Overeating is not always the prime factor in the development of obesity. In many instances, the energy imbalance is due to a depressed level of daily physical activity. Consequently, the obese must not only relearn or modify existing eating behaviors, but also reverse an existing syndrome of insufficient energy output from a sedentary lifestyle.
5. After a detailed physical activity profile is established for an individual, behavioral techniques are applied to substitute more strenuous physical activities for those that rate low on energy expenditure.
6. A variety of techniques are available to maximize success and provide positive reinforcement to a person's efforts to increase daily physical activity.

RELATED READINGS

Atkinson, R.L., et al.: Combination of very-low-calorie diet and behavior modification in the treatment of obesity. *Am. J. Clin. Nutr.*, 56:199S, 1992.

Bjorvell, H., and Rossner, S.: Long term treatment of severe obesity: four year follow-up of results of combined behavioral modification programme. *Br. Med. J.*, 291:379, 1985.

Brownell, K.D.: Behavioral, psychological, and environmental predictors of obesity and success at weight reduction. *Int. J. Obesity*, 8:543, 1984.

Brownell, K.D., and Kaye, F.S.: A school-based behavior modification, nutrition education, and physical activity program for obese children. *Am. J. Clin. Nutr.*, 35:277, 1982.

Drewnowski, A., et al.: Taste preferences in human obesity: environmental and familial factors. *Am. J. Clin. Nutr.*, 54:635, 1991.

Eilmore, J.A.: Eating and weight disorders in the female athlete. *Int. J. Sports Nutr.*, 1:104, 1991.

Epstein, L.H., et al.: A comparison of lifestyle exercise, aerobic exercise, and calisthenics on weight loss in obese children. *Behav. Ther.*, 16:345, 1985.

Epstein, L.H., et al.: Ten-year follow-up of behavioral, family-based treatment for obese children. *JAMA*, 264:2519, 1990.

Garner, D.M., et al.: Development and validation of multidimensional eating disorder inventory for anorexia nervosa and bulimia. *Int. J. Eat. Disorders*, 2:15, 1983.

Graham, L.E., et al.: Five-year follow-up to a behavioral weight-loss program. *J. Consult. Clin. Psychol.*, 51:322, 1983.

James, W.P.T., et al.: Dietary recommendations after weight loss: how to avoid relapse of obesity. *Am. J. Clin. Nutr.*, 45:1135, 1987.

Jeffery, R.W., et al.: Behavioral treatment of obesity with monetary contracting: two year follow up. *Addictive Behav.*, 9:311, 1984.

Johnson, M.L., et al.: Relative importance of inactivity and overeating in the energy balance of obese high school girls. *Am. J. Clin. Nutr.*, 4:37, 1956.

Kurtzman, F.D., et al.: Eating disorders among selected female student populations at UCLA. *J. Am. Dietet. Assoc.* 89:45, 1989.

Leon, G.R.: The behavior modification approach to weight reduction. *Contemp. Nutr.*, 4(8): 1979.

Palgi, A., et al.: Multidisciplinary treatment of obesity with a protein-sparing modified fast: results in 668 outpatients. *Am. J. Publ. Health*, 75:1190, 1985.

Perri, M.G., et al.: Maintenance strategies for the treatment of obesity: an evaluation of relapse prevention training and post-treatment contact by mail and telephone. *J. Consult. Clin. Psychol.*, 52:404, 1985.

Phinney, S.D.: Exercise during and after very-low-calorie dieting. *Am. J. Clin. Nutr.*, 56:190S, 1992.

Prentice, A.M., et al.: Effects of weight cycling on body composition. *Am. J. Clin. Nutr.*, 56:209S, 1992.

Schotte, D.E., and Stunkard, A.J.: Bulimia versus bulimic behaviors on a college campus. *JAMA* 258:1213, 1987.

Stunkard, A.J.: Conservative treatments for obesity. *Am. J. Clin. Nutr.*, 45:1142, 1987.

Stunkard, A.J., and Penick, S.B.: Behavior modification in the treatment of obesity: the problem of maintaining weight loss. *Arch. Gen. Psychiatry*, 36:801, 1979.

Wadden, T.A., and Stunkard, A.J.: Social and psychological consequences of obesity. *Ann. Intern. Med.*, 103:1062, 1985.

Wadden, T.A., et al.: Treatment of obesity by very-low calorie diet and behavior therapy. *J. Consult. Clin. Psychol.*, 52:692, 1984.

Wilmore, J.H.: Eating and weight disorders in the female athlete. *Int. J. Sport Nutr.*, 1:104, 1991.

Wilson, G.T., Brownel, K.D.: Behavior therapy for obesity: an evaluation of treatment outcome. *Adv. Behav. Res. Ther.*, 3:49, 1980.

Zuckerman, D.M., et al.: The prevalence of bulimia among college students. *Am. J. Publ. Health*, 76:1135, 1986.

PHYSIOLOGIC CONDITIONING FOR TOTAL FITNESS

III

Physical fitness to some reflects the trim legs and waist of the model who demonstrates stretching exercises in the popular glamour magazines or videos. To others, fitness means superior strength with its accompanying large muscular development. In the past, the popularity of health clubs, spas, and other exercise facilities has flourished in this image. At the other extreme, the fit individual is exemplified by the lean, rather frail-looking competitive marathoner who runs at a 5-minute per mile pace for 26 miles.

The housewife, business executive, or college student may take a more moderate view. They may consider themselves physically fit by successfully completing a set of tennis, round of golf, or game of racquetball, or by climbing several flights of stairs without fatigue. This perspective places fitness on a continuum, with the necessary level of fitness determined only by one's daily physical requirements. While this may be a practical view, medical evidence suggests that our bodies need regular aerobic exercise, especially if our jobs are sedentary and our lifestyles inactive.

THE CONCEPT OF TOTAL FITNESS

An important goal. The primary objective of physiologic training is to cause biologic adaptations to improve performance in specific tasks.

While it is difficult to formulate a precise definition of fitness, it is appropriate to view **total fitness** as a state of physical well-being that incorporates a balance between several fitness components. More specifically, total physical fitness requires adequate muscular strength and endurance, reasonable joint flexibility, an efficient cardiovascular system with a good level of aerobic fitness, and favorable body composition with acceptable control of body weight. Within this framework, exercise programs should be designed based on research-proven training principles and techniques with regular adjustments to keep pace with one's improving fitness. *The approach to physiologic conditioning for men is basically the same as for women regardless of age; they both respond and adapt to physical training in essentially the same manner.*

GENERAL PRINCIPLES OF PHYSIOLOGIC CONDITIONING

The term **physiologic conditioning** refers to a planned program of exercise directed toward improving the functional capacity of a particular body system. This improvement does not occur haphazardly, but requires adherence to carefully planned and executed activities. Attention is focused on factors such as frequency and length of workouts, type of training, speed, intensity, and repetition of the activity, and appropriate competition.

OVERLOAD PRINCIPLE

Although exercise programs differ considerably depending on a person's specific goals and expectations, an effective program must be based on the proper application of physiologic stress or *overload.* A major tenet of the **overload principle** is that by exercising a body system at a level above which it normally operates, that system will adapt so as to function more efficiently. Overload can be accomplished in several ways:

- Increase the *frequency* of exercise
- Increase the *intensity* of exercise within a given time period
- Increase the *duration* of exercise at a specified intensity

Consider the following example of a sedentary woman who uses jogging to train her cardiovascular system and improve aerobic exercise capacity. If this woman jogged one block twice a week at a slow pace for 1 year, undoubtedly there would be some increase in fitness. However, the improvement would be slight. To improve fitness above some minimal level, a person must select one of the preceding three methods to implement an overload. The jogger could elect to speed up her running pace to increase the intensity of exercise. Other alternatives for progressive overload would be to periodically extend the distance run or to increase the frequency of exercise from 2 to 5 days a week. The relative importance of frequency, duration, and intensity in physiologic conditioning is developed more fully in the sections that follow. *The important point is that to ensure continued improvement during training, the relative degree of overload must keep pace with the adaptive changes that occur in both physiology and performance.*

A good example of the positive results of **progressive overload** is the cardiac patient who completely recovered from a heart attack and, through a planned training program, was eventually able to complete a 26-mile marathon in 4 hours. This impressive capability for exercise did not occur within a few months. At first, walking for just a few minutes was strenuous. Soon, functional capacity improved and the patient walked longer distances. In a short time, a plateau was reached at which further improvement did not occur until additional overload was applied. Walking was replaced by slow jogging, which in turn was replaced by jogging at faster speeds. Simultaneously, distance gradually and systematically increased from a few yards to several blocks, to miles, and finally to a point that became personally rewarding. Of course, this can be carried to spectacular extremes. The world record for the longest-duration swim is 168 hours; the record for walking on hands is 871 miles (55 daily 10-hour stints, from Vienna to Paris, in 1900); for running nonstop, the record is 121 hours, 54 minutes (352.9 miles); the winner in the longest foot race (3665 miles from Los Angeles to New York City) averaged 6.97 mph in an elapsed time of 525 hours, 57 minutes, 20 seconds over 79 days; for ice skating, the winner of the longest race completed 124 miles, 483 yards in 6 hours, 5 minutes, 12 seconds.

The fundamental training principle. The concept of individualized and progressive overload applies to the athlete, the sedentary person, the disabled, and even the cardiac patient.

SPECIFICITY PRINCIPLE

In general, the **training specificity principle** refers to adaptations in metabolism and physiology that depend on the type of overload imposed. Exercise that develops one aspect of fitness generally contributes little to other fitness components. It is known that a specific exercise stress such as strength-power training induces specific strength-power adaptations. However, such strengthening exercises per se offer little stimulus for increasing blood flow through the body and provide only a minimal effect in terms of calories expended.

Research indicates that there is also a high degree of specificity in terms of improving a particular physiologic capacity. Evidence from these studies dictates that a person should train in a manner as close as possible to the way he or she wishes to use the improved capacity. Developing the aerobic system for swimming, skiing, bicycling, or rowing, for example, can be achieved most readily when the exerciser trains using the specific muscles required by the activity. Consequently, fitness for bicycling is best achieved through cycling exercise, those desiring fitness for swimming should swim, while the runner is best conditioned through specific programs of run training. The same is true for improving the muscular system: performing an exercise with the arms in one pattern of movement, as in lifting a weight with two hands from the waist to a position above the head, does not necessarily mean that this improved specific lifting strength "transfers" to another arm movement such as the shot put, even though both movements may use the *same* muscles.

World's fittest man—specificity in action. Steve Sokol, a specialist in fitness training and education from San Jose, California, holds the following world records for a variety of fitness activities:

- 52,003 situps in 32 hours, 17 minutes
- 3,336 situps in 1 hour
- 13,013 leg lifts in 5 hours, 45 minutes
- 3,522 leg lifts in 1 hour
- 30,000 jumping jacks in 7 hours, 30 minutes
- 4,412 jumping jacks in 1 hour
- 3,333 squat thrusts in 4 hours
- Rode 500.2 miles in 24 hours on a stationary bicycle
- Rode 500 miles from San Francisco to Los Angeles in 43 hours without sitting down on the seat of the bicycle!

Training specificity means that specific exercises elicit specific adaptations, creating specific training effects.

INDIVIDUAL DIFFERENCES PRINCIPLE

Genetics play a role. Genetic factors clearly interact to influence the training response. Simply stated, some people are more "trainable" than others.

Many factors contribute to individual variation in the training response. Of considerable importance is the person's fitness level at the start of training. It is unrealistic to expect different people to be in the same state of training at the same time. Consequently, it is counterproductive to insist that all individuals train the same way or at the same work rate. It is also unrealistic to expect all individuals to respond to a given training dosage in precisely the same manner. According to the **individual differences principle,** *training benefits are optimized when programs are planned to meet the individual needs and capacities of the participants.*

REVERSIBILITY PRINCIPLE

The functional capacity of a body system is determined by the current level of overload. Once a person reaches a certain fitness level, regular physical activity must be continued to prevent deconditioning, or loss in functional capacity. When the normal level of exercise can no longer be applied, as occurs when an arm or leg is placed in a cast or when someone adopts a sedentary lifestyle, physiologic capacity will regress to a lower level. This is an example of the **reversibility principle.** For this reason the muscles of a limb immobilized in a cast will atrophy, or shrink, to a size smaller than the weight-bearing or opposite limb.

Because the effects of training are transient and reversible, athletes in various sports begin a reconditioning program a month or two before the start of the competitive season. Many ex-athletes are in poorer physiologic condition several years after they retire from active participation than the 50-year-old business executive who has played handball 1 hour a day, 3 days a week, since college days.

Deconditioning. Only 1 or 2 weeks after stopping training, significant reductions in physiologic and exercise capacity are noted, and many of the training improvements are lost within several months.

An optimal state of functional capacity can be developed and maintained through activities such as tennis, handball, swimming, bicycling, volleyball, vigorous dancing, or backpacking, as well as through organized programs of jogging, aerobic dance, and calisthenics. In fact, the simple activity of skipping rope or exercising to music can be easily adapted for a program of aerobic conditioning. Many programs will work; the important point is to select activities that blend with your personality and lifestyle.

A WORD OF CAUTION BEFORE YOU BEGIN

There is no evidence that participation in intense physical exercise will damage a normal heart. In fact, the circulatory system adapts to exercise by an increase in its functional capacity. *Before beginning an exercise program, however, a medical checkup is recommended.* A sudden burst of vigorous exercise could be dangerous to some people. For example, intense physical activity coupled with certain environmental conditions may aggravate an existing asthmatic condition. People with a tendency toward high blood pressure should refrain from heavy lifting or straining exercises that may cause temporary, yet rapid increases in heart rate and blood pressure above a safe level. Those over the age of 35 and certain **"coronary-prone"** younger people who possess a cluster of risk factors such as obesity, hypertension, diabetes, sedentary lifestyle, cigarette smoking, and a family history of early heart disease are urged to obtain an electrocardiogram, preferably one administered during increasing levels of exercise.

The exercise or stress electrocardiogram may pick up subtle changes in the heart muscle that indicate early development of coronary heart disease. Seemingly healthy people may seriously harm themselves if, after years of sedentary living, they decide suddenly to become active by running a mile, climbing a mountain, or shoveling the snow from the front walk. This does not mean that the coronary-prone or those with existing coronary heart disease should avoid exercise. On the contrary, with objective medical advice, exercise can be prescribed to improve exercise capacity. Such programs may reduce risk factors and retard the progression of the degenerative process. For this reason exercise "cardiac clubs" flourish throughout the country. Such groups engage in regular aerobic exercise at the proper intensity for the purpose of improving overall health and fitness.

18

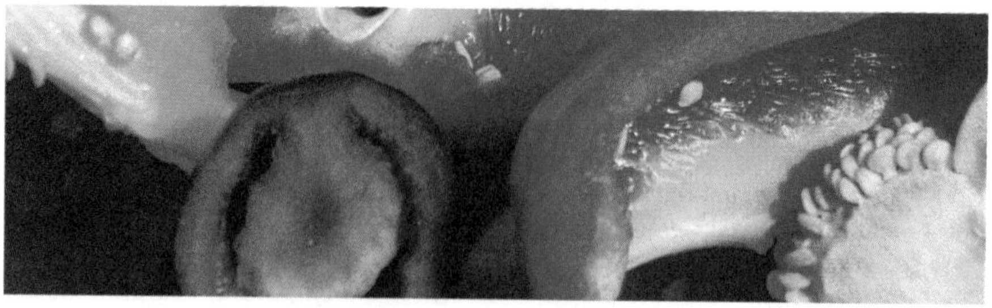

CONDITIONING FOR MUSCULAR STRENGTH

In training for muscular strength, the overload principle is applied by the use of weights (dumbbells or barbells), immovable bars, straps, pulleys, springs, water, air, and oil hydraulic devices. There is nothing unique in the use of a barbell or spring, or any heavy object, to improve muscular strength. In each case the muscle responds to the *intensity* of the overload rather than to the actual form it takes.

In general, muscular overload is applied by either increasing the load or *resistance,* increasing the number of times or *repetitions* the exercise is performed, increasing the *speed* of muscular contraction, or by various combinations of these factors.

DIFFERENT FORMS OF MUSCULAR CONTRACTION

There are three basic types of muscular contraction: concentric, eccentric, and isometric.

Concentric contraction is the most common type of muscular contraction and occurs in rhythmic activities in which the muscle *shortens* as it develops tension. The muscles contract concentrically in most sport activities. Figure 18–1A illustrates a concentric muscular contraction during the raising of a dumbbell from the extended to the flexed elbow position.

Eccentric contraction occurs when external resistance exceeds muscle force and the muscle *lengthens* while developing tension. As shown in Figure 18–1B, the weight is slowly lowered against the force of gravity. The muscles of the upper arm increase in length as they contract eccentrically to prevent the weight from crashing to the floor.

Isometric contraction occurs when a muscle attempts to shorten but is unable to overcome resistance. Considerable muscular force can be generated during an isometric contraction with *no noticeable lengthening or shortening* of the muscle. Figure 18–1C illustrates an isometric muscular contraction.

Both concentric and eccentric muscle contractions are commonly referred to as isotonic because in both cases movement occurs. With such contractions, muscular force is developed either to overcome or to control the

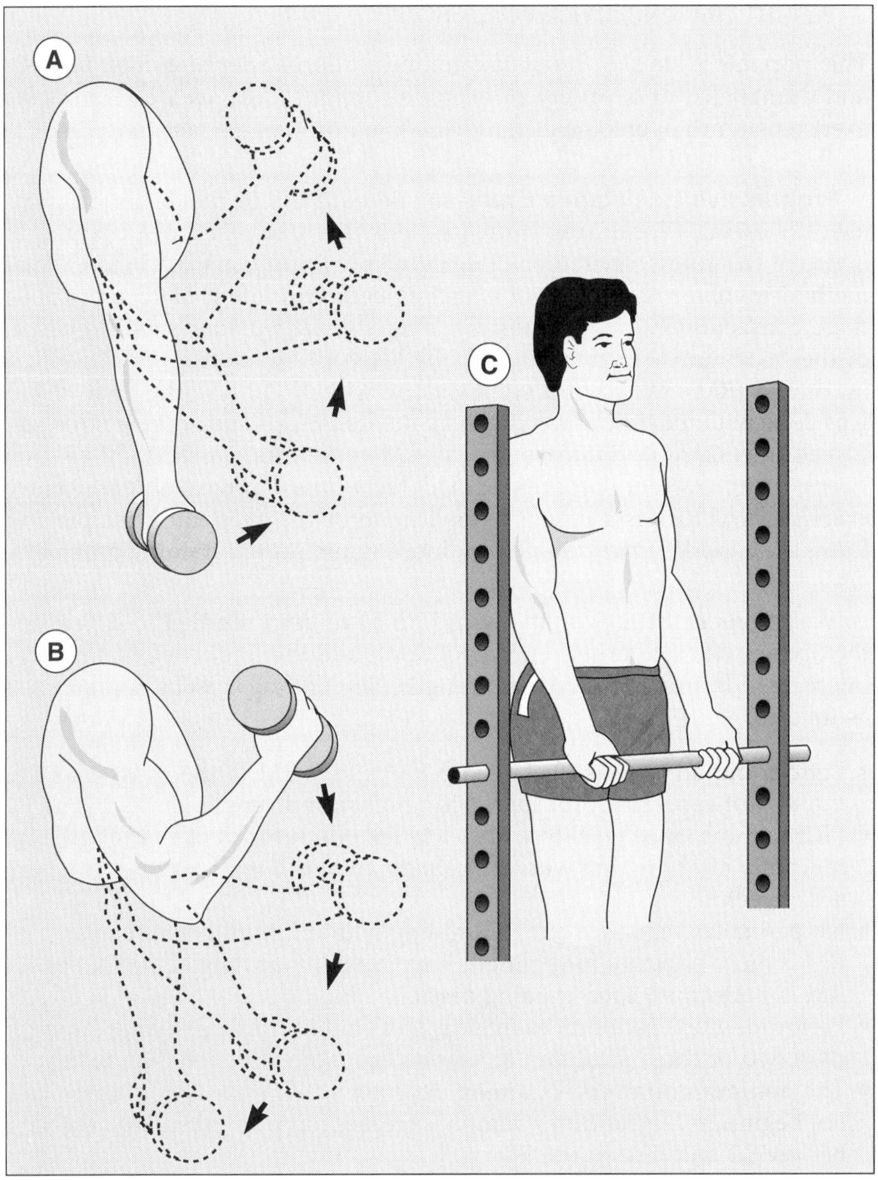

FIG. 18–1. (A) Concentric (shortening) contraction, (B) eccentric (lengthening) contraction, and (C) isometric (static) contraction.

resistance during movement. The term *isotonic* is derived from the Greek word *isotonos* (*iso* meaning the same or equal; *tonos*, tension or strain). Actually, this term is imprecise when applied to most muscular actions that involve movement because muscle tension varies as the joint angle changes; thus, the tension does not remain constant through the range of motion.

TYPES OF RESISTANCE TRAINING

Three exercise systems are commonly used to develop muscular strength: weight training, isometric training, and isokinetic training.

WEIGHT TRAINING: DYNAMIC EXERCISE

This popular system of resistance training utilizes weight plates, barbells and dumbbells, or a variety of exercise machines against which muscles exert tension to overcome and move a fixed or variable resistance.

Progressive Resistance Exercise. Researchers in rehabilitation medicine following World War II devised a method of resistance training to improve the force-generating capacity of previously injured limbs. Their method involved three sets of exercises each consisting of 10 repetitions done consecutively without resting. The first set was done with one-half of the maximum weight that could be lifted 10 times or ½, 10-repetition maximum (RM); the second set was done with ¾, 10-RM; the final 10-RM was done with maximum weight. As patients trained and became stronger, it was necessary to increase the 10-RM resistance periodically so that strength improvement progressed. This technique of **progressive resistance exercise,** or (PRE), is a practical application of the overload principle and forms the basis of most strength conditioning and muscle training programs.

Variations of PRE. Variations of PRE have been studied to determine the optimal number of sets and repetitions, and the frequency and relative intensity of training to improve strength. The findings can be summarized as follows.

- Performing an exercise between 3-RM and 9-RM is the most effective number of repetitions for increasing muscular strength.
- PRE training once weekly with 1-RM for one set increases strength significantly after the first week of training and each week up to at least the sixth week.
- No particular sequence of PRE training with different percentages of 10-RM is more effective for strength improvement, as long as one set of 10-RM is performed each training session.
- Performing one set of an exercise is less effective for increasing strength than two or three sets, and three sets are more effective than two.
- The optimum number of training days per week with PRE is unknown. For beginners, significant strength increases have occurred with training between 1 and 5 days weekly.
- When PRE training uses several different exercises, training 4 or 5 days a week may be less effective for increasing strength than training 2 or 3 times. The more frequent training may prevent sufficient recuperation between exercise sessions, which could retard progress in neuromuscular adaptation and strength development.
- For a given resistance or load, a fast rate of movement may generate greater strength improvement than lifting at a slower rate. Furthermore, neither free weights (barbells or dumbbells) nor concentric-eccentric-type weight machines are inherently superior to the other for strength development.

ISOMETRIC TRAINING (STATIC EXERCISE)

The system of **isometric strength training** was most popular between 1955 and 1965. Research in Germany during this time showed that an increase in isometric strength of about 5% a week could be achieved by performing a single, maximum contraction of only 1 second duration each day! Repeating this contraction between 5 and 10 times daily produced even greater increases in isometric strength.

Limitations of Isometrics. There are several **limitations of isometric training.** A major drawback of the isometric method is the difficulty in obtaining knowledge of training results. Because there is essentially no movement, it is difficult to determine objectively if the person's strength is actually improving and whether an appropriate overload force is being exerted during training. Furthermore, the measurement of isometric force requires specialized equipment not available at most exercise facilities. Another limitation is that isometric strength is developed specific to the angle at which the force is applied. For example, pushing against an immovable object, as illustrated in Figure 18–1C, will develop isometric strength at the particular joint angle at which the force is applied. There is little, if any, transfer of isometric strength developed at one joint angle to other angles or body positions, even when the same muscles are involved! *Thus, the muscle trained isometrically is stronger when measured isometrically, and particularly when measured at the specific joint angle at which the isometric overload was applied.*

Isometric strength training is not ideal for sports training. Isometric training can provide a relatively quick and convenient method for overloading and strengthening muscles, especially in rehabilitation medicine. Because of the specificity of the training response, however, this means of strength training is less than optimal for most sports activities that require dynamic rather than static muscle action.

Specificity of isometric training. The greatest increase in isometric strength occurs when strength is measured in the exact position at which isometric training took place.

Benefits of Isometrics. There are several **benefits of isometric training.** Isometric training is effective for developing the "total" strength of a particular muscle or group of muscles if the isometric force is applied at four or five angles through the range of motion. This can be time-consuming, especially if conventional dynamic training methods are available. Isometric training is desirable for special orthopedic applications that require specific strength assessment and rehabilitation. With isometric training, the exact area of muscle weakness can be isolated and strengthening exercises administered at the proper joint angle.

WHICH ARE BETTER, STATIC OR DYNAMIC METHODS?

Both static and dynamic resistance training produce significant increases in muscular strength. The training method selected, however, must be determined by the individual's particular needs and governed by the specificity of the training response.

Specificity of the Training Response. The isometrically trained muscle is stronger when measured isometrically, while the muscle trained dynamically is stronger when evaluated during the movement of resistance. The **specificity of resistance training** occurs because strength improvements result from favorable adaptations within the muscle itself, as well as in the neural organization required for a particular movement. Even when muscles are trained in a limited range of motion, they show the greatest strength improvement when evaluated in that specific range of motion. The angle-specific training response is observed for both static *and* dynamic resistance training.

A coordinated integration of neuromuscular factors. The effective application of force in relatively complex, learned movements such as the tennis serve or the shot put depends on a series of coordinated neuromuscular patterns, and not simply the strength of the muscle groups required for the movement.

Practical Implications. The complex interaction between the nervous and muscular systems provides some explanation for why the leg muscles, when strengthened using squats or deep knee bends, do not show the same improvement in another leg movement such as jumping. Consequently, strengthening muscles for use in a specific activity such as golf, rowing, swimming, or football requires more than just identifying and overloading the muscles involved in the movement. Rather, training should be specific to the exact movement. There is little transfer of newly acquired strength to other patterns of movement, even though the same muscles are involved. This was clearly shown in a recent study in which a 227% increase in leg extension strength occurred through standard weight training. When peak torque of the leg extensors was evaluated in the same subjects with an isokinetic dynamometer (see next section), however, there was only a 10 to 17% improvement!

As a general rule, to improve specific muscular performance, the muscles must be trained with movements as similar as possible to the desired movement or actual skill. Within this framework of training specificity, isokinetic-type methods are effective for improving strength at different speeds of movement.

ISOKINETIC TRAINING

Advantage of isokinetic training. Theoretically, isokinetic training makes it possible to activate muscles maximally at all points through the range of motion.

Isokinetic resistance training is different from both conventional dynamic and static methods. Recall that dynamic training occurs against an external load that generally remains constant throughout the movement, while static training is performed at a constant angle against an immovable load. *In contrast, isokinetic training generates force during movement at a preset, fixed speed. This enables the muscle to mobilize its maximum force-generating capacity through the full range of movement while shortening.* This is done with the aid of an electromechanical device, the isokinetic dynamometer, containing a mechanism that accelerates to a preset speed when force is applied. Once a constant speed is attained, the isokinetic loading mechanism accommodates to provide a counterforce in relation to the force generated by the muscle.

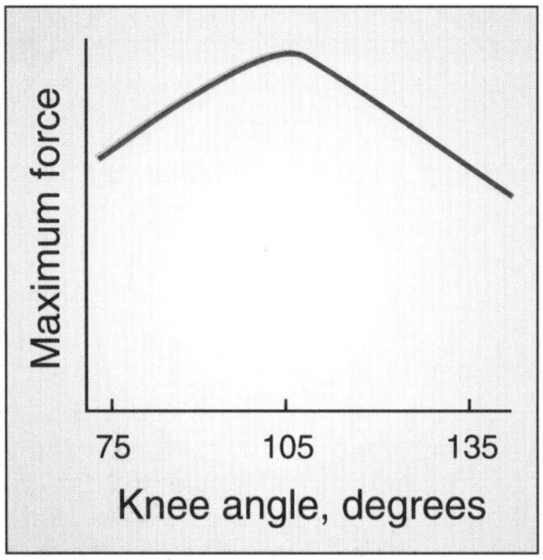

FIG. 18–2. Peak force generated by knee extensor muscles in relation to the joint angle of the knee.

A distinction can be made between a muscle loaded isotonically and one loaded isokinetically. Figure 18–2 shows the relationship between maximal force generated by the knee extensor muscles at various knee-joint angles. As with all joints in the body, the maximal muscle force exerted against an external resistance varies with the bony lever configuration as the joint moves through its normal range of motion. In weight-lifting exercises, for example, the inertia of the load must first be overcome; then execution of the movement progresses. The weight lifted can be no heavier than the maximum force capacity of the muscle at the "weakest" point in the range of motion; otherwise the movement would not be completed. Consequently, the amount of force generated by the muscles during a dynamic contraction cannot be maximum through all phases of the movement. In an isokinetically loaded muscle, however, the desired speed of movement occurs almost immediately, and the muscle is able to generate its peak power output throughout the movement and at a specific speed of contraction.

ADAPTATIONS WITH STRENGTH TRAINING

"Sticking point." Weight lifters frequently refer to the weakest point in their range of motion as the "sticking point."

Figure 18–3 displays six factors that impact on the development and maintenance of muscle mass. Without doubt, genetics provides the governing frame of reference that influences the effect of each of the other factors on the ultimate training outcome. However, muscle activity contributes little to tissue growth without appropriate nutrition to provide essential building

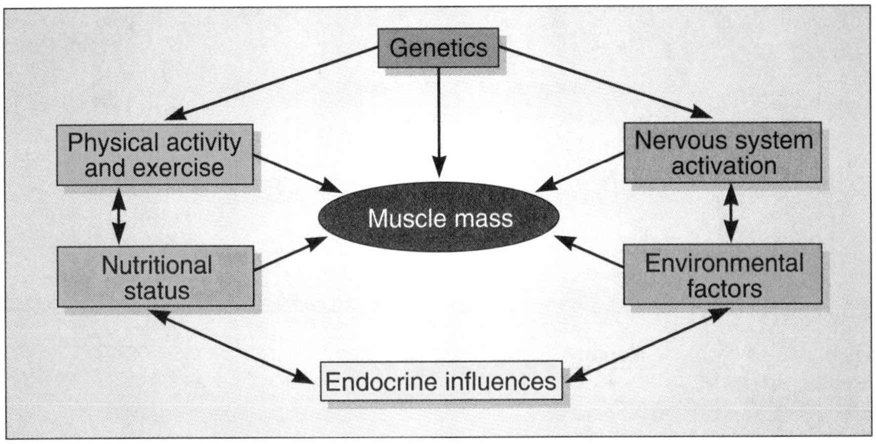

FIG. 18–3. Six factors that impact on the development and maintenance of total muscle mass.

Isokinetics is widely used for rehabilitation. Isokinetic equipment is used widely in sports medicine and athletic training. Many rehabilitation programs apply isokinetic training to evaluate and improve the muscular strength and power of injured limbs over their full range of motion.

blocks. Similarly, specific hormones and patterns of nervous system activation are crucial to the outcome. Without tension overload, however, each of the other factors is relatively ineffective to produce improvement.

FACTORS THAT MODIFY THE EXPRESSION OF HUMAN STRENGTH

The gross structural and microscopic changes that occur within muscle tissue as a result of overload training are fairly well documented. Considerable attention has also focused on the role of psychological and learning factors in determining and modifying the expression of muscular strength. As shown in Figure 18–4, factors broadly classified as psychological (neural) and muscular influence the expression of human strength. Many of these factors are readily modified by a resistance training program, whereas others appear to be training resistant; these are probably determined by natural endowment or are fixed early in life.

PSYCHOLOGICAL FACTORS

A unique series of experiments illustrates clearly the importance of **"psychological" factors** in the acquisition of muscular strength. The strength of the arm muscles was determined for 17 male and 8 female subjects prior to various treatments. These strength scores served as the baseline for all subsequent comparisons. In one series of experiments, the researchers measured arm strength while intermittent gunshots were fired behind the subjects just before their exertions. At another time they instructed the subjects to shout or scream loudly at the moment force was exerted. Following the "shoot and shout" experiments, the experimenters measured subjects' strength under the influence of two disinhibitory drugs, alcohol and amphetamines or "pep pills." They also measured strength while subjects were in a posthypnotic state and were told their strength would be greater than ever before and they should have no fear of injury. In almost all of the psychological conditions, arm strength was significantly greater

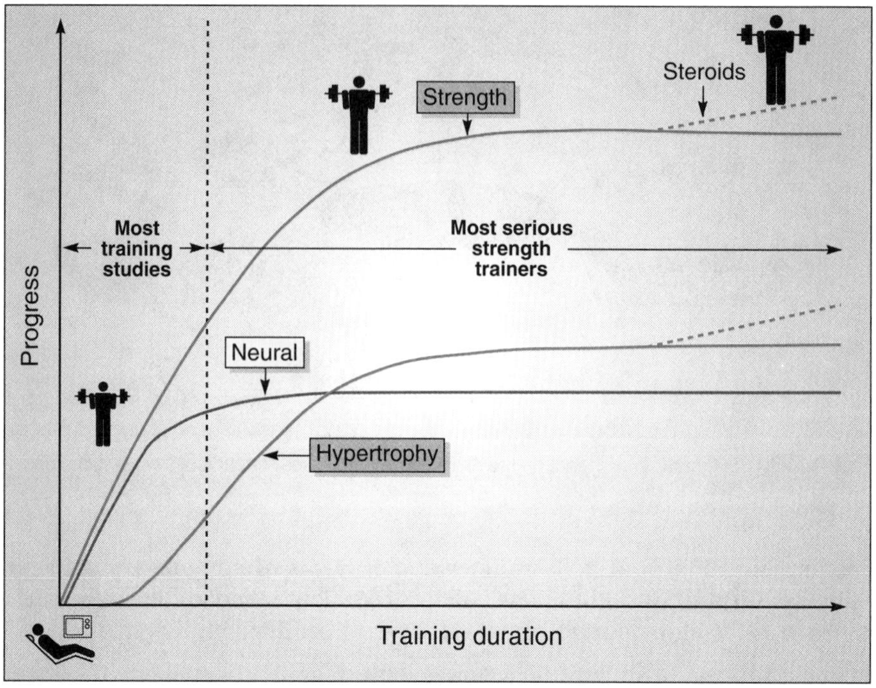

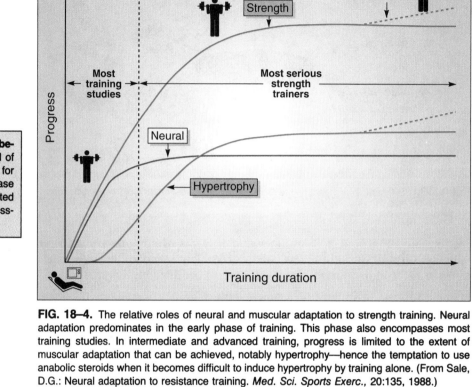

FIG. 18–4. The relative roles of neural and muscular adaptation to strength training. Neural adaptation predominates in the early phase of training. This phase also encompasses most training studies. In intermediate and advanced training, progress is limited to the extent of muscular adaptation that can be achieved, notably hypertrophy—hence the temptation to use anabolic steroids when it becomes difficult to induce hypertrophy by training alone. (From Sale, D.G.: Neural adaptation to resistance training. *Med. Sci. Sports Exerc.*, 20:135, 1988.)

Strength increases rapidly when beginning training. An enhanced level of neural facilitation probably accounts for the rapid and significant strength increase early in training, which is not associated with an increase in muscle size and cross-sectional area.

than under normal conditions. The greatest strength increases were observed under hypnosis, the most "mental" of all the treatments.

Mind over matter. Mental factors can have a significant impact on the expression of human strength.

To explain these observations, the researchers suggested that physical factors such as the size and type of muscle fibers and the anatomic lever arrangement of bone and muscle ultimately determine a person's capacity for muscular strength. They took the position that psychological or mental factors within the central nervous system exert neural influences that prevent most people from achieving their strength capacity. Neural inhibitions might be the result of social conditioning, unpleasant past experiences with physical activity, or an overprotective home environment. When performing under intense emotional conditions, such as athletic competition, an emergency situation, or posthypnotic suggestion, the inhibitory neural mechanisms are considerably reduced so the person is often capable of a "super performance" that more closely matches the physiologically determined capacity.

Observations such as these help to explain the apparent beneficial effects of "psyching," the almost self-induced hypnosis of athletes before competition. Excellent examples of such disinhibition can be observed in weight lifters, high jumpers and other track and field competitors, and self defense experts who perform nontraditional skills such as smashing cement bricks with their hands and feet. The great feats of strength observed during emotionally laden emergency situations also fit nicely with this explanation. In addition, the rapid improvements in muscular strength made during the first few weeks of a strength training program may be largely the result of a learning phenomenon as well as lessening of fear and psychological inhibition as the person becomes more accustomed to performing in the strength activity.

MUSCULAR FACTORS

Although psychological inhibitions as well as learning factors greatly modify ability to express muscular strength, the ultimate limit of strength development is determined by anatomic and physiologic factors within the muscle. As shown in Table 18–1, these **muscular factors** are not immutable but

TABLE 18–1. PHYSIOLOGIC ADAPTATIONS THAT OCCUR IN RESPONSE TO RESISTANCE TRAINING

SYSTEM/VARIABLE	RESPONSE
Muscle Fibers	
Number	Equivocal
Size	Increase
Type	?
Capillary Density	
In body builders	No change
In power lifters	Decrease
Mitochondrial	
Volume	Decrease
Density	
Twitch Contraction Time	Decrease
Enzymes	
Creatine phosphokinase	Increase
Myokinase	Increase
Enzymes of Glycolysis	
Phosphofructokinase	Increase
Lactate dehydrogenase	No change
Aerobic Metabolism Enzymes	
Carbohydrate metabolism	Increase
Triglycerides	No known
Intramuscular Fuel Stores	
Adenosine triphosphate	Increase
Phosphocreatine	Increase
Glycogen	Increase
Triglycerides	Not known
max $\dot{V}O_2$	
Circuit resistance training	Increase
Heavy resistance training	No change
Connective Tissue	
Ligament strength	Increase
Tendon strength	Increase
Collagen content of muscle	No change
Bone	
Mineral content	Increase
Cross-sectional area	No change

Modified from Fleck, S.J., and Kramer, W.J.: Resistance training: physiological responses and adaptions (Part 2 of 4). Phys. Sportsmed., 16:108, 1988.

can be modified considerably with strength training. The gross structural and microscopic changes in muscles that occur as a result of strength training are generally limited to adaptations in the contractile mechanisms and are usually accompanied by substantial increases in muscular strength and power.

Muscle Hypertrophy. *Increases in muscle size with resistance training for both men and women can be viewed as a fundamental biologic adaptation.* The large muscle size of weight lifters and body builders results from enlargement or **hypertrophy** of individual muscle cells, particularly the fast-twitch fibers. This growth results from synthesis of biologic compounds: there is an increase in the contractile proteins *actin* and *myosin* as well as in enzymes and stored nutrients.

Muscle Hyperplasia: Are new muscle fibers made? A question frequently raised is whether the actual number of muscle cells increases with resistance training in humans, a response called **hyperplasia.** Researchers have reported that some muscle fibers from trained animals undergo a process of longitudinal splitting which results in the development of new fibers. This response may be species specific, however, because most animals do not undergo the massive hypertrophy observed in humans with resistance training. Recent studies of body builders with a relatively large muscle mass have failed to show that these athletes possess significant hypertrophy of individual muscle fibers. *This certainly leaves open the possibility that hyperplasia occurs in humans with resistance training.* It suggests either an inherited difference in fiber number or that muscle cells may adapt differently to the high-volume, high-intensity training used by body builders compared with the typical low-repetition, heavy-load system favored by strength and power athletes.

Hyperplasia in humans. Individual muscle fibers increase in thickness; whether they increase in number remains a question. Even if hyperplasia is replicated in other human studies (and even if the response is a positive adjustment), the greatest contribution to muscular size with overload training is made by the enlargement of existing individual muscle cells.

Aside from enlarging existing muscle fibers, resistance training also stimulates an increase in bone mineral content as well as proliferation of connective tissue surrounding the individual muscle fibers. This thickens and strengthens the muscles' connective tissue harness. Resistance training also improves the structural and functional integrity of both tendons and ligaments. These adaptations provide protection from joint and muscle injury, which supports the use of resistance exercise as preventive and rehabilitative training.

Fast-twitch fibers are most responsive to resistance training. Fast-twitch muscle fibers of weight lifters are about 45% larger than similar fibers in healthy untrained people and endurance athletes.

MUSCULAR STRENGTH OF MEN AND WOMEN

When strength is compared on an absolute basis (i.e., total force applied or weight lifted), women generally possess about 70% of the force-generating capacity of men. This difference is magnified in comparisons of upper body strength, where the female is about 50% weaker than the male. This **gender characterization of muscular strength** is true regardless of the device used to measure strength. Certainly there are exceptions to this generalization, especially for women involved in resistance training programs. Variations in body size and composition largely account for the large differences between genders. Men generally develop a larger muscle mass than women; thus their absolute strength is greater. Differences in body composition, however, may totally account for differences in muscular strength between the genders.

In a recent experiment in which men and women were matched for total body mass, lean body mass, and prior training status, males were still significantly "stronger" by 14 to 35% than females in the squat and bench press. Attempting to equalize the differences in strength between men and women by expressing a woman's strength score in relation to her body mass or lean body mass probably will not totally eliminate the observed differences in strength. Considered in total, males are stronger than females independent of the method used to express strength. This includes the absolute strength score as well as strength expressed per unit of body mass, lean body mass, or muscle cross-sectional dimension. True biologic factors may be at the heart of such gender differences.

STRENGTH TRAINING FOR WOMEN

One of the more vivid illustrations of the redefining of women's roles in society has been their present participation in a wide range of competitive sports and physical activities. Although muscular strength is an important factor in achieving optimum sports performance, many women have shied away from strengthening exercises for fear of developing the enlarged muscles so common in men. This is unfortunate because the failure of many women to learn skills and improve in activities such as tennis, golf, dance, and gymnastics can be attributed to lack of muscular strength, especially upper-body strength. A proper program of resistance training can usually improve such muscular weakness.

Gender differences. A basic **gender difference in the response to resistance training** appears to be the absolute amount of muscle hypertrophy.

Muscular Strength and Hypertrophy. Despite similar percentage improvements in strength with resistance training, increases in muscle girth have been reported to be less for women. Researchers have speculated that this is because of hormonal differences between the genders, especially the 20 to 30 times higher **testosterone** level in men, which exerts a strong anabolic or tissue-building effect. It should be noted, however, that testosterone levels are on a continuum for men and women, with some females normally possessing high levels of this hormone.

Testosterone. Testosterone is the major male sex hormone responsible for promoting growth and development of the reproductive organs and secondary sex characteristics.

Recent experiments using computed axial tomography (CAT) scans to directly evaluate muscle cross-sectional area indicated that the hypertrophic response to resistance training was *similar* for men and women. The absolute change in muscle size was certainly greater for men (because their total muscle mass is greater), but the enlargement of muscle on a percentage basis was the same between genders. Other comparisons between elite male and female body builders have verified these observations. More research is needed before definitive statements can be made concerning similarities and differences in the resistance training responses of men and women. The limited data from relatively short-term studies do suggest that women can utilize conventional resistance training without developing overly large muscles.

METABOLIC STRESS OF RESISTANCE TRAINING

Numerous claims have been made concerning the physical benefits to be derived from various forms of resistance training. These include the promise

Strength training and blood lipids. Although resistance training programs significantly improve muscular strength and increase lean body mass, they have essentially no effect on total cholesterol or other aspects of the blood lipid profile.

of improved "organic vigor," reduced body fat, and better aerobic and cardiovascular function. Undoubtedly, a properly planned program of resistance training is highly effective for developing and maintaining muscular strength. It does not appear, however, that traditional methods of resistance training are especially effective for programs of aerobic fitness or weight control, or for modifying risk factors related to cardiovascular disease.

ISOMETRIC AND WEIGHT-LIFTING EXERCISE

Energy expenditure. The number of calories expended in weight training is not very high. The rate of oxygen consumed during standard barbell resistance training is equivalent to walking on level ground at 4 miles per hour, gardening, or swimming slowly.

In a series of experiments to evaluate the **metabolic stress of standard resistance exercises,** we studied the immediate physiologic effects of isometric and resistance exercises. The resistance exercises were performed with a weight that enabled the person to complete eight repetitions of a particular movement. Isometric exercise involved a 6-second contraction performed against a bar placed in a position halfway through the range of motion of the corresponding weight-lifting exercise. In this experiment we studied the two-arm curl, two-arm press, bench press, and squat.

The results for heart rate and oxygen uptake indicated that both forms of exercise would be classified as only light to moderate in terms of energy expenditure, even though considerable stress is placed on the involved muscle groups. Although a person may perform 15 or 20 different resistance exercises during a 1-hour training session, the time devoted to actual exercise is short, usually no longer than 6 or 7 minutes. This brief activity period, which produces only a moderate expenditure of energy, indicates that traditional resistance training programs would not improve endurance capacity for activities such as running or swimming. Furthermore, they would be of limited value as major activities in weight-reducing programs because the caloric expenditure is low during an exercise session.

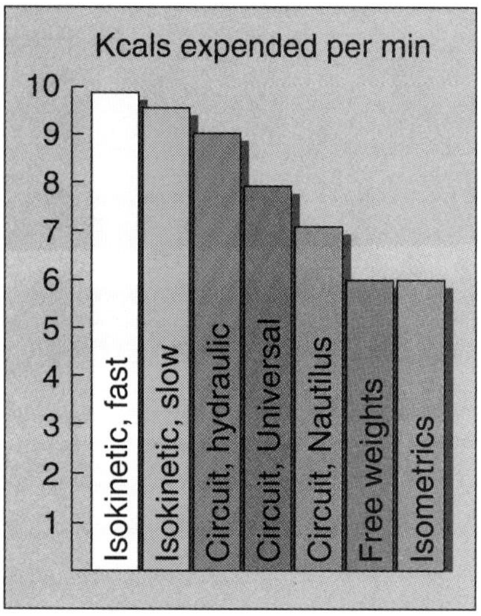

Calories expended per minute for different modes of resistance exercise. Values are based on a body mass of 68 kg.

CIRCUIT RESISTANCE TRAINING

By modifying standard resistance training so that heavy overload is deemphasized, it is possible to increase the caloric cost of exercise and improve more than one aspect of fitness. Current research has focused on the energy cost and **cardiorespiratory demands of circuit resistance training** (CRT). In CRT, resistance exercises are performed in a preestablished exercise-rest sequence. In most programs, the circuit consists of 8 to 12 different exercise stations with a prescribed number of repetitions, usually 15 to 20, performed for each exercise. Such exercise requires between 40 and 50% of a person's maximum strength. After a 15-second rest, the participant moves to the next exercise station and so on until the circuit is completed.

In one experiment, the energy expended during CRT was determined for 20 men and 20 women. They performed three exercise circuits (10 stations per circuit utilizing weight machines) with a 15-second rest between exercises. The total time to perform the three circuits was 22.5 minutes. The net amount of energy expended (excluding resting metabolism), was 129 kcal for the men and 95 kcal for the women over the total exercise period. Heart rate averaged 142 beats per minute (72% of maximum) for the men and 158 (82% of maximum) for the women. This corresponded to about 40% of maximum oxygen uptake (max $\dot{V}O_2$) for the men and 45% for the women. Because the energy expended during the circuit was related to the participant's body mass, the results in Table 18–2 are presented in terms of body mass. On average, the continuous level of energy expended in CRT

Circuit resistance training. CRT deemphasizes the heavy muscle overload of standard resistance training to provide more general conditioning that improves body composition, muscular strength and endurance, and aerobic fitness.

TABLE 18–2. NET ENERGY EXPENDITURE DURING CRT TRAINING FOR MEN AND WOMEN												
KCAL EXPENDED PER MINUTE*												
Body Weight, Pounds	100	110	120	130	140	150	160	170	180	190	200	210
Men			4.1	4.4	4.8	5.1	5.4	5.7	6.0	6.4	6.7	7.0
Women	3.4	3.6	3.7	3.9	4.1	4.3	4.4	4.6	4.8			

* Calculated from data of Wilmore, J.H., et al.: Energy cost of circuit weight training. *Med. Sci. Sports* 10:75, 1978. To determine the total number of calories expended during workouts (over and above rest), multiply the value in the column that corresponds to your body weight by the duration of the circuit. For example, a 160-pound male who exercises on the circuit for 43 minutes would expend 232 kcal (5.4 kcal/min × 43 min), excluding resting metabolism.

was equivalent to a slow jog, hiking in the hills at a moderate pace, playing basketball or tennis, or leisurely swimming the crawl stroke.

This modification of standard resistance training is an attractive alternative for those fitness enthusiasts desiring a general conditioning program. It may also be a good supplemental off-season fitness program for athletes involved in sports that require a high level of strength, power, and muscular endurance.

ORGANIZING A RESISTANCE TRAINING PROGRAM

People without previous resistance training experience should follow a program designed to produce all-around strength improvements.

THE WARM-UP

The value of **preliminary warm-up exercise** to reduce the chances for muscle and joint injuries, as well as to improve subsequent performance, has been challenged over the years. Although the scientific basis for recommending a warm-up is not conclusive, we feel it would be unwise to completely ignore warming up. Furthermore, evidence indicates that moderate preliminary exercise improves the cardiovascular response to subsequent strenuous exercise. Adjustments in blood flow within the heart muscle to a sudden, vigorous bout of exercise are not instantaneous, and even healthy individuals may show a transient poor oxygen supply to the myocardium under such conditions. However, with a prior warm-up of several minutes of easy jogging, for example, adjustments in myocardial blood flow and oxygen supply are more favorable. Any sequence of calisthenic and flexibility exercises, as well as running in place or other moderate rhythmic exercises, can be used as a warm-up. The general warm-up exercises illustrated in Figure 18–5 serve this purpose and can be completed in a few minutes. These exercises will gradually increase joint flexibility and general circulation, and may help deter muscle and joint discomfort.

Stretching exercises should be done slowly and smoothly until you feel mild tension on your muscles. The goal is not to complete many repetitions of the particular movement, but rather to *hold* the stretch. A reasonable

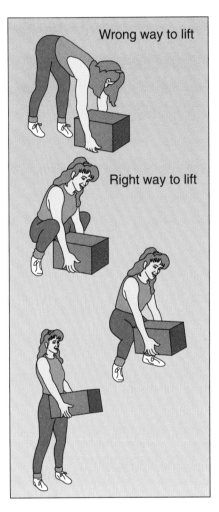

Proper lifting mechanics avoids musculoskeletal injuries. (Top) The wrong way to lift an object. (Bottom) The right way to lift an object. Maintain a wide base of support by keeping the feet wider apart than than shoulder width. After you grasp the object, stand up using the power of the leg muscles and keeping the head up and back straight as you straighten up.

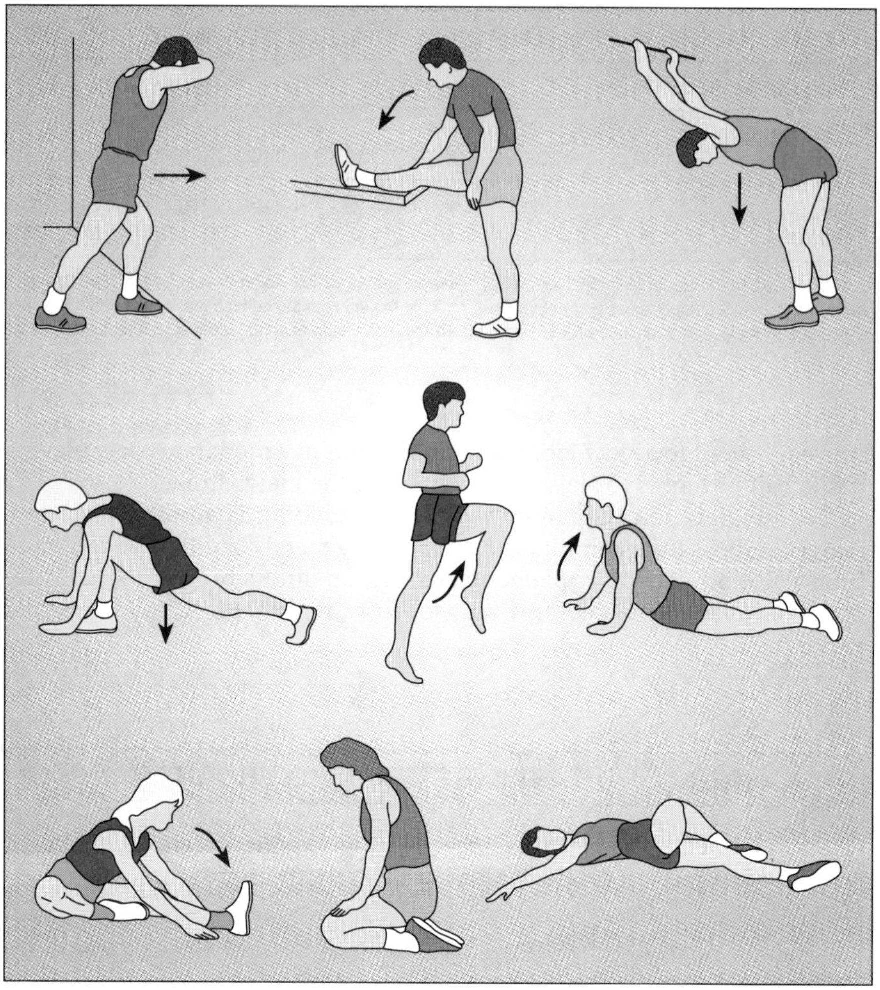

FIG. 18–5. Examples of calisthenic and flexibility exercises that can be performed as part of a warm-up.

Hold that stretch! Stretching that employs fast bouncing and jerky movement that uses the body's momentum can strain or tear muscles and may create a reflex action that actually resists the muscle's stretching.

goal is to hold the stretch for 10 seconds in the beginning; as flexibility improves, increase the duration of the static stretch to 30 seconds.

THE LOWER BACK

The lower back is susceptible to injury. Many people lose considerable time at work, suffer chronic discomfort, and spend large amounts of money on orthopedists and chiropractors attempting to alleviate low back pain. In fact, it has been estimated that one-half of the work force in the United States will suffer from back problems at some point in their career! The causes for this malady are not always apparent and a cure is elusive. However, many orthopedists feel the prime factors in "low back syndrome" are *muscular weakness*, especially in the abdominal region, and *poor joint flexibility* in the back and legs. Both strengthening and flexibility exercises are commonly prescribed for prevention of and rehabilitation from chronic low back strain.

The use of resistance training exercises poses a dilemma. If done properly, such training provides an excellent means to strengthen the muscles of the abdomen and lower back to support and protect the spine. As is often the case, however, many people, attempting to create too much force, perform an exercise improperly. As a result, additional muscle groups are recruited, the spinal column is placed in improper alignment, especially with arching of the back, and lower back strain results. A seemingly simple exercise such as a sit-up, if done improperly with legs stiff, back arched, and head thrown back, can place tremendous strain on the lower spine (sit-ups should always be done with the knees flexed and chin tucked to the chest). Pressing and curling exercises with weights, if performed with excessive hyperextension or arch to the back, may cause muscle strain or spinal pressure that can trigger low back pain. For these reasons, those who begin a program of strenghtening exercises are urged to do all exercises correctly in the manner described.

Anti-inflamatory compounds for muscle pain. An anti-inflamatory drug that contains 400 mg of ibuprofen reduces postexercise swelling, stiffness, joint pain, and sore muscles by up to 75% if taken 4 hours before exercise and then twice more at 8-hour intervals after the workout. The regimen may work best for people beginning an exercise program because it is in these people that soreness is most prevalent. Caution is recommended, however, in taking ibuprofen before exercise because the drug can cause significant stomach irritation.

Always use proper technique. Never sacrifice proper execution to lift a heavier load or "squeeze out" an additional repetition. The extra weight lifted through improper technique will not facilitate muscle strengthening, and may precipitate lower back injury.

SELECTING THE PROPER WEIGHT

In the beginning stages of training, you should not attempt to see how much weight can be lifted. This serves little purpose in improving strength and greatly increases the likelihood of muscle or joint injury. *It is unnecessary to exercise at maximum levels to develop muscular strength.* A load that represents between 60 and 80% of a muscle's maximum strength is **sufficient overload for improvement.** This resistance permits completion of between 6 and 10 repetitions of a particular exercise when using barbells or exercise machines. Our experience has shown that beginners should aim to complete 12 repetitions of an exercise. If the weight selected for the 12 repetitions feels "too easy," a heavier weight should be used; if the exerciser cannot do 12 repetitions, the weight is too heavy. This is a trial-and-error process, and it may take several exercise sessions before a proper starting weight is selected.

Go easy when starting out. The amount of weight lifted during 12 repetitions will not place excessive strain on the muscles during the beginning phase of resistance training.

After 5 or 6 training sessions, the muscles will begin to adapt and the exerciser will have learned the correct lifting movements. The number of repetitions should now be reduced to between 6 and 8 and the resistance increased accordingly. When the exerciser can complete 8 repetitions, add more weight. The additional weight will undoubtedly reduce the number of repetitions. This is exactly the desired outcome. Eight repetitions should be achieved within several exercise sessions, and again, more weight will have to be added.

The exercises are performed in the same order on each workout day. This is because many exercises involve more than one muscle group, and some fatigue may result from a previous exercise. By maintaining the same order of exercise, the cumulative fatigue effect should remain relatively constant. In scheduling workouts, consistency is the key to successful training. This does not mean that workouts should be scheduled every day. At least 2 or 3 exercise sessions each week are necessary to continue strength improvements. Some people exercise 5 or 6 days a week. With this protocol, different muscle groups are usually exercised on alternate days so, in reality, a specific muscle group is still trained only 2 or 3 days a week.

SIX STEPS IN PLANNING THE WORKOUT

Organization and structure are important components when formulating a program to develop muscular strength.

Step 1. Establish the primary aims and objectives of the strength training program. Strengthening exercises are performed for many different reasons: improved sports performance, development and maintenance of muscle tone or firmness, aesthetic enhancement, or fun and pleasure. Whatever the reason, include exercises that will meet personal objectives. Use a variety of exercises for an all-around strength conditioning program; include exercises for the neck, arms, forearms, shoulders, abdomen, back, chest, buttocks, and legs.

Step 2. Determine the length of time available for exercise. Work schedules and other restraints often limit the number of exercises a person can complete in a workout. A minimum of about 20 minutes is usually required to complete a series of basic exercises. This includes rest intervals as well as the time spent in actual exercise.

Step 3. Determine the available facilities and equipment. It is not necessary to purchase expensive equipment; many household items can be used to provide muscular overload, and often people can construct equipment with minimal expense. The exercises shown in Figure 18–6 rely on common household and store-bought items. Weights can be made by filling plastic containers with water or filling socks and other clothes with sand. A broom or mop handle can serve as a bar to which these objects are attached. Ski boots, telephone books, bricks wrapped in a towel, and other objects can also provide resistance to muscular contraction. Of course, barbells and dumbbells are the easiest to use and are relatively inexpensive. Chairs, table tops, and other stable furniture items can take the place of standard gymnasium equipment. A piece of clothesline can be used as a jump rope.

Step 4. Selection of the exercises. A variety of exercises can be done for strengthening the large muscle groups of the body. Such exercises can meet the needs of most people interested in toning and strengthening muscles.

Step 5. Arrange an **exercise circuit** similar to that described for CRT. When arranging the exercises in a proper sequence, it is important not to perform consecutively two exercises that involve the same muscle groups. This way the possible transfer of fatigue effects will be minimized. For example, two exercises for the chest should be separated by another exercise that does not use the the chest musculature. Figure 18–7 illustrates the basic model of the circuit for hydraulic resistance exercise. In this example, there are 8 different exercise stations with one exercise performed at each station. The type of equipment used in the circuit is not the crucial element. Any

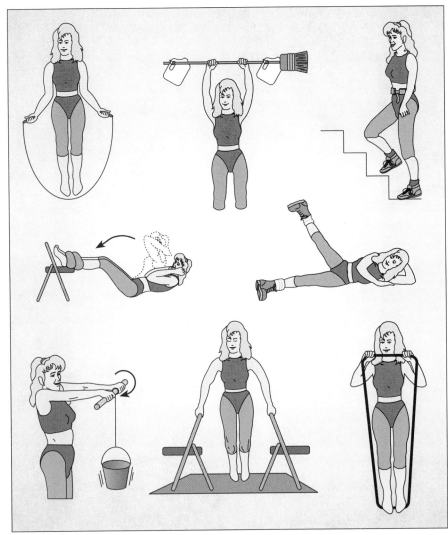

FIG. 18–6. Household items incorporated into a strength training program.

equipment can be used, from homemade items to cement "barbells" to the latest resistance machines that are interfaced with computer-controlled audio, laser disc, and interactive video.

Modifications to an Exercise Circuit. Each exercise can consist of any number of repetitions desired. Initially, when working with weights, 12 repetitions of each exercise are done until the proper load or resistance is established. After several weeks, additional weight is added until a target number of 6 to 8 repetitions is achieved. The goal of this circuit could be simply to complete the desired exercises in the time available for the workout. When the *target number* of repetitions is achieved, more weight is added. Another objective might be to perform the required number of repetitions of each exercise within a previously established *target time.* For example, suppose the 10 exercise stations, each with one exercise performed 12 times, are to be completed twice. Initially, it may require 20 minutes to complete two circuits. This would then become the target time, and during each workout the objective would be to complete two circuits within this time.

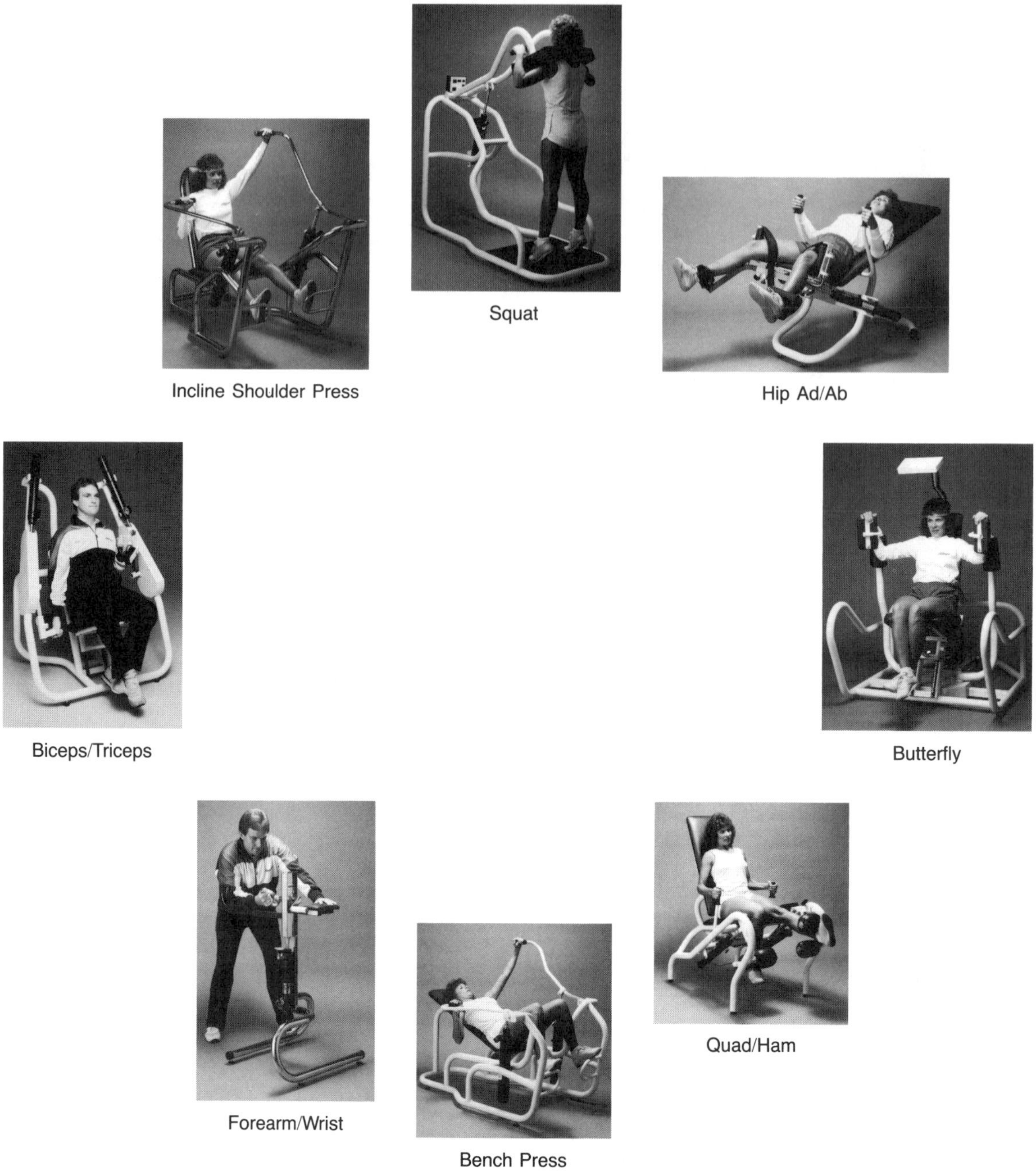

FIG. 18–7. Arrangement of an exercise circuit. Each exercise should be designed for a different group of muscles. After completing an exercise at one station, the exerciser performs the next exercise in the circuit. To provide variety, music can be used to signal the start and end of each exercise and rest break. Louder volume can signal the start of exercise, and softer volume the end of the rest period before proceeding to the next exercise. A reasonable exercise time is 20 to 30 seconds with a 20 to 40 second rest. People usually complete 2 circuits during the workout.

Once this occurs, several methods can be used to maintain a *progressive overload*. For example, a faster target time might be set. Other modifications could include the use of heavier weights while maintaining the 20-minute target time, or attempting to complete one additional circuit during the 20-minute exercise period. Thus, circuits for strength development can achieve overload by manipulating three variables:

- Load or resistance
- Repetitions of each exercise in the circuit
- Target time to complete the circuit

Each variable can be manipulated separately or in combination to ensure progressive overload.

The overload principle can be applied to exercises that require little or no equipment. This is done by increasing the difficulty of the exercise. For example, the conventional push-up can be made more difficult by changing the body position from horizontal (starting position on the level) to a slant by placing the feet on a 12- to 16-inch bench. The same can be done for sit-ups. To do this, place the feet on the seat of a chair, hands clasped behind the neck and chin to chest. Curl up until the elbows touch the knees, and then return to the starting position. This type of "incline" sit-up can be made even more strenuous if a weight is held across the chest.

Step 6. The last step in planning the workout involves the most efficient use of available facilities. This is usually not a problem in gymnasiums or health clubs where specialized equipment is available. For those who exercise at home, the situation is different and necessitates other solutions. In small or confined areas, it may not be possible to progress from one station to the next. In this case, one can exercise in several small areas. Sometimes, however, the constraints of exercising in a limited space make a person more aware of the potential for using other available facilities, such as hallways, staircases or stairwells, washrooms, dorm lounges, garages, or nearby parks and walkways.

We are aware of a CRT program arranged by a man who lived in a high-rise apartment building. He exercised 4 days a week completing three circuits, each consisting of 8 stations and 20 repetitions per station. Station 1 was sit-ups, done on the bedroom floor with knees bent and feet supported under the bed. He performed these holding a 10-pound weight across his chest. Station 2 consisted of modified pull-ups (feet supported on a chair) from a bar secured in the bathroom doorway. Station 3 was rope skipping in the hallway. To increase the intensity of this cardiovascular exercise, the exerciser wore ski boots while jumping at a rate of 100 skips a minute. Station 4 involved raising and lowering the body with the arms supported between two kitchen chairs while wearing a jacket filled with 20 pounds of sand. Station 5 was performed on the living room floor. The exercise consisted of raising and lowering each leg while lying supported on the side, with a knee-high sock filled with 15 pounds of sand attached around the ankle. Station 6 was a chest press performed while lying supine on the floor, using a broom barbell with weights of plastic containers filled with 26 pounds of cement. Station 7 consisted of back extensions, performed while lying face down over the edge of a coffee table with the feet secured under a rope tied around the table top and a 10-pound weight held behind the head. Station 8 involved quickly descending and then ascending five flights of stairs. On the first and second circuit, stair climbing was done as fast as possible. Going up the stairs on the last circuit, the man hopped up each stair keeping his feet together, with only a minimal rest between floors!

SUMMARY

1. Muscles become stronger in response to overload training. Overload is created by increasing the load, the number of repetitions, or the speed of muscular contraction, or by a combination of these factors.
2. There are three basic types of muscle contraction: (1) concentric contraction, in which the muscle shortens as it develops tension; (2) eccentric contraction, in which external resistance exceeds muscle force and the muscle lengthens while developing tension; and (3) isometric contraction, in which no noticeable shortening of the muscle occurs as it generates force but is unable to overcome external resistance.
3. The three major systems for developing strength are progressive resistance weight training, isometrics, and isokinetic-type training. Each system results in strength gains that are highly specific to the type of training.
4. Isokinetic-type training, because of the possibility for generating maximum force throughout the full range of motion at different velocities of limb movement, appears to offer a unique method for resistance training.
5. Genetic, exercise, nutritional, hormonal, environmental, and neural factors interact to regulate skeletal muscle mass and corresponding strength development.
6. A person's capacity for muscular strength is largely determined by physiologic factors such as size and type of muscle fibers, as well as by the anatomic-lever arrangement of bone and muscle. This strength capacity is probably greatly affected by neural influences from the central nervous system that activate the prime movers in a specific muscular action.
7. Increases in strength with resistance training result from improved efficiency and capacity for neuromuscular contraction as well as significant alterations in the contractile elements within the muscle cell itself.
8. As muscles are overloaded and become stronger, they normally hypertrophy, or grow larger. This process involves increased protein synthesis for the contractile elements within the muscle cell and proliferation of connective tissue cells that thickens and strengthens the muscle's connective tissue harness.
9. In short-term training studies, strength improvements for women on a percentage basis are similar to those for men. Recent research also indicates that women are capable of significant increases in muscle mass as a result of resistance training.
10. Conventional resistance-training exercises contribute little to cardiovascular-aerobic fitness. Because of their relatively low caloric cost, they would not be effective major activities in weight-reducing programs.
11. By use of lower resistance and higher repetitions, circuit resistance training offers an effective alternative for combining the muscle-training benefits of resistance exercise with the cardiovascular benefits of more continuous dynamic exercise.

12. A load that represents 60 to 80% of a muscle's force-generating capacity is usually sufficient overload to produce strength gains.

RELATED READINGS

Bembem, M.G., et al.: Isometric muscle force production as a function of age in healthy 20- to 74-year-old men. *Med. Sci. Sport Exerc.*, 23:1302, 1992.

Gettman, L.R., and Pollock, M.L.: Circuit weight training: a critical review of its physiological benefits. *Phys. Sportsmed.*, 9:44, 1980.

Gettman, L.R., et al.: A comparison of combined running and weight training with circuit weight training. *Med. Sci. Sports Exerc.*, 14:229, 1982.

Goldberg, A.L., et al.: Mechanism of work induced hypertrophy. *Med. Sci. Sports*, 7:185, 1975.

Hortobagyi, T., and Katch, F.: Role of concentric force in limiting improvement in muscular strength. *J. Appl. Physiol.*, 68:650, 1990.

Hortobagyi, T., and Katch, F.: Transfer of cycling-induced fatigue to performance in vertical jump and isokinetic squat strength. *J. Hum. Muscle Perform.*, 1:32, 1992.

Hortobagyi, T., et al.: Effects of simultaneous training for strength and endurance on upper and lower body strength and running performance. *J. Sports Med. Phys. Fit.*, 31:20, 1991.

Hurley, B.F., et al.: Effects of high intensity strength training on cardiovascular function. *Med. Sci. Sports Exerc.*, 16:483, 1984.

Ikai, M., and Steinhaus, A.H.: Some factors modifying the expression of human strength. *J. Appl. Physiol.*, 16:157, 1961.

Katch, F.I., et al.: Evaluation of acute cardiorespiratory responses to hydraulic resistance exercise. *Med. Sci. Sports Exerc.*, 17:168, 1985.

Kokkinos, P.F., et al.: Strength training does not improve lipoprotein-lipid profiles in men at risk for CHD. *Med. Sci. Sports Exerc.*, 23:1134, 1991.

Larson, L., and Tesch, P.A.: Motor unit fibre density in extremely hypertrophied skeletal muscles in man. Electrophysiological signs of muscle fibre hyperplasia. *Eur. J. Appl. Physiol.*, 55:130, 1986.

Lortie, G., et al.: Relationships between skeletal muscle characteristics and aerobic performance in sedentary and active subjects. *Eur. J. Appl. Physiol.*, 54:471, 1985.

Luthi, J.M., et al.: Structural changes in skeletal muscle tissue with heavy-resistance exercise. *Int. J. Sports Med.*, 7:123, 1986.

MacDougall, J.D., et al.: Muscle ultrastructural characteristics of elite power lifters and bodybuilders. *Eur. J. Appl. Physiol.*, 48:117, 1982.

MacDougall, J.D., et al.: Muscle fiber number in biceps brachii in body builders and control subjects. *J. Appl. Physiol.*, 57:1399, 1984.

McArdle, W.D., and Foglia, G.F.: Energy cost and cardiorespiratory stress of isometric and weight training exercise. *J. Sports Med. Phys. Fit.*, 9:23, 1969.

McArdle, W.D., et al.: Exercise Physiology: Energy, Nutrition, and Human Performance, 3rd ed. Philadelphia, Lea & Febiger, 1991.

Weltman, A.W., et al.: The effects of hydraulic resistance strength training in pre-pubertal males. *Med. Sci. Sports Exerc.*, 18:629, 1986.

19

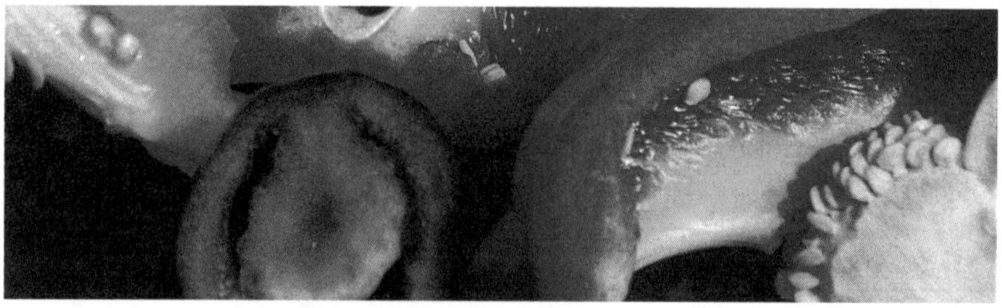

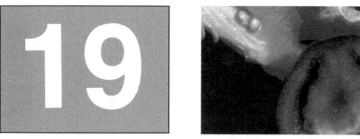

CONDITIONING FOR ANAEROBIC AND AEROBIC POWER

Energy needs to be generated rapidly in many forms of physical activity. Because energy release is required almost instantaneously, sufficient oxygen cannot be delivered to the muscles quickly enough to match energy requirements. Even if oxygen was immediately available, it could not be utilized fast enough to be of much use. Consequently, the anaerobic energy capacity determines success in ploughing through the line in football, spiking in volleyball, or runnning out an infield hit in softball. The apparent steady-state sports such as basketball, tennis, field hockey, lacrosse, and soccer also involve sprinting, dashing, darting, and stop-and-go, in which the capacity to generate short bursts of anaerobic power plays an important role. Too often, coaches of these sports place considerable emphasis on the development of aerobic capacity at the sacrifice of vigorous anaerobic conditioning. It is true that these sports do require a relatively steady release of energy for a considerable period of time. However, in those crucial situations that demand an all-out effort, the relative capacity of the athlete's ***anaerobic energy system*** may be poor and the player or team will be unable to perform at full potential. On the other hand, training the anaerobic capacity of endurance athletes such as marathon runners or channel swimmers would be wasteful because the contribution of this energy system to this type of performance is minimal. Success in endurance activities necessitates a highly trained ***aerobic energy system*** that depends upon a well-conditioned heart and vascular system capable of delivering a large quantity of blood for an extended time.

ENERGY FOR EXERCISE: IT'S THE BLEND THAT'S IMPORTANT

Figure 19–1 summarizes the relative involvement of the systems of anaerobic and aerobic energy transfer during "all-out" exercise of varying durations. Keep in mind that the three energy systems—the adenosine triphosphate–creatine phosphate (ATP-CP) system, the lactic acid system, and the aerobic system—are often operating simultaneously during physical activity. However, their relative contributions to the total energy requirement can differ markedly depending on the *duration* and *intensity* of the activity.

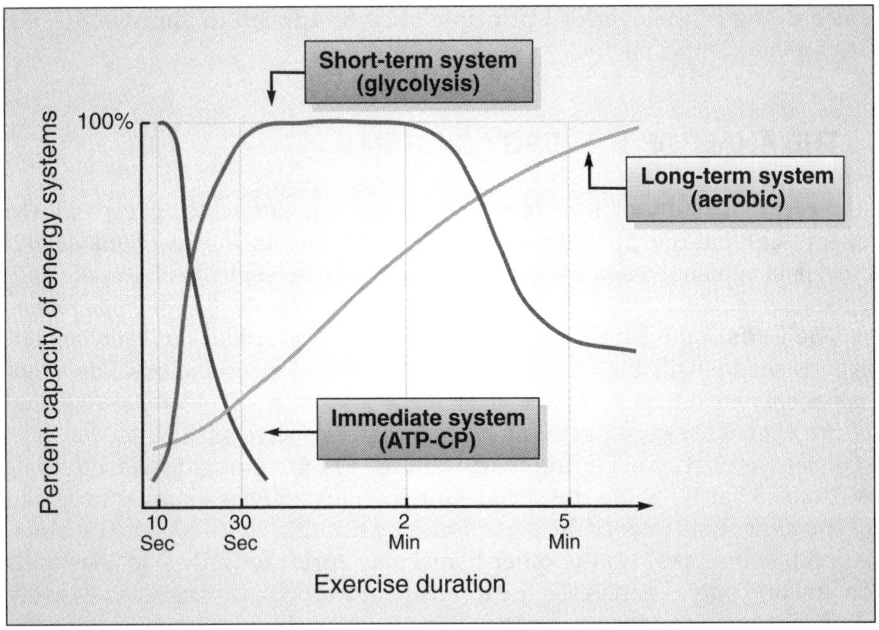

FIG. 19–1. The various energy systems and their involvement during all-out exercise of different durations.

Energy continuum. All activity and sports performance can be classified on an **anaerobic-to-aerobic continuum.** These activities use some percentage from each of the energy systems, depending on the intensity and duration of the effort.

With an immediate, maximum burst of effort as in the tennis serve, golf swing, volleyball spike, and even the 60- or 100-yard dash, energy is provided anaerobically almost exclusively by the stored high-energy phosphates ATP and CP. In a performance that lasts between 10 and 90 seconds, as in a 100-yard swim or 220-yard run, energy is still supplied predominantly by anaerobic reactions. In this case, however, the primary role is played by energy from the initial phase of carbohydrate breakdown with lactic acid formation. Training for such activities must be of sufficient intensity and duration to overload this specific anaerobic energy system. In wrestling, boxing, ice hockey, a 400- or 1500-meter run, or a fullcourt press in basketball, the magnitude of energy generated from anaerobic sources depends on the person's capacity and tolerance for lactic acid accumulation. In these activities, however, aerobic energy metabolism also plays an important role. As exercise intensity diminishes somewhat and the duration extends between 2 and 4 minutes, dependence on energy from the anaerobic pathways decreases while energy release from oxygen-consuming reactions predominates. With continuous exercise beyond 4 minutes, the activity becomes progressively more dependent on aerobic energy; in a marathon run or long-distance swim, the body is powered almost exclusively by the energy from aerobic reactions.

In training for a particular sport or performance goal, the activity must be carefully evaluated in terms of its energy components. As a result of this analysis, an appropriate amount of time is then devoted to the specific training of each energy system.

ANAEROBIC CONDITIONING

The capacity to perform all-out exercise of up to 90 seconds depends mainly on anaerobic energy metabolism. As was the case with training to improve muscular strength, the overload principle must be applied to improve this energy-generating capacity.

THE ANAEROBIC ENERGY SYSTEM

Recall from Chapter 11 that anaerobic energy is generated from breakdown of the high-energy phosphates ATP and CP, and in the reactions of glycolysis in which glucose is transformed into lactic acid.

Bursts of energy. Sports such as football, weight lifting, and various other brief, sprint-type activities requiring rapid energy release rely almost exclusively on energy derived from the muscle's pool of high-energy phosphates.

The Phosphate Pool. During the first 6 seconds of all-out exercise, energy is made available almost immediately from anaerobic breakdown of the energy currency, ATP, and the energy reservoir, CP. *Maximum overload of* ***the phosphate pool*** *in specific muscles can be achieved with all-out bursts of effort for 5 to 10 seconds.* During swim training, a sprinter might swim intervals of 20 to 25 yards, while the sprint runner could achieve a similar **overload of the phosphate pool** of the leg muscles by running 60- to 100-yard sprints. A football lineman, on the other hand, may sprint for only 2 to 3 seconds on any one play. To increase the intensity of overload during this relatively short but intense exercise period, the player could practice running with a weighted belt or vest, or sprint up hills or stairs. Because high-energy phosphates supply the energy for such brief, intermittent exercise, only a small amount of lactic acid is produced and recovery is quite rapid. Thus, a subsequent exercise bout can begin after only a 30- to 60-second recovery.

As a general rule, in training to enhance a muscle's ATP-CP energy capacity, the individual should undertake repetitive bouts of intense, very short duration exercise. *The training activities selected must engage the muscles in the movement patterns for which the person desires this improved anaerobic power.* This will enhance the metabolic capacity of the specifically trained muscle fibers, and also facilitate neuromuscular adaptations to the specific rate and pattern of movement.

Interval training. The use of brief, all-out work periods interspersed with recovery represents a specific application of interval training. This approach is excellent for anaerobic conditioning.

Lactic Acid. As the duration of all-out effort extends beyond 10 seconds, dependence on energy from phosphates decreases, while the quantity of anaerobic energy generated from the formation of lactic acid increases. To improve capacity for energy release by the lactic acid system, training must overload this specific form of energy metabolism.

Anaerobic **training of the lactic acid system** is physiologically and psychologically taxing and requires considerable motivation. Bouts of up to 1 minute of intense running, swimming, or cycling, stopped 30 to 40 seconds before exhaustion, will cause large increases in lactic acid. To assure that maximum levels of lactic acid are produced during each training session, the exercise bout should be repeated several times interspersed with 3 to 5 minutes' recovery. Each successive work interval will cause a **"lactate stacking"** that results in higher levels of lactic acid than would occur with just one bout of all-out effort to the point of voluntary exhaustion. Of course, it is critical to use the specific muscle groups that require enhanced anaerobic capacity.

Recovery time can be considerable with exercises that produce large amounts of lactic acid. For this reason, intervals of anaerobic power training should occur at the end of the workout. Otherwise, fatigue from this high-intensity training would carry over and perhaps hinder the effectiveness of subsequent aerobic training.

AEROBIC CONDITIONING

The current interest in exercise training results largely from the desire of many people to improve their ability to sustain physical activity without undue fatigue. Often this desire is directed toward sports participation, although a variety of recreational, leisure, household, and occupational activities require a continuous and fairly high level of aerobic energy expenditure. In the following discussion we present a relatively simple method to evaluate one's present physiologic status for aerobic exercise. We also outline the principles that govern effective overload of the aerobic energy system.

THE AEROBIC ENERGY SYSTEM

Vigorous exercise for longer than 3 or 4 minutes is powered mainly by aerobic energy transfer. Under aerobic conditions, pyruvic acid from carbohydrate metabolism, as well as the food fragments from lipid and protein, enter the Krebs cycle for oxidation. The energy released from the complete breakdown of the macronutrients is used to resynthesize ATP. If the supply and utilization of oxygen are adequate to meet energy requirements, then exercise continues in a steady state and feelings of fatigue are minimal. On the other hand, if aerobic metabolism is inadequate, an excess of anaerobic energy transfer will cause lactic acid to accumulate and fatigue will set in. *The intensity at which exercise can be sustained beyond several minutes depends on the body's capability for aerobic metabolism.* This in turn depends on the functional capacity of the support systems for oxygen transport—the heart, lungs, and vascular system—as well as the muscles' ability to process oxygen as it is delivered.

Different terms but the same fitness component. The terms *stamina*, *endurance fitness*, *cardiovascular fitness*, and *aerobic fitness* refer to the body's ability to generate ATP aerobically.

A USEFUL METHOD TO EVALUATE CARDIOVASCULAR CAPACITY

A low heart rate because of a large stroke volume during submaximal exercise generally reflects a high level of cardiovascular fitness (Chapter 12). If a large quantity of blood is pumped with each heart beat, then only a small increase in heart rate is required to deliver blood with its complement of oxygen to the exercising muscles. *A **step test** provides a convenient means to use heart rate to evaluate the efficiency of the cardiovascular response to aerobic exercise.*

Suppose three people perform 3 minutes of step-up exercise on a bench to the cadence of a metronome. Figure 19–2 illustrates the heart rate response of each person during the 3 minutes of stepping. Heart rate increases rapidly during the first minute and then starts to level off. Subject A, a varsity basketball player, attains a heart rate of 120 beats per minute at the end of 3 minutes, while the heart rate of subject B, an exercise science major, is 142 beats per minute. For subject C, a sedentary college student, the heart rate response to this exercise is 170 beats per minute. Clearly, the cardiovascular stress of bench stepping for student C is considerably greater than for the other two students, especially student A, whose heart rate increase is minimal. It is reasonable to conclude that cardiovascular capacity is greatest for the athlete, less for the exercise science major, and relatively poor for the sedentary student.

Lower heart rate indicates a training effect. As the heart's stroke volume increases and the circulatory system becomes more efficient in delivering blood as a result of training, there will be a decrease in exercise heart rate as well as the heart rate in recovery.

The step test is a practical test. While the step test prediction method certainly does not possess the accuracy required for use in research, it does provide a valid method for classification purposes.

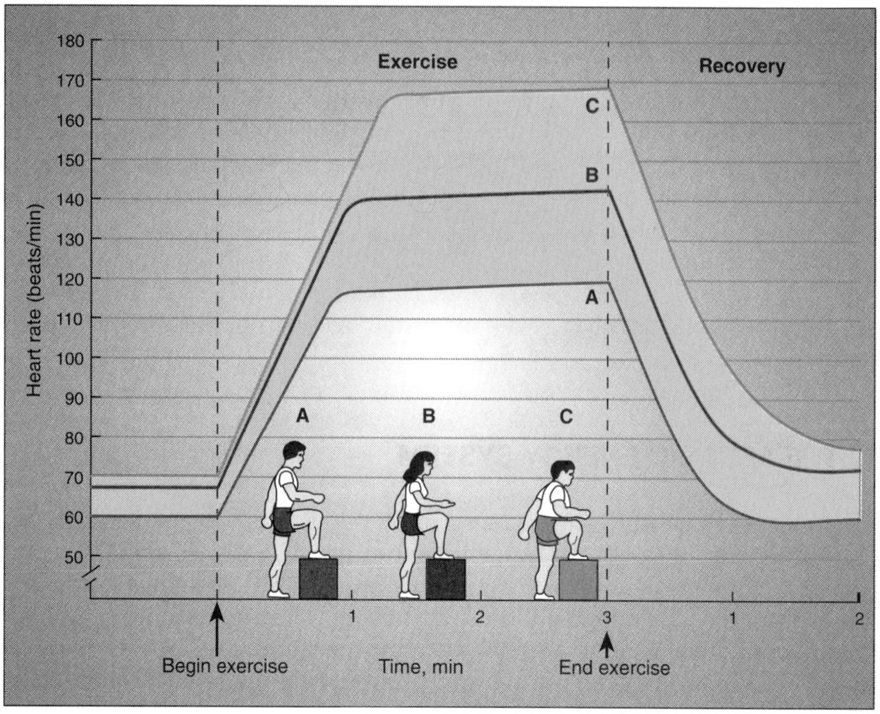

FIG. 19–2. Heart rate response of three students during stepping exercise and in recovery.

Figure 19–2 also illustrates the **pattern of heart rate recovery** for the three students in the 2 minutes immediately following bench stepping. Notice that on completion of exercise, heart rate decreases rapidly during the first 30 seconds; it then continues to decline but at a much slower rate. After 2 minutes, heart rates have essentially returned to resting values. The most noticeable differences between students A, B, and C are observed in the period immediately following exercise. Thus, if recovery heart rate is measured as soon as exercise stops, it is still possible to discriminate among subjects in terms of their heart rate response to the stress of exercise.

The Queens College Step Test. Using the **Queens College Step Test**, we have measured cardiovascular response in thousands of male and female students. To measure large numbers at the same time, stepping was done using the bottom step of the gymnasium bleachers, which was 41.3 cm ($16\frac{1}{4}$ inches) high. For women, the stepping cadence was set by a metronome at 88 beats per minute, or 22 complete step-ups; for men, it was set at 96 beats or 24 steps per minute. One complete stepping cycle on the bench represented 4 beats on the metronome, "up-up, down-down." Following a demonstration, students were given 15 seconds of practice stepping to adjust to the cadence of the metronome. The test was then begun and continued for 3 minutes. On completion of stepping, the students remained standing while the pulse was counted for a 15-second interval beginning 5 seconds after the end of stepping (5 seconds to 20 seconds postexercise). This 15-second pulse rate value was then multiplied by 4 to express the heart rate score in beats per minute. Table 19–1 presents percentile rankings for the various heart rate scores for men and women. Accompanying these scores are the corresponding values for maximal oxygen uptake (max $\dot{V}O_2$)

TABLE 19–1. PERCENTILE RANKINGS FOR RECOVERY HEART RATE AND PREDICTED MAXIMAL OXYGEN UPTAKE FOR MALE AND FEMALE COLLEGE STUDENTS

PERCENTILE RANKING	RECOVERY HR, FEMALE	PREDICTED MAX $\dot{V}O_2$ (ML/KG/MIN)	RECOVERY HR, MALE	PREDICTED MAX $\dot{V}O_2$ (ML/KG/MIN)
100	128	42.2	120	60.9
95	140	40.0	124	59.3
90	148	38.5	128	57.6
85	152	37.7	136	54.2
80	156	37.0	140	52.5
75	158	36.6	144	50.9
70	160	36.3	148	49.2
65	162	35.9	149	48.8
60	163	35.7	152	47.5
55	164	35.5	154	46.7
50	166	35.1	156	45.8
45	168	34.8	160	44.1
40	170	34.4	162	43.3
35	171	34.2	164	42.5
30	172	34.0	166	41.6
25	176	33.3	168	40.8
20	180	32.6	172	39.1
15	182	32.2	176	37.4
10	184	31.8	178	36.6
5	196	29.6	184	34.1

Source: From McArdle, W.D., et al.: Percentile norms for a valid step test in college women. Res. Q. 44:498, 1973.

that were *predicted* from the heart rate values (see the section Prediction of Maximal Oxygen Uptake).

In comparing heart rate response on the stepping exercise to the standards of the New York students, you must follow the exact procedures for administering the test. The stepping cadence *must* be 22 steps per minute for women and 24 steps per minute for men. The bench height *must* be 41.3 cm, and recovery heart rate *must* be measured during the 5- to 20-second interval at the end of exercise.

Measurement of Pulse Rate. Accurate **measurement of heart rate** is essential in evaluating the response to the step test and comparing scores to normative standards. As we will explain shortly, it is also important in establishing the appropriate exercise intensity for aerobic training. Locating the pulse at rest requires some practice. After exercise, however, the pulse can be easily located by pressing *softly* at the carotid artery along the trachea in the neck. Do not press too hard because this can cause your heart rate to slow. The recovery pulse rate can also be used to estimate the heart rate during exercise. In this case, use the *immediate* 10-second recovery period. Then multiply the number of beats counted during this interval by 6 to express the heart rate per minute.

Prediction of Maximal Oxygen Uptake. It is reasonable to expect that a person with a low heart rate during the step test and in recovery is in better aerobic condition than someone whose heart rate on the same test is relatively high. To evaluate the validity of this expectation, laboratory studies were conducted on a sample of men and women who were part of the larger study of the Queens College step test. Maximal oxygen uptake was measured for all subjects using treadmill test procedures. Each subject's max $\dot{V}O_2$ was then plotted in relation to the corresponding recovery heart rate score obtained on the step test. Figure 19–3 illustrates these results for the sample of women.

It was clear that a definite relationship existed. Subjects with a higher max $\dot{V}O_2$ tended to have lower heart rate recovery scores on the step test. Although the relationship was not a perfect one, significant information about aerobic capacity was obtained by knowing an individual's heart rate score. We therefore derived the mathematical equation to describe the "best fit" line that passed through the scores for recovery heart rate and max $\dot{V}O_2$. Based on these equations, a max $\dot{V}O_2$ value was predicted from heart rate with the value expressed in relation to body mass as milliliters of oxygen per kilogram of body mass per minute (ml/kg·min). Table 19–1 also presents the predicted max $\dot{V}O_2$s for college-aged men and women. For example, if the step test recovery heart rate for a woman was 156 beats per minute, the predicted max $\dot{V}O_2$ would be 37.0 ml/kg·min; a heart rate of 172 beats per minute for a man results in a value of 39.1 ml/kg/min.

Ideally, the most accurate measurement of max $\dot{V}O_2$ takes place in the laboratory, where sophisticated equipment is used (Chapter 11). This type of test also requires near-maximal effort from the subject. Although not possessing the accuracy required for research, the step test gives as good an **estimate of max $\dot{V}O_2$** as that obtained with other submaximal prediction tests that require a bicycle ergometer or treadmill, or performance in a running test on a track.

How do you rate? You can evaluate your predicted max $\dot{V}O_2$ score against the **aerobic capacity classifications** in Table 19–2. Although such classifi-

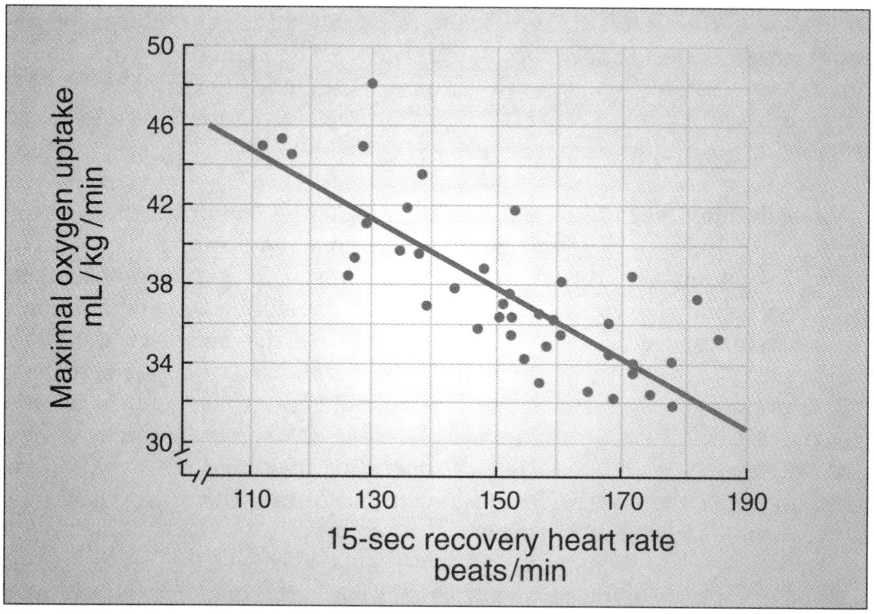

FIG. 19–3. Scattergram and line of "best fit" relating step-test heart rate score and maximal oxygen uptake in college women.

TABLE 19–2. AEROBIC CAPACITY CLASSIFICATION BASED ON GENDER AND AGE

AGE	MAXIMAL OXYGEN UPTAKE (ML/KG · MIN) LOW	FAIR	AVERAGE	GOOD	HIGH
Women					
20–29	28	29–34	35–40	41–46	47
30–39	27	38–41	34–38	39–45	46
40–49	25	26–31	30–37	38–43	44
50–65	21	22–28	27–34	35–40	41
Men					
20–29	37	38–41	42–50	51–55	56
30–39	33	34–37	38–42	43–50	51
40–49	29	30–35	36–40	41–46	47
50–59	25	26–30	31–38	39–42	43
60–69	21	22–25	26–33	34–37	38

cations are subjective, they have been constructed from average max $\dot{V}O_2$ values for hundreds of trained and sedentary men and women measured in the United States and abroad.

The Tecumseh Step Test: A Valid Alternative. The **Tecumseh Step Test** has been developed for use with adult men and women of all ages. While a heart rate score on this test cannot be transposed into a max $\dot{V}O_2$ value, the recovery heart rates are valid for showing relative fitness for aerobic exercise. The fitness classifications were constructed from average values based on a large sample from Tecumseh, Michigan, a representative midwestern community. The norms are applicable to a broad age range. The test is also attractive from a practical standpoint because the exercise level is relatively moderate and the stepping surface is the approximate height of most stairs.

The test can be performed alone, but it is much easier with a partner. Find a stair or stool *8 inches high* (20.3 cm). The correct stepping height is important and can easily be achieved by adjusting the stepping or floor surface with a board or similar hard, flat object. As with all standardized step tests, the correct stepping cadence is crucial, so practice briefly to make sure that you step up and down *twice* within a 5-second span, or *24 complete step-ups each minute for 3 minutes.* You can have a partner chant "Up-up, down-down, up-up, down-down" within a 5-second span to establish the proper cadence. Each new sequence starts at 5, 10, 15, 20, and so on. For more precision, set a metronome at *96 beats per minute,* giving one footstep per beat.

Once you master the cadence, either time yourself or have someone else signal you when to begin and stop. At the completion of 3 minutes of stepping, remain standing and locate your pulse. Exactly 30 seconds after stopping, measure your pulse for 30 more seconds. The number of pulse beats from 30 seconds after stepping to 1 minute postexercise is your heart rate score. Refer to Table 19–3 to obtain the cardiovascular fitness classification for your age and gender.

The heart rate response to a step test can serve as the frame of reference for evaluating cardiovascular adaptation to a particular program of aerobic

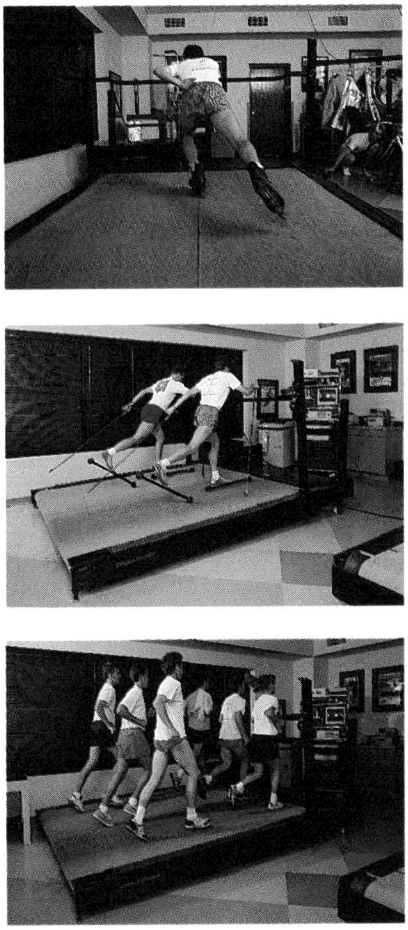

Hi-tech aerobic and anaerobic specific sports training. At the Baylor/UT Southwestern Sports Science Research Center in Dallas, Texas, specific sports training is done on the world's largest treadmill mainly for rollerblading, rollerskiing, wheelchair, running, and bicycling. Maximum speed is 25 mph and maximum grade is 25%. The treadmill is 8 feet wide and 9 feet long. A computer can be programmed to provide up to 40 different combinations of specific speed, grade, and time sequences for optimizing workouts. (Photos courtesy of Dr. James Stray-Gundersen and Bob Lukeman.)

TABLE 19–3. STEP TEST CLASSIFICATIONS BASED ON 30-SECOND RECOVERY HEART RATE FOR MEN AND WOMEN

	NUMBER OF BEATS*			
CLASSIFICATION AGE:	20–29	30–39	40–49	50 & OLDER
Men				
Outstanding	34–36	35–38	37–39	37–40
Very good	37–40	39–41	40–42	41–43
Good	41–42	42–43	43–44	44–45
Fair	43–47	44–47	45–49	46–49
Low	48–51	48–51	50–53	50–53
Poor	52–59	52–59	54–60	54–62
Women				
Outstanding	39–42	39–42	41–43	41–44
Very good	43–44	43–45	44–45	45–47
Good	45–46	46–47	46–47	48–49
Fair	47–52	48–53	48–54	50–55
Low	53–56	54–56	55–57	56–58
Poor	57–66	57–66	58–67	59–66

* Thirty-second heart rate is counted beginning 30 seconds after exercise stops.

Based on information in Montoye, H.J.: Physical Activity and Health: An Epidemiologic Study of an Entire Community. Englewood Cliffs, N.J., Prentice-Hall, 1975.

conditioning. *The important consideration is that the procedures for administering a step test must be identical each time the test is taken.*

FACTORS THAT AFFECT AEROBIC CONDITIONING

As shown in Figure 19–4, there are two major **goals of aerobic conditioning:** to enhance the capacity of the central circulation to deliver blood, and to develop the "metabolic machinery" to consume oxygen within the active muscles. This in essence embodies the specificity principle as applied to aerobic training.

Five factors influence aerobic conditioning:

- Initial level of cardiovascular fitness
- Frequency of training
- Duration of training
- Intensity of training
- Specificity of training

Initial Level of Cardiovascular Fitness. As a general rule, the amount of improvement through training depends on a person's **initial fitness level.** In simple terms, if you rate low at the start, there is room for considerable improvement. If aerobic capacity is already high, then naturally there will be relatively less improvement. Of course, a 5% improvement in physiologic function for an elite athlete is just as important to that person as a 40% increase is for a sedentary person. As a broad guideline, individuals classified as average for max $\dot{V}O_2$ generally can expect to improve from 5 to 25% following a 12-week program of aerobic training.

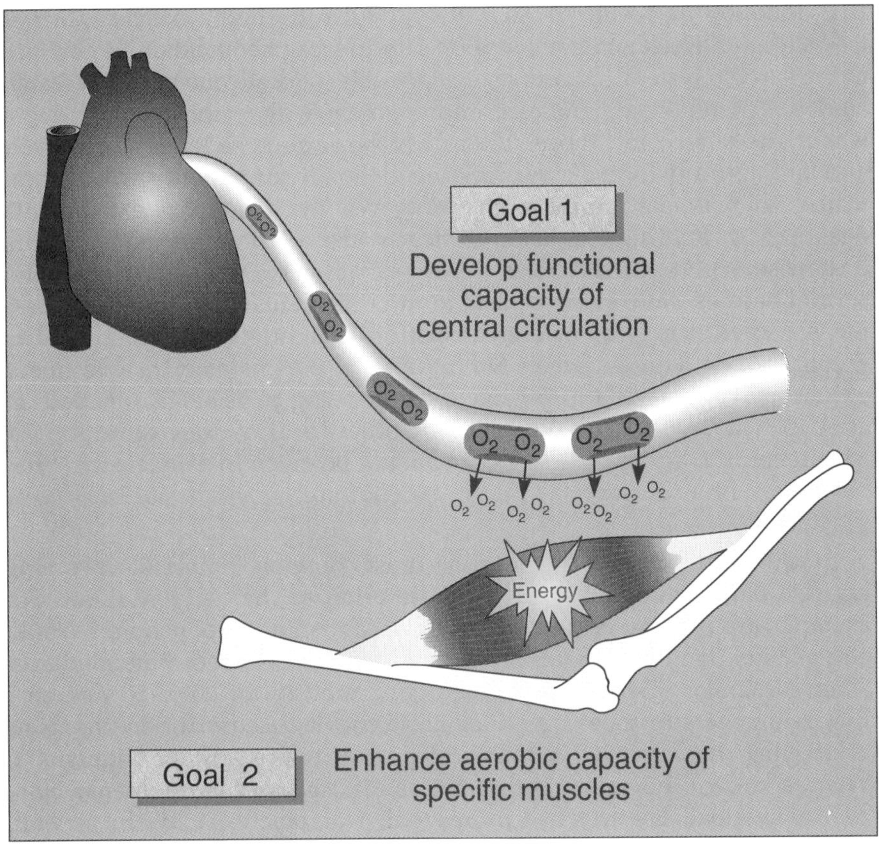

FIG. 19–4. Two major goals of aerobic conditioning.

How much improvement? Initial fitness and activity level influence the training response. In studies of previously sedentary middle-aged men with heart disease, max $\dot{V}O_2$ improved by 50% compared to 10 to 15% for the same training in healthy, active counterparts. Training improvements generally occur rapidly and continue in a steady fashion provided exercise intensity is regularly adjusted.

How Long before Improvement Occurs? Positive adaptations in cardiovascular fitness and aerobic capacity occur rapidly, often being noted within several weeks. Figure 19–5 shows absolute and percentage improvements in max $\dot{V}O_2$ for men who trained 6 days a week for 10 weeks. Training consisted of 30 minutes of bicycling 3 days a week combined with running up to 40 minutes on alternate days. As illustrated, there was a continuous week-by-week improvement in aerobic capacity. Of course, these adaptive responses eventually begin to level off as a person reaches the "genetically determined" maximum. Although fewer studies have been conducted with women, it appears that their amount and rate of improvement in aerobic capacity with training is similar to men's.

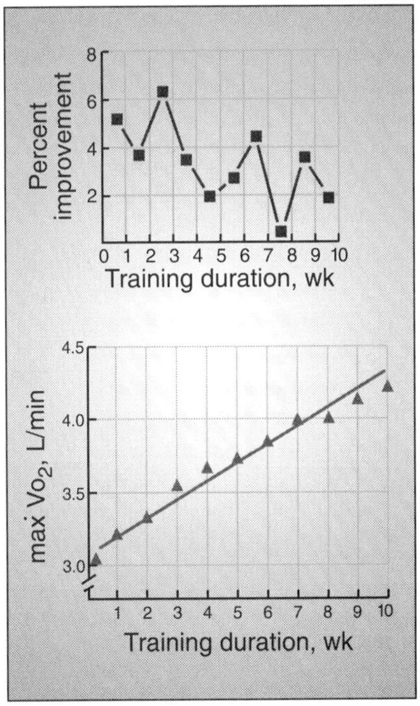

FIG. 19–5. Improvements in max $\dot{V}O_2$ over 8 weeks of high-intensity training. (From Hickson, R.C., et al.: Linear increases in aerobic power induced by a program of endurance exercise. *J. Appl. Physiol.*, 42:373, 1977.)

Genetics Plays a Role. Genetic factors play an important role in influencing the amount of improvement with training. This makes it difficult to predict exactly how much improvement can be expected based on a subject's pretraining test results. Because of inherited traits, some people possess a relatively high aerobic capacity without having had any previous training experience. In addition, some individuals are more "training responsive" than others. Dr. Per Olaf Åstrand, a renowned Swedish physiologist, contends that a highly developed aerobic capacity is as much determined by who one's parents are as by participation in vigorous conditioning programs.

Frequency of Training. As with muscular strength, exercising for at least 3 days a week generally is necessary to bring about adaptive changes in the aerobic system. Of course, it is possible to locate one or two research studies that report a significant improvement with training only 1 day a week. The subjects in those studies had been quite sedentary, however, and for them, any form of overload—even though infrequent—would stimulate cardiovascular improvement. However, the majority of experiments dealing with **training frequency** indicates that a training response occurs if exercise is performed 3 times weekly for at least 6 weeks. Interestingly, several studies have shown that the improvements from training 4 or 5 times a week were either no greater or only slightly greater compared to exercising only 3 times a week. For the average person, an extra investment of time may not be that profitable for improving physiologic function, at least as measured by max $\dot{V}O_2$. On the other hand, if exercise is used for weight control, strong consideration should be given to daily exercise that can represent a considerable caloric expenditure.

Duration of Training. One of the most common inquiries concerning exercise participation deals with the **duration of the daily workout.** For example, are 10 minutes twice as beneficial as 5 minutes of jogging? Would a run of 2 or 3 minutes that is repeated 8 to 10 times be recommended over a run at similar intensity performed continuously for 20 to 30 minutes? Precise answers to these questions are difficult because the mechanisms underlying the improvement in aerobic capacity are still not understood. What is known, however, is that both *continuous* and more intense *intermittent* overload are effective in improving aerobic capacity. In general, however, performing less exhaustive, moderate-paced exercise for 20 to 30 minutes per session is a realistic recommendation for exercising in terms of both intensity of effort and time commitment. This may be far from optimal, however, as most competitive endurance runners and swimmers spend from 2 to 3 hours or more per training session in activities geared to enhance the functional capacity of their physiologic systems.

Intensity of Training. *Intensity of training is the most critical factor related to successful aerobic conditioning.* Intensity of exercise reflects both the energy requirements of the activity and the specific energy systems activated. Intensity can be expressed in several ways:

- As calories expended per unit time
- As a percentage of max $\dot{V}O_2$
- As a particular heart rate or some percentage of maximum heart rate
- As multiples of the resting metabolic rate required to perform the work

How to improve aerobic capacity. As a general rule, aerobic capacity improves if exercise is of sufficient intensity to increase the heart rate to about 70% of maximum.

By far, the most practical means to assess the strenuousness of exercise is the exercise heart rate. Researchers frequently use exercise heart rate to structure a training program and evaluate the effectiveness of various training intensities. In general, for college-age men and women, the exercise must be of sufficient intensity to increase heart rate to at least 130 to 140 beats per minute. *This is equivalent to about 50 to 55% of max $\dot{V}O_2$,* or 70% of the maximum exercise heart rate. This exercise intensity represents the minimal stimulus to cardiovascular improvement. Although this level of cardiovascular stress is the **threshold for aerobic improvement,** more intense exercise is even more effective. Conversely, intensity of effort below the threshold level can also induce fitness improvements if the duration of the exercise session is extended.

Exercise Need Not Be Overly Strenuous. An exercise heart rate of 70% maximum (140 beats per minute for young adults) represents only moderate exercise that can be continued for long duration with little or no discomfort. This training level is frequently referred to as **"conversational exercise"**; it is sufficiently intense to stimulate a training effect, yet not so strenuous that it limits a person from talking during the workout. *It is unnecessary to exercise above this heart rate to improve physiologic capacity.*

Figure 19–6 shows that as aerobic fitness improves, heart rate at a given submaximal level of exercise or oxygen uptake gradually becomes reduced. Consequently, to keep pace with improving fitness, the exercise level will have to increase periodically to achieve the *same* threshold heart rate, or whatever target rate has been selected. A person who began training by walking would have to walk more briskly; this would be gradually replaced by jogging for periods of the workout. Eventually, continuous running would be required to achieve the same relative strenuousness at the desired training heart rate.

Aerobic conditioning reduces exercise heart rate. It is common for the submaximal exercise heart rate to be lowered by 10 to 20 beats per minute as a result of an aerobic conditioning program.

Within the framework of available research, as well as the **recommendations of the American College of Sports Medicine,** an aerobic training program for most people should be conducted at least 3 days a week utilizing 30 to 60 minutes of continuous exercise of sufficient intensity to expend about 300 kcal. This is usually assured by exercising at a pulse rate of about 70% of maximum. However, if the goal of exercise training is weight control,

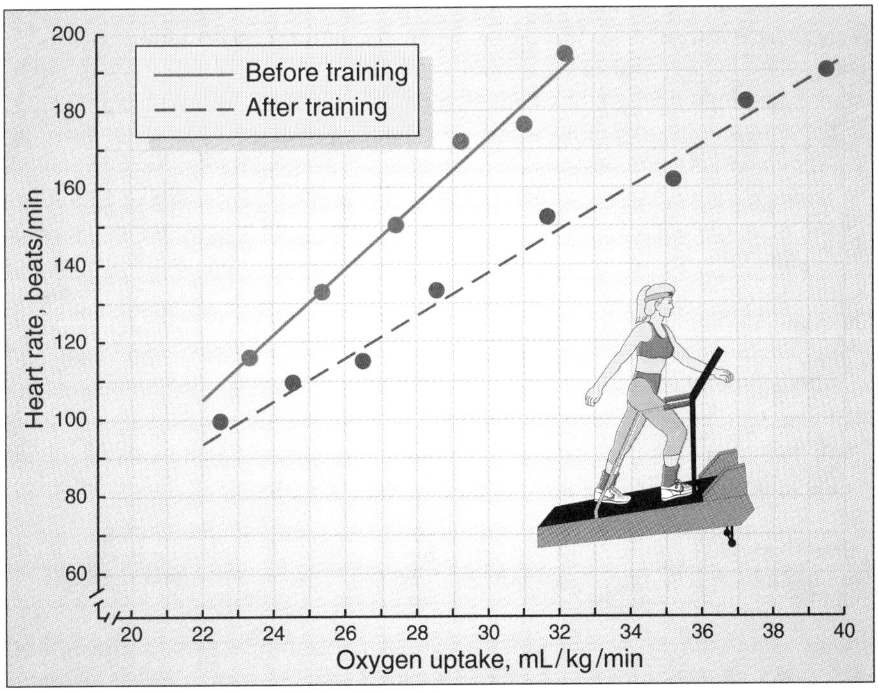

FIG. 19–6. Improvements in heart rate response in relation to oxygen uptake resulting from training.

then serious consideration should be given to performing 1-hour workouts, at an intensity of 60 to 70% of maximum, 7 days a week!

Step training—the new kid on the bench. Step training has become the current craze in the fitness marketplace. Nearly a dozen step benches have been designed and a variety of videos are on the market or in preparation. This form of training involves stepping to music on and off a bench platform between 4 and 12 inches high using a variety of foot, arm, and leg movements. Intensity of effort is generally regulated by bench height and body movements, although speeding up the beat of the music can also contribute to the cardiovascular demands of this low-impact exercise.

Specificity of Training. Another common inquiry concerning exercise participation deals with the question of whether swimming, cycling, or running is most effective in developing aerobic capacity. The proper answer concerning **specificity of training** is that each is equally effective, since all three are **"big muscle" activities** that can provide sufficient cardiovascular overload. In fact, champion athletes in the distance events in each activity are noted for their high level of aerobic fitness. Recall that for improving exercise performance, however, two physiologic capacities must be developed through aerobic conditioning. The first is the central circulation (heart and vascular system), which can be trained in a variety of activities performed at threshold heart rate. The second and perhaps equally important factor is to develop the metabolic capacity of the specific muscles to be used in exercise. Walking, running, and stepping broadly meet the aerobic training thresholds for those activities that require predominant use of the legs. One could question, however, if training by running would improve one's aerobic fitness for swimming, or vice versa. Although the answers are far from definitive, research has shown that improvement from aerobic training is not as general as once believed.

In one of our laboratories, 20 men trained on a bicycle ergometer 20 minutes a day, 3 times a week, for 8 weeks. The training intensity was set at 85% of maximum heart rate. Each subject's max $\dot{V}O_2$, measured on both the treadmill and bicycle ergometer before and after the training program, improved 7.8% as a result of the conditioning program of bicycle exercise when the subjects were measured on the bicycle test. However, when the same subjects were measured during treadmill running, the improvement in aerobic capacity averaged only 2.6%. These results indicated that aerobic training improvement was specific to the mode of exercise; there was little improvement when measured during running, but significant improvement when the test apparatus was the same as that used during training.

In a similar experiment, swimming was used for aerobic conditioning. Fifteen men trained 1 hour a day, 3 days a week, for 10 weeks. Training heart rates averaged between 85 and 95% of each subject's maximum. All subjects were measured during treadmill running, an exercise involving predominantly the leg muscles, and swimming, which uses the muscles of the arms and upper body. The results indicated *complete specificity* for the improvement in aerobic capacity with swim training. While improvements in max $\dot{V}O_2$ averaged 11% when the subjects were measured while swimming, they showed no change while running on the treadmill. This was surprising, since we had expected at least a minimal improvement on the running test from the intense nature of the "general" cardiovascular overload during swim training. Apparently, there was no "transfer" in the improved aerobic capacity from swim training to running.

The training response is highly specific. In aerobic training for a specific activity such as rowing, swimming, running, or cycling, the mode of training must overload the appropriate muscles as well as provide an exercise stress for the heart and vascular system. In each of these examples, the appropriate overload consists of training in the actual activity.

DEVELOPING AN AEROBIC CONDITIONING PROGRAM

In this section we present **guidelines for initiating aerobic training** and describe a method for gauging the intensity of that training. We also discuss the advantages and possible limitations of aerobic conditioning through intermittent or continuous training procedures.

GUIDELINES

Regardless of your present physical condition, there are some *basic guidelines* to follow as you begin an aerobic exercise program. These are based on both research and common sense, and are designed to help you improve fitness effectively and enjoyably. The person who "pulls" a muscle or develops painful cramps early in an exercise program usually has violated one of the rules of intelligent physical conditioning.

Swimming tops the list of sports participation. In 1989, 70.4 million people went swimming at least once during the year. This was followed closely by exercise walking (66.6 million); aerobics and volleyball were last with 25.1 million participants.

- **Start slowly.** Any sudden burst of vigorous activity following a few years of sedentary living can cause injury. While it is normal to feel minor muscle aches and twinges of joint pain when starting an exercise program, it is not normal to experience severe muscular discomfort or excessive cardiovascular strain. Anyone who has felt such discomfort knows that there is no greater discouragement to continuing a program of regular exercise.
- **Warm up.** Before you start exercising, it is prudent to stretch gently and limber up. There are numerous warm-up and calisthenic exercises to limber joints and stretch muscles (see Chapter 18). You should also run in place, jog on a treadmill, skip rope, or cycle on a stationary bicycle for several minutes immediately prior to the aerobic phase of the workout. The important point is to perform a variety of big muscle exercises in a rhythmic, moderate, and continuous manner so your pulse attains between 50 and 60% of its maximum.
- **Dress sensibly.** Except in cold weather, wear loose-fitting, light cotton exercise attire and the most comfortable, lightweight shoes you can afford.
- **Allow a cool-down period.** After exercising for 30 minutes or so, allow 5 to 10 minutes to slow down gradually before you stop. This allows your metabolism to progress to resting levels. More importantly, a gradual cool down prevents blood from pooling in the large veins of the previously exercised muscles. **Venous pooling** could bring about a drop in blood pressure and cause less blood to circulate to the heart and brain. This can cause dizziness, nausea, and even fainting, while a reduction in blood to the heart muscle itself may precipitate a series of irregular heart beats that could trigger a dangerous cardiac episode. It's simply not a good idea to just "lie down and rest."

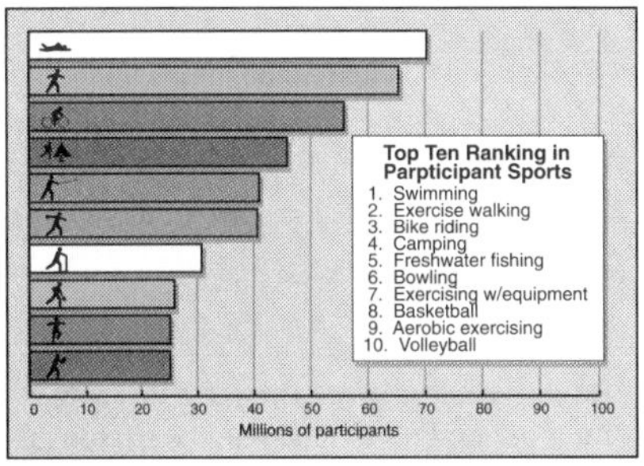

DETERMINING THE TRAINING INTENSITY

The term *intensity* is quite relative in terms of establishing an appropriate level of exercise for a specific individual. What could pose a considerable exercise stress for one person might well be below the threshold intensity of 70% maximum heart rate for an elite athlete. Thus, it is necessary to evaluate exercise in terms of the stress it places on each person's aerobic system. Several methods have been proposed to **individualize exercise training.**

Training intensity. The intensity of training is the most important factor for improving aerobic capacity.

Train at a Percentage of max $\dot{V}O_2$. In one method, the actual oxygen uptake is determined during exercise so that an individual can **train at a percentage of max $\dot{V}O_2$.** For example, if jogging at 5.5 miles per hour requires an oxygen uptake of 33 ml O_2/kg min and the jogger's max $\dot{V}O_2$ is 60 ml O_2/kg min, this exercise would represent an aerobic stress of 55% of aerobic capacity. For another person with a lower aerobic capacity of 40 ml O_2/kg min, the oxygen cost of jogging at 5.5 miles per hour would still be approximately 33 ml O_2/kg min, yet this person would be exercising at 83% of maximum. To provide a similar overload of 83% of max $\dot{V}O_2$ for the first jogger, the pace would have to be increased to a run requiring about 48 ml O_2/kg min or an increase in pace to about 8.6 miles per hour.

A personal evaluation. The strenuousness of any exercise is relative and depends upon one's present level of physiologic condition.

Although the assessment of exercise intensity by direct measurement of oxygen uptake is quite accurate, it is impractical without a fairly extensive laboratory. An alternative is to use heart rate to classify exercise in terms of its intensity or strenuousness for a specific individual. This makes it possible to personalize an exercise program and regulate the intensity of exercise to keep pace with improving fitness.

Train at a Percentage of Maximum Heart Rate. To **train at a percentage of maximum heart rate** requires knowledge of what the heart rate would be during near-exhausting exercise. A person's actual maximum heart rate can be determined immediately following 3 or 4 minutes of all-out running or swimming. This procedure is inadvisable, however, because such intense exercise requires considerable motivation and could be dangerous for people predisposed to coronary heart disease. *For this reason, we recommend that people consider themselves "average" and use the* ***age-predicted maximum heart rates*** *shown in Figure 19–7.* In addition to the average maximum heart rates by age, Figure 19–7 illustrates the **"training-sensitive zone"** that represents the threshold level of 70% and the upper level of 90% of maximum heart rate for each age group. *Conditioning of the aerobic systems will occur as long as the exercise heart rate is within this zone.*

How to estimate maximum heart rate? As a general rule, maximum heart rate is approximately 220 beats per minute minus a person's age in years.

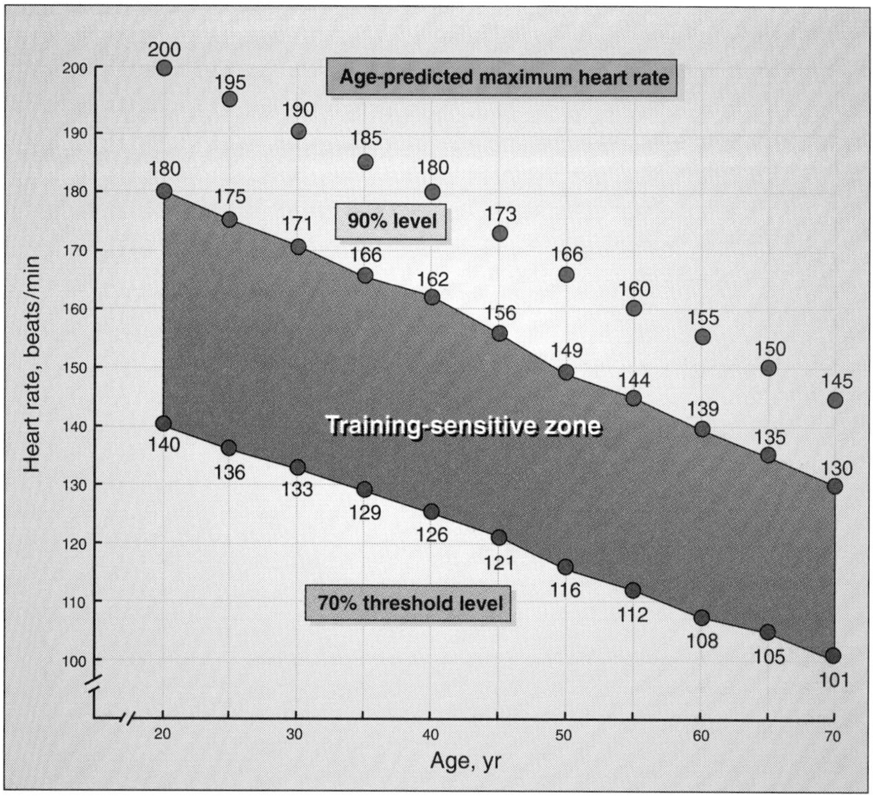

FIG. 19–7. Maximal heart rates and training-sensitive zone for use in aerobic training programs for people of different ages.

To help combat obesity, increase exercise duration. The ideal aerobic prescription for the individual who needs to reduce excess fat is approximately 60 minutes daily, seven days a week! Walking is a preferred mode of exercise. The daily exercise can be split into 10-, 20-, or 30-minute sessions, as long as the daily total is 60 minutes or more. For an individual who weighs 216 pounds, the caloric expenditure during slow walking on the level would be approximately 7.8 calories a minute or 470 calories an hour. In one month, this would equal 14,400 calories (480 kcal × 30 days), or the equivalent of 4.1 pounds of body fat (14,400 kcal/3500 kcal a pound). In one year, as long as caloric intake remains constant, fat loss *without* dieting would translate to a fat loss of about 50 pounds! Consult Appendix A for the caloric expenditure for various household, sport, and recreational activities.

If a 30-year-old man wishes to train at moderate intensity, yet still be at the threshold level, the training heart rate selected would be equal to 70% of his age-predicted maximum (190 beats/min), or a target exercise heart rate of 133 beats per minute (0.70 × 190). For a 40-year-old woman, on the other hand, the target heart rate would be 126 beats per minute (0.70 × 180). By trial and error using progressive increments of exercise, each person can arrive at a walking, jogging, or cycling speed to produce the desired target heart rate.

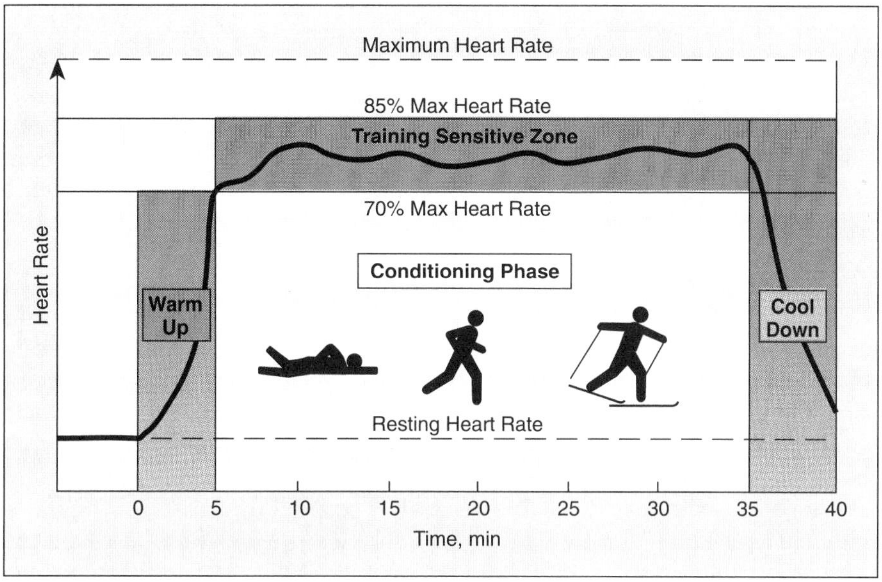

The ideal aerobic workout. The ideal workout to improve cardiovascular fitness consists of a 5-minute warm-up, a minimum of 30 minutes of large muscle activity at an intensity between 70 and 85% of maximum heart rate, and a recovery period of less intense exercise. Exercise during the 30-minute workout is known as the conditioning phase of the regimen.

In carrying out this procedure, the person should exercise moderately for 3 to 5 minutes and count the pulse rate for 10 seconds immediately afterward. If the exercise is not intense enough to produce the desired target heart rate, the same exercise is repeated but at a faster pace—jogging instead of walking, pedaling faster or switching to a lower gear while cycling, or swimming faster to cover a greater distance within a specified time. If the 30-year-old man wishes to train at 85% of maximum heart rate, exercise intensity would be increased to produce a heart rate of 161 beats per minute (0.85 × 190).

Exercise need not be exhausting. It is now clear that even less intense exercise below the 70% of maximum heart rate level will produce meaningful fitness gains for many men and women. Researchers at Stanford University concluded that low-intensity exercise in 30-minute sessions 5 times a week was just as good for improving the physical fitness of sedentary older adults as high-intensity exercise—and there were fewer injuries with the low-intensity workout.

Adjust for Swimming and Other Upper Body Exercise. In one of our laboratories, we compared the cardiovascular response to running and swimming in trained and untrained subjects. In both activities the cardiovascular and metabolic adjustments to exercise were quite similar. The **maximum heart rate for swimming,** however, averaged about *13 beats per minute lower* than for running. This occurred in both trained and untrained subjects, and is probably the result of using the arms primarily during swimming exercise. Therefore, if you select swimming or other forms of upper body exercise such as arm cranking as your training exercise, consider the decrease in maximum heart rate in this form of work when establishing your exercise intensity. We recommend that 13 beats per minute be subtracted from the age-predicted maximum heart rate values in Figure 19–7. Consequently, a 25-year-old person wishing to swim at 80% of maximum heart rate would select a swimming speed that produces a heart rate of

Aerobic training in elite athletes. It is not uncommon for elite distance runners to train twice a day year round and to run between 100 and 150 miles each week.

RPE scale

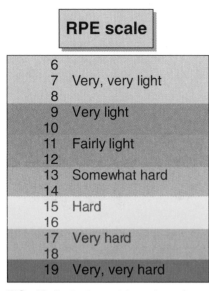

6	
7	Very, very light
8	
9	Very light
10	
11	Fairly light
12	
13	Somewhat hard
14	
15	Hard
16	
17	Very hard
18	
19	Very, very hard

FIG. 19–8. Scale used for ratings of perceived exertion (RPE). (From Borg, G.A.: Psychological basis of physical exertion. *Med. Sci. Sports Exerc.*, 14:377, 1982.)

about 146 beats per minute (0.80 × ([195 − 13]). This represents more accurately the appropriate training heart rate for swimming.

Is Less Intense Exercise Effective? The recommendation for training at 70% of maximum heart rate as the threshold for aerobic improvement should be viewed as a *general guideline* for establishing an effective, yet comfortable exercise level. While 20 to 30 minutes of continuous exercise at the 70% level will stimulate a training effect, exercise at a lower intensity of 60% for 45 minutes will also prove beneficial. *In general, lower exercise intensity is offset by longer exercise duration.* The important point is that, regardless of the exercise level you select, more is not necessarily better. Excessive exercise increases your chance for bone, joint, and muscle injury. In Chapter 20 we point out that the health benefits from regular exercise do not require heroic levels of physical activity. Unfortunately, far too many people push themselves, adhering to the slogan, "no pain, no gain." As a general guideline, 30 minutes of regular exercise performed within the training-sensitive zone 3 times a week is probably all that is required.

Train at a Perception of Effort. In addition to oxygen uptake and heart rate as indicators of exercise intensity, one can also use the ***rating of perceived exertion*** (*RPE*). With this approach, the exerciser rates on a numerical scale how he or she feels in relation to the level of exertion. The levels of exercise that correspond to higher levels of energy expenditure and physiologic strain result in higher ratings. For example, an RPE of 13 or 14 ("somewhat hard"), illustrated in Figure 19–8, coincides with an exercise heart rate of about 70% maximum. This is the generally accepted threshold for the training-sensitive zone. Individuals can quickly learn to exercise at a specific RPE based on their subjective feeling of exertion. These subjective measures coincide nicely with objective measures of exercise intensity. In this sense, it is appropriate to consider the axiom, "listen to your body."

CONTINUOUS VS. INTERMITTENT AEROBIC CONDITIONING

CONTINUOUS EXERCISE TRAINING

Continuous or *long slow distance* (*LSD*) training involves steady-state aerobic exercise performed at either moderate or high intensity for a sustained period. By its nature, **continuous exercise training** is submaximal and can be performed for considerable time in relative comfort. Such training is suitable for people just beginning an exercise program or desiring to expend considerable calories for purposes of weight control. It is certainly a more pleasant method of training the aerobic system than the more intense interval training discussed in the next section. Continuous exercise training can be maintained at the threshold intensity of 70% maximum heart rate or increased to the 85% or even 90% level.

Continuous exercise training is desirable for endurance athletes because it allows them to train at nearly the same intensity as in actual competition. A champion middle-distance runner may run 5 miles continuously in 26 minutes during workouts at a heart rate of 180 beats per minute; this pace would not be exhausting but would still nearly duplicate race conditions. By finishing each exercise session with several all-out sprints stopped 30 to 40 seconds before exhaustion, the athlete can also train the anaerobic system that does play a small role in such middle-distance events, especially at the race's finish. The marathon runner will train at a slightly slower pace than the middle-distance athlete because a much longer distance must be run in both practice and competition.

INTERVAL EXERCISE TRAINING

Many daily activities and sports are intermittent, characterized by periods of intense activity interspersed with periods requiring only a moderate to low level of energy expenditure. The basis of **interval exercise training** requires correct spacing of exercise and rest periods so a person can accomplish a tremendous amount of exercise with minimal fatigue. The rest-to-exercise intervals can vary from a few seconds to several minutes or more. The training prescription is formulated in terms of the intensity and duration of the exercise interval, the length of recovery, and the number of repetitions. For example, running continuously at a "4-minute mile" pace would exhaust most people within a minute. However, running at this speed for only 15 seconds followed by a 30-second rest period would enable many people to run 4 minutes at this near-record pace. Of course, this is not equivalent to a 4-minute mile; but during 4 minutes of actual running, 1 mile would have been run even though the combined work and rest intervals would have taken 11 minutes 30 seconds.

The rationale for interval training has a sound basis in physiology. In the example of the continuous run at a 4-minute mile pace, a major portion of energy would be supplied through anaerobic production of lactic acid. The level of this acid metabolite rises rapidly and causes exhaustion. On the other hand, intermittent exercise performed for repeated intervals of 15 seconds or less would allow a severe load to be imposed on the muscles before appreciable accumulation of lactic acid. Recovery from these brief, yet intense work intervals would be predominantly "alactic" in nature and would take place quickly. The subsequent exercise interval could then begin again after only a brief rest period. These repetitive exercise intervals will eventually place considerable demand on the aerobic system.

In interval training, as in other forms of physiologic conditioning, the intensity of exercise should be geared to the particular energy systems the person desires to train. A practical system for determining interval training exercise rates is presented in Table 19–4.

- Exercise interval. To determine the **exercise interval,** 1.5 to 5.0 seconds is added to the exerciser's "best time" for training distances between 60 and 220 yards for running and 15 to 55 yards for swimming. If a person can run 60 yards from a running start in 8 seconds, the training time for each repeat would therefore be 8 + 1.5 or 9.5 seconds. For interval training distances of 110 and 220 yards, 3 and 5 seconds are added, respectively, to the best running times. This particular application of interval training is suited for training the high-energy phosphate component of the anaerobic energy system.

  For training distances of 440 yards running or 110 yards swimming, the exercise rate is determined by subtracting 1 to 4 seconds from the average 440-yard portion of a mile run or 110-yard portion of a 440-yard swim. If a person runs a 7-minute mile (averaging 105 seconds per 440

TABLE 19–4. GUIDELINES FOR DETERMINING INTERVAL-TRAINING EXERCISE RATE FOR RUNNING AND SWIMMING DIFFERENT DISTANCES

INTERVAL TRAINING DISTANCES (YARDS)		WORK RATE FOR EACH EXERCISE INTERVAL OR REPEAT
Run	Swim	
55	15	1.5 seconds *slower* than best times from running (or swimming) start for each distance
110	25	3 seconds *slower* than best times from running (or swimming) start for each distance
220	55	5 seconds *slower* than best times from running (or swimming) start for each distance
440	110	1 to 4 seconds *faster* than the average 440-yard run or 110-yard swim times recorded during a mile run or 440-yard swim
660–1320	165–320	3 to 4 seconds *slower* than the average 440-yard run or 100-yard swim times recorded during a mile run or 440-yard swim

Source: From Fox, E.L., and Mathers, D.K., Interval Training. Philadelphia, W.B. Saunders, 1974.

yards), the interval time for each 440-yard repeat would be between 104 seconds (105 − 1) and 101 seconds (105 − 4). For training intervals beyond 440 yards, 3 to 4 seconds is added for each 440-yard portion of the interval distance. In running an interval of 880 yards, the 7-minute miler would thus run each interval at about 216 seconds ([105 + 3] × 2 = 216).

- Relief interval. The **relief interval** can be either passive (rest-relief) or active (exercise-relief). The recommended duration of relief is usually expressed as a ratio of exercise duration to recovery duration. The ratio of 1 to 3 is generally recommended for training the immediate energy system. Thus, for a sprinter who runs 10-second intervals, the relief interval is usually about 30 seconds. For training the short-term glycolytic energy system, the relief interval is twice as long as the exercise interval, an exercise-relief ratio of 1 to 2. These specific ratios of exercise to relief for anaerobic training provide for sufficient restoration of the high energy phosphate pools or lactic acid removal so that the next exercise bout can proceed without undue fatigue.

At present, there is insufficient evidence to claim superiority for either continuous or interval training for aerobic fitness. Both methods will provide results; they probably can be used interchangeably.

MAINTAINING AEROBIC FITNESS

An interesting question concerning **fitness maintenance** is the optimal frequency, duration, and intensity of exercise required to retain the improved aerobic fitness attained through training. Studies reveal that if exercise *intensity* is maintained, the frequency and duration of training can be reduced considerably without any decrements in aerobic performance (e.g., 6 day a week training reduced to 2 days; 40 minutes a day training reduced to 13 minutes). However, a small reduction in exercise intensity, keeping training frequency and duration constant, causes a significant decline in aerobic fitness.

EXERCISING DURING PREGNANCY

With a considerable number of women involved in physically demanding occupations and maintaining an active lifestyle, there is growing interest in these topics as they relate to **exercise and pregnancy;** specifically, the degree to which pregnancy affects the energy cost and physiologic demands of exercise, the effects of exercise on the fetus, and the effects of regular exercise on the course of pregnancy, including final outcome and ease of delivery.

Energy Cost. The cardiovascular responses during exercise in pregnancy follow normal patterns. In addition, other than the strain provided by the additional weight gain and possible encumbrance of fetal tissue, an uncomplicated pregnancy offers no greater physiologic strain to the mother during moderate exercise. This means that as pregnancy progresses, the increase in maternal body mass adds significantly to the exercise effort in weight-bearing activities such as walking, jogging, and stair climbing. On the other hand, if body weight is supported during exercise, as in stationary bicycling, the exercise response for heart rate and oxygen uptake during pregnancy is essentially identical to that observed in the nonpregnant state.

Fetal Blood Supply. Studies of uterine blood flow during exercise in various species of mammals indicate that for healthy animals, oxygen supply to the developing fetus is maintained during moderate to heavy levels of maternal exercise. However, in animals with one umbilical artery tied off to restrict circulation to the placenta, oxygen supply to the fetus is significantly reduced. The researchers concluded that vigorous maternal exercise is well tolerated by the fetus during a normal pregnancy, but could be potentially harmful to a fetus with some limitation of the umbilical circulation.

Because vigorous exercise probably diverts some blood from the uterus, and this could pose a hazard to a fetus with restricted placental blood flow, it is prudent for a pregnant woman to exercise in *moderation* especially if the pregnancy is compromised to any degree. In addition, an elevation in maternal core temperature could hinder heat dissipation from the fetus through the placenta. During warm weather, it is therefore prudent for pregnant women to exercise in the cool part of the day and for shorter intervals while maintaining regular fluid intake.

Outcome of Pregnancy. Although regular aerobic exercise can serve an important role in maintaining the physical fitness, optimal body weight, and general well-being of a pregnant woman, it remains unclear whether extremes of maternal exercise are beneficial to the developing fetus and whether exercise enhances the course of pregnancy, including labor, delivery, and outcome.

Exercise moderation during pregnancy. For a previously active, healthy woman during an uncomplicated pregnancy, moderate aerobic exercise does not produce circulatory alterations that compromise fetal oxygen supply.

Milk production during pregnancy. There is no apparent adverse effect of vigorous exercise on lactation.

Pregnancy, a form of training. Pregnancy-related factors appear to offset the required level of physical exercise during pregnancy. As a result, pregnancy leads to a small increase in aerobic capacity in women who maintain only moderate levels of exercise during and after pregnancy.

Pregnancy and weight gain. In a recent study of 2000 young pregnant women, researchers found that failure of the mother to gain adequate weight in the first and second trimesters of pregnancy was a major cause of low birth weight. The infant mortality rate in the United States is one of the highest in the world—nearly 11 of 1000 babies die as newborns—and low birth weight is a major factor in early infant death. A weight gain of about 30 pounds is "normal" if the woman was not obese before pregnancy. A weight gain of 9 to 10 pounds is recommended during the second trimester except in teenagers, who should gain more weight because their growth is not yet complete. Failure to "eat right" during pregnancy and concern about "getting too fat" are major factors why many women don't gain weight.

SUMMARY

1. Activities can be classified in terms of their predominant activation of a specific system of energy transfer, either aerobic or anaerobic. An

effective training program is one that allocates a proportionate time commitment to training the specific energy system(s) involved in the activity.

2. The contribution of anaerobic and aerobic energy transfer depends largely on the intensity and duration of exercise. During sprint-power activities, the primary means for energy transfer involves the immediate and short-term energy systems. The long-term aerobic system becomes progressively more important in activities that last longer than 2 minutes.
3. Proper physical conditioning is based on sound principles that produce optimum improvements. Of crucial importance are the overload principle, the specificity of exercise principle, the individual difference principle, and the reversibility principle.
4. Aerobic training brings about both functional and dimensional changes in the cardiovascular system. These include decreases in resting and submaximal exercise heart rate, enhanced stroke volume and cardiac output, and improved ability of the specifically trained muscles to process oxygen.
5. The step test provides a convenient means by which heart rate can be used to evaluate the efficiency of the cardiovascular response to aerobic exercise and training.
6. Aerobic training must be geared to enhance both circulatory function and the metabolic capacity of specific muscles. Peripheral adaptations in active muscle may have a profound effect on exercise performance.
7. The major factors that affect training improvement are initial fitness level, frequency of training, exercise intensity, duration of exercise, and type (mode) of training. Of these, intensity is most crucial.
8. Training intensity can be applied either on an absolute basis in terms of exercise load, or relative to an individual's physiologic response. It is practical and effective to set exercise intensity to a percentage of a person's maximum heart rate response. Training levels that correspond to 70 to 90% of maximum heart rate are most desirable for inducing aerobic fitness changes.
9. Training duration and intensity are intimately related. Nevertheless, 30 minutes per session seems to be desirable in terms of exercise duration. Extending the duration can compensate somewhat for reduced intensity.
10. Frequency for optimum aerobic training appears to be a minimum of 3 days per week. Optimal frequency levels have not been established.
11. If intensity, duration, and frequency are held constant, training improvements are similar regardless of training mode, as long as large muscle groups are exercised.
12. The level of physical activity required to maintain an improved level of aerobic fitness is less than that required to improve it.

RELATED READINGS

American College of Sports Medicine: The recommended quantity and quality of exercise for developing and maintaining fitness in healthy adults. *Med. Sci. Sports Exerc.*, 10:7, 1978.

Åstrand, P.O., and Rodahl, K.: Textbook of Work Physiology, 3rd ed. New York, McGraw-Hill, 1986.

Ballor, D.L., et al.: Resistance weight training during caloric restriction enhances lean body weight maintenance. *Am. J. Clin. Nutr.*, 47:19, 1988.

Clapp, J.F., III, and Capeless, E.: The $\dot{V}O_2$max of recreational athletes before and after pregnancy. *Med. Sci. Sports Exerc.*, 23:1128, 1991.

Costill, D.L.: Inside Running: Basics of Sports Physiology. Indianapolis, Benchmark Press, 1986.

Cowan, M.M., and Gregory, L.W.: Responses of pre- and post-menopausal females to aerobic conditioning. *Med. Sci. Sports Exerc.*, 17:138, 1985.

Coyle, E.F., et al.: Time course of loss of adaptations after stopping prolonged intense endurance training. *J. Appl. Physiol.*, 57:1857, 1984.

Daniels, J., and Scardinia, N.: Interval training and performance. *Sports Med.*, 1:327, 1984.

Fox, E.L., and Matthews, D.K.: Interval Training: Conditioning for Sports and General Fitness. Philadelphia, W.B. Saunders, 1974.

Gergley, T., et al.: Specificity of arm training on aerobic power during swimming and running. *Med. Sci. Sports Exerc.*, 16:349, 1984.

Gettman, L.R., et al.: Physiological responses of men to 1, 3, and 5 day per week training programs. *Res. Q.*, 47:638, 1976.

Gorski, J.: Exercise during pregnancy: maternal and fetal responses. A brief review. *Med. Sci. Sports Exerc.*, 17:407, 1985.

Greer, N.L., and Katch, F.I.: Validity of palpation recovery pulse following four intensities of bench step exercise. *Res. Q. Exerc. Sport*, 53:340, 1982.

Gregg, S.G., et al.: Interactive effects of anemia and muscle oxidative capacity on exercise endurance. *J. Appl. Physiol.*, 67:765, 1989.

Hickson, R.C., et al.: Time course of adaptive responses of aerobic power and heart rate to training. *Med. Sci. Sports Exerc.*, 13:17, 1981.

Hickson, R.C., et al.: Reduced training intensities and loss of aerobic power, endurance, and cardiac growth. *J. Appl. Physiol.*, 58:492, 1985.

Holloszy, J.O.: Metabolic consequences of endurance exercise training. In: Exercise, Nutrition, and Energy Metabolism. Edited by E.S. Horton and R.L. Terjung. New York, Macmillan, 1988.

Jacobs, I.: Sprint training effects on muscle myoglobin, enzymes, fiber types, and blood lactate. *Med. Sci. Sports Exerc.*, 19:368, 1987.

King, A.C., et al.: Group- vs. home-based exercise training in healthy older men and women. *JAMA*, 266:1535, 1991.

Kohrt, W.M., et al.: Longitudinal assessment of responses of triathletes to swimming, cycling, and running. *Med. Sci. Sports Exerc.*, 21:569, 1989.

Kulpa, P.J., et al.: Aerobic exercise in pregnancy. *Am. J. Obstet. Gynecol.*, 156:1395, 1987.

Londeree, B.R., and Moeschberger, M.L.: Effect of age and other factors on maximal heart rate. *Res. Q. Exerc. Sport*, 53:297, 1982.

Lovelady, C.A., et al.: Lactation performance of exercising women. *Am. J. Clin. Nutr.*, 52:103, 1990.

Magel, J.R., et al.: Specificity of swim training on maximum oxygen uptake. *J. Appl. Physiol.*, 38:151, 1975.

Magel, J.R., et al.: Metabolic and cardiovascular adjustment to arm training. *J. Appl. Physiol.*, 45:75, 1978.

McArdle, W.D., et al.: Specificity of run training on $\dot{V}O_2$ max and heart rate changes during running and swimming. *Med. Sci. Sports*, 10:16, 1978.

McArdle, W.D., et al.: Exercise Physiology: Energy, Nutrition, and Human Performance, 3rd ed. Philadelphia, Lea & Febiger, 1991.

Örlander, J., and Aniansson, A.: Effects of physical training on skeletal muscle metabolism and ultrastructure in 70- to 75-year-old men. *Acta Physiol. Scand.*, 109:149, 1980.

Pechar, G.S., et al.: Specificity of cardiorespiratory adaptation to bicycle and treadmill training. *J. Appl. Physiol.*, 36:753, 1974.

Pollock, M.L., et al.: Effects of mode of training on cardiovascular function and body composition of adult men. *Med. Sci. Sports*, 7:139, 1975.

Powell, K.E., et al.: An epidemiological perspective on the causes of running injuries. *Phys. Sportsmed.*, 14:100, 1986.

Riviere, D., et al.: Lipolytic response of fat cells to catecholamines in sedentary and exercise-trained women. *J. Appl. Physiol.*, 66:330, 1989.

Ruten Franz, J.: Longitudinal approach for assessing maximal aerobic power during growth: the European experience. *Med. Sci. Sports Exerc.*, 18:270, 1986.

Saavedra, C., et al.: Maximal anaerobic performance of the knee extensor muscles during growth. *Med. Sci. Sports Exerc.*, 23:1083, 1991.

Seals, D.R., et al.: Endurance training in older men and women. I. Cardiovascular responses to exercise. *J. Appl. Physiol.*, 57:1024, 1984.
Treadway, J.L., and Young, J.C.: Decreased glucose uptake in fetus after maternal exercise. *Med. Sci. Sports Exerc.*, 21:140, 1989.
Wilt, F.: Training for competitive running. In: Exercise Physiology. Edited by H. Falls. New York, Academic Press, 1968.

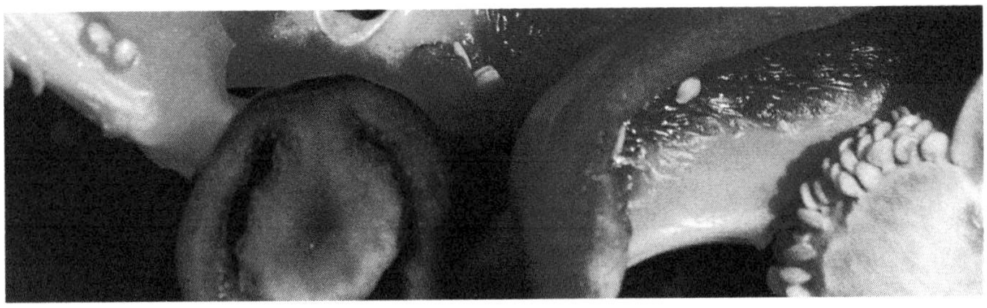

20

AGING, EXERCISE, AND CARDIOVASCULAR HEALTH

There is no question that the physiologic and exercise capacities of older people are generally below those of younger counterparts. What is uncertain is the degree to which these differences are caused by true biologic aging or are simply the result of environmental factors and disuse brought on by alterations in lifestyle and activity opportunities as people age. No longer can older men and women be stereotyped as sedentary with little or no initiative for active pursuits. There is currently a tremendous upswing in participation by "senior citizens" in a broad range of physical activity experiences and exercise programs. Research clearly demonstrates that if an active lifestyle is continued into later years, a relatively high level of function is retained and vigorous activities can be engaged in safely and successfully.

Senior citizens. The elderly represent the fastest growing segment of the American population with the average life expectancy for men and women rapidly approaching 80 years.

Despite the inherent problems in disease research in humans, there is considerable evidence that evolution has not kept pace with automation. Aside from the positive effects of exercise in maintaining physiologic function, it is clear that regular physical activity protects against the ravages of this nation's greatest killer, **coronary heart disease** (CHD). Individuals in physically active occupations have a two- to threefold lower risk of heart attack than those in sedentary jobs. Furthermore, the chances of surviving a heart attack are much greater for those with a physically demanding job or lifestyle. Regular physical activity can also favorably modify some of the important **CHD risk factors.** Elevated blood pressure can be lowered by regular aerobic exercise; similarly, body mass, body fat, and blood lipids are lowered with prudent exercise and diet. The blood clotting mechanism can be normalized with exercise training; this would reduce the chances of a blood clot forming on the roughened surface of a coronary artery. Research with animals has demonstrated an improved blood supply to the myocardium as a result of regular exercise. If this adaptation in coronary circulation takes place in humans, then regular exercise may retard the heart disease process, or at least maintain an adequate blood supply to the heart muscle to compensate for those channels already narrowed by fatty deposits on their vascular walls.

Inactivity is a disease. Considered alone, sedentary living probably is to blame for as many as 200,000 preventable cardiovascular deaths in the United States each year.

Now it's the Big Four. Physical inactivity has now joined high blood cholesterol, cigarette smoking, and hypertension on the American Heart Association's list of primary, yet modifiable, heart disease risks.

From a practical standpoint, an active lifestyle is often effective in blunting the cumulative effects of the highly atherogenic American diet and accompanying life of inactivity and stress. Regardless of genetics, age, and life circumstances, individuals can significantly enhance their chances for a healthy life by adapting sound habits that include regular exercise. In the sections that follow, we explore several aspects of the aging process with special emphasis on exercise and its relation to cardiovascular disease.

PARTICIPATION IN PHYSICAL ACTIVITY

Not enough of a good thing. At best, no more than 20% and possibly less than 10% of the adults in the United States obtain sufficient regular physical activity to impart discernible health and fitness benefits. Conservatively, 40% are completely sedentary, and 40% exercise below recommended levels.

The current status of exercise participation for American adults is not encouraging, as the "exercise boom" appears to be leveling off. According to data from the U.S. National Center for Health Statistics on the physical activity of noninstitutionalized adults aged 18 years and older, only 8% of men and 7% of women reported that they engaged in regular vigorous exercise. Regular but less intense activity was done by 36% of the men and 32% of the women, indicating that only about 44% of males and 39% of females engage in some regular physical activity. Furthermore, available data indicate that generally about half of those who start exercising give it up within the first 6 months.

Figure 20–1 illustrates the findings for **exercise participation** from a large-scale study of over 15,000 adults enrolled in exercise programs that included aerobic and muscle-strengthening activities. With increasing age there was a progressive decline in participation in fitness activities, with the smallest percentage of participation noted for the oldest group. Sadly, these are the men and women who might benefit the most from regular exercise. In fact, an alarmingly large number of older citizens have such poor functional capacity that they cannot do relatively simple physical tasks without assistance.

Many start but few continue. Data indicate that only 14% of American adults expend more than 1600 kcal per week in leisure-time physical activities. In terms of organized exercise, the drop-out rate for most health clubs is about 70%!

IS EXERCISING SAFE?

Many people have raised this question largely because of several well-publicized reports of sudden death during exercise. In actuality, sudden death rates during exercise have *declined* over the past 20 years even though

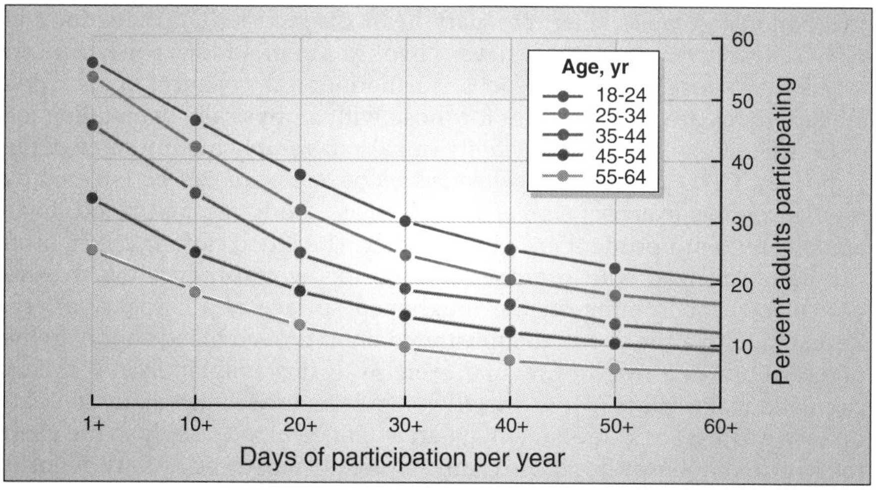

FIG. 20–1. Percentage of adults in the United States, grouped by age, who participate in fitness activities. (Courtesy of C. Brooks, Department of Sports Management and Communication, University of Michigan, Ann Arbor, 1989.)

there has been an overall *increase* in exercise participation. In one report of cardiovascular episodes during a little more than 5 years, 2935 exercisers recorded 374,798 hours of exercise that included 2,726,272 km (1.7 million miles) of running and walking. There were no deaths during this time and only 2 nonfatal cardiovascular complications. By gender, there were 3 complications per 100,000 hours of exercise for men and 2 for women. Certainly, there is a small increased risk of a cardiovascular episode during exercise compared to resting. However, the *total reduction* in heart disease risk to be derived from engaging in regular physical activity (compared to leading a sedentary life) far outweighs any slight increase in risk during the actual activity period.

Perhaps not surprisingly, the **most prevalent exercise complications** are musculoskeletal in nature. In a study of aerobic dance injuries for 351 participants and 60 instructors at six dance facilities, 327 medical complaints were reported during nearly 30,000 hours of activity. Only 84 of the injuries resulted in disability (2.8 per 1000 person-hours of participation), and just 2.1% of the injuries required medical attention. *For jogging and running activities, the orthopedic injury potential is greatest among those who exercise for extended periods of time.* In this sense, more is certainly not better!

AGING AND BODILY FUNCTION

Figure 20–2 shows that the various measures of bodily function generally improve rapidly during childhood to reach a maximum between age 20 and 30 years; thereafter, there is a gradual **decline in functional capacity with advancing years.** While the trend with age is generally similar for the physically active, physiologic function is about 25% higher for each age category, so that an active 50-year-old man or woman often maintains the functional level of a 20-year-old.

Although all measures eventually decline with age, not all decline at the same rate and there is considerable variation from person to person and

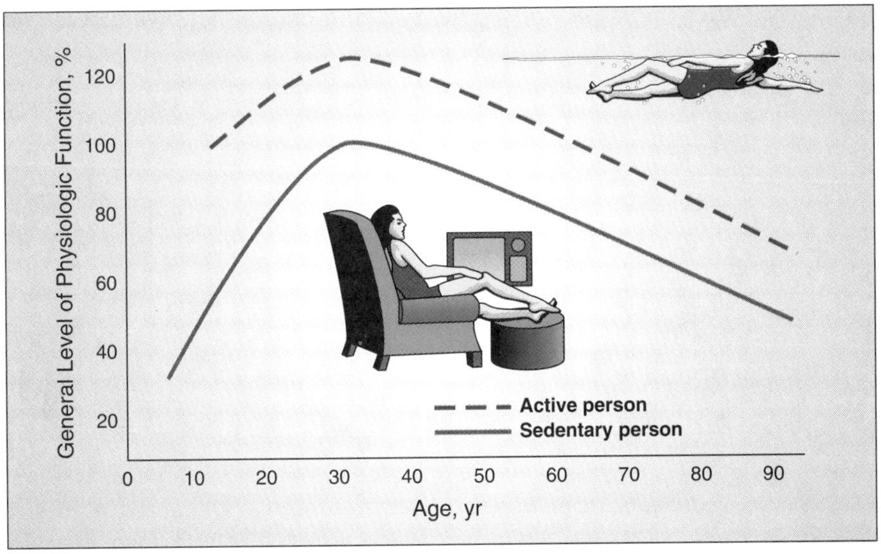

FIG. 20–2. Generalized curve to illustrate changes in physiologic function with age. All comparisons are made against the 100% value achieved by the 20- to 30-year-old sedentary person.

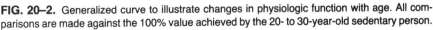

The body responds at any age. Research indicates impressive plasticity in physiologic, structural, and performance characteristics among the elderly. A marked and rapid improvement can occur with exercise training at least into the ninth decade of life!

from system to system within the same person. Nerve conduction velocity, for example, declines only 10 to 15% from 30 to 80 years of age, whereas resting cardiac index (ratio of cardiac output to surface area) and joint flexibility decline 20 to 30%; maximum breathing capacity at age 80 is about 40% that of a 30-year-old. Brain cells die at a constant rate until age 60, while the liver and kidneys lose about 40 to 50% of their function between ages 30 and 70, the average female has lost 30% of her bone mass, while men at this age have lost only about 15%.

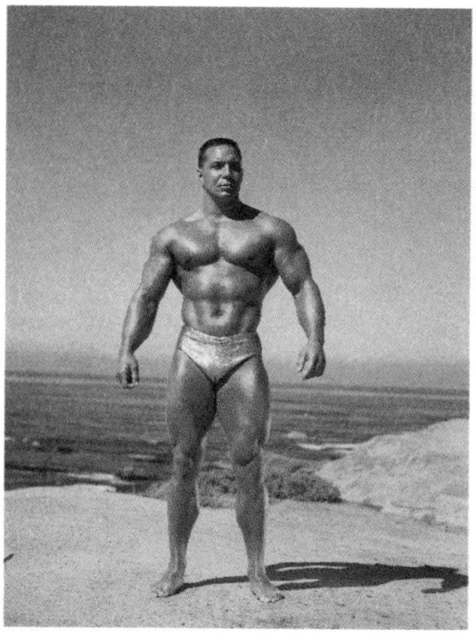

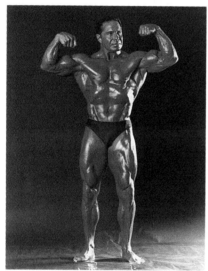

Fifty-one consecutive years of resistance training! Bill Pearl, currently age 62, is one of the greatest bodybuilding champions of all time. Holder of four Mr. Universe titles (1956, 1961, 1967, 1971), he still trains about 2.5 hours daily (beginning at 4:30 A.M.) with his training partner and wife Judy at their Talent, Oregon farmhouse. In 1974, the World Bodybuilding Guild named him the world's best built man. Top. 1967 Mr. Universe, age 37. Bottom. Last formal pose, age 59.

Muscular Strength. **Maximum strength of men and women** is generally achieved between 20 and 30 years of age, when muscular cross-sectional area is usually the largest. Thereafter, strength progressively declines for most muscle groups so that by age 70 there is 30% less overall strength.

Decrease in Muscle Mass. *Reduced muscle mass is a primary factor responsible for the age-associated strength decrease.* This reflects loss of total muscle protein brought about by inactivity, aging, or both. There is also probably some loss in the number of muscle fibers with aging. For example, the biceps muscle of a newborn contains about 500,000 individual fibers while the same muscle for a man in his 80s has about 300,000 fibers.

Muscle Trainability Among the Elderly. **Regular physical training facilitates protein retention** and delays the decrement in lean body mass and muscular strength with aging. Healthy men between the ages of 60 and 72 years were trained for 12 weeks with a standard resistance training program similar to that outlined in Chapter 18. As shown in Figure 20–3, muscle strength increased progressively throughout the training to average about 5% per training session—a training response similar to that noted for young adults. In addition, these dramatic strength improvements were accompanied by significant muscular hypertrophy.

Flexibility. With advancing age, connective tissue (cartilage, ligaments, and tendons) becomes stiffer and more rigid, which reduces **joint flexibility.** What is uncertain is whether these changes are the result of biologic aging per se or rather the impact of sedentary living or degenerative disease on

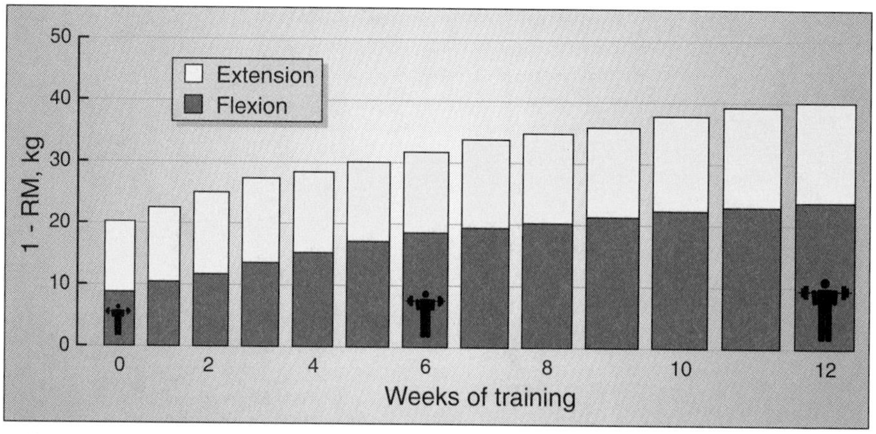

FIG. 20–3. Weekly measurements of dynamic muscle strength (1-RM) of left knee extension (yellow) and flexion (blue). (From Frontera, W.R., et al.: Strength conditioning in older men: skeletal muscle hypertrophy and improved function. *J. Appl. Physiol.*, 64:1038, 1988.)

the tissues that make up a specific joint. What is clear, however, is that appropriate exercises that move joints through their full range of motion can increase flexibility by as much as 20 to 50% in men and women at all ages.

Nervous System. The cumulative effects of aging on **central nervous system function** are exhibited by a 37% decline in the number of spinal cord axons, 10% decline in nerve conduction velocity, and significant loss in the elastic properties of connective tissue. Such changes partially explain the age-related decrements in neuromuscular performance. When reaction time is partitioned into central processing time and muscle contraction time, it is processing time that is most affected by the aging process. This suggests that aging mainly affects the ability to detect a stimulus and process the information to produce a response. Since reflexes such as the knee jerk reflex do not involve processing in the brain, they are less affected than voluntary responses by the aging process. While aging has a definite effect on the nervous system in terms of reaction and movement time, *physically active groups (be they young or old) move significantly faster than a corresponding age group that is less active.* It is tempting to speculate that the biologic aging of certain neuromuscular functions can be somewhat retarded by regular participation in physical activity.

Pulmonary Function. Measures of **lung function** generally deteriorate with age. How regular exercise throughout one's lifetime can override this "aging" of the pulmonary system is unknown, but older endurance-trained athletes do have greater pulmonary function capacity than sedentary peers. Such findings are encouraging because they indicate that regular physical activity may retard the decline in pulmonary function associated with aging.

Cardiovascular Function. Maximal oxygen uptake and endurance performance decline steadily after age 20, and aerobic fitness has decreased by about 35% at age 65. For both active and sedentary people, the **decline in aerobic capacity** is influenced by age-related decrements in central and peripheral functions linked to oxygen transport and utilization. One clear change is the progressive decline in maximum heart rate with age. A rough approximation of this decline is expressed by the relationship:

$$\textbf{Max HR (beats/min)} = 220 - \textbf{age (years)}$$

Also contributing to diminished blood flow capacity with age is a reduction in the heart's stroke volume that may reflect changes in myocardial contractility. Other age-related cardiovascular changes include reduction in blood flow capacity to peripheral tissues, narrowing of the arteries that supply blood to the heart (by middle age the coronary arteries are about 30% obstructed), and decrease in the elasticity of major blood vessels.

The Aerobic System Is Responsive to Training at Any Age. Research indicates a high degree of **trainability among older men and women,** with adaptations similar to those in younger individuals. Sedentary individuals have nearly a twofold faster rate of decline in aerobic capacity as they age compared to counterparts who remain physically active. Both low- and high-intensity regular exercise enables older individuals to retain a level of cardiovascular function much above that of age-paired sedentary subjects. In fact, when middle-aged men trained regularly over a 10-year period, the usual 10 to 15% decline in work capacity and aerobic fitness was forestalled. At age 55, these active men had maintained the same values for blood pressure, body mass, and max $\dot{V}O_2$ as at age 45.

Body Mass and Body Fat. The **accumulation of excess fat** usually begins in childhood or develops slowly during adulthood. Middle-aged men and women invariably weigh more than college-age counterparts of the same stature—and this weight difference is accounted for by differences in body fat. In the Western world, the average 20-year-old male will gain between 0.25 and 0.5 kg of fat each year until age 60. In one study, the fat content of 27 adult men increased an average of 6.5 kg (14 lb) over a 12-year period from ages 32 to 44. This was equal to the group's total gain in body mass for the duration of the study. What remains unknown is the extent to which such gains in body fat during adulthood represent a normal biologic pattern. However, observations of physically active older individuals suggest that although it is common to see most "normal" individuals grow fatter as they become older, those who remain physically active retain lean body mass and a reduced level of body fat.

TRUE AGING OR SEDENTARY LIFESTYLE?

The culprit, aging or lifestyle? Sedentary living often brings about losses in cardiovascular function that are as great as the effects of aging itself.

The more the body is used, the better it works—at any age. Regular exercise can blunt the progress of so-called age-related disorders, from diabetes to heart disease, and greatly increase the body's functional capacity:

- **Body composition.** Exercise reduces the percentage of body fat and contributes to maintenance of the lean or muscular component of the body
- **Cardiovascular system.** Regular physical activity can lower cholesterol and blood pressure, while improving the ability of the heart to pump blood throughout the body
- **Metabolism.** Exercise increases our ability to burn fat and improves the tissues' sensitivity to insulin
- **Skeleton.** For both men and women, regular exercise contributes to the maintenance of strong bones throughout life
- **Nervous system.** Active people of any age retain a higher level of neuromotor function compared to sedentary counterparts

REGULAR EXERCISE: A FOUNTAIN OF YOUTH?

While exercise may not necessarily be a "fountain of youth," researchers are finding that regular physical activity not only retards the decline in functional capacity associated with aging and disuse, but often reverses this loss regardless of when in life a person becomes active. Improvements have been noted in muscular strength, body composition, joint flexibility (stiff joints are often the result of disuse, not arthritis), aerobic capacity, pulmonary and neural function, heart disease risk, and resistance to mental depression. Evidence is also accumulating that regular exercise can conserve and actually increase bone mass in the elderly, thus staving off the ravages of osteoporosis that afflict both women and men.

DOES EXERCISE IMPROVE HEALTH AND EXTEND LIFE?

Over the years, medical experts have debated whether a lifetime of regular exercise contributes to good health and perhaps longevity compared to the sedentary "good life." Because older fit individuals have many of the functional characteristics of younger people, one could argue that **improved physical fitness and a vigorous lifestyle may retard the aging process** and confer some protection to health in later life. In an early study of exercise and longevity, former Harvard oarsmen exceeded their predicted longevity by 5.1 years per man. While other research supports these findings, the studies were plagued with methodologic problems including inadequate record keeping, small sample size, improper statistical procedures for estimating expected longevity, and inability to account for other important factors such as socioeconomic background, body type, cigarette smoking, and family background.

Keeping the cardiovascular system young. Researchers maintain that a 30-minute program of rapid walking performed by an older person 3 or 4 times a week can turn back the biologic clock some 10 years in terms of cardiovascular and aerobic function.

One group of researchers attempted to overcome the limitations of earlier research in their study of the diseases and **longevity of former college athletes.** Because collegiate athletes usually have a longer involvement in habitual physical activity prior to entering college than nonathletes, and since they may remain more physically active after college, this seemed to be an excellent group to study to provide insight concerning exercise and longevity.

Figure 20–4 shows there was essentially *no difference* in the longevity of the ex-athletes compared to nonathletes. Some degree of equality in genetic background existed between the groups because there was similarity in the average age at death of grandparents, parents, and siblings of ex-athletes and nonathletes. These and more recent findings suggest that participation in athletics as a young adult does not necessarily ensure longevity.

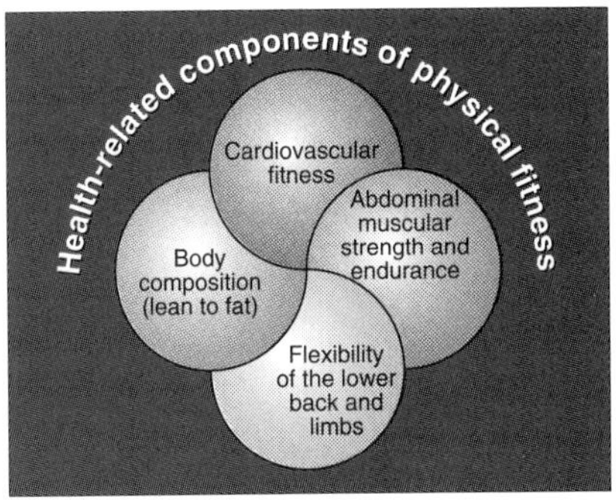

The components of health-related physical fitness.

ENHANCED QUALITY TO A LONGER LIFE: A STUDY OF HARVARD ALUMNI

Research concerning the current lifestyles and exercise habits of 17,000 **Harvard alumni** who entered college between 1916 and 1950 indicates that only moderate aerobic exercise, equivalent to jogging 3 miles a day, promotes good health and may actually add years to life. Men who expended

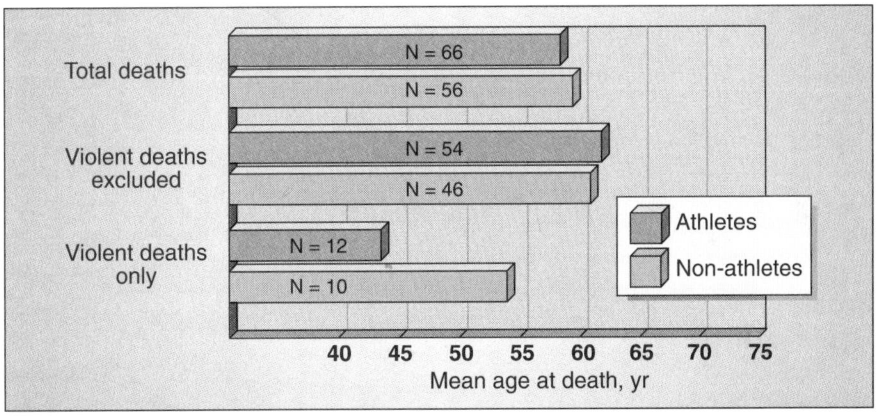

FIG. 20–4. Age at death of athletes and nonathletes. None of the differences between the groups are statistically significant. (From Montoye, H.J., et al.: The Longevity and Morbidity of College Athletes. Indianapolis, Phi Epsilon Kappa, 1957.)

about 2000 kcal in weekly exercise had death rates one-quarter to one-third lower than classmates who did little or no exercise. To achieve this 2000 kcal output weekly requires moderate activity such as a daily 30-minute brisk walk, run, cycle, swim, cross-country ski, or aerobic dance. The specific results of these long-term studies can be summarized as follows:

> Regular exercise counters the life-shortening effects of cigarette smoking and excess body weight. Even for people with high blood pressure (a primary heart disease risk), those who exercised regularly reduced their death rate by one-half. Moreover, genetic tendencies toward an early death were countered by regular exercise. For individuals who had one or both parents die before age 65 (another significant health risk), a lifestyle that included regular exercise reduced the risk of death by 25%. A 50% reduction in mortality rate was observed for those whose parents lived beyond 65 years.

Exercise is good medicine. In recent studies of the health and exercise habits of Harvard alumni, those men who were physically active had about half the risk of colon cancer as those who were inactive. The protection disappeared if the men stopped exercising. One mechanism proposed for this exercise benefit against one of the major American killers is that exercise speeds up the passage of food residues through the digestive tract. This would reduce the time that potential carcinogens in food would be exposed to the colon lining.

As shown in Figure 20–5, a person who exercises more has an improved health profile. For example, mortality rates were 21% lower for men who walked 9 or more miles a week than for those who walked 3 miles or less. Exercising in light sports activities increased life expectancy 24% over men who remained sedentary. From a perspective of energy expenditure, the life expectancy of Harvard alumni increased steadily from a weekly exercise energy output of 500 kcal to 3500 kcal, the equivalent of 6 to 8 hours of strenuous weekly exercise. In addition, active men lived an average of 1 to 2 years longer than sedentary classmates. Beyond weekly exercise of 3500 kcal, there were no additional health or longevity benefits. In fact, when exercise was carried to extremes, the men had higher death rates than their more active colleagues—another example of more not necessarily being better!

EPIDEMIOLOGIC EVIDENCE

A critique of 43 studies of the relationship between physical inactivity and CHD concluded that lack of regular exercise contributes to heart disease in a cause-and-effect manner, with the sedentary person at almost twice the risk as the most active individual. The strength of this protective as-

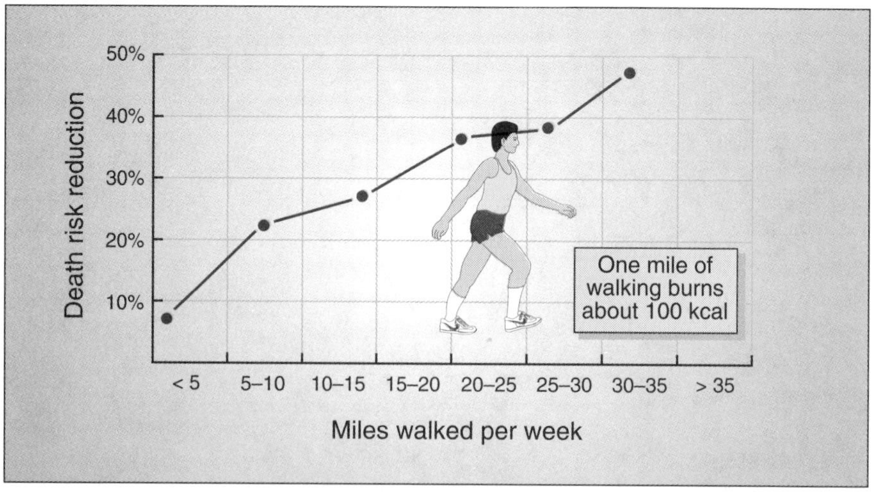

FIG. 20–5. Reduced risk of death with regular exercise. (Adapted from Paffenbarger, R.S., Jr., et al.: Physical activity, all-cause mortality, and longevity of college alumni. *N. Engl. J. Med.*, 314:605, 1986.)

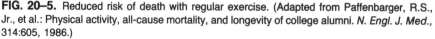

sociation was essentially the same as that observed between heart disease and hypertension, cigarette smoking, and high serum cholesterol. In the researchers' opinion, this placed physical inactivity as the greater heart disease risk, considering that more people lead sedentary lives than possess one or more of the other risks. Although vigorous exercise does entail a small risk of sudden death during the activity, the significant longer-term health benefits of regular activity far outweigh any potential acute risk.

From available data, it appears that if life-extending benefits of exercise exist, they are associated more with preventing early mortality than with improving overall life span. While the maximum life span may not be greatly extended, more active people tend to survive to a "ripe old age." That only moderate exercise is needed to achieve these benefits is further good news.

IMPROVED FITNESS: A LITTLE GOES A LONG WAY

A recent study of more than 13,000 men and women followed for an average of 8 years indicates that even modest amounts of exercise substantially reduce the risk of dying from heart disease, cancer, and other causes. This was one of the few studies that looked directly at fitness performance rather than verbal or written reports of regular physical activity habits. To isolate the effect of fitness per se, the study considered such factors as smoking, cholesterol and blood sugar levels, blood pressure, and family history of CHD. Based on age-adjusted death rates per 10,000 person-years, Figure 20–6 illustrates that the death rate of the least fit group was more than 3 times that of the most fit subjects. The most striking finding was that the greatest health benefit occurred in the group rated just above the most sedentary category. For men, the drop in death rate from the least fit to the next category was more than 38 (64.0 vs. 25.5 deaths per 10,000 person-years), whereas the drop in moving from the second group up to the most fit category was only 7. Similar benefits were found for women. The amount of exercise required to move from the most sedentary category to the next most fit—the jump that showed the greatest health benefits—occurred for

An all-around good thing. According to one prominent researcher, "Exercise seems to be good for almost everything—heart disease, weight loss, diabetes, bone loss, and cancer."

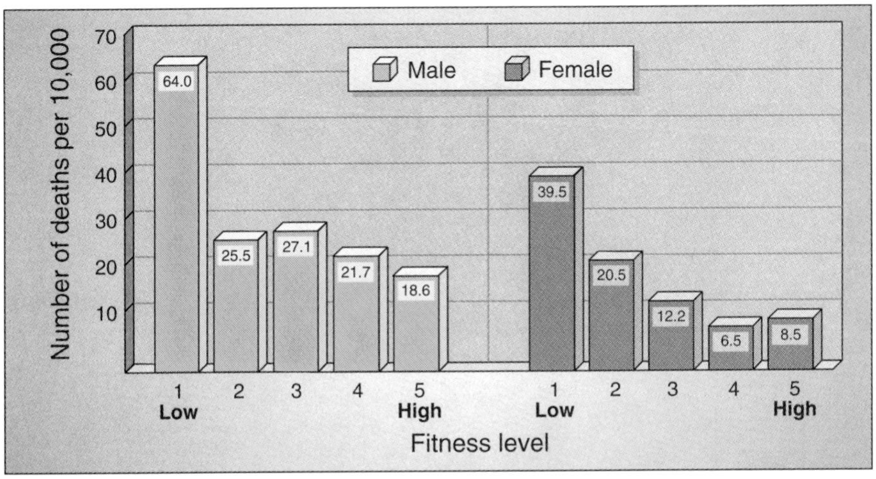

FIG. 20–6. Physical fitness and longevity: a little goes a long way. (From Blair, S.N., et al.: Physical fitness and all-cause mortality: a prospective study of healthy men and women. *JAMA*, 262:2395, 1989.)

moderate-intensity exercise such as walking briskly for 30 minutes several times a week.

CORONARY HEART DISEASE

Heart disease is an equal-opportunity killer. According to the American Heart Association, heart attack is the number one killer of women. Each year, women are struck down with just about half of the 520,000 heart attack deaths and more than 90,000 strokes, compared to 40,500 deaths from breast cancer and 41,000 from lung cancer.

Figure 20–7 illustrates that 50% of total deaths in the United States are caused by **diseases of the heart and blood vessels.** Stated somewhat more graphically, as many as 1.5 million Americans will have a heart attack this year and about one-third of them will die. While deaths from CHD have declined more than one-third since 1970, heart disease still remains the leading cause of death in the Western world. Between ages 55 and 65, about 13 of every 100 men and 6 of every 100 women die from CHD. Although the death rates for women lag about 10 years behind those for men, the gap is closing fast, especially with the upswing in cigarette smoking by women. For every American who dies of cancer, nearly 3 die of heart-related disease. The economic cost of this health disaster—medical costs, loss of earnings and productivity—is staggering ($120 billion in 1992). And this does not include the emotional impact of loss of a loved one in the prime of life!

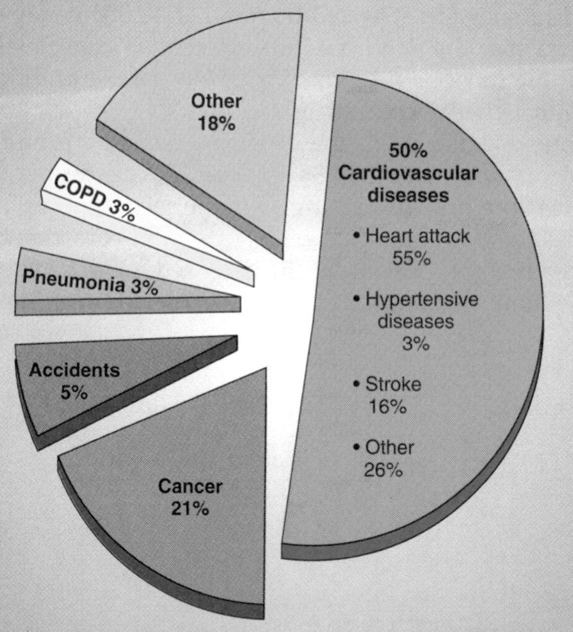

*Based on data from the American Heart Association, "1987 Heart Facts." The total cost of cardiovascular disease in 1987 is estimated at $85.2 billion

FIG. 20–7. Leading causes of death in the United States.

THE HEART'S BLOOD SUPPLY

Although literally tons of blood flow through the heart each day, none of its nourishment passes directly into the myocardium. This is because there

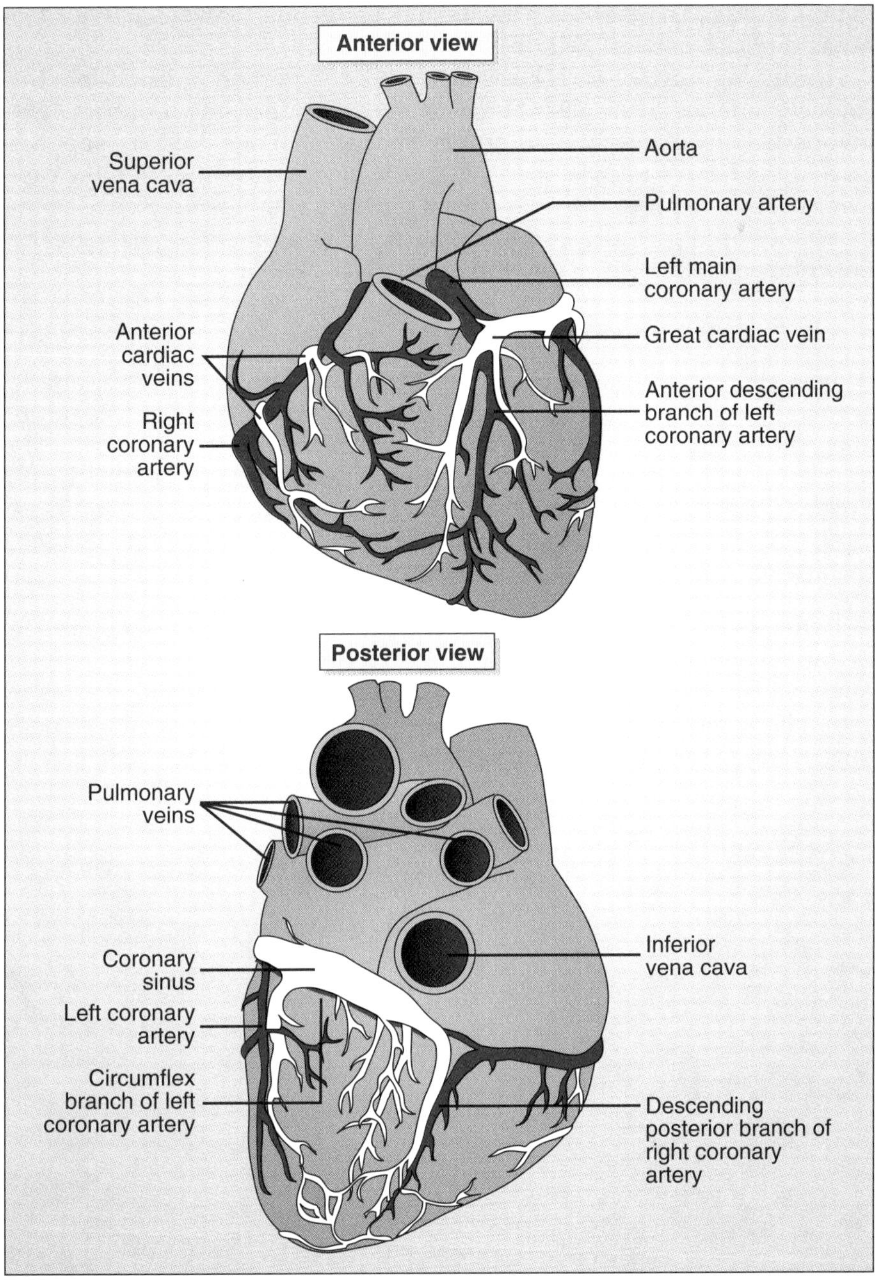

FIG. 20–8. The coronary circulation. Arteries are shaded darker than veins.

are no direct circulatory channels into the myocardium from within the heart's chambers. Instead, the heart muscle has an elaborate circulatory network of its own. As shown in Figure 20–8, these vessels form a visible, crown-like arterial network called the **coronary circulation.** Openings for the two coronary arteries are situated in the aorta at a point where the freshly oxygenated blood leaves the left ventricle to be distributed throughout the body. These arteries then curl around the heart's surface; the *right coronary artery* supplies predominantly the right atrium and ventricle, whereas the greatest volume of blood flows in the *left coronary artery* to supply the tissue of the left atrium and ventricle and a small part of the right ventricle. These vessels divide and proliferate to eventually form a dense capillary network within the myocardium.

The driving force of each heart beat pushes a portion of blood into the coronary arteries to be distributed to the individual muscle fibers. The myocardial blood supply is so profuse that at least one capillary supplies each of the heart's muscle fibers. After the blood passes through the capillaries, it empties into the right atrium via the *coronary veins.* Exercise produces increased pressure in the aorta that forces a proportionately greater flow of oxygenated blood into the coronary circulation.

Less than an aspirin a day keeps the doctor away! Daily ingestion of only 30 mg of aspirin, one-tenth of an adult aspirin or a little less than half a baby aspirin, is safer than higher doses and equally effective in warding off strokes and heart attacks in patients with cardiovascular disease. Lower-dose aspirin therapy was also associated with many fewer complications such as bleeding and undue gastrointestinal irritation. The beneficial effects of aspirin are related to its inhibiting effects on the formation of blood clots that can clog a blood vessel. Drug companies are in a fierce battle to perfect a hybrid type of aspirin to unblock coronary vessels clogged with blood clots. The new generation aspirin works by keeping blood platelets from binding to each other at special receptor sites at their surface, the process that causes blood to clot. At present, regular aspirin blocks only about 20% of the receptor sites on the platelets; the hope for the super aspirins is 100%.

A LIFE-LONG PROCESS

Almost all people show some evidence of CHD, and it can be severe in seemingly healthy young adults. Actually, this degenerative process probably starts early in life because fatty streaks are common in the coronary arteries of children by the age of 5 years! There seems to be little harm, however, unless the arteries are markedly narrowed. As shown in Figure 20–9, CHD involves long-term degenerative changes in the inner lining of the arteries that supply the heart muscle.

Changes on the Cellular Level. The action and chemical modification of various compounds, including the cholesterol in low-density lipoproteins, initiate a complex process that ultimately causes bulging lesions in the walls of the coronary arteries. These changes initially take the form of fatty streaks, the first signs of **atherosclerosis.** With further damage and

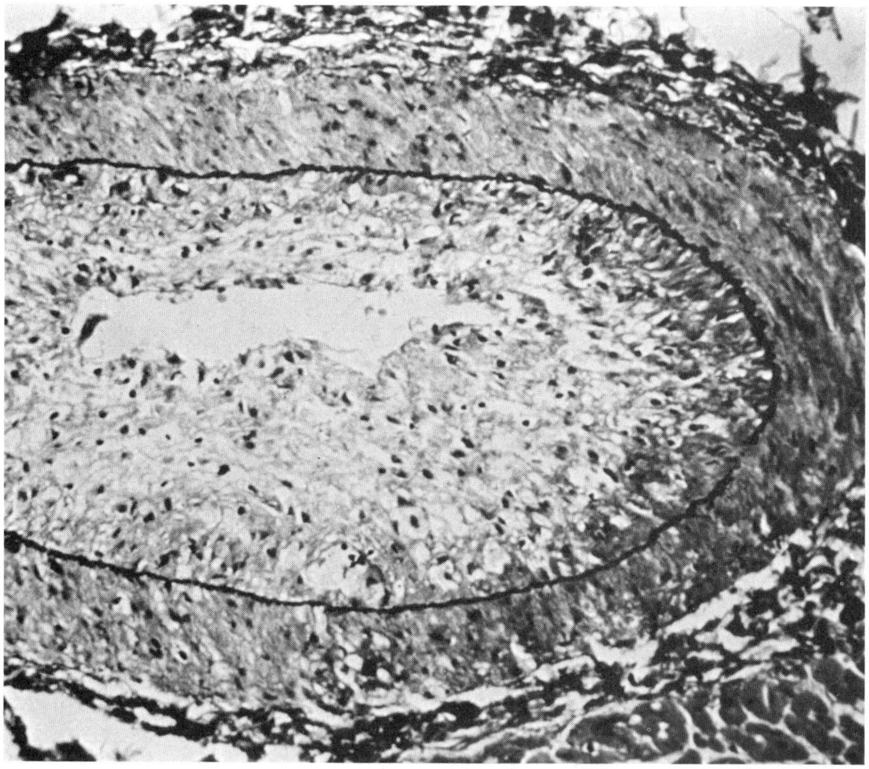

FIG. 20–9. Deterioration of a normal coronary artery is seen as atherosclerosis develops with the beginning of deposits of fatty substances that roughen the vessel's center. The clot then forms and plugs the artery, depriving the heart muscle of vital blood. The result is a myocardial infarction or heart attack.

A lifetime battle. Risk factors are also prevalent among children, as about 40% of kids age 5 to 8 years exhibit either obesity, hypertension, or elevated cholesterol.

proliferation of underlying cells, the vessel becomes progressively congested with lipid-filled plaques, fibrous scar tissue, or both. This change progressively reduces the capacity for blood flow and causes the myocardium to become **ischemic**—that is, poorly supplied with oxygen because of the reduced blood supply. The roughened, hardened lining of the coronary artery frequently causes the slowly flowing blood to clot. This blood clot, or **thrombus,** may plug one of the smaller coronary vessels. In such cases, a portion of the heart muscle dies and the person is said to have suffered a heart attack, or **myocardial infarction.** If the blockage is not too severe but blood flow is at times reduced below the heart's requirement, the person may experience temporary chest pains termed **angina pectoris.** These pains are usually felt during exertion, because this causes the greatest demand for myocardial blood flow. Anginal attacks provide vivid evidence of the importance of adequate oxygen supply to this vital organ.

> **Heart attack versus cardiac arrest.** The difference is:
> - Heart attack—caused by blockage in one or more arteries supplying the heart, thus cutting off the heart's blood supply, or sudden spasms or constrictions of a coronary vessel, causing part of the heart muscle to die (necrosis)
> - Cardiac arrest—caused by irregular neural-electrical transmission within the heart muscle, causing chaotic, unregulated beating in the heart's upper chambers (atrial fibrillation) or lower chambers (ventricular fibrillation)

RISK FACTORS FOR CORONARY HEART DISEASE

Various personal characteristics and environmental factors have been identified over the past 35 years that indicate a person's susceptibility to CHD. The relative importance of each of these factors has been established. *In general, the greater the risk factor, the more likely it is that the coronary arteries are diseased or will become diseased in the near future.* This is not to say that a specific risk factor is the cause of the disease, as numerous factors may be acting and interacting in a cause-and-effect manner. However, based on the total evidence presently available, it is prudent to assess these factors on a personal basis and make efforts to modify each within reasonable limits (see RISKO in Section 2H of the *Study Guide* to assess your own risk of heart disease).

> **Has the tide changed?** According to the U.S. Public Health Service, heart disease rates declined by 34% and stroke by 55% between 1970 and 1988. Part of the reason for this reduction in cardiovascular disease is that people are taking charge of their lifestyles and altering modifiable risk factors in favorable directions.

The significant heart disease risk factors, including those that can and cannot be modified as well as important contributing factors, are:

- Age and gender
- Elevated blood lipids
- Hypertension
- Cigarette smoking
- Physical inactivity
- Obesity
- Diabetes mellitus
- Diet
- Heredity
- Personality and behavior patterns
- High uric acid levels
- Pulmonary function abnormalities
- Race
- Electrocardiographic abnormalities during rest and exercise
- Tension and stress

> **A deadly habit in the Minuteman state.** In Massachusetts, smoking plays a role in at least 1 in 5 deaths among residents over age 35. It is a bigger killer than drug abuse, violence, car accidents, AIDS, and other preventable causes combined.

It is difficult to determine quantitatively the importance of a single CHD risk factor in comparison to any other, because many of the factors are interrelated. For example, blood lipid abnormalities, diabetes, heredity, and obesity often go hand-in-hand. Compounding such observations is the finding that physical training generally lowers body mass, body fat, blood lipids, and the risk of developing diabetes. Also, certain groups, inde-

> **"Super-mom" has increased CHD risk.** A study of women aged 50 to 70 with graduate nursing degrees revealed that those who experienced conflict and tension trying to balance family and job responsibilities had 9 times more heart disease than women without such conflicts. Similar research shows that high-demand, low-control jobs produce more heart attacks in women. Having to juggle career and family are two high-demand jobs; conflict between the two could mean the woman feels less in control because she perceives less ability to complete both tasks equally well.

pendent of other risk factors, are generally exposed to less psychological stress because of the nature of their occupation or cultural setting.

The risk factors of age, gender, and heredity are predetermined and cannot be controlled or remedied. However, four "treatable" factors—serum lipids, blood pressure, physical inactivity, and cigarette smoking—stand out as potent CHD risk factors. Of somewhat less predictive value than these **primary risk factors** are the risk factors of obesity and personality type. Although risk factors are closely associated with CHD, the associations do not necessarily infer causality. In many instances it remains to be shown that risk factor modification offers effective protection from the disease. Until definite proof is demonstrated, however, it is logical to assume that eliminating or reducing one or more risk factors will cause a corresponding decrease in the probability of contracting CHD.

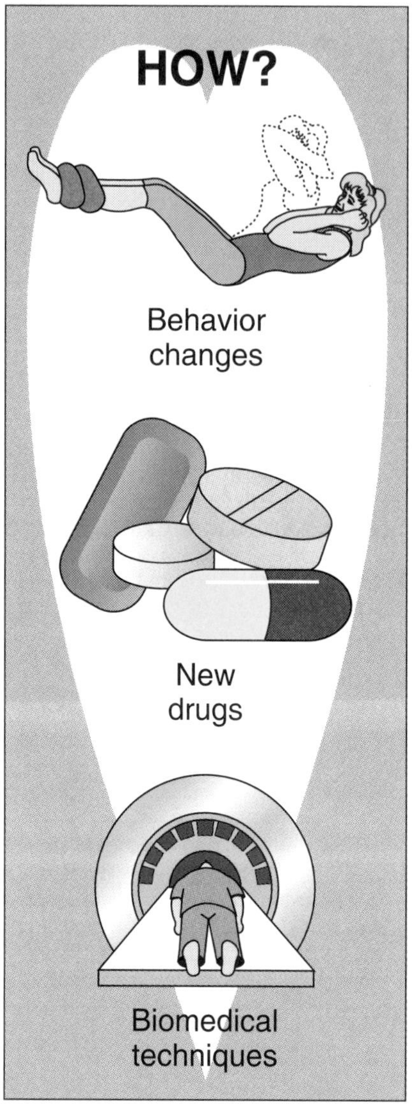

Looking ahead. By the year 2016, an estimated 31 million Americans will die from heart disease and strokes. The good news is that advances in science and healthy living could cut the toll in half. How? Behavior changes (50%), new drugs (40%), and biomedical techniques (10%).

AGE, GENDER, AND HEREDITY

Age is a risk factor largely because other **associated risk factors** such as hypertension, elevated blood lipids, and glucose intolerance become more prevalent in older years. As shown in Figure 20–10, after age 35 in males and age 45 in females, the chances of dying from CHD increase progressively and dramatically. Between ages 55 and 65, about 13 of every 100 men and 6 of 100 women die from CHD. At most ages women fare much better than men. For example, in middle age, a man stands about a sixfold greater chance of dying from a heart attack. However, American women still lead all other countries in heart disease and the specific **"gender advantage"** is greatly reduced after the age of menopause. This has led to speculation that some of the CHD protection for women is provided by hormonal differences between the genders. Although the cause is not known, heart attacks that strike at an early age appear to run in families.

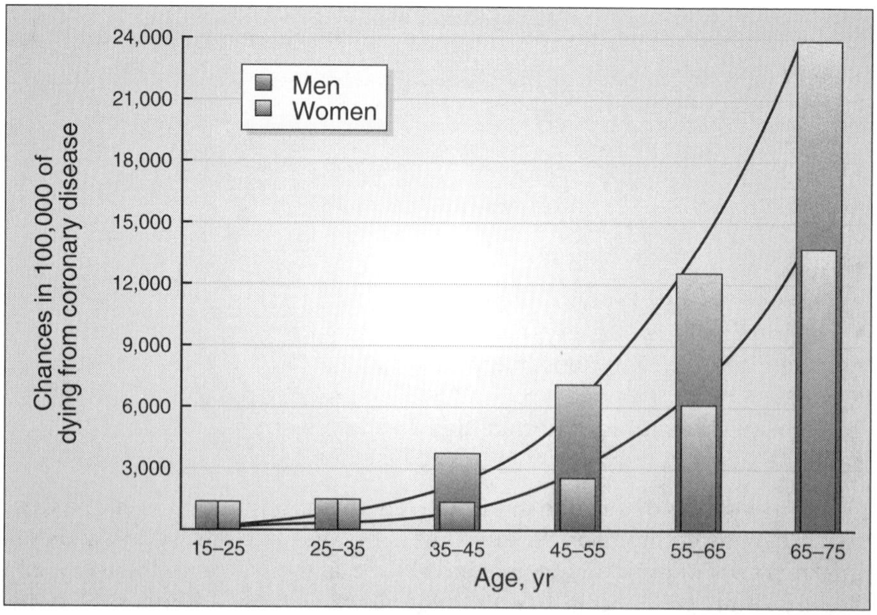

FIG. 20–10. The chance of a single individual dying from coronary atherosclerosis. (Data from the American Heart Association.)

The precise mechanism by which plasma lipids affect the development of CHD is not fully understood. Nevertheless, overwhelming evidence links high blood lipid levels with an increased heart disease risk.

Adding exercise to a low-fat, low-calorie diet enhances results. Men and women who combine regular aerobic physical activity with a low-fat, weight-loss diet have a significantly greater reduction in their risk for coronary heart disease compared with groups that only diet.

Cholesterol and Triglycerides. Table 20–1 presents levels of serum cholesterol above which young and older adults should seek advice on treatment. In general, a cholesterol level of 200 mg/dl or lower is considered desirable. A cholesterol value of 230 mg/dl increases the risk of heart attack to about twice that of a person with 180 mg/dl, and a value of 300 mg/dl increases the risk fourfold. An increased lipid level in the blood plasma is termed **hyperlipidemia.**

High cholesterol also increases risk of a second heart attack. For individuals recovering from heart attacks, those with high levels of blood cholesterol (275 mg/dl or above) were:

- At four times greater risk of having another heart attack than recovering patients with cholesterol less than 200
- Twice as likely to die from heart disease as patients with low cholesterol
- Nearly twice as likely to die from other causes

People of short stature at risk for heart disease. Research on the relation between stature and CHD risk indicates that the heart attack rate was 60% higher in men 5 feet 7 inches or shorter than in men taller than 6 feet 1 inch—and for every inch of added height the risk decreases by 3%. The researchers speculate that shorter people have relatively narrower arteries that might clog more quickly. This does not mean that short men and women are destined to early heart attack. Shortness holds about the same risk as obesity and family history, but less than hypertension, cigarette smoking, elevated cholesterol, or diabetes.

The French Paradox. In the Gascony region of southwestern France, where the average Frenchman consumes 40 pounds of high-fat cheeses a year and routinely dines on fatty foods from goose and duck, the death rate from cardiovascular diseases is the lowest in the country. Such eating habits, if practiced by Americans, would be akin to blasphemy, yet the death rate for middle-aged men in the Gascony region is only 80 per 100,000, whereas in the Paris region it is 145 and in the United States it is four times higher at 315! The explanation may lie in the cheeses' composition (natural fermentation may neutralize the fats from freely entering the circulation) and the daily consumption of two glasses of red wine. American and French researchers will continue the 10-year epidemiologic study for another 5 years; they will now focus on consumption of vegetables and fruits as well as alcohol.

Triglyceride levels in blood generally have been thought to have little effect on heart disease risk. Recent studies now indicate that for patients

Family history is important. Should children have their cholesterol measured? Guidelines issued by the National Cholesterol Education Program say yes if there is a family history of high cholesterol or heart disease (particularly if a parent suffered a heart attack before age 50). Shockingly, this parental "cardiac proneness" includes up to one-fourth the adult population of the United States!

TABLE 20–1. DESIRABLE LEVELS OF TOTAL CHOLESTEROL (MG/DL), INCLUDING HDL AND LDL CHOLESTEROL, AND LEVELS ABOVE WHICH ADULTS SHOULD RECEIVE TREATMENT

AGE	GOAL	MODERATE RISK (75TH PERCENTILE)	HIGH RISK (90TH PERCENTILE)
20–29	<180	>200	>220
30–39	<200	>220	>240
40 and over	<200	>240	>260

UNDESIRABLE LEVELS

HDL cholesterol < 35 mg/dl
LDL cholesterol > 130 mg/dl

Source: Adapted from National Institutes of Health Consensus Development Conference Statement: Lowering blood cholesterol to prevent heart disease. *JAMA*, 253:2080, 1985.

with high cholesterol levels, those with elevated triglycerides were at greatest risk for heart attack. And when triglycerides are elevated, the risk of developing diabetes is twice that of people with normal triglyceride levels.

Cholesterol-lowering drug shrinks fatty deposits in arteries. Lovastatin, a drug sold under the trade name Mevacor that is commonly used to lower blood cholesterol, halts the progression of plaque buildup in the coronary arteries and shrinks existing plaque deposits in patients with atherosclerotic damage to the coronary vessels. The technique of angiography was used to evaluate the extent of plaque regression following Mevacor treatment for up to 2 years in 270 men and women whose cholesterol ranged between 190 and 270 mg/dl. In angiography, a radiopaque dye is injected into the coronary vessels and x-rays are taken in rapid sequence to obtain an image of blood flowing through the arteries.

The Forms of Cholesterol Are Also Important. Cholesterol and triglycerides are the two most common lipids associated with CHD risk. These fats are not soluble in water so they do not circulate freely in the blood plasma. Rather, they are transported in combination with a carrier protein to form a **lipoprotein.** This lipoprotein can vary in size depending on how much protein and fat it contains. Although it is proper to refer to an elevation in blood lipids as hyperlipidemia, it is more meaningful to evaluate and discuss the different types of **hyperlipoproteinemia.** Table 20–2 lists the four different lipoproteins, their approximate density, and their percentage composition in the blood. Serum cholesterol represents a composite of the total cholesterol contained in the different lipoproteins.

The distribution of cholesterol among the various types of lipoproteins is a more powerful predictor of heart disease than simply the total quantity of plasma lipids (Figure 20–11). This partially explains how one person with a high total serum cholesterol may not develop CHD, while it develops in another with a lower cholesterol level. Specifically, a high level of **high-density lipoproteins** (HDL), which comprise the smallest portion of lipoproteins but contain the largest quantity of protein and least amount of cholesterol, is associated with a lower heart disease risk. In contrast, elevated levels of the cholesterol-rich **low-density lipoproteins** (LDL) represent an increased risk.

Although controversy exists concerning the role of the various lipoproteins in heart disease, it is generally believed that LDL is the means for transporting lipids throughout the body for delivery to the cells, including those of the smooth muscle walls of the arteries. Here it ultimately contributes to the artery-narrowing process of atherosclerosis. Whereas LDL carries cholesterol to the tissues and is associated with arterial damage, HDL acts as a scavenger, gathering cholesterol from cells (including those of the arterial wall) and returning it to the liver, where it is metabolized and excreted in the bile. It is also possible that HDL retards cholesterol buildup by interfering with the binding and subsequent uptake of LDL at the cell membrane of the various tissues.

Cholesterol ratios are also important. An effective way to evaluate lipoprotein status is to divide total cholesterol by HDL cholesterol. A ratio greater than 4.5 indicates a high heart disease risk, while a ratio of 3.5 or lower is considered optimal.

Research is progressing to clarify how HDL is protective and what factors can raise its levels. For one thing, cigarette smoking has adverse effects on the HDL pattern. This may account for the significant CHD risk with smoking. It is encouraging from an exercise perspective that HDL levels are

TABLE 20–2. APPROXIMATE COMPOSITION OF LIPOPROTEINS IN THE BLOOD

	CHYLOMICRONS	VERY LOW DENSITY LIPOPROTEINS (VLDL: PREBETA)	LOW-DENSITY LIPOPROTEINS (LDL: BETA)	HIGH-DENSITY LIPOPROTEINS (HDL: ALPHA)
Density, g/cc	0.95	0.95–1.006	1.006–1.019	1.063–1.210
Protein, %	0.5–1.0	5–15	25	45–55
Lipid, %	99	95	75	50
Cholesterol, %	2–5	10–20	40–45	18
Triglyceride, %	85	50–70	5–10	2
Phospholipid, %	3–6	10–20	20–25	30

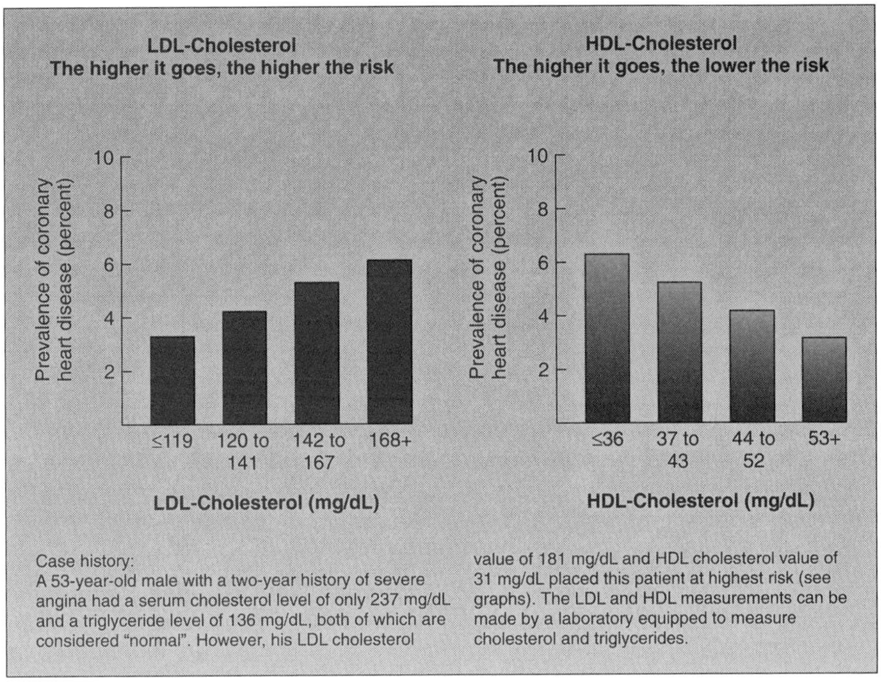
LDL-Cholesterol
The higher it goes, the higher the risk
HDL-Cholesterol
The higher it goes, the lower the risk
Prevalence of coronary heart disease (percent)
10
8
6
4
2
≤119
120 to 141
142 to 167
168+
LDL-Cholesterol (mg/dL)
≤36
37 to 43
44 to 52
53+
HDL-Cholesterol (mg/dL)
Case history:
A 53-year-old male with a two-year history of severe angina had a serum cholesterol level of only 237 mg/dL and a triglyceride level of 136 mg/dL, both of which are considered "normal". However, his LDL cholesterol value of 181 mg/dL and HDL cholesterol value of 31 mg/dL placed this patient at highest risk (see graphs). The LDL and HDL measurements can be made by a laboratory equipped to measure cholesterol and triglycerides.

FIG. 20–11. Coronary heart disease and lipoproteins. (Courtesy of CPC International, Best Foods Division.)

Aerobic exercise reduces risk of diabetes. Individuals who regularly perform moderate to vigorous aerobic exercise such as playing tennis, swimming laps, or jogging greatly reduce their risk of developing adult-onset diabetes, a disease that afflicts about 12 million Americans. The risk is reduced by about 6% for every 500 kcal of additional weekly exercise.

elevated in endurance athletes and are favorably altered in sedentary people who engage in either moderate or vigorous aerobic training. Concurrently, LDL is lowered with exercise so the net result is a considerably improved ratio of HDL to LDL or HDL to total cholesterol. This exercise effect appears to be independent of the lipid content of the diet or the leanness of the exerciser. A moderate consumption of alcohol (equivalent to about 2 oz or 30 g of 90 proof alcohol, three 6 oz glasses of wine, or a bit less than three 12 oz cans of beer) has been reported to significantly reduce an otherwise healthy person's risk of heart attack. Although the protective mechanism is unclear, it may be that moderate alcohol intake increases HDL and lowers LDL. Excessive alcohol consumption offered no lipoprotein benefit and greatly increased the risk of liver disease and cancer.

Heart attack. A moderate intake of red wine appears to lower the artery-clogging LDL cholesterol while at the same time raising the protective HDL cholesterol. Researchers suggest that a natural antifungal chemical in the skin of grapes is the protective agent.

The important factors that affect the level of blood cholesterol as well as the lipoprotein fractions are:

Favorable Effects

- Weight loss through food restriction
- Regular aerobic exercise
- Intake of high-fiber foods, particularly water-soluble fibers such as in beans, legumes, and oat bran
- Increased polyunsaturated to saturated fatty acid ratio in the diet as well as monounsaturated fat
- Increased intake of unique polyunsaturated fats in fish oils
- Moderate alcohol consumption

Unfavorable Effects

- Cigarette smoking
- Diet high in saturated fat and preformed cholesterol
- Emotionally stressful situations
- Certain oral contraceptives
- Sedentary lifestyle

HYPERTENSION

For individuals whose arteries have become "hardened" because fatty materials have deposited within their walls (or because the vessel's connective tissue layer has thickened), or whose arterial system offers excessive resistance to blood flow in the periphery from nervous strain or kidney malfunction, systolic blood pressure at rest may be as high as 300 mm Hg. The diastolic or runoff pressure also is often elevated. Such **hypertension** imposes a chronic strain on the normal functioning of the cardiovascular system.

It has been estimated that 1 of every 5 people will have abnormally high blood pressure sometime during their lives. Presently, more than 35 million Americans have systolic pressures over 140 mm Hg **(systolic hypertension)** or diastolic pressures that exceed 90 mm Hg **(diastolic hypertension).** These values form the lower *borderline* limit for the classification of **borderline high blood pressure.** Uncorrected chronic hypertension can lead to heart failure, heart attack, stroke, or kidney failure.

Hypertension is often called the "silent killer" because it generally progresses unnoticed for decades before it deals its deadly blow. It is also a mysterious killer because the origin of hypertension is unknown in more than 90% of cases. *Statistics indicate that the optimal blood pressure for longevity is about 110 mm Hg systolic and 70 mm Hg diastolic.* Anything higher results in an increased risk for disease. For example, a man with systolic blood pressure above 150 mm Hg has more than twice the heart disease risk as a man whose pressure is 120 mm Hg.

Blood pressure can often be reduced by altering factors over which we have direct control. If you are overweight, reduce; if you smoke, stop, because nicotine may constrict peripheral blood vessels, thus elevating blood pressure. Reduce salt intake, as sodium can cause the body to retain fluid that boosts blood pressure. High blood pressure can also be effectively treated by relatively safe drugs that either reduce fluid volume or decrease peripheral resistance to blood flow.

An inherited tendency for hypertension. Many people have a genetic predisposition toward hypertension that increases their tendency to retain salt, heightens the reactivity of their blood vessels to stress, and causes higher levels of chemicals that constrict the peripheral vasculature.

Try diet and exercise first. Before starting drug therapy to lower blood pressure, try four lifestyle changes to produce the desired effect: lose weight, reduce salt intake, drink less alcohol, and start exercising.

Even a small reduction is beneficial. Men and women aged 30 to 54 years with mild hypertension successfully reduced systolic (2.9 mm Hg) and diastolic (2.3 mm Hg) blood pressure when they reduced body weight and salt intake over an 18-month period. There were no changes in blood pressure for subjects who undertook only stress reduction and relaxation techniques, or who consumed dietary supplements of calcium, magnesium, phosphorus, and fish oil. Cutting daily salt intake from 10 g to 2 g achieved about one-half the improvement in blood pressure as weight loss alone. Experts estimate that a 2 point reduction in blood pressure decreases the rate of CHD by 4% and the chances of stroke by 6%.

Exercise Is Effective. In "borderline" hypertensive patients, exercise training is effective in reducing blood pressure. For middle-aged men, resting systolic pressure decreased from 139 to 133 mm Hg following 4 to 6 weeks of exercise training. In addition, during submaximal exercise, systolic pressure decreased from 173 to 155 mm Hg while diastolic pressure fell from 92 to 79 mm Hg. Consequently, the average blood pressure during a cardiac cycle of systole and diastole was reduced about 14% with training. Based on available evidence, a prudent recommendation is to have your blood pressure checked periodically and include regular exercise for both preventive and therapeutic management.

CIGARETTE SMOKING

In terms of health status, the more a person smokes, the less healthy he or she is likely to be in the future. **Cigarette smoking is one of the best predictors of CHD.** In fact, the probability of death from heart disease for smokers is almost twice as great as for nonsmokers. Essentially, the more you smoke, the deeper you inhale, and the stronger the cigarette in terms of tars and noxious by-products, the greater your risk. In addition, smokers are nearly 5 times as likely to have a stroke as nonsmokers—and those who smoke a pack or more a day have an 11 times greater chance of suffering a specific type of sudden, deadly stroke that tends to strike younger men and women. Surprisingly, this CHD risk for men and women is associated with 2 to 3 times more deaths than the excess mortality of cigarette smokers due to lung cancer!

Smoking and Pregnancy. Cigarette smoking during pregnancy negatively affects breast milk output and infant growth rate. A recent study compared 10 lactating women who had never smoked with 10 women who smoked at least 4 cigarettes every day during pregnancy and lactation. The results were clear: mothers who smoked produced 28% less breast milk and their babies weighed 38% less than nonsmoking counterparts. The reduced breast milk output was apparently insufficient to support the energy needs of the infants.

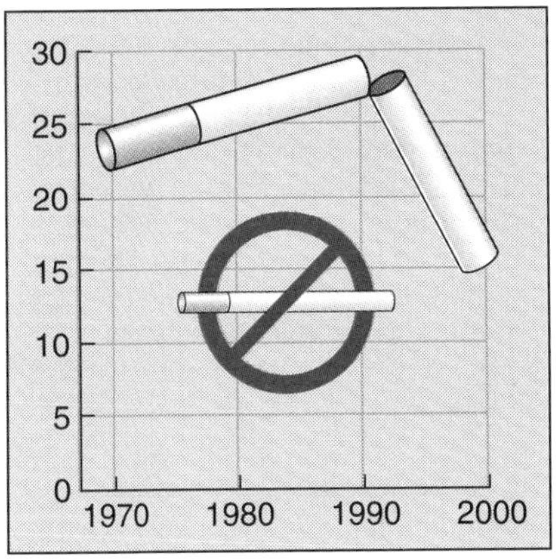

Smokers statistics. According to the Centers for Disease Control, the number of adult smokers has declined to the lowest level ever measured. The bad news is that 28% of the population still smokes. This includes 31% of men, 26% of women, 28% of whites, 32% of blacks, and 24% of Hispanic people. On further analysis, those who do smoke tend to be less educated or have marital troubles. While the overall smoking rate is dropping, those who smoke are starting at a younger age.

Smoking Is Bad for Bone Healing. Researchers at Emory University in Georgia have shown that the bones of habitual smokers take longer to heal than the bones of nonsmokers. Eleven smokers, 9 nonsmokers, and 9 ex-smokers with the bone disease osteomyelitis were followed for 3 years after corrective surgery to lengthen and repair the tibia (large bone of the lower leg). The results were clear: to achieve bone growth of 2 inches took smokers 15 months and ex-smokers 12.5 months, but only 10 months for non-smokers. The researchers believe that inadequate oxygen supply to the bone was the cause. Smoking for 10 minutes reduces tissue oxygen supply for 45 minutes, while the diminished oxygen flow for a pack-a-day smoker lasts 16 hours!

Lung Cancer vs. Heart Disease. Lung cancer has replaced heart disease as the main cause of death in smokers. Each year, about 400,000 Americans will die from smoking-related illnesses. This is almost 4 people every 5 minutes—about the time it takes to smoke a cigarette! The U.S. goal for the year 2000 is to cut smoking rates from the current 28% of the population—which includes 1 in 5 high school seniors who are frequent cigarette smokers—to 15%. According to the National Cancer Institute, this can be achieved by:

- Target school kids to prevent them from ever starting to smoke
- Use schools, churches, synagogues, and health groups to distribute antismoking materials
- Target major TV markets and increase public service announcements

Lung cancer has replaced heart disease as the main cause of death in smokers. Each year, about 400,000 Americans will die from smoking-related illnesses—almost 4 people every five minutes or about the time it takes to smoke a cigarette! The U.S. goal for the year 2000 is to cut smoking rates from the current 28% of the population to 15%. This includes 1 in 5 high school seniors who are frequent cigarette smokers. According to the National Cancer Institute, this can be achieved by:

- Target school kids to prevent them from ever starting to smoke
- Use schools, churches, and synagogues and health groups to distribute anti-smoking materials
- Target major and public service announcements.
- Regular exercise in nearly 60,000 college graduates significantly lowered colon cancer and heart disease risk.
- In animals, a combination of long-duration, high-intensity exercise and a low-fat diet appeared to modify hormone levels that reduce tumors similar to those found in human breast cancer.

OBESITY

Approximately 40% of all Americans are considered too heavy because their body mass is at least 10% above "ideal weight." The average male and female in the United States is about 4 kg heavier than their 1960 counterparts, even though the nation's per capita caloric intake has steadily decreased over this 30-year period. Such facts support the position that the "creeping obesity" in our society may be more the consequence of *physical inactivity* than of overeating.

It is difficult to determine quantitatively the importance of excess body fat per se as a risk to good health. However, the death rate for men who weigh 30% more than they should is nearly 70% higher than for those of normal weight. The overfat condition is often associated with multiple risk factors such as hypertension and elevated serum lipids. In addition, an obese person usually consumes a highly atherogenic diet that is rich in

Wisconsin's females rank first. The federal Centers for Disease Control reports that among 39 states surveyed in 1989, 33% of women between the ages of 18 and 44 years smoked. Wisconsin had the highest smoking rate, 39%, while Texas had the lowest, at 21%. The goal for the year 2000 is no more than 12% female smokers in this age range.

Being too fat is an expensive excess. The price tag for health problems related to obesity in 1989 was approximately $40 billion! This represents about 5.5% of the total cost of health care for that year and includes medical expenses related to gallbladder disease, adult-onset diabetes, cardiovascular disease, cancer, and hypertension.

saturated fats and cholesterol. The addition of extra pounds also increases the chance of developing impaired glucose tolerance and abnormal serum uric acid values.

Weight loss and accompanying fat reduction generally contribute to normalizing plasma cholesterol and triglycerides and have a beneficial effect on blood pressure and adult-onset diabetes. In fact, the normally observed increase in blood pressure with age is partially explained by the age-related gain in body mass. Although being too fat may not be a primary CHD risk factor, its role as a secondary and contributing factor in heart disease cannot be denied.

PERSONALITY AND BEHAVIOR PATTERNS

There appears to be a distinct personality that is susceptible to heart disease. The coronary-prone behaviors that typify what psychologists call the ***Type A personality*** are characterized as hard-driving, ambitious, impatient, short-tempered, hostile, and restless. Unrelenting pressures, drives, deadlines, anxieties, depression, and a constant struggle against the limitations of time are all part of this stress syndrome—with its accompanying excessive stimulation of the body's "fight or flight" hormonal response that may be detrimental to cardiovascular health. The opposite style of behavior, exemplified by the equally capable but easygoing, coronary-resistant **Type B personality,** is under no time pressure. This personality type is categorized by the absence of Type A behaviors. Generally, one is neither all Type A nor all Type B, but rather a blend of both types of behavior patterns.

The precise manner by which personality and behavior influence the development of CHD is unknown, let alone whether one's basic personality "type" can be significantly altered to influence a disease process. However, it is desirable to recognize, manage, and effectively channel the excess stress in daily life. To this end, exercise blended with the techniques of behavior modification is a positive step in channeling potentially harmful behaviors into ones that will produce positive "spin-off."

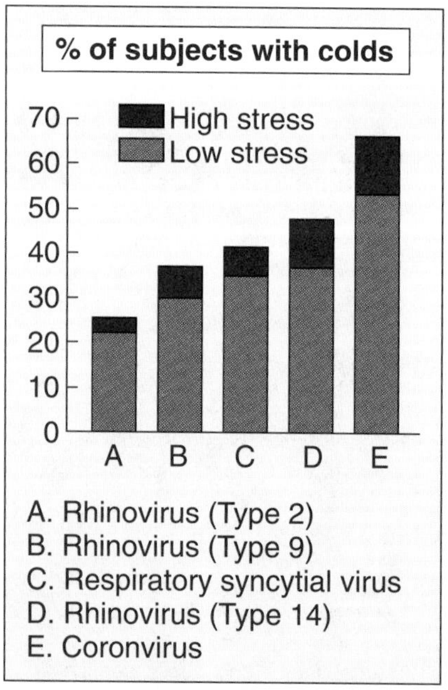

Psychological stress and clinical illness. Stress levels related to major life-altering events in the prior year, one's current stress level, and one's ability to cope with stress are linked to susceptibility to infection from five of the most common respiratory viruses. Suppression of the immune system is the likely cause.

PHYSICAL INACTIVITY

Poor physical fitness is bad medicine. The evidence relating sedentary habits to poor health is enough to classify physical inactivity as a major risk factor for early death. For both men and women, the maintenance of physical fitness throughout life provides significant protection from heart disease in terms of both risk factors and the occurrence of actual disease. In a 9-year study of Californians, sedentary men and women were more than twice as likely to die prematurely compared to those who exercised frequently. In terms of health status, people who reported even mild exercise were better off than those who were completely sedentary.

While the results from the latest studies argue strongly for regular physical activity, "critical or absolute proof" is still lacking of the protective role of exercise against premature cardiovascular disease in humans. However, the major weight of research on animals and humans indicates that regular exercise may operate against CHD in a variety of beneficial ways. These include:

- Improving myocardial circulation and metabolism to protect the heart from lack of oxygen; this includes possible enhanced vascularization as well as modest increases in cardiac glycogen stores and anaerobic capacity

that could be beneficial when the heart's oxygen supply is compromised
- Enhancing contractile properties of the myocardium; this may enable the conditioned heart to maintain or increase contractility during a specific challenge
- Providing for more favorable blood clotting characteristics
- Normalizing the blood lipid profile, especially via an increase in HDL and lowering of LDL
- Favorably altering heart rate and blood pressure so the work of the heart is reduced at rest and during exercise
- Achieving a more desirable body composition (higher lean to fat ratio)
- Establishing a more favorable neural hormonal balance that may conserve oxygen for the myocardium and improve the mixture of carbohydrate and fat metabolized by the body
- Providing a favorable outlet for psychological stress and tensions

A cancer-prevention workout? The results are preliminary, but if you exercise more and eat less fat, your risk for cancer may drop.

INTERACTION OF RISK FACTORS

Many **risk factors are associated with each other** as well as with CHD itself. Generally, the smoking risk acts independently of other risk factors. At the same time, however, if other risk factors are present, the multiple risks interact in an additive way and cigarette smoking may even accentuate the influence of other risks. The interaction of the three primary CHD risk factors when elevated in the same person is shown in Figure 20–12. With one risk factor, a 45-year-old man's chance of CHD during the year is about 2 times greater than that of a man with no risks. With three risk factors,

Passive smoking can kill. Smoking risk is not only for the smoker. Researchers now estimate that up to 53,000 nonsmokers will die each year from lung cancer and heart disease due to exposure to second-hand cigarette smoke.

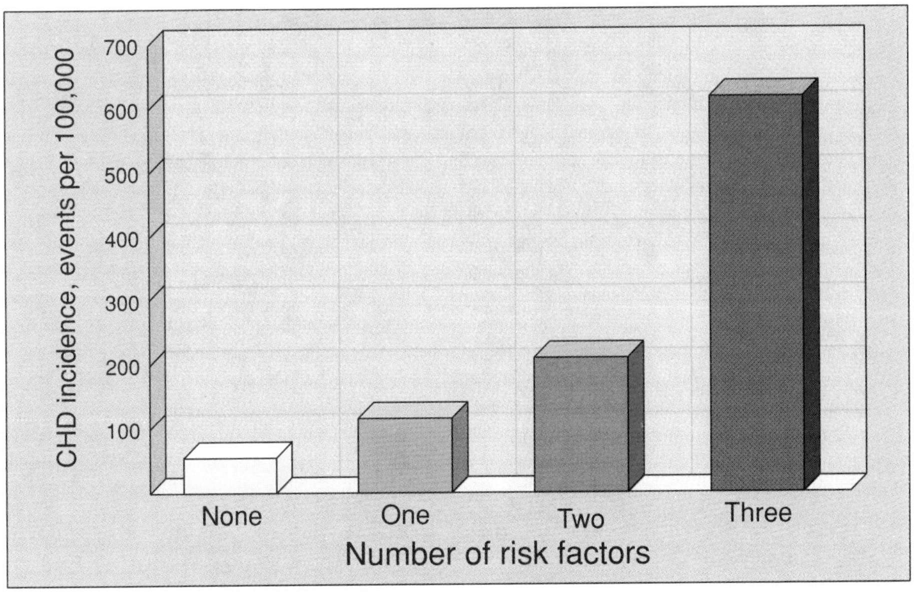

FIG. 20–12. Relationship between a combination of abnormal risk factors (cholesterol > 250 mg · dl; systolic blood pressure > 160 mmHg; smoking > 1 pack a day), and incidence of coronary heart disease. (Adapted from Kannel, W.B., and Gordon, T.: *The Framingham Study: An epidemiologic investigation of cardiovascular disease.* Section 30. Washington, DC, Public Health Service, NIH, DHEW Publication #74–599, Feb. 1974.)

It's never too late to stop smoking! The good news is that it's never too late to quit smoking. Even if you've smoked for 40 years, if you stop, your CHD risk returns to that of a "never smoker" within 5 years, no matter how old you are. As for cancer, the risk decline takes longer but it is still substantial.

TABLE 20–3. PREVENTING MAJOR DISEASES: A CHECKLIST OF HEALTH-SAVING TACTICS

	NO TOBACCO	LOW-FAT DIET	HIGH-FIBER DIET	AVOID ALCOHOL	AVOID SALTED, PICKLED FOODS	DIET HIGH IN VEGETABLES AND FRUITS	EXERCISE, WEIGHT CONTROL
Cancer							
Lung	√√√	√				√	
Breast		√√√	√			√√	√
Colon		√√√	√√√			√√√	√
Liver				√√√	√	√√	
Heart attack	√√√	√√√				√√	√√√
Stroke	√				√√√	√√	√√
Adult diabetes		√√√	√			√√	√√

Modified from American Medical Foundation.
√√√ Highly effective; √√ Moderately effective; √ Somewhat effective.

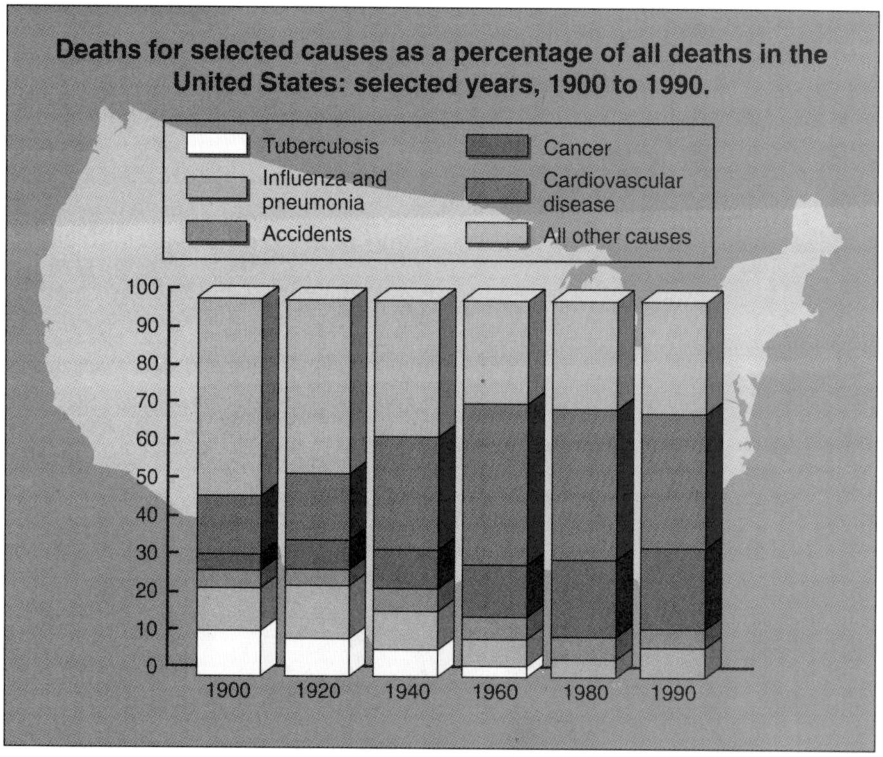

Deaths for selected causes as a percentage of all deaths in the United States: selected years, 1900 to 1990.

the man's chance for chest pain, heart attack, or sudden death is 5 times higher than if he had no risk factors. An important consideration is that many risk factors have a common root in health behavior patterns, and consequently can be influenced by similar, and in some cases identical, interventions. For example, regular physical activity exerts a positive influence on the risk factors of obesity, hypertension, glucose metabolism, and elevated lipid profiles.

BEHAVIORAL CHANGES THAT CAN IMPROVE YOUR OVERALL HEALTH PROFILE

Health-promoting habits can be effective in areas other than related to one's risk for heart attack. Table 20–3 ranks the value of several health-saving tactics that reduce risk or bolster resistance to the major diseases of cancer, heart attack, stroke, and diabetes. For example, a low-fat diet is highly effective in protecting against adult-onset diabetes, heart attack, and cancers of the breast and colon (and moderately effective in preventing other cancers as well). A diet rich in vegetables and fruits is most effective against colon cancer, as well as throat cancer, and offers some protection against diabetes and cardiovascular disease. Smoking is our country's single deadliest habit and is the primary cause of lung cancer and a major factor in heart attacks. Regular exercise and weight control are most effective in reducing the risk of heart disease, stroke, and adult-onset diabetes, and they offer some protection against certain cancers.

Clearly, the prudent use of nutrition, weight control, and exercise can greatly enhance a person's chances for good health. We encourage you to develop a healthy lifestyle so it can contribute to your enjoyment and fulfillment of the things you care most about. *You* truly can make a difference!

SUMMARY

1. Physiologic and performance capability generally declines after about 30 years of age. The rates of decline in the various functions differ and are significantly influenced by many factors, including level of physical activity. Regular physical training enables older persons to retain higher levels of functional capacity, especially cardiovascular function.
2. Regardless of age, regular vigorous physical activity produces measurable physiologic improvements. The magnitude of these improvements depends on many factors including initial fitness status, age, and type and amount of training.
3. Participation in vigorous activity early in life probably contributes little to increased longevity or health in later life. However, a physically active lifestyle throughout life confers significant health benefits.
4. Coronary heart disease is the single largest cause of death in the Western world. The pathogenesis of this disease involves degenerative changes in the inner lining of the arterial wall that result in progressive occlusion. The mechanism for the development of coronary atherosclerosis is not fully understood.
5. Numerous factors have been identified that make individuals more susceptible to developing CHD. The major risk factors are age and gender, elevated blood lipids, hypertension, cigarette smoking, obesity, physical inactivity, diet, heredity, and ECG abnormalities during rest and exercise.
6. In general, a cholesterol level of 200 mg or lower is considered desirable with many experts recommending the lower values as being most healthful.
7. The distribution of the various lipoproteins, especially HDL and LDL cholesterol, is a more powerful predictor of heart disease risk than simply the total quantity of plasma cholesterol.

8. The risk of death from heart disease is almost twice as great for smokers as for nonsmokers. One mechanism for risk may be the adverse effect of smoking on lipoprotein levels.
9. The interaction of CHD risk factors significantly magnifies their individual effect in predicting one's chances for disease.
10. Many CHD risk factors can be modified by proper programs of nutrition, exercise, and weight control. This "risk intervention" generally improves an individual's health outlook.

RELATED READINGS

Blair, S.N., et al.: Physical activity and health: a lifestyle approach. Med. Exerc. Nutr. Health, 1:54, 1992.

Blair, S.N., et al.: Physical fitness and all-cause mortality: a prospective study of healthy men and women. JAMA, 262:2395, 1989.

Burke, G.L., et al.: Trends in serum cholesterol levels from 1980 to 1987—the Minnesota Heart Survey. *N. Engl. J. Med.*, 324:941, 1991.

Clapp, J.F., et al.: Exercise in pregnancy. Med. Sci. Sports Exerc., 24:S294, 1992.

Cohen, S., et al.: Psychological stress and susceptibility to the common cold. *N. Engl. J. Med.*, 325:606, 1991.

Corbin, C.B., and Pangrazi, R.B.: Are American children and youth fit? Res. Quart. Exerc. Sport, 63:96, 1992.

Costill, D.L.: Inside Running: Basics of Sports Physiology. Indianapolis, Benchmark Press, 1986.

Douglas, P.S., et al.: Exercise and atherosclerotic heart disease in women. Med. Sci. Sport Exerc., 24:S266, 1992.

Helmrich, S.P., et al.: Physical activity and reduced occurrence of non-insulin-dependent diabetes mellitus. *N. Engl. J. Med.*, 325:147, 1991.

Jones, N.L., et al. (eds.): Human Muscle Power. Champaign, Human Kinetics Publishers, 1986.

King, A.C., et al.: Group- vs. home-based exercise training in healthy older men and women. *JAMA*, 266:1535, 1991.

Lacroix, A.Z., et al.: Smoking and mortality among older men and women in three communities. *N. Engl. J. Med.*, 324:169, 1991.

Levin, S.: Can older be better? Phys. Sports Med., 20:139, 1992.

Manson, J.E., et al.: A prospective study of exercise and incidence of diabetes among US male physicians. JAMA, 268:63, 1992.

McArdle, W.D., et al.: Exercise Physiology: Energy, Nutrition, and Human Performance, 3rd ed. Philadelphia, Lea & Febiger, 1991.

McGinnis, J.M.: The public health burden of a sedentary lifestyle. Med. Sci. Sport Exerc., 24:S196, 1992.

Montoye, H.J.: Physical Activity and Health: An Epidemiologic Study of an Entire Community. Englewood Cliffs, NJ, Prentice-Hall, 1975.

Morris, J.N., et al.: Exercise in leisure time: coronary attack and death rates. Br. Heart J., 63:325, 1990.

Morris, J.N., et al.: Vigorous exercise in leisure time: protection against coronary heart disease. *Lancet*, 2:1207, 1980.

NIH Consensus Development Conference: Lowering blood cholesterol to prevent heart disease. *JAMA*, 253:2080, 1985.

Oster, G., and Epstein, A.M.: Primary prevention and coronary heart disease: the economic benefits of lowering serum cholesterol. *Am. J. Publ. Health.* 76:647, 1986.

Paffenbarger, R.S., Jr., et al.: Energy expenditure, cigarette smoking and blood pressure level as related to death from specific diseases. *Am. J. Epidemiol.*, 108:12, 1978.

Paffenbarger, R.S., Jr., et al.: Physical activity, all-cause mortality, and longevity of college alumni. *N. Engl. J. Med.*, 314:605, 1986.

Posner, J.D.: Exercise capacity in the elderly. *Am. J. Cardiol.*, 57:52C, 1986.

Pyörälä, K.: Dietary cholesterol in relation to plasma cholesterol and coronary heart disease. *Am. J. Clin. Nutr.*, 45:1176, 1987.

Rayssiguier, Y., and Gueux, E.: Magnesium and lipids in cardiovascular disease. *Am. Coll. Nutr.*, 5:507, 1986.

Ross, R.: The pathogenesis of atherosclerosis—an update. *N. Engl. J. Med.*, 314:488, 1986.
Seals, D.R., et al.: Endurance training in older men and women. I. Cardiovascular response to exercise. *J. Appl. Physiol.*, 57:1024, 1984.
Smith, E.L.: Exercise for prevention of osteoporosis: a review. *Phys. Sportsmed.*, 3:72, 1982.
Spirduso, W.W.: Physical fitness, aging, and psychomotor speed: a review. *J. Gerontol.*, 35:850, 1980.
Stampfer, M.J., et al.: A prospective study of cholesterol, apolipoproteins, and the risk of myocardial infarction. *N. Engl. J. Med.*, 325:373, 1991.
Wallberg-Henriksson, J.H.: Exercise and diabetes mellitus. In: Exercise and Sport Science Reviews. Vol. 20. Edited by J.O. Holloszy. Baltimore, Williams & Wilkins, 1992.
Wasserman, K., et al.: Principles of Exercise Testing and Interpretation. Philadelphia, Lea & Febiger, 1987.

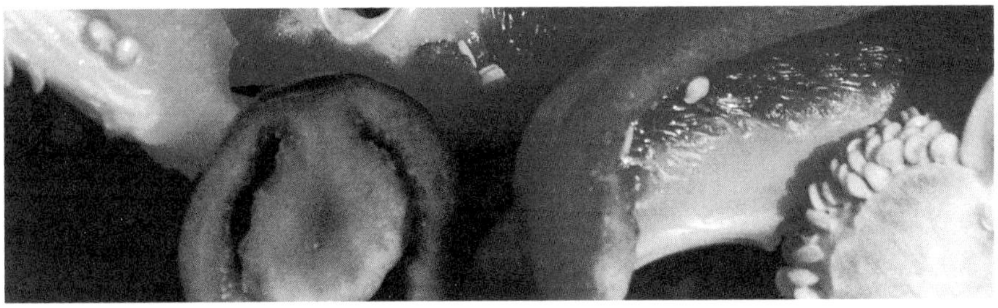

A

ENERGY EXPENDITURE IN HOUSEHOLD, RECREATIONAL, AND SPORTS ACTIVITIES (IN KCAL/MIN)

Your Body Weight

Activity	kg / lb	47 / 104	50 / 110	53 / 117	56 / 123	59 / 130	62 / 137	65 / 143	68 / 150
Archery		3.1	3.3	3.4	3.6	3.8	4.0	4.2	4.4
Backpacking									
without load		5.7	6.1	6.4	6.8	7.1	7.5	7.9	8.2
with 11 pound load		6.1	6.5	6.8	7.2	7.6	8.0	8.4	8.8
with 22 pound load		6.6	7.0	7.4	7.8	8.3	8.7	9.1	9.5
with 44 pound load		7.0	7.4	7.8	8.2	8.7	9.1	9.6	10.0
Badminton									
leisure		4.6	4.9	5.1	5.4	5.7	6.0	6.3	6.6
tournament		7.0	7.3	7.7	8.1	8.6	9.0	9.4	9.9
Baking, general (F)		1.6	1.8	1.9	2.0	2.1	2.2	2.3	2.4
Baseball									
fielder		2.8	3.0	3.2	3.4	3.6	3.8	4.0	4.1
pitcher		4.2	4.5	4.8	5.0	5.3	5.6	5.9	6.2
Basketball									
competition		7.1	7.4	7.9	8.3	8.7	9.2	9.6	10.1
practice		6.5	6.9	7.3	7.7	8.1	8.6	9.0	9.4
Baton twirling		6.3	6.8	7.3	7.6	8.1	8.5	8.9	9.3
Billiards ("pool")		2.0	2.1	2.2	2.4	2.5	2.6	2.7	2.9
Bookbinding		1.8	1.9	2.0	2.1	2.2	2.4	2.5	2.6
Bowling		4.4	4.8	5.2	5.4	5.7	6.0	6.3	6.6
Boxing									
in ring, match		10.4	11.1	11.8	12.4	13.1	13.8	14.4	15.1
sparring, practice		6.5	6.9	7.3	7.7	8.1	8.6	9.0	9.4
Calisthenics, warm-ups		3.4	3.7	4.0	4.2	4.4	4.7	4.9	5.1
Canoeing									
leisure (2.5 mph)		2.1	2.2	2.3	2.5	2.6	2.7	2.9	3.0
racing ("fast")		4.8	5.2	5.5	5.8	6.1	6.4	6.7	7.0
Car washing		3.3	3.5	3.7	3.9	4.1	4.3	4.5	4.8
Card playing		1.2	1.3	1.3	1.4	1.5	1.6	1.6	1.7
Carpentry, general		2.4	2.6	2.8	2.9	3.1	3.2	3.4	3.5
Carpet sweeping (F)		2.2	2.3	2.4	2.5	2.7	2.8	2.9	3.1
Carpet sweeping (M)		2.3	2.4	2.5	2.7	2.8	3.0	3.1	3.3
Circuit weight training									
Free weights		4.0	4.3	4.5	4.8	5.0	5.3	5.5	5.8
Hydra-Fitness		6.2	6.6	7.0	7.4	7.8	8.2	8.6	9.0
Nautilus		4.3	4.6	4.9	5.2	5.5	5.8	6.0	6.3
Universal		5.3	5.8	6.2	6.5	6.9	7.2	7.5	7.9
Cleaning (F)		2.9	3.1	3.3	3.5	3.7	3.8	4.0	4.2
Cleaning (M)		2.7	2.9	3.1	3.2	3.4	3.6	3.8	3.9
Coal mining									
drilling coal, rock		4.4	4.7	5.0	5.3	5.5	5.8	6.1	6.4
erecting supports		4.1	4.4	4.7	4.9	5.2	5.5	5.7	6.0
shoveling coal		5.1	5.4	5.7	6.0	6.4	6.7	7.0	7.3
Cooking (F)		2.1	2.3	2.4	2.5	2.7	2.8	2.9	3.1
Cooking (M)		2.3	2.4	2.5	2.7	2.8	3.0	3.1	3.3
Cricket									
batting		3.9	4.2	4.4	4.6	4.9	5.1	5.4	5.6
bowling		4.2	4.5	4.8	5.0	5.3	5.6	5.9	6.1
fielding		3.7	3.9	4.1	4.3	4.8	4.8	5.0	5.3
Croquet		2.8	3.0	3.1	3.3	3.5	3.7	3.8	4.0

Note: Symbols (M) and (F) denote experiments for males and females, respectively. See p. 224 for instructions on how to use this appendix.

71 157	74 163	77 170	80 176	83 183	86 190	89 196	92 203	95 209	98 216
4.6	4.8	5.0	5.2	5.4	5.6	5.8	6.0	6.2	6.4
8.6	9.0	9.3	9.7	10.0	10.4	10.8	11.1	11.5	11.9
9.2	9.5	9.9	10.3	10.7	11.1	11.5	11.9	12.3	12.6
9.9	10.4	10.8	11.2	11.6	12.0	12.5	12.9	13.3	13.7
10.4	10.9	11.3	11.8	12.2	12.6	13.1	13.5	14.0	14.4
6.9	7.2	7.5	7.8	8.1	8.3	8.6	8.9	9.2	9.5
10.4	10.8	11.2	11.6	12.1	12.5	12.9	13.4	13.8	14.3
2.5	2.6	2.7	2.8	2.9	3.0	3.1	3.2	3.3	3.4
4.3	4.5	4.7	4.9	5.1	5.2	5.4	5.6	5.8	6.0
6.4	6.7	7.0	7.2	7.5	7.8	8.0	8.3	8.6	8.9
10.5	10.9	11.4	11.8	12.3	12.7	13.1	13.6	14.0	14.5
9.8	10.2	10.6	11.0	11.5	11.9	12.3	12.7	13.1	13.5
9.5	9.7	9.9	10.1	10.4	10.6	10.8	11.0	11.2	11.4
3.0	3.1	3.2	3.4	3.5	3.6	3.7	3.9	4.0	4.1
2.7	2.8	2.9	3.0	3.2	3.3	3.4	3.5	3.6	3.7
6.9	7.2	7.5	7.7	8.1	8.4	8.6	8.9	9.2	9.5
15.8	16.4	17.1	17.8	18.4	19.1	19.8	20.4	21.1	21.8
9.8	10.2	10.6	11.0	11.5	11.9	12.3	12.7	13.1	13.5
5.3	5.5	5.8	6.0	6.2	6.5	6.7	6.9	7.1	7.3
3.1	3.3	3.4	3.5	3.7	3.8	3.9	4.0	4.2	4.3
7.3	7.6	7.9	8.2	8.5	8.9	9.2	9.5	9.8	10.1
5.0	5.2	5.5	5.7	5.7	5.9	6.1	6.3	6.5	6.9
1.8	1.9	1.9	2.0	2.1	2.2	2.2	2.3	2.4	2.5
3.7	3.8	4.0	4.2	4.3	4.5	4.6	4.8	4.9	5.1
3.2	3.3	3.5	3.6	3.7	3.9	4.0	4.1	4.3	4.4
3.4	3.6	3.7	3.8	4.0	4.1	4.3	4.4	4.6	4.7
6.1	6.3	6.6	6.8	7.1	7.4	7.6	7.9	8.1	8.4
9.4	9.7	10.2	10.5	10.9	11.4	11.7	12.1	12.5	12.9
6.6	6.8	7.1	7.4	7.7	8.0	8.2	8.5	8.8	9.1
8.3	8.6	8.9	9.3	9.6	10.0	10.3	10.7	11.0	11.4
4.4	4.6	4.8	5.0	5.1	5.3	5.5	5.7	5.9	6.1
4.1	4.3	4.5	4.6	4.8	5.0	5.2	5.3	5.5	5.7
6.7	7.0	7.2	7.5	7.8	8.1	8.4	8.6	8.9	9.2
6.2	6.5	6.8	7.0	7.3	7.6	7.8	8.1	8.4	8.6
7.7	8.0	8.3	8.6	9.0	9.3	9.6	9.9	10.3	10.6
3.2	3.3	3.5	3.6	3.7	3.9	4.0	4.1	4.3	4.4
3.4	3.6	3.7	3.8	4.0	4.1	4.3	4.4	4.6	4.7
5.9	6.1	6.4	6.6	6.9	7.1	7.4	7.6	7.9	8.1
6.4	6.7	6.9	7.2	7.5	7.7	8.0	8.3	8.6	8.8
5.6	5.9	6.2	6.5	6.8	7.1	7.4	7.7	8.0	8.3
4.2	4.4	4.5	4.7	4.9	5.1	5.3	5.4	5.6	5.8

Your Body Weight

Activity	kg / lb	47 / 104	50 / 110	53 / 117	56 / 123	59 / 130	62 / 137	65 / 143	68 / 150
Cycling									
leisure, 5.5 mph		3.0	3.2	3.4	3.6	3.8	4.0	4.2	4.4
leisure, 9.4 mph		4.8	5.0	5.3	5.6	5.9	6.2	6.5	6.8
racing, fast		8.0	8.5	9.0	9.5	10.0	10.5	11.0	11.5
Dancing									
aerobic, easy		4.3	4.8	5.2	5.6	5.9	6.2	6.4	6.7
aerobic, medium		4.8	5.2	5.5	5.8	6.1	6.4	6.7	7.0
aerobic, intense		6.3	6.7	7.1	7.5	7.9	8.3	8.7	9.2
ballroom		2.4	2.6	2.7	2.9	3.0	3.2	3.3	3.5
choreographed		5.0	5.2	5.5	5.8	6.1	6.4	6.7	7.0
"twist," "lambada"		8.0	8.4	8.9	9.4	9.9	10.4	10.9	11.4
modern		3.4	3.6	3.8	4.0	4.3	4.5	4.7	4.9
Digging trenches		6.8	7.3	7.7	8.1	8.6	9.0	9.4	9.9
Drawing (standing)		1.7	1.8	1.9	2.0	2.1	2.2	2.3	2.4
Eating (sitting)		1.1	1.2	1.2	1.3	1.4	1.4	1.5	1.6
Electrical work		2.7	2.9	3.1	3.2	3.4	3.6	3.8	3.9
Farming									
barn cleaning		6.3	6.8	7.2	7.6	8.0	8.4	8.8	9.2
driving harvester		1.9	2.0	2.1	2.2	2.4	2.5	2.6	2.7
driving tractor		1.8	1.9	2.0	2.1	2.2	2.3	2.4	2.5
feeding cattle		4.2	4.3	4.5	4.8	5.0	5.3	5.5	5.8
feeding animals		3.1	3.3	3.4	3.6	3.8	4.0	4.2	4.4
forking straw bales		6.7	6.9	7.3	7.7	8.1	8.6	9.0	9.4
milking by hand		2.5	2.7	2.9	3.0	3.2	3.3	3.5	3.7
milking by machine		1.1	1.2	1.2	1.3	1.4	1.4	1.5	1.6
shoveling grain		4.2	4.3	4.5	4.8	5.0	5.3	5.5	5.8
Fencing									
competition		7.2	7.6	8.1	8.5	9.0	9.4	9.9	10.8
practice		3.6	3.9	4.2	4.4	4.6	4.9	5.1	5.3
Field hockey		6.5	6.7	7.1	7.5	7.9	8.3	8.7	9.1
Fishing		3.0	3.1	3.3	3.5	3.7	3.8	4.0	4.2
Food shopping (F)		3.0	3.1	3.3	3.5	3.7	3.8	4.0	4.2
Football, competition		6.2	6.6	7.0	7.4	7.8	8.2	8.6	9.0
Forestry									
ax chopping, fast		14.0	14.9	15.7	16.6	17.5	18.4	19.3	20.2
ax chopping, slow		4.0	4.3	4.5	4.8	5.0	5.3	5.5	5.8
barking trees		5.8	6.2	6.5	6.9	7.3	7.6	8.0	8.4
carrying logs		8.7	9.3	9.9	10.4	11.0	11.5	12.1	12.6
felling trees		6.2	6.6	7.0	7.4	7.8	8.2	8.6	9.0
hoeing		4.2	4.6	4.8	5.1	5.4	5.6	5.9	6.2
planting by hand		5.1	5.5	5.8	6.1	6.4	6.8	7.1	7.4
sawing by hand		5.7	6.1	6.5	6.8	7.2	7.6	7.9	8.3
sawing, power		3.5	3.8	4.0	4.2	4.4	4.7	4.9	5.1
stacking firewood		4.2	4.4	4.7	4.9	5.2	5.5	5.7	6.0
trimming trees		6.1	6.5	6.8	7.2	7.6	8.0	8.4	8.8
weeding		3.4	3.6	3.8	4.0	4.2	4.5	4.7	4.9
Frisbee		4.7	5.0	5.3	5.5	5.9	6.2	6.4	6.8
Furriery		3.9	4.2	4.4	4.6	4.9	5.1	5.4	5.6

71 157	74 163	77 170	80 176	83 183	86 190	89 196	92 203	95 209	98 216
4.5	4.7	4.9	5.1	5.3	5.5	5.7	5.9	6.1	6.3
7.1	7.4	7.7	8.0	8.3	8.6	8.9	9.2	9.5	9.8
12.0	12.5	13.0	13.5	14.0	14.5	15.0	15.5	16.1	16.6
6.9	7.2	7.5	7.8	8.1	8.4	8.8	9.1	9.4	9.7
7.3	7.6	7.9	8.2	8.5	8.9	9.2	9.5	9.8	10.1
9.6	10.0	10.4	10.8	11.2	11.6	12.0	12.4	12.8	13.2
3.6	3.8	3.9	4.1	4.2	4.4	4.5	4.7	4.8	5.0
7.3	7.6	7.9	8.2	8.5	8.9	9.2	9.5	9.8	10.1
11.9	12.4	12.9	13.4	13.9	14.4	15.0	15.5	16.0	16.5
5.1	5.3	5.6	5.8	6.0	6.2	6.4	6.7	6.9	7.1
10.3	10.7	11.2	11.6	12.0	12.5	12.9	13.3	13.8	14.2
2.6	2.7	2.8	2.9	3.0	3.1	3.2	3.3	3.4	3.5
1.6	1.7	1.8	1.8	1.9	2.0	2.0	2.1	2.2	2.3
4.1	4.3	4.5	4.6	4.8	5.0	5.2	5.3	5.5	5.7
9.6	10.0	10.4	10.8	11.2	11.6	12.0	12.4	12.8	13.2
2.8	3.0	3.1	3.2	3.3	3.4	3.6	3.7	3.8	3.9
2.6	2.7	2.8	3.0	3.1	3.2	3.3	3.4	3.5	3.6
6.0	6.3	6.5	6.8	7.1	7.3	7.6	7.8	8.1	8.3
4.6	4.8	5.0	5.2	5.4	5.6	5.8	6.0	6.2	6.4
9.8	10.2	10.6	11.0	11.5	11.9	12.3	12.7	13.1	13.5
3.8	4.0	4.2	4.3	4.5	4.6	4.8	5.0	5.1	5.3
1.6	1.7	1.8	1.8	1.9	2.0	2.0	2.1	2.2	2.3
6.0	6.3	6.5	6.8	7.1	7.3	7.6	7.8	8.1	8.3
11.2	11.7	12.1	12.6	13.1	13.5	14.0	14.4	14.9	15.5
5.6	5.8	6.1	6.3	6.5	6.8	7.0	7.2	7.4	7.7
9.5	9.9	10.3	10.7	11.1	11.5	11.9	12.3	12.7	13.1
4.4	4.6	4.8	5.0	5.1	5.3	5.5	5.7	5.9	6.1
4.4	4.6	4.8	5.0	5.1	5.3	5.5	5.7	5.9	6.1
9.4	9.8	10.2	10.6	11.0	11.4	11.7	12.1	12.5	12.9
21.1	22.0	22.9	23.8	24.7	25.5	26.4	27.3	28.2	29.1
6.0	6.3	6.5	6.8	7.1	7.3	7.6	7.8	8.1	8.3
8.7	9.1	9.5	9.8	10.2	10.6	10.9	11.3	11.7	12.1
13.2	13.8	14.3	14.9	15.4	16.0	16.6	17.1	17.7	18.2
9.4	9.8	10.2	10.6	11.0	11.4	11.7	12.1	12.5	12.9
6.5	6.7	7.0	7.3	7.6	7.8	8.1	8.4	8.6	8.9
7.7	8.1	8.4	8.7	9.0	9.4	9.7	10.0	10.4	10.7
8.7	9.0	9.4	9.8	10.1	10.5	10.9	11.2	11.6	12.0
5.3	5.6	5.8	6.0	6.2	6.5	6.7	6.9	7.1	7.4
6.2	6.5	6.8	7.0	7.3	7.6	7.8	8.1	8.4	8.6
9.2	9.5	9.9	10.3	10.7	11.1	11.5	11.9	12.3	12.6
5.1	5.3	5.5	5.8	6.0	6.2	6.4	6.6	6.8	7.1
7.1	7.4	7.7	8.0	8.2	8.5	8.8	9.1	9.4	9.7
5.9	6.1	6.4	6.6	6.9	7.1	7.4	7.6	7.9	8.1

Your Body Weight

Activity	kg lb	47 104	50 110	53 117	56 123	59 130	62 137	65 143	68 150
Gardening									
digging		5.9	6.3	6.7	7.1	7.4	7.8	8.2	8.6
hedging		3.3	3.9	4.1	4.3	4.5	4.8	5.0	5.2
mowing		5.3	5.6	5.9	6.3	6.6	6.9	7.3	7.6
raking		2.5	2.7	2.9	3.0	3.2	3.3	3.5	3.7
Golf		4.0	4.3	4.5	4.8	5.0	5.3	5.5	5.8
Gymnastics		3.0	3.3	3.5	3.7	3.9	4.1	4.3	4.5
Handball		6.9	7.2	7.7	8.1	8.5	9.0	9.4	9.8
Horse-grooming		6.0	6.4	6.8	7.2	7.6	7.9	8.3	8.7
Horseback riding									
galloping		6.4	6.9	7.3	7.7	8.1	8.5	8.9	9.3
trotting		5.2	5.5	5.8	6.2	6.5	6.8	7.2	7.5
walking		1.9	2.1	2.2	2.3	2.4	2.5	2.7	2.8
Horseshoes		3.3	3.4	3.5	3.7	3.9	4.1	4.3	4.5
Housework									
mopping floors		2.8	3.1	3.3	3.5	3.7	3.8	4.0	4.2
dusting		3.0	3.3	3.4	3.6	3.8	4.0	4.2	4.4
laundry		3.1	3.4	3.5	3.7	3.9	4.1	4.3	4.5
washing windows		3.2	3.5	3.6	3.8	4.0	4.2	4.4	4.6
vacuuming		3.0	3.3	3.4	3.6	3.8	4.0	4.2	4.4
Hunting		4.1	4.4	4.7	4.9	5.2	5.5	5.7	6.0
Ice hockey		7.4	7.7	8.2	8.6	9.1	9.6	10.0	10.5
Ironing clothes		1.6	1.7	1.7	1.8	1.9	2.0	2.1	2.2
Judo		9.2	9.8	10.3	10.9	11.5	12.1	12.7	13.3
Jumping rope									
70 per min		7.6	8.1	8.6	9.1	9.6	10.0	10.5	11.0
80 per min		7.7	8.2	8.7	9.2	9.7	10.2	10.7	11.2
125 per min		8.3	8.9	9.4	9.9	10.4	11.0	11.5	12.0
145 per min		9.3	9.9	10.4	11.0	11.6	12.2	12.8	13.4
Karate		9.5	9.8	10.3	10.9	11.5	12.1	12.7	13.3
Kendo		9.3	9.7	10.2	10.8	11.4	12.0	12.6	13.2
Knitting, sewing		1.1	1.1	1.2	1.2	1.3	1.4	1.4	1.5
Lacrosse		7.0	7.4	7.9	8.3	8.7	9.2	9.6	10.1
Locksmith		2.8	2.9	3.0	3.2	3.4	3.5	3.7	3.9
Lying at ease		1.0	1.1	1.2	1.2	1.3	1.4	1.4	1.5
Machine-tooling									
machining		2.3	2.4	2.5	2.7	2.8	3.0	3.1	3.3
operating lathe		2.5	2.6	2.8	2.9	3.1	3.2	3.4	3.5
operating punch press		4.2	4.4	4.7	4.9	5.2	5.5	5.7	6.0
tapping and drilling		3.2	3.3	3.4	3.6	3.8	4.0	4.2	4.4
welding		2.4	2.6	2.8	2.9	3.1	3.2	3.4	3.5
working sheet metal		2.3	2.4	2.5	2.7	2.8	3.0	3.1	3.3
Marching, rapid		6.7	7.1	7.5	8.0	8.4	8.8	9.2	9.7
Mountain climbing		7.4	7.9	8.4	8.9	9.4	9.9	10.3	10.8
Motorcycle riding		6.5	6.9	7.3	7.7	8.1	8.5	8.9	9.3

71	74	77	80	83	86	89	92	95	98
157	163	170	176	183	190	196	203	209	216
8.9	9.3	9.7	10.1	10.5	10.8	11.2	11.6	12.0	12.3
5.5	5.7	5.9	6.2	6.4	6.6	6.9	7.1	7.3	7.5
8.0	8.3	8.6	9.0	9.3	9.6	10.0	10.3	10.6	11.0
3.8	4.0	4.2	4.3	4.5	4.6	4.8	5.0	5.1	5.3
6.0	6.3	6.5	6.8	7.1	7.3	7.6	7.8	8.1	8.3
4.7	4.9	5.1	5.3	5.5	5.7	5.9	6.1	6.3	6.5
10.3	10.7	11.2	11.5	12.0	12.5	12.9	13.3	13.7	14.2
9.1	9.5	9.9	10.2	10.6	11.0	11.4	11.8	12.2	12.5
9.7	10.1	10.6	11.0	11.4	11.8	12.2	12.6	13.0	13.4
7.8	8.1	8.5	8.8	9.1	9.5	9.8	10.1	10.5	10.8
2.9	3.0	3.2	3.3	3.4	3.5	3.6	3.8	3.9	4.0
4.7	4.9	5.1	5.3	5.5	5.7	5.9	6.1	6.3	6.5
4.4	4.6	4.8	5.0	5.2	5.4	5.6	5.8	6.0	6.2
4.6	4.7	4.9	5.1	5.3	5.5	5.7	5.9	6.1	6.3
4.7	4.9	5.1	5.3	5.5	5.7	5.9	6.1	6.3	6.5
4.8	5.0	5.2	5.4	5.6	5.8	6.0	6.2	6.4	6.6
4.6	4.8	5.0	5.2	5.4	5.6	5.8	6.0	6.2	6.4
6.2	6.5	6.7	7.0	7.2	7.5	7.8	8.0	8.2	8.5
11.0	11.5	12.0	12.5	13.1	13.6	14.1	14.6	15.1	15.7
2.3	2.4	2.5	2.6	2.7	2.8	2.9	3.0	3.1	3.2
13.8	14.4	15.0	15.6	16.2	16.8	17.4	17.9	18.5	19.1
11.5	12.0	12.5	13.0	13.4	13.9	14.4	14.9	15.4	15.9
11.6	12.1	12.6	13.1	13.6	14.1	14.6	14.6	15.6	16.1
12.6	13.1	13.6	14.2	14.7	15.2	15.8	16.3	16.8	17.3
14.0	14.6	15.2	15.8	16.4	16.9	17.5	18.1	18.7	19.3
13.8	14.4	15.0	15.6	16.2	16.8	17.4	17.9	18.5	19.1
13.7	14.3	14.9	15.5	16.1	16.7	17.3	17.8	18.4	19.0
1.6	1.6	1.7	1.8	1.8	1.9	2.0	2.0	2.1	2.2
10.4	10.7	11.0	11.2	11.5	11.8	12.1	12.4	12.7	13.0
4.0	4.2	4.4	4.6	4.7	4.9	5.1	5.2	5.4	5.6
1.6	1.6	1.7	1.8	1.8	1.9	2.0	2.0	2.1	2.2
3.4	3.6	3.7	3.8	4.0	4.1	4.3	4.4	4.6	4.7
3.7	3.8	4.0	4.2	4.3	4.5	4.6	4.8	4.9	5.1
6.2	6.5	6.8	7.0	7.3	7.6	7.8	8.1	8.4	8.6
4.6	4.8	5.0	5.2	5.4	5.6	5.8	6.0	6.2	6.4
3.7	3.8	4.0	4.2	4.3	4.5	4.6	4.8	4.9	5.1
3.4	3.6	3.7	3.8	4.0	4.1	4.3	4.4	4.6	4.7
10.1	10.5	10.9	11.4	11.8	12.2	12.6	13.1	13.5	13.9
11.3	11.7	12.2	12.7	13.2	13.7	14.1	14.6	15.0	15.6
9.7	10.1	10.5	10.9	11.3	11.7	12.1	12.5	12.9	13.3

Your Body Weight

Activity	kg / lb	47 / 104	50 / 110	53 / 117	56 / 123	59 / 130	62 / 137	65 / 143	68 / 150
Music playing									
accordion (sitting)		1.5	1.6	1.7	1.8	1.9	2.0	2.1	2.2
cello (sitting)		2.0	2.1	2.2	2.3	2.4	2.5	2.7	2.8
conducting		1.9	2.0	2.1	2.2	2.3	2.4	2.5	2.7
drums (sitting)		3.1	3.3	3.5	3.7	3.9	4.1	4.3	4.5
flute (sitting)		1.7	1.8	1.9	2.0	2.1	2.2	2.3	2.4
horn (sitting)		1.4	1.5	1.5	1.6	1.7	1.8	1.9	2.0
organ (sitting)		2.6	2.7	2.8	3.0	3.1	3.3	3.4	3.6
piano (sitting)		1.9	2.0	2.1	2.2	2.4	2.5	2.6	2.7
trumpet (standing)		1.5	1.6	1.6	1.7	1.8	1.9	2.0	2.1
violin (sitting)		2.2	2.3	2.4	2.5	2.7	2.8	2.9	3.1
woodwind (sitting)		1.5	1.6	1.7	1.8	1.9	2.0	2.1	2.2
Paddleball		8.5	8.9	9.4	10.0	10.5	11.0	11.6	12.1
Paddle tennis		8.4	8.6	9.1	9.6	10.1	10.7	11.1	11.7
Painting									
inside projects		1.6	1.7	1.8	1.9	2.0	2.1	2.2	2.3
outside projects		3.7	3.9	4.1	4.3	4.5	4.8	5.0	5.2
scraping		3.1	3.2	3.3	3.5	3.7	3.9	4.1	4.3
Planting seedlings		3.3	3.5	3.7	3.9	4.1	4.3	4.6	4.8
Plastering		3.7	3.9	4.1	4.4	4.6	4.8	5.1	5.3
Printing press work		1.7	1.8	1.9	2.0	2.1	2.2	2.3	2.4
Racquetball		8.4	8.9	9.4	10.0	10.5	11.0	11.6	12.1
Roller skating, leisure		5.3	5.8	6.2	6.5	6.9	7.3	7.3	8.0
Rope jumping									
110 rpm			7.1	7.5	7.9	8.4	8.8	9.2	9.7
120 rpm			6.8	7.3	7.7	8.1	8.5	8.9	9.3
130 rpm			6.4	6.8	7.1	7.5	7.7	8.3	8.7
Rowing									
machine, moderate		5.7	6.0	6.3	6.7	7.0	7.4	7.7	8.1
machine, race pace		8.6	8.9	9.4	10.0	10.5	11.0	11.6	12.1
skull, leisure		4.7	5.0	5.3	5.5	5.9	6.2	6.4	6.8
skull, race pace		8.7	8.9	9.4	10.0	10.5	11.0	11.6	12.1
Running, cross-country		7.8	8.2	8.6	9.1	9.6	10.1	10.6	11.1
Running, on flat surface									
11 min, 30 s per mile		6.3	6.8	7.2	7.6	8.0	8.4	8.8	9.2
9 min per mile		9.1	9.7	10.2	10.8	11.4	12.0	12.5	13.1
8 min per mile		9.8	10.8	11.3	11.9	12.5	13.1	13.6	14.2
7 min per mile		10.7	12.2	12.7	13.3	13.9	14.5	15.0	15.6
6 min per mile		11.8	13.9	14.4	15.0	15.6	16.2	16.7	17.3
5 min, 30 s per mile		13.6	14.5	15.3	16.2	17.1	17.9	18.8	19.7
Sailing, leisure		2.1	2.2	2.3	2.5	2.6	2.7	2.9	3.0
Scrubbing floors		5.1	5.5	5.8	6.1	6.4	6.8	7.1	7.4
Scuba diving		10.9	11.2	11.5	11.8	12.1	12.4	12.7	13.0
Shoe repair, general		2.2	2.3	2.4	2.5	2.7	2.8	2.9	3.1
Sitting quietly		1.0	1.1	1.1	1.2	1.2	1.3	1.4	1.4
Skateboarding		5.6	5.8	6.2	6.5	6.9	7.2	7.5	7.9
Skiing, hard snow									
level, moderate speed		5.6	6.0	6.3	6.7	7.0	7.4	7.7	8.1
level, walking speed		6.7	7.2	7.6	8.0	8.4	8.9	9.3	9.7
uphill, "fast" speed		12.9	13.7	14.5	15.3	16.2	17.0	17.8	18.6
Skiing, soft snow									
leisure (F)		4.6	4.9	5.2	5.5	5.8	6.1	6.4	6.7
leisure (M)		5.2	5.6	5.9	6.2	6.5	6.9	7.2	7.5

71	74	77	80	83	86	89	92	95	98
157	163	170	176	183	190	196	203	209	216
2.3	2.4	2.5	2.6	2.7	2.8	2.8	2.9	3.0	3.1
2.9	3.0	3.2	3.3	3.4	3.5	3.6	3.8	3.9	4.0
2.8	2.9	3.0	3.1	3.2	3.4	3.5	3.6	3.7	3.8
4.7	4.9	5.1	5.3	5.5	5.7	5.9	6.1	6.3	6.6
2.5	2.6	2.7	2.8	2.9	3.0	3.1	3.2	3.3	3.4
2.1	2.1	2.2	2.3	2.4	2.5	2.6	2.7	2.8	2.8
3.8	3.9	4.1	4.2	4.4	4.6	4.7	4.9	5.0	5.2
2.8	3.0	3.1	3.2	3.3	3.4	3.6	3.7	3.8	3.9
2.2	2.3	2.4	2.5	2.6	2.7	2.8	2.9	2.9	3.0
3.2	3.3	3.5	3.6	3.7	3.9	4.0	4.1	4.3	4.4
2.3	2.4	2.5	2.6	2.7	2.8	2.8	2.9	3.0	3.1
12.6	13.2	13.7	14.2	14.8	15.3	15.8	16.4	16.9	17.4
12.2	12.7	13.2	13.7	14.2	14.2	15.2	15.8	16.3	16.8
2.4	2.5	2.6	2.7	2.8	2.9	3.0	3.1	3.2	3.3
5.5	5.7	5.9	6.2	6.4	6.6	6.9	7.1	7.3	7.5
4.5	4.7	4.9	5.0	5.2	5.4	5.6	5.8	6.0	6.2
5.0	5.2	5.4	5.6	5.8	6.0	6.2	6.4	6.7	6.9
5.5	5.8	6.0	6.2	6.5	6.7	6.9	7.2	7.4	7.6
2.5	2.6	2.7	2.8	2.9	3.0	3.1	3.2	3.3	3.4
12.6	13.2	13.7	14.2	14.8	15.3	15.8	16.4	16.9	17.4
8.3	8.6	9.0	9.3	9.7	10.1	10.4	10.8	11.1	11.4
10.1	10.5	10.5	11.3	11.8	12.2	12.6	13.1	13.5	13.9
9.8	10.1	10.6	10.9	11.4	11.8	12.2	12.6	13.0	13.4
9.1	9.4	9.8	10.2	10.6	11.0	11.3	11.7	12.1	12.5
8.5	8.9	9.3	9.7	10.1	10.6	11.1	11.6	12.1	12.6
12.6	13.2	13.7	14.2	14.8	15.3	15.8	16.4	16.9	17.4
7.2	7.6	8.0	8.4	8.8	9.2	9.6	10.0	10.4	10.8
12.6	13.2	13.7	14.2	14.8	15.3	15.8	16.4	16.9	17.4
11.6	12.1	12.6	13.0	13.5	14.0	14.5	15.0	15.5	16.0
9.6	10.0	10.5	10.9	11.3	11.7	12.1	12.5	12.9	13.3
13.7	14.3	14.9	15.4	16.0	16.6	17.2	17.8	18.3	18.9
14.8	15.4	16.0	16.5	17.1	17.7	18.3	18.9	19.4	20.0
16.2	16.8	17.4	17.9	18.5	19.1	19.7	20.3	20.8	21.4
17.9	18.5	19.1	19.6	20.2	20.8	21.4	22.0	22.5	23.1
20.5	21.4	22.3	23.1	24.0	24.9	25.7	26.6	27.5	28.3
3.1	3.3	3.4	3.5	3.7	3.8	3.9	4.1	4.2	4.3
7.7	8.1	8.4	8.7	9.0	9.4	9.7	10.0	10.4	10.7
13.3	13.6	13.9	14.2	14.5	14.8	15.1	15.4	15.7	16.0
3.2	3.3	3.5	3.6	3.7	3.9	4.0	4.1	4.3	4.4
1.5	1.6	1.6	1.7	1.7	1.8	1.9	1.9	2.0	2.1
8.3	8.6	8.9	9.3	9.6	10.0	10.3	10.7	11.0	11.4
8.4	8.8	9.2	9.5	9.9	10.2	10.6	10.9	11.3	11.7
10.2	10.6	11.0	11.4	11.9	12.3	12.7	13.2	13.6	14.0
19.5	20.3	21.1	21.9	22.7	23.6	24.4	25.2	26.0	26.9
7.0	7.3	7.5	7.8	8.1	8.4	8.7	9.0	9.3	9.6
7.9	8.2	8.5	8.9	9.2	9.5	9.9	10.2	10.5	10.9

Your Body Weight

Activity	kg 47 lb 104	50 110	53 117	56 123	59 130	62 137	65 143	68 150
Skindiving								
considerable motion	13.0	13.8	14.6	15.5	16.3	17.1	17.9	18.8
moderate motion	9.7	10.3	10.9	11.5	12.2	12.8	13.4	14.0
Snorkeling	4.3	4.6	4.9	5.2	5.5	5.8	6.0	6.3
Snowshoeing, soft snow	7.8	8.3	8.8	9.3	9.8	10.3	10.8	11.3
Snowmobiling	3.4	3.7	4.0	4.2	4.4	4.7	4.9	5.1
Soccer	6.5	6.8	7.3	7.7	8.1	8.5	8.9	9.3
Softball	3.3	3.5	3.7	3.9	4.1	4.3	4.5	4.7
Squash	10.0	10.6	11.2	11.9	12.5	13.1	13.8	14.4
Standing quietly (M)	1.3	1.4	1.4	1.5	1.6	1.7	1.8	1.8
Steel mill, working in								
fettling	4.3	4.5	4.7	5.0	5.3	5.5	5.8	6.1
forging	4.7	5.0	5.3	5.6	5.9	6.2	6.5	6.8
hand rolling	6.4	6.9	7.3	7.7	8.1	8.5	8.9	9.3
merchant mill rolling	6.8	7.3	7.7	8.1	8.6	9.0	9.4	9.9
removing slag	8.4	8.9	9.4	10.0	10.5	11.0	11.6	12.1
tending furnace	5.9	6.3	6.7	7.1	7.4	7.8	8.2	8.6
tipping molds	4.3	4.6	4.9	5.2	5.4	5.7	6.0	6.3
Surfing		4.1	4.3	4.5	4.8	5.0	5.3	5.5
Stock clerking	2.5	2.7	2.9	3.0	3.2	3.3	3.5	3.7
Swimming, fitness swims								
back stroke	7.9	8.5	9.0	9.5	10.0	10.5	11.0	11.5
breast stroke	7.6	8.1	8.6	9.1	9.6	10.0	10.5	11.0
butterfly		8.6	9.1	9.6	10.1	10.7	11.1	11.7
crawl, fast	7.3	7.8	8.3	8.7	9.2	9.7	10.1	10.6
crawl, slow	6.0	6.4	6.8	7.2	7.6	7.9	8.3	8.7
side stroke	5.7	6.1	6.5	6.8	7.2	7.6	7.9	8.3
treading, fast	8.0	8.5	9.0	9.5	10.0	10.5	11.1	11.6
treading, normal	2.9	3.1	3.3	3.5	3.7	3.8	4.0	4.2
Table tennis (ping pong)	3.2	3.4	3.6	3.8	4.0	4.2	4.4	4.6
Tailoring								
cutting	2.0	2.1	2.2	2.3	2.4	2.5	2.7	2.8
hand-sewing	1.5	1.6	1.7	1.8	1.9	2.0	2.1	2.2
machine-sewing	2.2	2.3	2.4	2.5	2.7	2.8	2.9	3.1
pressing	2.9	3.1	3.3	3.5	3.7	3.8	4.0	4.2
Tennis								
competition	6.9	7.3	7.8	8.2	8.7	9.1	9.5	9.9
recreational	5.1	5.5	5.8	6.1	6.4	6.8	7.1	7.4
Typing								
electric (computer)	1.3	1.4	1.4	1.5	1.6	1.7	1.8	1.8
manual	1.5	1.6	1.6	1.7	1.8	1.9	2.0	2.1
Volleyball								
competition	5.9	7.3	7.8	8.2	8.7	9.1	9.5	10.0
recreational	2.4	2.5	2.7	2.8	3.0	3.1	3.3	3.4
Walking, leisure outdoors								
asphalt road	3.8	4.0	4.2	4.5	4.7	5.0	5.2	5.4
fields and hillsides	3.9	4.1	4.3	4.6	4.8	5.1	5.3	5.6
grass track	3.8	4.1	4.3	4.5	4.8	5.0	5.3	5.5
plowed field	3.6	3.9	4.1	4.3	4.5	4.8	5.0	5.2

71 157	74 163	77 170	80 176	83 183	86 190	89 196	92 203	95 209	98 216
19.6	20.4	21.3	22.1	22.9	23.7	24.6	25.4	26.2	27.0
14.6	15.2	15.9	16.5	17.1	17.7	18.3	19.0	19.6	20.2
6.6	6.8	7.1	7.4	7.7	8.0	8.2	8.5	8.8	9.1
11.8	12.3	12.8	13.3	13.8	14.3	14.8	15.3	15.8	16.3
5.3	5.5	5.8	6.0	6.2	6.5	6.7	6.9	7.1	7.3
9.8	10.1	10.6	10.9	11.4	11.8	12.2	12.6	13.0	13.4
4.9	5.1	5.3	5.5	5.7	5.9	6.1	6.3	6.5	6.7
15.1	15.7	16.3	17.0	17.6	18.2	18.9	19.5	20.1	20.8
1.9	2.0	2.1	2.2	2.2	2.3	2.4	2.5	2.6	2.6
6.3	6.6	6.9	7.1	7.4	7.7	7.9	8.2	8.5	8.7
7.1	7.4	7.7	8.0	8.3	8.6	8.9	9.2	9.5	9.8
9.7	10.1	10.6	11.0	11.4	11.8	12.2	12.6	13.0	13.4
10.3	10.7	11.2	11.6	12.0	12.5	12.9	13.3	13.8	14.2
12.6	13.2	13.7	14.2	14.8	15.3	15.8	16.4	16.9	17.4
8.9	9.3	9.7	10.1	10.5	10.8	11.2	11.6	12.0	12.3
6.5	6.8	7.1	7.4	7.6	7.9	8.2	8.5	8.7	9.0
5.7	6.0	6.3	6.5	6.8	7.0	7.2	7.4	7.6	7.9
3.8	4.0	4.2	4.3	4.5	4.6	4.8	5.0	5.1	5.3
12.0	12.5	13.0	13.5	14.0	14.5	15.0	15.5	16.1	16.6
11.5	12.0	12.5	13.0	13.4	13.9	14.4	14.9	15.4	15.9
12.2	12.7	13.2	13.7	14.2	14.2	15.2	15.8	16.3	16.8
11.1	11.5	12.0	12.5	12.9	13.4	13.9	14.4	14.8	15.3
9.1	9.5	9.9	10.2	10.6	11.0	11.4	11.8	12.2	12.5
8.7	9.0	9.4	9.8	10.1	10.5	10.9	11.2	11.6	12.0
12.1	12.6	13.1	13.6	14.1	14.6	15.1	15.6	16.2	16.7
4.4	4.6	4.8	5.0	5.1	5.3	5.5	5.7	5.9	6.1
4.8	5.0	5.2	5.4	5.6	5.8	6.1	6.3	6.5	6.7
2.9	3.0	3.2	3.3	3.4	3.5	3.6	3.8	3.9	4.0
2.3	2.4	2.5	2.6	2.7	2.8	2.8	2.9	3.0	3.1
3.2	3.3	3.5	3.6	3.7	3.9	4.0	4.1	4.3	4.4
4.4	4.6	4.8	5.0	5.1	5.3	5.5	5.7	5.9	6.1
10.2	10.6	11.1	11.5	11.9	12.4	12.8	13.2	13.7	14.1
7.7	8.1	8.4	8.7	9.0	9.4	9.7	10.0	10.4	10.7
1.9	2.0	2.1	2.2	2.2	2.3	2.4	2.5	2.6	2.6
2.2	2.3	2.4	2.5	2.6	2.7	2.8	2.9	2.9	3.0
3.6	3.7	3.9	4.0	4.2	4.3	4.5	4.6	4.8	4.9
10.5	10.9	11.4	11.8	12.3	12.7	13.1	13.6	14.0	14.5
5.7	5.9	6.2	6.4	6.6	6.9	7.1	7.4	7.6	7.8
5.8	6.1	6.3	6.6	6.8	7.1	7.3	7.5	7.8	8.0
5.8	6.0	6.2	6.5	6.7	7.0	7.2	7.5	7.7	7.9
5.5	5.7	5.9	6.2	6.4	6.6	6.9	7.1	7.3	7.5

Your Body Weight

Activity	kg / lb	47 / 104	50 / 110	53 / 117	56 / 123	59 / 130	62 / 137	65 / 143	68 / 150
Walking, treadmill level									
2.0 mph		2.4	2.6	2.8	3.0	3.1	3.3	3.4	3.6
2.5 mph		3.0	3.2	3.4	3.6	3.8	4.0	4.2	4.4
3.0 mph		3.6	3.8	4.0	4.2	4.4	4.6	4.8	5.0
3.5 mph		4.0	4.3	4.6	4.8	5.1	5.3	5.6	6.1
4.0 mph		4.6	4.9	5.2	5.4	5.7	6.0	6.3	6.6
Wallpapering		2.3	2.4	2.5	2.7	2.8	3.0	3.1	3.3
Water-skiing		5.6	6.0	6.4	6.7	7.1	7.5	7.8	8.2
Watch repairing		1.2	1.3	1.3	1.4	1.5	1.6	1.6	1.7
Window cleaning		2.9	3.0	3.1	3.3	3.5	3.7	3.8	4.0
Wrestling, competition			9.7	10.3	10.8	11.4	12.0	12.6	13.2
Writing (sitting)		1.4	1.5	1.5	1.6	1.7	1.8	1.9	2.0
Yoga		2.9	3.1	3.3	3.5	3.7	3.8	4.0	4.2

71	74	77	80	83	86	89	92	95	98
157	163	170	176	183	190	196	203	209	216
3.7	3.9	4.1	4.2	4.4	4.5	4.7	4.9	5.0	5.2
4.5	4.7	4.9	5.1	5.3	5.5	5.7	5.9	6.1	6.3
5.3	5.5	5.7	5.9	6.2	6.5	6.7	6.9	7.1	7.3
6.1	6.4	6.6	6.9	7.1	7.4	7.7	7.9	8.2	8.4
6.9	7.2	7.5	7.8	8.1	8.4	8.7	8.9	9.2	9.5
3.4	3.6	3.7	3.8	4.0	4.1	4.3	4.4	4.6	4.7
8.7	9.1	9.4	9.8	10.1	10.5	10.9	11.2	11.6	12.0
1.8	1.9	1.9	2.0	2.1	2.2	2.2	2.3	2.4	2.5
4.2	4.4	4.5	4.7	4.9	5.1	5.3	5.4	5.6	5.8
13.8	14.3	14.9	15.5	16.1	16.7	17.2	17.8	18.4	19.0
2.1	2.1	2.2	2.3	2.4	2.5	2.6	2.7	2.8	2.8
4.4	4.6	4.8	5.0	5.1	5.3	5.5	5.7	5.9	6.1

B

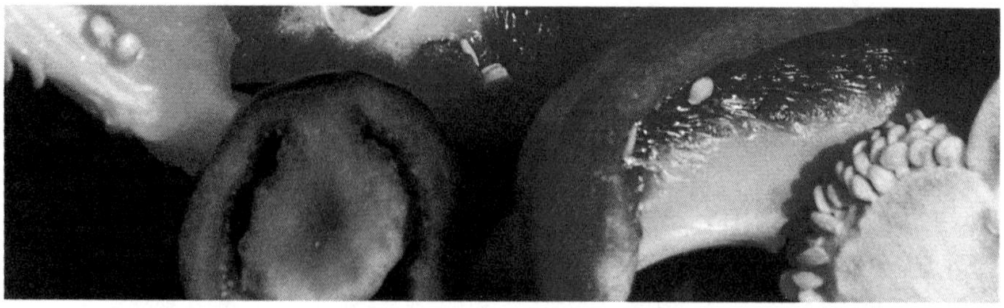

NUTRITIVE VALUES FOR COMMON FOODS, ALCOHOLIC AND NONALCOHOLIC BEVERAGES, AND SPECIALITY AND FAST-FOOD ITEMS

This appendix has three parts. Part 1 lists nutritive values for common foods, Part 2 lists nutritive values for alcoholic and nonalcoholic beverages, and Part 3 presents nutritive values for specialty and fast-food items. The nutritive values of foods and alcoholic and nonalcoholic beverages are expressed in 1-ounce (28.4 g) portions so comparisons can readily be made among and between the different food categories. Thus, for example, the protein content of 1.55 g for 1 ounce of banana nut bread can be compared directly to the protein content of 6.28 g for 1 ounce of processed American cheese.

PART 1. NUTRITIVE VALUES FOR COMMON FOODS*

The foods are grouped into categories and are listed in alphabetical order within each category. The categories include breads, cakes and pies, cookies, candy bars, chocolate, desserts, cereals, cheese, fish, fruits, meats, eggs,

* The information about the nutritive value of the foods was taken from a variety of sources. This includes primarily data from Watt, B.K., and Merrill, A.L.: *Composition of Foods—Raw, Processed and Prepared.* U.S. Department of Agriculture, Washington, DC, 1963; Adams, C., and Richardson, M.: *Nutritive Value of Foods.* Home and Garden Bulletin No. 72, rev, Government Printing Office, Washington, DC, 1981; and Pennington, J.A.T., and Church, H.N.: *Food Values of Portions Commonly Used,* 14th ed. New York, Harper & Row, 1985. Other sources included a comprehensive database on the Cyber mainframe computer at the University of Massachusetts, the consumer relations departments of manufacturers, and journal articles that evaluated specific food items. *NA indicates data not available.*

dairy products, vegetables, and typical salad bar entries. An additional section labeled Variety consists of food items such as soups, sandwiches, salad dressings, oils, some condiments, and other "goodies." The nutritive value for each food is expressed per ounce or 28.4 g of that food item. The specific values for each food include the caloric content (kcal) for 1 ounce, protein, total fat, carbohydrate, calcium, iron, vitamin B_1, vitamin B_2, fiber content, and cholesterol.

Breads	kcal	Protein (g)	Fat (g)	CHO (g)	Ca (mg)	Fe (mg)	B_1 (mg)	B_2 (mg)	Fiber (g)	Cholesterol (mg)
Banana nut	91	1.55	4.00	12.7	10.0	0.470	0.054	0.046	0.66	18.3
Boston brown—canned	60	1.26	0.39	13.2	25.8	0.567	0.038	0.025	1.34	1.9
Cornmeal muffin—recipe	91	1.89	3.15	13.2	41.6	0.567	0.069	0.069	1.00	14.5
Croutons—dry	105	3.69	1.04	20.5	35.0	1.020	0.099	0.099	0.09	0
Cracked wheat—slice	74	2.63	0.99	14.2	18.1	0.755	0.108	0.108	1.50	0
Cracked wheat—toast	88	3.00	1.17	16.9	21.6	0.899	0.100	0.128	1.82	0
French—chunk	81	2.67	1.10	14.3	31.6	0.875	0.130	0.097	0.57	0
Italian	78	2.55	0.25	16.0	4.7	0.756	0.116	0.066	0.47	0
Mixed grain—slice	74	2.27	1.05	13.6	30.6	0.907	0.113	0.113	1.78	0
Mixed grain—toast	80	2.47	1.15	14.8	33.3	0.986	0.099	0.123	1.97	0
Oatmeal—slice	74	2.37	1.25	13.6	17.0	0.794	0.130	0.075	1.10	0
Oatmeal—toast	80	2.47	1.36	14.8	18.5	0.863	0.110	0.081	1.20	0
Pita pocket	78	2.94	0.42	15.6	23.2	0.685	0.129	0.061	0.45	0
Pumpernickel—slice	71	2.60	0.98	13.6	20.4	0.777	0.097	0.147	1.67	0
Pumpernickel—toast	78	2.86	1.08	15.0	22.5	0.857	0.088	0.162	1.87	0
Raisin—slice	77	2.15	1.12	15.0	28.4	0.879	0.093	0.176	0.68	0
Raisin—toasted	92	2.57	1.34	17.6	33.8	1.080	0.081	0.209	0.81	0
Rye—light—piece	74	2.40	1.04	13.6	22.7	0.771	0.116	0.090	1.87	0
Rye—light—toast	84	2.73	1.18	15.5	25.8	0.876	0.107	0.103	2.15	0
Vienna—slice	79	2.72	1.10	14.4	31.2	0.873	0.130	0.100	0.91	0
White—slice	76	2.35	1.10	13.8	35.7	0.806	0.133	0.088	0.54	0
White—toast	84	2.67	1.26	15.7	40.6	0.915	0.121	0.103	0.64	0
Whole wheat—slice	69	2.84	1.22	12.9	20.2	0.964	0.100	0.059	2.10	0
Whole wheat—toasted	79	3.42	1.47	14.4	22.5	1.090	0.090	0.066	2.74	0
Bread crumbs—dry grated	111	3.69	1.42	20.7	34.6	1.160	0.099	0.099	1.15	1.4
Bread crumbs—soft	76	2.35	1.10	13.9	35.9	0.806	0.134	0.088	0.54	0
Bread sticks wo/salt	109	3.40	0.82	21.3	7.9	0.255	0.017	0.020	0.43	0
Bread sticks w/salt	86	2.67	0.89	16.4	13.0	0.243	0.016	0.024	0.41	0

Cakes and Pies	kcal	Protein (g)	Fat (g)	CHO (g)	Ca (mg)	Fe (mg)	B_1 (mg)	B_2 (mg)	Fiber (g)	Cholesterol (mg)
Cakes										
Angel food cake	67	1.71	0.09	15.2	23.5	0.123	0.014	0.057	0	0
Boston cream pie	61	0.59	1.89	10.4	6.1	0.142	0.002	0.043	0	4.7
Carrot cake	103	1.05	5.32	13.2	6.9	0.304	0.030	0.035	0	14.6
Cheesecake	86	1.54	5.45	8.1	15.9	0.136	0.009	0.037	0	52.4
Choc cupcake/choc frosting	97	1.24	3.29	16.5	16.9	0.575	0.029	0.041	0	15.2
Coffee cake	91	1.78	2.70	14.8	17.3	0.480	0.054	0.059	0	18.5
Dark fruitcake	109	1.32	4.62	16.5	27.0	0.791	0.053	0.053	0	13.2
Gingerbread cake	91	1.15	2.86	15.2	12.2	0.706	0.042	0.038	0	7.8
Pound cake	113	1.89	4.72	14.2	18.9	0.472	0.047	0.057	0	30.2
Sheet cake—plain	104	1.32	3.96	15.8	18.1	0.429	0.046	0.049	0	20.1
Sheet cake—white frosting	104	0.94	3.28	18.0	14.3	0.281	0.030	0.037	0	16.4

Cakes and Pies (cont.)	kcal	Protein (g)	Fat (g)	CHO (g)	Ca (mg)	Fe (mg)	B_1 (mg)	B_2 (mg)	Fiber (g)	Cholesterol (mg)
Sponge cake	83	2.01	1.27	16.0	10.8	0.524	0.043	0.046	0	58.8
White cake/coconut	109	1.30	4.05	17.0	13.7	0.454	0.041	0.053	0	1.2
White cake/white frosting	104	1.20	3.59	16.8	13.2	0.399	0.080	0.052	0	1.2
Yellow cake/choc frosting	101	1.03	4.48	15.9	9.5	0.509	0.020	0.058	0	15.6
Pies										
Apple pie	73	0.66	3.14	10.7	5.0	0.300	0.031	0.023	0	0
Apple pie—fried	85	0.73	4.67	10.7	4.0	0.312	0.030	0.020	0	4.7
Banana cream pie	46	0.90	1.85	6.7	21.0	0.156	0.022	0.042	0	2.2
Blueberry pie	68	0.72	3.05	9.9	4.7	0.377	0.031	0.025	0	0
Boston cream pie	61	0.59	1.89	10.4	6.1	0.142	0.002	0.043	0	4.7
Cherry pie	74	0.77	3.19	10.9	6.6	0.569	0.034	0.025	0	0
Cherry pie—fried	83	0.68	4.74	10.7	3.7	0.233	0.020	0.020	0	4.3
Chocolate cream pie	50	1.20	2.04	6.9	25.9	0.175	0.024	0.049	0	2.4
Coconut cream pie	57	1.03	2.79	7.2	24.0	0.198	0.021	0.042	0	2.5
Coconut custard pie	66	1.69	3.85	6.3	25.0	0.304	0.029	0.055	0	31.4
Cream pie	85	0.56	4.29	11.0	8.6	0.205	0.011	0.028	0	1.5
Custard pie	55	1.43	2.65	6.3	23.1	0.269	0.026	0.050	0	27.6
Lemon meringue pie	72	0.95	2.90	10.7	5.1	0.283	0.020	0.028	0	27.7
Mincemeat pie	70	0.65	2.13	12.8	6.9	0.360	0.028	0.024	0	0
Peach pie	73	0.63	3.14	10.9	4.8	0.340	0.031	0.028	0	0
Pecan pie	120	1.30	4.87	18.9	7.2	0.380	0.045	0.034	0	28.1
Pumpkin pie	52	1.28	2.23	7.3	30.0	0.373	0.019	0.042	0	15.5
Strawberry chiffon pie	65	0.85	3.46	8.0	7.7	0.254	0.022	0.023	0	7.1

Cookies	kcal	Protein (g)	Fat (g)	CHO (g)	Ca (mg)	Fe (mg)	B_1 (mg)	B_2 (mg)	Fiber (g)	Cholesterol (mg)
Animal cookies	120	1.90	2.89	22.0	3.0	0.918	0.080	0.130	0	0.1
Brownies w/nuts	135	1.84	8.93	15.6	12.8	0.567	0.070	0.070	0	25.5
Butter cookies	130	1.76	4.82	20.2	36.3	0.170	0.011	0.017	0	4.1
Fig bars	106	1.02	1.93	21.4	20.2	0.689	0.039	0.037	0	13.7
Lady fingers	102	2.19	2.19	18.3	11.6	0.515	0.019	0.039	0	101.0
Oatmeal raisin cookies	134	1.64	5.45	19.6	9.8	0.600	0.049	0.044	0	1.1
Peanut butter cookies	145	2.36	8.27	16.5	12.4	0.650	0.041	0.041	0	13.0
Sandwich type cookies	138	1.42	5.67	20.6	8.5	0.992	0.064	0.050	0	0
Shortbread cookies	137	1.77	7.09	17.7	11.5	0.709	0.089	0.080	0	23.9
Sugar cookies	139	1.18	7.09	18.3	29.5	0.532	0.053	0.035	0	17.1
Vanilla wafers	131	1.42	4.96	20.6	11.3	0.567	0.050	0.070	0	17.7

Candy Bars	kcal	Protein (g)	Fat (g)	CHO (g)	Ca (mg)	Fe (mg)	B_1 (mg)	B_2 (mg)	Fiber (g)	Cholesterol (mg)
Almond Joy	151	1.69	7.82	18.5	2.0	0.778			0	0
Sugar-coated almonds	146	3.10	9.12	14.6	39.6	0.775	0.042	0.156	0	0
Bittersweet chocolate	141	1.90	9.73	15.7	13.0	1.040	0.015	0.050	0	0
Caramel—plain or choc	115	1.00	2.99	22.0	41.9	0.399	0.010	0.050	0	1.0
Chocolate candy kisses	154	2.10	8.98	15.9	52.9	0.499	0.020	0.080	0	0
Chocolate-coated almonds	161	3.92	12.70	8.0	47.8	1.090	0.052	0.186	0	0
Chocolate-covered coconut	133	0.91	7.10	17.5	8.4	0.614	0.008	0.016	0	0
Chocolate-covered mints	116	0.50	2.99	23.0	16.0	0.299	0.010	0.020	0	0

Candy Bars (cont.)	kcal	Protein (g)	Fat (g)	CHO (g)	Ca (mg)	Fe (mg)	B_1 (mg)	B_2 (mg)	Fiber (g)	Cholesterol (mg)
Chocolate-covered peanuts	159	5.00	11.70	9.8	32.9	0.689	0.086	0.043	0	0
Chocolate-covered raisins	111	1.06	2.71	20.6	12.2	0.663	0.034	0.025	0	0
Chocolate fudge	115	0.56	2.78	21.0	22.0	0.299	0.010	0.030	0	1.0
Chocolate fudge with nuts	114	1.06	4.99	18.8	22.0	0.299	0.016	0.030	0	7.4
English toffee	195	0.89	16.90	9.8	0	0.177	0.470	0.044	0	0
Gum drops	98	0	0.20	24.8	2.0	0.100	0	0	0	0
Hard candy	109	0	0	27.6	6.0	0.100	0	0	0	0
Jelly beans	104	0	0.10	26.4	1.0	0.299	0	0	0	0
Kit Kat	138	1.98	7.25	16.5	42.9	0.369	0.020	0.073	0	0
Krackle	149	2.00	8.09	16.9	50.0	0.400	0.017	0.075	0	0
Malted milk balls	135	2.30	6.99	17.8	62.9	0	0	0	0	0
M&M's plain chocolate	140	1.95	6.08	19.5	46.7	0.449	0.015	0.073	0	0
M&M's peanut chocolate	144	3.23	7.25	16.5	35.4	0.402	0.016	0.056	0	0
Mars bar	136	2.27	6.24	17.0	48.2	0.312	0.014	0.093	0	0
Milk chocolate—plain	145	2.00	8.98	16.0	49.9	0.399	0.020	0.100	0	6.0
Milk chocolate w/almonds	150	2.90	10.40	15.0	60.9	0.559	0.030	0.130	0	4.5
Milk chocolate w/peanuts	155	4.89	11.70	10.0	31.9	0.679	0.112	0.065	0	3.0
Milk chocolate + rice cereal	140	2.00	6.99	18.0	47.9	0.200	0.010	0.080	0	6.0
Milky Way	123	1.53	4.25	20.3	40.6	0.232	0.013	0.070	0	6.6
Mr. Goodbar	151	3.62	9.05	13.9	39.2	0.567	0.030	0.072	0	4.2
Reese's peanut butter cup	151	3.65	9.07	13.9	21.7	0.430	0.020	0.032	0	1.6
Snickers—2.2 oz	134	3.08	6.62	17.0	32.4	0.227	0.013	0.050	0	0
Vanilla fudge	118	0.70	3.15	22.0	29.9	0.030	0.006	0.025	0	10.0
Vanilla fudge with nuts	122	1.00	5.01	18.3	25.0	0.159	0.017	0.026	0	8.5

Chocolate	kcal	Protein (g)	Fat (g)	CHO (g)	Ca (mg)	Fe (mg)	B_1 (mg)	B_2 (mg)	Fiber (g)	Cholesterol (mg)
Baking chocolate	145	3.49	15.00	7.5	22.0	1.900	0.015	0.099	0	0
Bittersweet chocolate	141	1.90	9.73	15.7	13.0	1.040	0.015	0.050	0	0
Milk chocolate—plain	145	2.00	8.98	16.0	49.9	0.399	0.020	0.100	0	6.0
Semi-swt chocolate chips	143	1.17	10.20	16.2	8.5	0.967	0.017	0.023	0	0
Dark chocolate—sweet	150	1.00	9.98	16.0	7.0	0.599	0.010	0.040	0	0
Choc cupcake/choc frosting	97	1.24	3.29	16.5	16.9	0.575	0.029	0.041	0	15.2
Chocolate candy kisses	154	2.10	8.98	15.9	52.9	0.499	0.020	0.080	0	0
Chocolate chip cookies	122	1.54	5.94	18.9	11.0	0.540	0.068	0.155	0	3.4
Chocolate coated almonds	161	3.92	12.70	8.0	47.8	1.090	0.052	0.186	0	0
Chocolate coated peanuts	159	5.00	11.70	9.8	32.9	0.689	0.086	0.043	0	0
Chocolate covered mints	116	0.50	2.99	23.0	16.0	0.299	0.010	0.020	0	0
Chocolate covered raisins	111	1.06	2.71	20.6	12.2	0.663	0.034	0.025	0	0
Chocolate cream pie	50	1.20	2.04	6.9	25.9	0.175	0.024	0.049	0	2.4
Chocolate fudge	115	0.56	2.78	21.0	22.0	0.299	0.010	0.030	0	1.0
Chocolate fudge with nuts	114	1.06	4.99	18.8	22.0	0.299	0.016	0.030	0	7.4
Cake flour-baked value	103	2.08	0.28	22.4	4.5	1.250	0.154	0.096	0	0
Reese's peanut butter cup	151	3.65	9.07	13.9	21.7	0.430	0.020	0.032	0	1.6
Chocolate pudding/recipe	42	0.88	1.25	7.3	27.3	0.142	0.005	0.039	0	4.3
Chocolate pudding—instant	34	0.85	0.818	5.9	28.4	0.065	0.009	0.039	0	3.1

Desserts and Breakfast Pastries	kcal	Protein (g)	Fat (g)	CHO (g)	Ca (mg)	Fe (mg)	B_1 (mg)	B_2 (mg)	Fiber (g)	Cholesterol (mg)
Apple brown betty	43	0.30	1.60	7.40	5.4	0.130	0.016	0.012	0	3.8
Apple cobbler	55	0.53	1.74	9.57	8.8	0.206	0.023	0.019	0	0.3
Apple crisp	53	0.33	1.93	9.09	7.4	0.278	0.018	0.013	0	0
Apple dumpling	55	0.32	2.37	8.64	7.1	0.253	0.012	0.013	0	0
Banana nut bread	91	1.60	4.00	12.70	10.0	0.470	0.054	0.046	0	18.3
Bread + raisin pudding	60	1.20	2.47	8.54	27.7	0.304	0.030	0.048	0	24.4
Cheesecake	86	1.50	5.45	8.10	15.9	0.136	0.009	0.037	0	52.4
Cherry cobbler	44	0.53	1.37	7.52	8.5	0.391	0.019	0.021	0	0.3
Cherry&cream cheese torte	79	1.28	3.96	10.00	28.5	0.266	0.015	0.052	0	11.2
Vanilla milkshake	32	0.98	0.841	5.09	34.5	0.026	0.013	0.052	0	3.2
Cream puff w/custard fill	72	1.24	4.54	6.83	16.4	0.276	0.015	0.040	0	58.8
Choc eclair w/custard fill	79	1.20	4.43	8.96	18.6	0.258	0.019	0.041	0	50.4
Gelatin salad	17	0.43	0	3.99	0.5	0.024	0.002	0.002	0	0
Peach cobbler	28	0.50	1.35	7.96	7.6	0.197	0.018	0.017	0	0.3
Peach crisp	34	0.31	1.06	6.18	4.8	0.203	0.010	0.010	0	0
Crepe, unfilled	49	2.06	1.32	7.07	25.0	0.475	0.045	0.070	0.21	43.0
Pancakes—plain	63	2.10	2.10	9.45	28.4	0.525	0.063	0.074	0.42	16.8
Croissant	117	2.32	6.02	13.40	10.0	1.040	0.085	0.065	0.54	6.5
Danish pastry—plain	109	1.99	5.97	12.90	29.8	0.547	0.080	0.085	0	24.4
Danish pastry w/fruit	102	1.74	5.67	12.20	7.41	0.567	0.070	0.061	0	24.4
Doughnut—cake type	119	1.33	6.75	13.90	13.0	0.454	0.068	0.068	0	11.3
Doughnut—jelly filled	99	1.48	3.84	13.00	12.2	0.349	0.052	0.044	0	0
Doughnut—yeast-raised	111	1.89	6.28	12.30	8.0	0.661	0.132	0.057	0	9.9
Chocolate pudding	42	0.88	1.25	7.28	27.3	0.142	0.005	0.039	0	4.3
Tapioca pudding	38	1.43	1.44	4.85	29.7	0.120	0.012	0.052	0	27.3
Vanilla pudding	32	0.99	1.10	4.50	33.1	0.089	0.009	0.046	0	4.1
Chocolate pudding—instant	34	0.85	0.82	5.89	28.4	0.065	0.009	0.039	0	3.1
Rice pudding	33	0.86	0.86	5.80	28.6	0.107	0.021	0.039	0	3.2
Butterscotch pudding pop	47	1.19	1.29	7.80	37.8	0.020	0.015	0.055	0	0.5
Chocolate pudding pop	49	1.34	1.34	8.20	42.8	0.179	0.015	0.055	0	0.5
Vanilla pudding pop	46	1.19	1.29	7.80	37.8	0.020	0.015	0.055	0	0.5

Cereals (without milk)	kcal	Protein (g)	Fat (g)	CHO (g)	Ca (mg)	Fe (mg)	B_1 (mg)	B_2 (mg)	Fiber (g)	Cholesterol (mg)
All-Bran	70	3.99	0.50	21.0	23.00	4.49	0.369	0.429	8.490	0
Alpha Bits	111	2.20	0.60	24.6	7.99	1.80	0.399	0.399	0.650	0
Apple Jacks	110	1.50	0.10	25.7	2.99	4.49	0.399	0.399	0.200	0
Bran Buds	73	3.95	0.68	21.6	18.90	4.52	0.371	0.439	7.860	0
Bran Chex	90	2.95	0.81	22.6	16.80	4.51	0.347	0.150	5.200	0
Buc Wheats	110	2.00	1.00	24.0	59.90	8.09	0.674	0.764	2.000	0
C.W. Post—plain	126	2.54	4.44	20.3	13.70	4.50	0.380	0.438	0.643	0
C.W. Post w/raisins	123	2.45	4.05	20.3	14.00	4.51	0.358	0.413	0.660	0
Cap'n Crunch	120	1.46	2.60	22.9	4.60	7.53	0.506	0.544	0.709	0
Cap'n Crunchberries	118	1.46	2.35	23.0	8.91	7.32	0.478	0.543	0.324	0
Cap'n Crunch—pnut butter	125	2.03	3.64	21.5	5.67	7.37	0.486	0.567	0.324	0
Cheerios	110	4.24	1.77	19.4	47.30	4.44	0.394	0.394	3.000	0
Cocoa Krispies	109	1.50	0.39	25.2	4.73	1.81	0.394	0.394	0.354	0
Cocoa Pebbles	117	1.35	1.49	24.7	5.40	1.75	0.405	0.405	0.312	0
Corn Bran	98	1.97	1.02	23.9	32.30	9.60	0.299	0.551	5.390	0
Corn Chex	111	2.00	0.10	24.9	2.99	1.80	0.399	0.070	0.499	0
Corn flakes—Kellogg's	110	2.30	0.09	24.4	1.00	1.80	0.367	0.424	0.594	0
Corn flakes—Post Toasties	110	2.30	0.09	24.4	1.00	0.70	0.367	0.424	0.594	0
Corn grits—enr yellow dry	105	2.49	0.33	22.5	0.55	1.10	0.182	0.107	3.270	0

Cereals (without milk) (cont.)	kcal	Protein (g)	Fat (g)	CHO (g)	Ca (mg)	Fe (mg)	B_1 (mg)	B_2 (mg)	Fiber (g)	Cholesterol (mg)
Corn grits—enr yellow ckd	17	0.41	0.06	3.7	0.12	0.18	0.028	0.018	0.527	0
Cracklin' Oat Bran	108	2.60	4.16	19.4	18.90	1.80	0.378	0.425	4.280	0
Cream of Rice	15	0.24	0.01	3.3	0.93	0.05	0.012	0	0.163	0
Cream of Wheat	16	0.42	0.07	3.4	6.27	1.27	0.028	0.008	0.395	0
Crispy Wheat 'n Raisins	99	2.00	0.46	23.1	46.80	4.48	0.396	0.396	1.320	0
Farina—cooked	14	0.41	0.02	3.0	0.49	0.14	0.023	0.015	0.389	0
Fortified Oat Flakes	105	5.32	0.41	20.5	40.20	8.09	0.354	0.413	0.827	0
40% Bran Flakes—Kellogg's	91	3.60	0.54	22.2	13.80	8.14	0.369	0.430	0.850	0
40% Bran Flakes—Post	92	3.20	0.45	22.3	12.70	4.50	0.374	0.435	3.800	0
Froot Loops	111	1.70	1.00	25.0	2.99	4.49	0.399	0.399	0.299	0
Frosted Mini-Wheats	102	2.93	0.27	23.4	9.15	1.83	0.366	0.457	2.160	0
Frosted Rice Krispies	109	1.30	0.10	25.7	1.00	1.80	0.399	0.399	0.998	0
Fruit & Fiber w/apples	90	2.99	1.00	22.0	9.98	4.49	0.374	0.424	4.190	0
Fruit & Fiber w/dates	90	2.99	1.00	21.0	9.98	4.49	0.374	0.424	4.190	0
Fruitful Bran	92	2.50	0	22.5	8.34	6.75	0.313	0.354	4.170	0
Fruity Pebbles	115	1.10	1.50	24.4	2.99	1.80	0.399	0.399	0.226	0
Golden Grahams	109	1.60	1.09	24.1	17.40	4.50	0.363	0.436	1.670	0
Granola—homemade	138	3.49	7.69	15.6	17.70	1.12	0.170	0.072	2.970	0
Granola—Nature Valley	126	2.89	4.92	18.9	17.80	0.95	0.098	0.048	2.960	0
Grape Nuts	100	3.28	0.11	23.2	10.90	1.22	0.398	0.398	1.840	0
Grape Nuts Flakes	102	2.99	0.30	23.2	11.00	4.49	0.399	0.399	1.900	0
Honey & Nut Corn Flakes	113	1.80	1.50	23.3	2.99	1.80	0.399	0.399	0.299	0
Honey Bran	96	2.51	0.57	23.2	13.00	4.54	0.405	0.405	3.160	0
Honey Comb	111	1.68	0.52	25.3	5.15	1.80	0.387	0.387	0.387	0
Honey Nut Cheerios	107	3.09	0.69	22.8	19.80	4.47	0.344	0.430	0.790	0
King Vitamin	115	1.49	1.62	24.0	NA	17.10	0.124	1.430	0.135	0
Kix	109	2.49	0.70	23.3	34.80	8.06	0.398	0.398	0.398	0
Life	104	5.22	0.52	20.3	99.20	7.47	0.612	0.644	0.902	0
Lucky Charms	111	2.57	1.06	23.1	31.90	4.52	0.354	0.443	0.624	0
Malt-O-Meal	14	0.43	0.03	3.1	0.59	1.13	0.057	0.028	0.354	0
Maypo—cooked	1	0.02	0.01	0.1	0.52	0.04	0.003	0.003	0.012	0
Nutri-Grain—barley	106	3.11	0.21	23.4	7.60	1.00	0.346	0.415	1.660	0
Nutri-Grain—corn	108	2.30	0.68	24.0	0.68	0.60	0.338	0.405	1.750	0
Nutri-Grain—rye	102	2.48	0.21	24.0	5.67	0.80	0.354	0.425	2.160	0
Nutri-Grain—wheat	102	2.45	0.32	24.0	7.73	0.80	0.387	0.451	1.800	0
Oatmeal—prepared	18	0.73	0.29	3.1	2.42	0.19	0.032	0.006	0.497	0
Rolled Oats	109	4.55	1.78	19.0	14.70	1.19	0.206	0.038	3.090	0
Instant Oatmeal w/apples	26	0.74	0.30	5.0	30.00	1.15	0.091	0.053	0.552	0
Inst Oatmeal w/bran/raisn	23	0.71	0.28	4.4	25.20	1.10	0.081	0.092	0.480	0
Inst Oatmeal w/maple	30	0.84	0.35	5.8	29.60	1.16	0.097	0.059	0.530	0
Inst Oatmeal w/cinn/spice	31	0.85	0.34	6.2	30.30	1.17	0.099	0.060	0.510	0
Inst Oatmeal w/rais/spice	29	0.77	0.32	5.7	29.60	1.18	0.092	0.065	0.556	0
100% Bran	77	3.57	1.42	20.7	19.80	3.49	0.687	0.773	8.380	0
100% Natural	135	3.02	6.02	18.0	48.90	0.83	0.085	0.150	3.390	0
100% Natural—w/apples	130	2.92	5.32	19.0	42.80	0.79	0.090	0.158	1.300	0
100% Natural—w/rais/dates	128	2.89	5.23	18.7	41.20	0.80	0.077	0.165	1.080	0
Product 19	108	2.75	0.17	23.5	3.44	18.00	1.460	1.720	0.369	0
Puffed Rice	111	1.79	0.20	25.5	2.03	0.30	0.030	0.028	0.227	0
Puffed Wheat	104	4.25	0.24	22.4	7.09	1.35	0.047	0.070	5.430	0
Quisp	117	1.42	2.08	23.6	8.50	5.96	0.510	0.718	0.378	0
Raisin Bran—Kellogg's	91	3.07	0.46	21.4	14.50	13.90	0.293	0.332	3.410	0
Raisin Bran—Post	86	2.68	0.55	21.4	13.70	4.56	0.373	0.430	3.190	0
Raisins, Rice & Rye	96	1.60	0.06	24.2	6.16	3.45	0.308	0.370	0.308	0
Ralston—cooked	15	0.62	0.09	3.2	1.57	0.18	0.022	0.020	0.370	0
Rice Chex	112	1.49	1.00	25.2	3.88	1.79	0.400	0.298	1.840	0
Rice Krispies	109	1.86	0.20	24.2	3.91	1.76	0.391	0.391	0.312	0
Roman Meal—dry	91	4.07	0.60	20.4	18.40	1.31	0.142	0.069	0.905	0

Cereals (without milk) (cont.)	kcal	Protein (g)	Fat (g)	CHO (g)	Ca (mg)	Fe (mg)	B_1 (mg)	B_2 (mg)	Fiber (g)	Cholesterol (mg)
Roman Meal—cooked	17	0.77	0.11	3.9	3.45	0.25	0.028	0.014	0.877	0
Shredded Wheat	102	3.09	0.71	22.5	11.00	1.20	0.070	0.080	3.100	0
Shredded wheat	97	3.06	0.45	16.4	11.20	0.89	0.082	0.075	2.900	0
Special K	111	5.58	0.10	21.3	7.97	4.48	0.399	0.399	0.266	0
Sugar Corn Pops	108	1.40	0.10	25.6	0.10	1.80	0.399	0.399	0.100	0
Sugar Frosted Flakes	108	1.46	0.08	25.7	0.81	1.78	0.405	0.405	0.446	0
Sugar Smacks	106	2.00	0.50	24.7	2.99	1.80	0.369	0.429	0.319	0
Super Golden Crisp	106	1.80	0.26	25.6	6.01	1.80	0.344	0.430	0.430	0
Team	111	1.82	0.48	24.3	4.05	1.73	0.371	0.425	0.270	0
Total	105	2.84	0.60	22.3	172.00	18.00	1.460	1.720	2.060	0
Trix	108	1.50	0.40	24.9	5.99	4.49	0.399	0.399	0.184	0
Wheat & Raisin Chex	97	2.68	0.21	22.6	NA	4.04	0.263	0.315	1.890	0
Wheat Chex	104	2.77	0.68	23.3	11.00	4.50	0.370	0.105	2.100	0
Wheat germ—toasted	108	8.25	3.09	14.0	12.50	2.19	0.474	0.233	3.910	0
Wheat germ w/brn sgr, honey	107	6.19	2.30	17.2	8.98	1.93	0.349	0.180	3.390	0
Wheatena—cooked	16	0.58	0.13	3.4	1.28	0.16	0.002	0.006	0.385	0
Wheaties	99	2.74	0.51	22.6	43.00	4.50	0.391	0.391	2.540	0
Whole wheat berries	16	0.54	0.11	3.2	1.70	0.17	0.023	0.006	0.680	0
Whole wheat cereal—cooked	18	0.58	0.11	3.9	1.99	0.18	0.020	0.014	0.457	0

Cheese	kcal	Protein (g)	Fat (g)	CHO (g)	Ca (mg)	Fe (mg)	B_1 (mg)	B_2 (mg)	Fiber (g)	Cholesterol (mg)
American—processed	106	6.28	8.84	0.45	174	0.110	0.008	0.111	0	27.0
American cheese food—cold pack	94	5.23	6.78	2.36	145	0.240	0.009	0.274	0	18.0
American cheese spread	82	5.16	6.00	2.48	159	0.090	0.014	0.380	0	16.0
Blue	100	6.09	8.14	0.66	150	0.090	0.008	0.395	0	21.0
Brick	105	6.40	8.40	0.79	191	0.130	0.004	0.159	0	27.0
Brie	95	5.87	7.84	0.13	52	0.140	0.020	0.147	0	28.0
Camembert	85	5.60	6.86	0.13	110	0.094	0.008	0.138	0	20.0
Caraway	107	7.13	8.27	0.87	191	0.100	0.009	0.196	0	25.0
Cheddar	114	7.05	9.38	0.36	204	0.197	0.008	0.106	0	29.9
Cheshire	110	6.60	8.66	1.36	182	0.060	0.013	0.198	0	28.9
Colby	112	6.73	9.08	0.73	194	0.216	0.004	0.171	0	27.0
Cottage	29	3.54	1.20	0.76	17	0.040	0.006	0.115	0	4.2
Cottage—lowfat 2%	26	3.90	0.55	1.03	20	0.045	0.007	0.052	0	2.4
Cottage—lowfat 1%	21	3.51	0.29	0.77	18	0.040	0.006	0.115	0	1.3
Cottage—dry curd	24	4.89	0.12	0.52	9	0.065	0.007	0.004	0	2.0
Cottage—w/fruit	35	2.80	0.96	3.78	14	0.031	0.005	0.115	0	3.1
Cream	99	2.10	9.87	0.75	23	0.337	0.005	0.056	0	30.9
Edam	101	7.07	7.79	0.40	207	0.125	0.010	0.274	0	25.0
Feta	75	4.49	6.19	1.16	140	0.180	0.040	0.315	0	25.0
Fontina	110	7.25	8.62	0.44	156	0.060	0.006	NA	0	32.9
Gjetost	132	2.74	8.32	12.00	113	0.130	0.009	0.170	0	25.0
Gorgonzola	111	6.99	8.98	0	149	0.120	0.010	0.512	0	25.0
Gouda	101	7.06	7.72	0.63	198	0.070	0.009	0.232	0	31.9
Gruyere	117	8.44	9.05	0.10	286	0.060	0.017	0.095	0	30.9
Liederkranz	87	4.99	7.99	0	110	0.120	0.010	0.389	0	21.0
Limburger	93	5.67	7.59	0.14	141	0.040	0.023	0.227	0	26.0
Monterey jack	106	6.93	8.56	0.19	212	0.200	0.004	0.119	0	26.0
Mozzarella—skim, low moist	80	7.60	4.67	0.89	207	0.076	0.006	0.150	0	15.0
Mozzarella—whl milk, reg	80	5.50	5.75	0.63	147	0.050	0.004	0.106	0	22.0
Mozzarella—whl mlk, low moist	90	6.10	7.19	0.43	163	0.060	0.005	0.119	0	25.0

Cheese (cont.)	kcal	Protein (g)	Fat (g)	CHO (g)	Ca (mg)	Fe (mg)	B_1 (mg)	B_2 (mg)	Fiber (g)	Cholesterol (mg)
Muenster	104	6.40	8.42	0.32	203	0.125	0.004	0.178	0	27.0
Neufchatel	74	2.82	6.70	0.83	21	0.080	0.004	0.113	0	22.0
Parmesan—hard	111	10.00	7.30	0.91	335	0.230	0.010	0.453	0	19.0
Parmesan—grated	129	11.80	8.50	1.06	389	0.270	0.013	0.527	0	22.0
Pimento processed	106	6.26	8.82	0.49	174	0.120	0.008	0.404	0	27.0
Port du salut	100	6.73	7.99	0.16	84	0.140	0.004	0.151	0	34.9
Provolone	100	7.13	7.54	0.61	214	0.146	0.005	0.248	0	20.0
Ricotta—part skim	39	3.23	2.25	1.45	77	0.126	0.006	0.052	0	8.8
Ricotta—whole milk	49	3.19	3.68	0.86	59	0.108	0.004	0.024	0	14.3
Romano	110	9.00	7.63	1.03	301	0.230	0.010	0.339	0	28.9
Romano—grated	128	10.50	8.86	1.20	350	0.270	0.013	0.394	0	32.9
Roquefort	105	6.10	8.93	0.57	188	0.172	0.010	0.512	0	26.0
Swiss	107	8.03	7.79	0.96	272	0.050	0.006	0.074	0	26.0
Swiss processed	95	7.00	6.97	0.60	219	0.170	0.004	0.078	0	24.0

Fish	kcal	Protein (g)	Fat (g)	CHO (g)	Ca (mg)	Fe (mg)	B_1 (mg)	B_2 (mg)	Fiber (g)	Cholesterol (mg)
Bass—freshwater raw	32	5.36	1.05	0	22.7	0.422	0.028	0.009	0	19.3
Bluefish—baked/broiled	45	7.43	1.42	0	2.6	0.174	0.022	0.030	0	17.9
Bluefish—fried in crumbs	58	6.44	2.78	1.33	2.3	0.151	0.017	0.023	0	17
Bluefish—raw	35	5.67	1.20	0	2.0	0.136	0.016	0.023	0	16.7
Carp—raw	36	5.05	1.59	0	11.6	0.352	0.013	0.011	0	18.7
Catfish—Channel—raw	33	5.16	1.20	0	11.3	0.275	0.013	0.030	0	16.4
Cod—baked w/butter	37	6.46	0.94	0	5.7	0.139	0.025	0.022	0	17.0
Cod—batter-fried	56	5.56	2.92	2.13	22.7	0.142	0.011	0.011	0	15.6
Cod—baked/broiled	30	6.46	0.24	0	4.0	0.139	0.025	0.022	0	15.6
Cod—poached	29	6.24	0.24	0	4.0	0.139	0.025	0.022	0	15.6
Cod—steamed	29	6.24	0.24	0	4.0	0.139	0.025	0.022	0	15.9
Cod—smoked	22	5.19	0.17	0	4.0	0.113	0.023	0.020	0	14.2
Cod—Atlantic—raw	23	5.05	0.19	0	4.5	0.108	0.022	0.018	0	12.2
Cod liver oil	255	0	28.40	0	0	0	0	0	0	162.0
Eel—smoked	94	5.27	7.88	0.23	26.9	0.198	0.040	0.099	0	19.8
Haddock—breaded/fried	58	5.67	3.00	2.33	11.3	0.384	0.020	0.033	0.01	18.3
Haddock—smoked	33	7.14	0.27	0	13.9	0.397	0.013	0.014	0	21.8
Haddock—raw	22	5.36	0.20	0	9.4	0.298	0.010	0.010	0	16.2
Herring—pickled	74	4.03	5.10	2.73	21.8	0.346	0.010	0.039	0	3.7
Herring—smoked/kippered	62	6.97	3.52	0	23.8	0.428	0.036	0.090	0	22.7
Herring—canned w/liquid	59	5.64	3.86	0	41.7	0.879	0.007	0.051	0	27.5
Mackerel—fried	49	7.00	2.35	0	4.3	0.445	0.045	0.116	0	19.8
Mackerel—Atlantic—bkd/brld	74	6.78	5.05	0	4.3	0.445	0.045	0.117	0	21.3
Mackerel—Atlantic—raw	58	5.27	3.94	0	3.4	0.462	0.050	0.088	0	19.8
Mackerel—Pacific—raw	45	6.12	2.84	0	2.3	0.567	0.043	0.096	0	22.7
Northern pike—raw	25	5.47	0.20	0	16.2	0.156	0.017	0.018	0	11.0
Ocean perch—breaded/fried	62	5.34	3.67	2.33	30.7	0.400	0.033	0.037	0.03	15.3
Pollock—baked/broiled	28	6.60	0.31	0	19.3	0.149	0.014	0.057	0	19.8
Pollock—poached	36	6.60	0.31	0	17.0	0.149	0.010	0.050	0	19.8
Salmon—broiled/baked	61	7.74	3.10	0	2.0	0.157	0.061	0.048	0	24.7
Coho salmon—steamed/poached	52	7.77	2.14	0	8.22	0.252	0.057	0.031	0	13.9
Smoked salmon—Chinook	33	5.17	1.22	0	3.0	0.240	0.007	0.029	0	6.7
Atlantic salmon—small can	36	5.05	1.62	0	3.1	0.204	0.057	0.097	0	17.0
Pink salmon—raw	33	5.64	0.98	0	11.3	0.218	0.040	0.057	0	14.7
Sardines	59	7.00	3.24	0	108.0	0.826	0.023	0.064	0	40.4

Fish (cont.)	kcal	Protein (g)	Fat (g)	CHO (g)	Ca (mg)	Fe (mg)	B_1 (mg)	B_2 (mg)	Fiber (g)	Cholesterol (mg)
Seatrout/steelhead—raw	30	4.73	1.02	0	4.8	0.077	0.023	0.057	0	23.5
Seatrout/steelhead—cooked	37	6.07	1.42	0	5.7	0.088	0.024	0.064	0	32.3
Shad—baked with bacon	57	6.58	3.20	0	6.8	0.170	0.037	0.074	0	17.0
Smelt—rainbow—raw	28	4.99	0.69	0	17.0	0.255	0.016	0.034	0	19.8
Snapper—baked or broiled	36	7.46	0.49	0	11.3	0.068	0.015	0.021	0	13.3
Snapper—raw	28	5.81	0.38	0	9.1	0.051	0.013	0.017	0	10.5
Sole/flounder—bkd w/butter	40	5.34	2.00	0	5.3	0.093	0.023	0.032	0	22.7
Sole/flounder—bkd/ broiled	33	6.84	0.43	0	5.3	0.093	0.023	0.032	0	19.3
Sole/flounder—battr-fried	83	4.47	5.10	4.07	16.7	0.239	0.057	0.042	0.01	15.0
Sole/flounder—brd-fried	53	4.96	2.55	2.54	11.3	0.128	0.037	0.034	0	15.0
Sole/flounder—steamed	26	5.67	0.33	0	4.5	0.079	0.017	0.027	0	14.7
Sole/flounder—raw	26	5.33	0.34	0	5.1	0.102	0.025	0.022	0	13.6
Lemon sole—raw	23	4.85	0.21	0	4.8	0.088	0.026	0.023	0	17.0
Lemon sole—fried w/ crumbs	56	4.56	3.12	2.64	26.9	0.176	0.020	0.023	0	18.4
Lemon sole—steamed	26	5.84	0.26	0	6.0	0.147	0.026	0.026	0	17.0
Swordfish—raw	34	5.61	1.14	0	1.1	0.230	0.010	0.027	0	11.0
Swordfish—broiled/baked	44	7.20	1.46	0	1.7	0.295	0.012	0.033	0	14.2
Trout—baked/broiled	43	7.47	1.22	0	24.3	0.690	0.024	0.064	0	20.7
Tuna—oil pack	56	8.26	2.34	0	3.8	0.395	0.010	0.030	0	5.0
Tuna—water pack	37	8.38	0.14	0	3.4	0.409	0.010	0.033	0	16.0
Tuna—raw	31	6.63	0.27	0	4.5	0.207	0.123	0.013	0	12.8
Whiting—flour/bread-fried	54	5.13	1.56	1.98	11.3	0.198	0.023	0.020	0	18.4

Fruits	kcal	Protein (g)	Fat (g)	CHO (g)	Ca (mg)	Fe (mg)	B_1 (mg)	B_2 (mg)	Fiber (g)	Cholesterol (mg)
Apple w/peel	16	0.055	0.100	4.31	2.05	0.051	0.005	0.004	0.709	0
Apple slices w/peel—frsh	17	0.054	0.100	4.33	2.06	0.052	0.005	0.004	0.709	0
Apple juice—cannd/bottld	13	0.017	0.032	3.32	1.94	0.105	0.006	0.005	0.034	0
Apple juice—frozen conc	47	0.144	0.105	11.60	5.78	0.258	0.003	0.015	0.089	0
Applesauce—sweetened	22	0.052	0.052	5.67	1.11	0.111	0.003	0.008	0.397	0
Apricot—fresh halves	14	0.397	0.110	3.15	4.02	0.154	0.009	0.011	0.538	0
Apricot halves—light syrup	18	0.150	0.013	4.67	3.34	0.110	0.005	0.006	0.319	0
Apricot nectar—canned	16	0.104	0.025	4.08	2.03	0.108	0.003	0.004	0.170	0
Avocado—average	46	0.563	0.340	2.10	3.07	0.284	0.030	0.035	2.720	0
Banana—fresh slices	26	0.293	0.136	6.63	1.74	0.088	0.013	0.028	0.578	0
Blackberries—canned	26	0.370	0.040	6.54	5.98	0.184	0.008	0.011	1.011	0
Blackberries—fresh	15	0.205	0.110	3.62	9.06	0.158	0.008	0.011	1.910	0
Blackberries—frozen	18	0.334	0.122	4.45	8.26	0.173	0.008	0.013	1.460	0
Blueberries—fresh	16	0.190	0.108	4.00	1.76	0.047	0.014	0.014	0.763	0
Blueberries–fzn un-sweetnd	14	0.119	0.181	3.46	2.19	0.051	0.009	0.010	0.658	0
Boysenberries—frozen	14	0.314	0.075	3.46	7.73	0.240	0.015	0.010	1.100	0
Sour cherries—frozen	13	0.260	0.124	3.13	3.66	0.150	0.012	0.010	0.384	0
Sweet cherries—fresh	20	0.340	0.272	4.69	4.10	0.110	0.014	0.017	0.430	0
Sweet cherries—frozen	25	0.325	0.037	6.34	3.39	0.099	0.008	0.013	0.224	0
Cranberries—whole—raw	14	0.110	0.057	3.58	2.09	0.057	0.009	0.006	1.190	0
Cranberry/apple juice	19	0.015	0.090	4.82	2.02	0.017	0.001	0.006	0.070	0
Cranberry juice cocktail	16	0.009	0.015	4.03	0.90	0.043	0.002	0.002	0.085	0
Date—whole—each	78	0.557	0.127	20.80	9.22	0.342	0.026	0.028	2.300	0
Figs—medium—fresh	21	0.215	0.085	5.44	10.20	0.102	0.017	0.014	1.050	0

Fruits (cont.)	kcal	Protein (g)	Fat (g)	CHO (g)	Ca (mg)	Fe (mg)	B_1 (mg)	B_2 (mg)	Fiber (g)	Cholesterol (mg)
Fig—dried—each	72	0.864	0.330	18.50	40.80	0.634	0.020	0.025	3.140	0
Fruit cocktail—hvy syrup	21	0.111	0.020	5.36	1.78	0.081	0.005	0.005	0.280	0
Fruit cocktail—lite syrup	16	0.114	0.020	4.23	1.80	0.082	0.005	0.005	0.284	0
Grapefruit half—pink/red	9	0.157	0.028	2.18	3.00	0.034	0.010	0.006	0.369	0
Grapefruit half—white	10	0.195	0.029	2.38	3.36	0.017	0.010	0.006	0.368	0
Grapefruit sections—fresh	9	0.179	0.028	2.29	3.33	0.025	0.010	0.006	0.370	0
Grapefruit sections—cnd	17	0.160	0.028	4.38	4.02	0.114	0.010	0.006	0.313	0
Grapefruit juice—fresh	11	0.142	0.029	2.60	2.53	0.056	0.011	0.006	0.113	0
Grapefruit juice—sw	13	0.164	0.026	3.15	2.27	0.102	0.011	0.007	0.076	0
Grapefruit juice—unsw	11	0.148	0.028	2.54	1.95	0.057	0.012	0.006	0.077	0
Grapefruit juice—frzn conc	41	0.548	0.137	9.86	7.67	0.140	0.041	0.022	0.383	0
Grapes—Thompson	20	0.188	0.163	5.03	3.01	0.073	0.026	0.016	0.333	0
Grape juice—bottled/cnd	17	0.158	0.021	4.25	2.47	0.068	0.007	0.010	0.141	0
Grape juice—frzn conc	51	0.184	0.088	12.60	3.68	0.102	0.015	0.026	0.492	0
Grape juice—prep frozn	15	0.053	0.026	3.62	1.13	0.029	0.004	0.007	0.142	0
Kiwi fruit	17	0.280	0.127	4.22	7.46	0.112	0.007	0.015	0.962	0
Lemon—fresh wo/peel	8	0.313	0.083	2.64	7.33	0.171	0.011	0.006	0.582	0
Lemon juice—fresh	7	0.107	0.081	2.45	2.09	0.009	0.008	0.003	0.099	0
Lemon juice—bottled	6	0.114	0.081	1.84	3.02	0.036	0.012	0.003	0.085	0
Lime—fresh	9	0.199	0.055	2.99	9.30	0.169	0.008	0.006	0.228	0
Lime juice—fresh	8	0.124	0.029	2.56	2.54	0.009	0.006	0.003	0.113	0
Lime juice—bottled	6	0.115	0.115	1.84	3.46	0.069	0.009	0.001	0.099	0
Loganberries—fresh	20	0.430	0.088	3.69	8.50	0.181	0.014	0.010	1.760	0
Loganberries—frozen	16	0.430	0.089	3.68	7.33	0.181	0.014	0.010	1.760	0
Mango—fresh—slices	19	0.146	0.077	4.83	2.92	0.360	0.016	0.016	0.997	0
Mango—fresh—whole	19	0.145	0.078	4.82	2.88	0.356	0.016	0.016	1.010	0
Cantaloupe—cubes	10	0.250	0.079	2.37	3.19	0.060	0.006	0.006	0.284	0
Casaba melon—cubes	8	0.255	0.028	1.75	1.50	0.113	0.017	0.006	0.284	0
Honeydew melon—cubes	10	0.128	0.028	2.60	1.67	0.020	0.022	0.005	0.307	0
Melon balls—mixed—frozen	9	0.239	0.023	2.25	2.79	0.008	0.005	0.006	0.295	0
Mixed fruit—dried	69	0.697	0.139	18.20	10.60	0.767	0.012	0.045	1.220	0
Mixed fruit—frozen—thawed	28	0.397	0.052	6.87	2.04	0.079	0.005	0.010	0.386	0
Nectarine	14	0.267	0.129	3.34	1.25	0.044	0.005	0.012	0.554	0
Orange	13	0.266	0.035	3.33	11.30	0.029	0.025	0.011	0.680	0
Orange sections—fresh	13	0.266	0.035	3.34	11.30	0.029	0.025	0.011	0.680	0
Mandarin oranges—canned	17	0.113	0.011	4.61	2.03	0.101	0.015	0.012	0.478	0
Orange juice—fresh	13	0.199	0.057	2.95	3.09	0.057	0.025	0.008	0.113	0
Orange juice—frozen conc	45	0.679	0.059	10.80	9.05	0.099	0.079	0.018	0.313	0
Orange juice—prep frzn	13	0.191	0.016	3.05	2.50	0.031	0.023	0.005	0.057	0
Papaya—whole fresh	11	0.173	0.040	2.78	6.71	0.028	0.008	0.009	0.482	0
Papaya—slices fresh	12	0.174	0.040	2.77	6.68	0.060	0.008	0.009	0.482	0
Papaya nectar—canned	16	0.049	0.043	4.12	2.72	0.098	0.002	0.001	0.170	0
Peaches—fresh	12	0.199	0.026	3.14	1.30	0.031	0.005	0.012	0.489	0
Peach slices—frozen/thawd	27	0.177	0.037	6.80	0.91	0.105	0.004	0.010	0.467	0
Peach halves—heavy syrup	21	0.130	0.028	5.67	1.05	0.077	0.003	0.007	0.315	0
Peach halves—light syrup	15	0.126	0.010	4.13	1.05	0.101	0.002	0.007	0.402	0
Peach halves—dried	68	0.020	0.216	17.40	8.07	1.150	0	0.060	2.330	0
Peach nectar—canned	15	0.076	0.006	3.95	1.48	0.054	0	0.004	0.170	0
Pears—Bartlett	17	0.111	0.113	4.29	3.24	0.070	0.006	0.011	0.779	0
Pear halves—heavy syrup	21	0.057	0.036	5.42	1.44	0.061	0.004	0.006	0.395	0
Pear halves—lite syrup	16	0.054	0.007	4.30	1.44	0.082	0.003	0.005	0.395	0
Pear nectar—canned	17	0.030	0.003	4.47	1.25	0.073	0	0.004	0.204	0

Fruits (cont.)	kcal	Protein (g)	Fat (g)	CHO (g)	Ca (mg)	Fe (mg)	B_1 (mg)	B_2 (mg)	Fiber (g)	Cholesterol (mg)
Pineapple slices—hvy syrup	22	0.098	0.034	5.72	3.91	0.108	0.025	0.007	0.270	0
Pineapple slices—lite syrp	15	0.103	0.034	3.81	3.91	0.110	0.026	0.007	0.268	0
Pineapple—frozen—sweetened	24	0.113	0.029	6.29	2.55	0.113	0.028	0.009	0.496	0
Pineapple juice—frzn conc	51	0.369	0.029	12.60	11.00	0.255	0.065	0.017	0.255	0
Plums	16	0.223	0.176	3.69	1.29	0.030	0.012	0.027	0.550	0
Plums—cnd—hvy syrup	25	0.102	0.028	6.59	2.53	0.238	0.005	0.010	0.434	0
Plums—cnd—lite syrup	18	0.105	0.029	4.61	2.70	0.243	0.005	0.011	0.444	0
Prunes—dried	68	0.739	0.145	17.80	14.50	0.702	0.023	0.046	2.700	0
Prune juice—bottled	20	0.172	0.009	4.95	3.43	0.334	0.005	0.020	0.310	0
Raisins—seedless	85	0.914	0.130	22.50	13.90	0.594	0.044	0.025	1.670	0
Raspberries—fresh	14	0.256	0.157	3.27	6.22	0.162	0.009	0.026	1.770	0
Raspberries—canned w/liq	26	0.235	0.034	6.62	2.99	0.120	0.006	0.009	1.200	0
Raspberries—frozen	29	0.197	0.044	7.42	4.30	0.184	0.005	0.013	1.300	0
Rhubarb—raw—diced	6	0.253	0.056	1.29	39.50	0.062	0.006	0.009	0.737	0
Rhubarb—cooked w/sugar	33	0.111	0.013	8.85	41.10	0.060	0.005	0.006	0.624	0
Strawberries—fresh	9	0.173	0.105	2.00	4.00	0.108	0.006	0.019	0.736	0
Strawberries—frozen	10	0.120	0.030	2.59	4.38	0.213	0.006	0.010	0.736	0
Tangerine—fresh	13	0.179	0.054	3.17	4.05	0.028	0.030	0.006	0.574	0
Tangerines—cnd—lite syrup	17	0.127	0.028	4.61	2.03	0.105	0.015	0.012	0.453	0
Watermelon	9	0.175	0.121	2.04	2.24	0.048	0.023	0.006	0.114	0

Meats	kcal	Protein (g)	Fat (g)	CHO (g)	Ca (mg)	Fe (mg)	B_1 (mg)	B_2 (mg)	Fiber (g)	Cholesterol (mg)
Beef chuck—pot rstd	108	7.20	8.64	0	3.67	0.840	0.020	0.065	0	29.0
Beef chuck—pot rstd—lean	77	8.80	4.34	0	3.67	1.040	0.024	0.080	0	30.0
Beef round—pot rstd—lean & fat	74	8.44	4.20	0	1.67	0.920	0.020	0.069	0	27.0
Beef round—pot rstd lean	63	8.97	2.74	0	1.33	0.980	0.021	0.074	0	27.0
Ground beef—lean	77	7.00	5.34	0	3.00	0.600	0.013	0.060	0	24.7
Ground beef—regular	82	6.67	5.94	0	3.00	0.700	0.010	0.053	0	25.3
Sirloin steak—lean	57	8.10	2.53	0	2.33	0.700	0.026	0.056	0	21.7
T-bone steak—lean & fat	92	6.80	6.97	0	2.67	0.720	0.026	0.059	0	23.7
Beef lunchmt—thin-sliced	50	7.96	1.09	1.62	2.99	0.759	0.023	0.054	0	12.0
Beef lunchmeat—loaf/roll	87	4.06	7.42	0.82	2.99	0.659	0.030	0.062	0	18.0
Beef rib—oven rstd—lean	68	7.70	3.90	0	3.34	0.740	0.023	0.060	0	22.7
Beef round—oven rstd—lean	54	8.14	2.12	0	1.67	0.834	0.028	0.076	0	23.0
Beef rump roast—lean only	51	8.40	1.89	0	1.13	0.567	0.026	0.049	0	19.6
Beef brains—pan-fried	56	3.57	4.50	0	2.67	0.630	0.037	0.074	0	566.0
Beef heart	47	8.17	1.59	0.12	1.67	2.130	0.040	0.436	0	54.7
Beef kidney	41	7.23	0.97	0.27	5.00	2.070	0.054	1.150	0	110.0
Beef liver—fried	61	7.57	2.27	2.23	3.00	1.780	0.060	1.170	0	137.0
Beef tongue—cooked	80	6.27	5.87	0.09	2.00	0.960	0.009	0.009	0	30.4
Beef tripe—raw	28	4.14	1.12	0	36.00	0.553	0.002	0.047	0	26.9
Beef tripe—pickled	17	3.29	0.40	0	25.00	0.389	0	0.028	0	15.0
Corned beef—canned	71	7.67	4.24	0	5.67	0.590	0.006	0.042	0	24.3
Corned beef hash—canned	49	2.35	1.29	2.82	3.74	0.567	0.016	0.052	0.153	17.0

Meats (cont.)	kcal	Protein (g)	Fat (g)	CHO (g)	Ca (mg)	Fe (mg)	B_1 (mg)	B_2 (mg)	Fiber (g)	Cholesterol (mg)
Beef—dried/cured	47	8.24	1.10	0.44	2.00	1.280	0.050	0.230	0	45.9
Beef & veg stew	26	1.85	1.27	1.74	3.36	0.336	0.017	0.020	0.393	8.2
Beef stew—canned	22	1.64	0.88	2.06	2.66	0.368	0.008	0.014	0.150	1.7
Burrito—beef & bean	63	3.40	2.84	6.48	26.70	0.437	0.042	0.047	0.810	8.4
Tostada w/beans & beef	49	2.72	3.06	2.98	27.50	0.319	0.012	0.036	0.583	9.1
Beef + macaroni + tom	24	1.25	0.73	3.16	3.81	0.300	0.024	0.021	0.291	2.8
Beef enchilada	69	3.09	3.26	3.69	60.20	0.418	0.017	0.039	0.465	8.9
Frankfurter—beef	92	3.20	8.36	0.68	3.48	0.378	0.014	0.029	0	13.4
Frankfurter—beef & pork	91	3.20	8.26	0.73	2.98	0.328	0.056	0.034	0	14.4
Beef pot pie—fr/frozen	52	1.99	2.73	4.77	2.42	0.436	0.022	0.018	0.109	5.0
Beef pot pie—recipe	70	2.84	4.05	5.27	3.92	0.513	0.039	0.039	0.155	5.7
Beef taco	75	4.94	4.80	3.67	30.90	0.469	0.010	0.049	0.407	16.2
Chicken meat—all-fried	62	8.67	2.59	0.48	4.86	0.383	0.024	0.056	0.002	26.5
Chicken meat—all-roasted	54	8.20	2.10	0	4.25	0.342	0.020	0.050	0	25.3
Chicken meat—all-stewed	50	7.74	1.90	0	4.05	0.330	0.014	0.046	0	23.5
Boned chicken w/broth	47	6.17	2.26	0	3.99	0.439	0.004	0.037	0	17.6
Chicken—dark meat—fried	68	8.22	3.30	0.74	5.06	0.423	0.026	0.070	0.002	27.3
Chicken—dark meat—roasted	58	7.76	2.75	0	4.25	0.377	0.020	0.064	0	26.3
Chicken—dark meat—stewed	55	7.37	2.55	0	4.05	0.385	0.016	0.057	0	24.9
Chicken—light meat—fried	54	9.31	1.57	0.12	4.45	0.322	0.020	0.036	0	25.3
Chicken—light meat—roastd	49	8.77	1.28	0	4.25	0.302	0.018	0.033	0	23.9
Chicken—light meat—stewed	45	8.18	1.17	0	3.64	0.265	0.012	0.033	0	21.7
Chick breast—no skin	47	8.80	0.99	0	4.29	0.295	0.020	0.032	0	24.0
Chick breast meat—stewed	43	8.20	0.86	0	3.58	0.250	0.012	0.034	0	21.8
Chick drumstick—battr frd	76	6.22	4.45	2.36	4.73	0.382	0.032	0.061	0.008	24.4
Chick drumstick—roasted	61	7.69	3.16	0	3.27	0.376	0.020	0.061	0	26.2
Chick wing—batter-fried	92	5.64	6.19	3.10	5.79	0.365	0.030	0.043	0.012	22.6
Chick wing—flour-fried	91	7.40	6.28	0.67	4.43	0.354	0.017	0.039	0.009	23.0
Chick wing—roasted	83	7.48	5.53	0	4.17	0.359	0.012	0.037	0	24.2
Chicken gizzards—simmered	44	7.73	1.04	0.32	2.58	1.180	0.008	0.070	0	54.9
Chicken hearts—simmered	52	7.49	2.23	0.03	5.27	2.560	0.017	0.206	0	68.7
Chicken livers—simmered	44	6.90	1.55	0.25	4.05	2.400	0.043	0.496	0	179.0
Chicken roll—light meat	45	5.52	2.08	0.69	11.90	0.274	0.018	0.037	0	13.9
Chicken frankfurter	73	3.67	5.52	1.93	27.00	0.567	0.019	0.033	0	28.4
Chicken a la king	54	3.12	3.93	1.39	14.70	0.289	0.012	0.049	0.154	25.6
Chicken + noodles	43	2.60	2.13	3.07	3.07	0.278	0.006	0.020	0.142	12.2
Chicken chow mein	29	2.60	1.25	1.13	6.58	0.284	0.009	0.026	0.466	8.5
Chicken curry	26	2.21	1.53	0.64	2.52	0.170	0.009	0.019	0.033	5.3
Chicken frankfurter	72	3.67	5.52	1.93	27.00	0.567	0.019	0.033	0	28.4
Chicken pot pie—fr/frozen	53	1.84	2.84	5.08	3.70	0.382	0.020	0.020	0.210	4.9
Chicken roll—light meat	45	5.52	2.08	0.69	11.90	0.274	0.018	0.037	0	13.9
Chicken salad w/celery	97	3.82	8.90	0.47	5.92	0.239	0.012	0.028	0.109	17.3
Chicken patty sandwich	79	4.48	4.06	6.10	7.95	0.338	0.052	0.047	0.244	12.3
Chicken broth—from dry	2	0.16	0.13	0.17	1.74	0.009	0	0.004	0.001	0.1
Chicken broth—from cube	2	0.11	0.04	0.18	0.04	0.014	0.001	0.003	0	0.1
Chicken noodle soup	9	0.48	0.29	1.10	2.00	0.092	0.006	0.007	0.085	0.8
Tostada w/beans/chicken	45	3.50	2.06	3.38	29.30	0.305	0.013	0.034	0.668	9.6
Chicken taco	63	5.60	3.03	3.67	31.60	0.327	0.014	0.043	0.407	16.5
Chicken enchilada	64	3.38	2.48	3.69	60.50	0.359	0.018	0.036	0.465	9.1

Meats (cont.)	kcal	Protein (g)	Fat (g)	CHO (g)	Ca (mg)	Fe (mg)	B_1 (mg)	B_2 (mg)	Fiber (g)	Cholesterol (mg)
Turkey dark meat—roasted	53	8.10	2.05	0	9.11	0.662	0.018	0.070	0	24.0
Turkey white meat—roasted	44	8.48	0.91	0	5.47	0.380	0.017	0.037	0	19.6
Turkey breast—barbecued	40	6.39	1.40	0	2.00	0.120	0.010	0.030	0	16.0
Turkey gizzards	46	8.34	1.10	0.17	4.32	1.540	0.009	0.093	0	65.6
Turkey hearts	50	7.58	1.73	0.58	3.72	1.950	0.019	0.250	0	64.0
Turkey livers	48	6.80	1.69	0.97	3.02	2.210	0.015	0.404	0	177.0
Turkey loaf	31	6.38	0.45	0	2.00	0.113	0.011	0.030	0	11.6
Turkey roll	41	5.27	2.03	0.15	11.40	0.358	0.025	0.064	0	11.9
Turkey bologna	56	3.86	4.27	0.27	23.40	0.432	0.015	0.047	0	28.0
Turkey frankfurter	64	4.05	5.22	0.42	36.50	0.485	0.023	0.050	0	24.6
Turkey ham	36	5.37	1.49	0.42	2.49	0.776	0.020	0.075	0	15.9
Turkey pastrami	37	5.22	1.75	0.43	2.49	0.403	0.022	0.075	0	14.9
Turkey salami	55	4.62	3.89	0.15	5.47	0.463	0.029	0.075	0	22.9
Turkey pot pie—frozen	51	1.80	2.75	4.65	7.79	0.256	0.020	0.020	0.110	2.4

Eggs	kcal	Protein (g)	Fat (g)	CHO (g)	Ca (mg)	Fe (mg)	B_1 (mg)	B_2 (mg)	Fiber (g)	Cholesterol (mg)
Egg white, cooked	13	2.68	0	0.33	3.20	0.008	0.002	0.072	0	0
Egg yolk, cooked	108	4.76	8.73	0.07	44.40	1.620	0.044	0.121	0	355.0
Egg, fried in butter	56	3.54	3.45	0.38	15.70	0.536	0.018	0.148	0	129.0
Egg, hard cooked	40	3.52	2.79	0.34	13.80	0.474	0.014	0.132	0	113.0
Egg, poached	40	3.50	2.79	0.34	13.80	0.474	0.014	0.132	0	113.0
Egg, scrambled milk + butter	40	2.88	2.57	0.61	23.90	0.412	0.013	0.106	0	93.9
Egg raw—large	40	3.52	2.79	0.34	13.80	0.474	0.017	0.139	0	113.0
Egg white—raw	13	2.68	0	0.33	3.20	0.008	0.002	0.075	0	0
Egg yolk, raw	108	4.76	8.73	0.07	44.40	1.620	0.051	0.126	0	355.0
Egg substitute, frozen	45	3.20	3.15	0.91	20.80	0.562	0.034	0.110	0	0.5
Egg substitute, powder	125	15.60	3.66	6.12	90.70	0.879	0.062	0.493	0	162.0

Dairy Products	kcal	Protein (g)	Fat (g)	CHO (g)	Ca (mg)	Fe (mg)	B_1 (mg)	B_2 (mg)	Fiber (g)	Cholesterol (mg)
Milk—1% lowfat	12	0.93	0.30	1.36	34.9	0.014	0.011	0.047	0	1.16
Milk—2% lowfat	14	0.94	0.56	1.36	34.5	0.012	0.011	0.047	0	2.56
Milk—skim	10	0.97	0.05	1.38	34.9	0.012	0.010	0.040	0	0.46
Milk—whole	17	0.93	0.95	1.32	33.8	0.014	0.010	0.046	0	3.83
Buttermilk	12	0.94	0.25	1.35	33.0	0.014	0.010	0.044	0	1.04
Milk—instant nonfat dry	102	9.96	0.21	14.80	349.0	0.088	0.117	0.496	0	5.00
Canned skim milk—evap	22	2.11	0.06	3.22	82.0	0.078	0.013	0.088	0	1.11
Canned whole milk—evap	38	1.91	2.20	2.81	73.9	0.054	0.014	0.090	0	8.33
Carob flavor mix—powder	106	0.47	0.05	26.50	0	1.300	0.002	0	4.020	0
Chocolate milk—1%	18	0.92	0.28	2.96	32.5	0.068	0.010	0.047	0.425	0.79
Chocolate milk—2%	20	0.91	0.57	2.95	32.2	0.068	0.010	0.046	0.425	1.93
Chocolate milk—whole	24	0.90	0.96	2.94	31.8	0.068	0.010	0.046	0.425	3.52
Hot cocoa—with whole milk	25	1.03	1.03	2.93	33.8	0.088	0.012	0.049	0.340	3.74
Inst breakfast w/2% milk	25	1.52	0.47	3.50	31.0	0.807	0.040	0.048	0	1.82
Inst breakfast w/1% milk	23	1.51	0.25	3.50	31.3	0.807	0.040	0.048	0	1.00
Inst breakfast w/skim milk	22	1.55	0.04	3.50	31.4	0.804	0.039	0.041	0	0.40
Inst breakfast w/whl milk	28	1.51	0.82	3.47	30.4	0.807	0.040	0.047	0	3.33
Egg nog	38	1.08	2.12	3.84	36.8	0.057	0.010	0.054	0	16.60

Dairy Products (cont.)	kcal	Protein (g)	Fat (g)	CHO (g)	Ca (mg)	Fe (mg)	B_1 (mg)	B_2 (mg)	Fiber (g)	Cholesterol (mg)
Kefir	20	1.13	0.55	1.07	42.6	0.060	0.055	0.054	0	1.22
Malt powder—choc flavored	107	1.49	1.08	24.80	17.6	0.648	0.049	0.057	0.540	1.35
Malted milk powder	117	3.12	2.30	21.50	85.0	0.209	0.143	0.260	0.405	5.40
Malted milk drink—choc	25	1.00	0.95	3.19	32.5	0.064	0.014	0.047	0.043	3.64
Chocolate milkshake	36	0.96	1.05	5.80	32.0	0.088	0.016	0.069	0.035	3.70
Strawberry milkshake	32	0.95	0.80	5.35	32.0	0.030	0.013	0.055	0.024	3.10
Vanilla milkshake	32	0.98	0.84	5.09	34.5	0.026	0.013	0.052	0.019	3.20
Ovaltine powder—choc flvr	102	2.00	0.85	23.70	134.0	6.190	0.719	0.772	0.013	0
Ovaltine powder—malt flvr	104	2.53	0.24	23.60	106.0	5.820	0.772	1.010	0.040	0
Ovaltine drink—choc flvr	24	1.02	0.94	3.12	41.9	0.510	0.067	0.104	0.001	3.53
Ovaltine drink—malt flvr	24	1.06	0.89	3.10	39.7	0.480	0.072	0.124	0.003	3.53
Milk—goat	20	1.00	1.17	1.27	37.9	0.014	0.014	0.039	0	3.25
Milk—sheep	31	1.70	1.99	1.52	54.8	0.028	0.018	0.100	0	0
Milk—soybean	9	0.78	0.54	0.51	1.2	0.163	0.046	0.020	0	0
Ice cream—regular-vanilla	57	1.02	3.05	6.76	37.5	0.026	0.011	0.070	0	12.60
Ice cream—rich-vanilla	67	0.79	4.54	6.13	28.9	0.019	0.008	0.054	0	16.90
Ice cream—soft-serve	62	1.15	3.69	6.28	38.7	0.070	0.013	0.073	0	25.00
Creamsicle ice cream bar	44	0.52	1.33	7.56	19.8	0	0.009	0.034	0	0
Drumstick ice cream bar	88	1.23	4.68	10.20	31.7	0.047	0.009	0.043	0	0
Fudgesicle ice cream bar	35	1.48	0.08	7.22	50.0	0.039	0.012	0.070	0	0
Ice milk	40	1.12	1.22	6.28	38.0	0.039	0.016	0.075	0	3.90
Ice milk—soft-serve—3% fat	36	1.30	0.75	6.22	44.4	0.045	0.019	0.088	0	2.10
Yogurt—coffee-vanilla	24	1.40	0.35	3.90	48.5	0.020	0.012	0.057	0	1.42
Yogurt—lowfat with fruit	29	1.24	0.31	5.37	43.0	0.020	0.010	0.050	0	1.25
Yogurt—lowfat-plain	18	1.49	0.43	2.00	51.8	0.022	0.012	0.060	0	1.75
Yogurt—nonfat milk	16	1.62	0.05	2.17	56.5	0.025	0.014	0.066	0	0.50
Yogurt—whole milk	17	0.98	0.92	1.32	34.3	0.014	0.008	0.040	0	3.68

Vegetables	kcal	Protein (g)	Fat (g)	CHO (g)	Ca (mg)	Fe (mg)	B_1 (mg)	B_2 (mg)	Fiber (g)	Cholesterol (mg)
Alfalfa sprouts	9	1.13	0.200	1.07	9.5	0.272	0.021	0.036	1.030	0
Artichoke hearts—marinated	28	0.680	0.250	2.18	6.5	0.270	0.010	0.029	1.780	0
Asparagus—raw spears	6	0.865	0.063	1.05	6.4	0.193	0.032	0.035	0.395	0
Asparagus—canned spears	5	0.606	0.184	0.70	3.9	0.177	0.017	0.025	0.454	0
Bamboo shoots—sliced—raw	8	0.738	0.088	1.47	3.8	0.143	0.043	0.020	0.738	0
Bamboo shoots—sliced, canned	5	0.489	0.113	0.91	2.2	0.090	0.007	0.007	0.706	0
Bean sprouts—fresh raw	9	0.861	0.050	1.68	3.8	0.258	0.024	0.035	0.736	0
Bean sprouts—boiled	6	0.576	0.025	1.19	3.4	0.185	0.014	0.029	0.572	0
Bean sprouts—stir fried	14	1.220	0.059	3.00	3.7	0.549	0.040	0.050	0.777	0
Black beans—cooked	37	2.500	0.152	6.72	7.8	0.593	0.069	0.017	2.540	0
Green beans—raw uncooked	9	0.515	0.034	2.02	10.6	0.363	0.024	0.030	0.644	0
Green beans—fresh—cooked	10	0.535	0.082	2.24	13.2	0.363	0.021	0.027	0.737	0
Green beans—frzn—cooked	8	0.386	0.038	1.73	12.8	0.233	0.014	0.021	0.880	0
Green beans—canned/draind	6	0.326	0.028	1.28	7.6	0.256	0.004	0.016	0.378	0

Vegetables (cont.)	kcal	Protein (g)	Fat (g)	CHO (g)	Ca (mg)	Fe (mg)	B_1 (mg)	B_2 (mg)	Fiber (g)	Cholesterol (mg)
Red kidney beans—dry	94	6.690	0.234	16.90	40.5	2.330	0.150	0.062	6.160	0
Lima beans—dry large	96	6.080	0.194	18.00	22.9	2.130	0.144	0.057	8.600	0
Lima beans—fresh-cooked	35	1.930	0.090	6.70	9.0	0.695	0.040	0.027	2.670	0
Lima beans—dry small	98	5.790	0.397	18.20	18.4	2.270	0.136	0.048	8.500	0
Lima beans—canned/drained	27	1.530	0.100	5.20	8.0	0.487	0.010	0.013	2.420	0
Beans w/franks—canned	40	1.900	1.860	4.37	13.6	0.490	0.016	0.016	1.950	1.7
Pork & beans—canned	32	1.500	0.413	5.95	17.4	0.470	0.013	0.017	1.560	1.9
Navy beans—dry, cooked	40	2.460	0.162	7.77	19.9	0.703	0.057	0.017	2.490	0
Pinto beans—dry, cooked	39	2.320	0.148	7.28	13.6	0.741	0.053	0.026	3.230	0
Refried beans—canned	30	1.770	0.303	5.24	13.2	0.500	0.014	0.016	2.470	0
Soybeans—dry	118	10.400	5.650	8.55	78.5	4.450	0.248	0.247	1.570	0
White beans—dry	95	5.990	0.334	17.70	36.0	2.190	0.210	0.059	0.766	0
White beans—dry, cooked	40	2.550	0.182	7.32	20.7	0.808	0.067	0.017	2.230	0
Yellow wax beans—raw	9	0.515	0.034	2.02	10.6	0.294	0.024	0.030	0.644	0
Yellow wax beans—raw	10	0.535	0.082	2.24	13.2	0.363	0.021	0.027	0.726	0
Yellow wax beans—frzn	8	0.386	0.038	1.73	12.8	0.233	0.014	0.021	0.880	0
Beets—cooked	9	0.300	0.014	1.90	3.1	0.176	0.009	0.004	0.539	0
Beets—pickled slices	18	0.227	0.028	4.63	3.1	0.116	0.006	0.014	0.587	0
Broccoli—raw chopped	8	0.844	0.097	1.49	13.5	0.251	0.019	0.034	0.934	0
Broccoli—raw spears	8	0.845	0.098	1.49	13.5	0.250	0.018	0.034	0.935	0
Broccoli—frzn ckd spears	8	0.879	0.034	1.51	14.5	0.173	0.015	0.023	0.826	0
Brussels sprouts—raw	12	0.960	0.084	2.54	11.6	0.396	0.039	0.026	1.260	0
Brussels sprouts—ckd	11	1.090	0.145	2.45	10.2	0.342	0.030	0.023	1.220	0
Brussels sprouts—frzn, ckd	12	1.030	0.112	2.36	7.0	0.210	0.029	0.032	1.230	0
Cabbage—raw, shredded	7	0.340	0.049	1.52	13.0	0.162	0.015	0.009	0.680	0
Cabbage—cooked	6	0.272	0.070	1.35	9.5	0.110	0.016	0.016	0.661	0
Bok choy—raw, shredded	4	0.425	0.057	0.62	30.0	0.227	0.011	0.020	0.486	0
Bok choy—cooked	3	0.442	0.045	0.51	26.3	0.295	0.009	0.018	0.454	0
Red cabbage—raw	8	0.393	0.073	1.74	14.6	0.142	0.018	0.009	0.648	0
Red cabbage—cooked	6	0.299	0.057	1.32	10.6	0.102	0.010	0.006	1.567	0
Carrot—whole, raw	12	0.291	0.055	2.87	7.5	0.142	0.028	0.017	1.906	0
Carrot—grated, raw	12	0.289	0.052	2.88	7.7	0.142	0.027	0.016	0.907	0
Carrots—sliced, cooked	13	0.309	0.050	2.97	8.7	0.176	0.010	0.016	0.992	0
Carrots—fr/frozen, cooked	10	0.338	0.031	2.34	8.2	0.136	0.008	0.010	1.050	0
Carrots—canned, drained	7	0.183	0.054	1.57	7.4	0.181	0.005	0.009	0.435	0
Carrot juice	11	0.267	0.041	2.63	6.7	0.130	0.026	0.015	0.385	0
Cauliflower—raw	7	0.561	0.051	1.39	7.9	0.164	0.022	0.016	0.720	0
Cauliflower—cooked	7	0.530	0.050	1.31	7.8	0.119	0.018	0.018	0.622	0
Cauliflower—frozen, cooked	5	0.457	0.061	1.06	4.9	0.116	0.010	0.015	0.535	0
Celery—raw—chopped	5	0.189	0.033	1.03	10.4	0.137	0.009	0.009	0.472	0
Swiss chard—raw	5	0.510	0.057	1.06	14.5	0.510	0.011	0.025	0.512	0
Swiss chard—cooked	6	0.533	0.023	1.17	16.5	0.642	0.010	0.024	0.616	0
Collards—fresh	5	0.445	0.062	1.07	33.0	0.299	0.009	0.018	0.590	0
Collards—fresh, cooked	4	0.313	0.043	0.75	22.0	0.116	0.005	0.012	0.798	0
Collards—frozen, cooked	10	0.840	0.115	2.02	59.5	0.317	0.013	0.033	0.794	0
Corn—kernels raw	24	0.913	0.335	5.38	0.6	0.147	0.057	0.017	1.220	0
Corn on cob—cooked	31	0.943	0.363	7.14	0.6	0.173	0.061	0.020	1.190	0
Corn—cooked from frozen	23	0.857	0.020	5.80	0.6	0.085	0.020	0.020	1.190	0
Corn—canned, drained	23	0.743	0.283	5.26	1.4	0.142	0.009	0.014	0.398	0
Corn—canned cream style	21	0.494	0.119	5.14	0.9	0.108	0.007	0.015	0.354	0
Cucumber slices w/peel	4	0.153	0.037	0.82	4.0	0.079	0.009	0.006	0.329	0
Eggplant—cooked	8	0.236	0.066	1.88	1.7	0.099	0.022	0.006	1.060	0

Vegetables (cont.)	kcal	Protein (g)	Fat (g)	CHO (g)	Ca (mg)	Fe (mg)	B_1 (mg)	B_2 (mg)	Fiber (g)	Cholesterol (mg)
Escarole/curly endive—chp	5	0.354	0.057	0.95	14.7	0.235	0.023	0.022	0.369	0
Garbanzo/chickpeas—dry	103	5.470	1.720	17.20	29.9	1.770	0.135	0.060	5.390	0
Garbanzo/chickpeas—cooked	47	2.500	0.735	7.78	13.8	0.819	0.033	0.018	1.920	0
Jerusalem artichoke—raw	22	0.567	0.004	4.95	4.0	0.964	0.057	0.017	0.369	0
Kale—fresh, chopped	14	0.935	0.198	2.84	38.0	0.482	0.031	0.037	1.650	0
Kohlrabi—raw slices	8	0.482	0.028	1.76	6.9	0.113	0.014	0.006	0.405	0
Kohlrabi—cooked	8	0.510	0.030	1.96	7.0	0.113	0.011	0.006	0.395	0
Leeks—chopped raw	17	0.425	0.085	4.00	16.7	0.594	0.017	0.008	0.668	0
Leeks—cooked, chopped	9	0.230	0.057	2.16	8.5	0.310	0.007	0.006	0.927	0
Lentils—dry	96	7.960	0.273	16.20	14.6	2.550	0.135	0.069	3.400	0
Lentils—cooked from dry	33	2.560	0.106	5.73	5.3	0.944	0.048	0.020	1.430	0
Lentils—sprouted, raw	30	2.540	0.156	6.30	7.0	0.909	0.065	0.036	1.150	0
Lettuce—butterhead	4	0.367	0.062	0.66	9.5	0.085	0.017	0.017	0.397	0
Lettuce—iceberg	4	0.286	0.054	0.59	5.4	0.142	0.013	0.009	0.347	0
Lettuce—romaine	5	0.459	0.057	0.67	10.2	0.312	0.028	0.028	0.482	0
Mushrooms—raw sliced	7	0.593	0.119	1.32	1.4	0.352	0.029	0.127	0.508	0
Mushrooms—cooked	8	0.614	0.134	1.46	1.7	0.494	0.020	0.085	0.625	0
Mushrooms—canned, drained	7	0.530	0.082	1.40	3.1	0.224	0.017	0.063	0.596	0
Mustard greens—fresh	7	0.764	0.057	1.39	29.4	0.414	0.023	0.031	0.764	0
Mustard greens—ckd	4	0.640	0.068	0.60	21.0	0.316	0.012	0.018	0.587	0
Okra pods—cooked	9	0.530	0.048	2.04	17.9	0.128	0.037	0.016	0.624	0
Okra slices—cooked	11	0.589	0.085	2.32	27.1	0.190	0.028	0.035	0.709	0
Onions—chopped, raw	10	0.335	0.074	2.07	7.1	0.105	0.017	0.003	0.454	0
Onion slices—raw	10	0.335	0.074	2.08	7.2	0.105	0.017	0.003	0.454	0
Onion—dehydrated flakes	91	2.530	0.122	23.70	72.9	0.446	0.022	0.018	2.510	0
Onion rings—frozen, heated	115	1.520	7.570	10.80	8.8	0.482	0.079	0.040	0.240	0
Parsley—freeze dried	81	8.910	1.420	11.90	40.5	15.200	0.304	0.648	22.000	0
Parsley—fresh chopped	9	0.624	0.085	1.96	36.9	1.760	0.023	0.031	1.550	0
Parsnips—sliced raw	21	0.341	0.085	5.09	10.0	0.167	0.026	0.014	1.280	0
Fresh peas—uncooked	23	1.530	0.113	4.10	7.0	0.416	0.075	0.037	1.380	0
Peas—cooked	24	1.520	0.060	4.43	7.8	0.438	0.073	0.042	1.360	0
Peas—frozen, cooked	22	1.460	0.078	4.04	6.7	0.443	0.080	0.050	1.280	0
Peas—edible pods—fresh	12	0.794	0.057	2.15	12.1	0.589	0.043	0.023	0.794	0
Split peas—dry	97	6.970	0.328	17.10	15.5	1.250	0.206	0.061	4.030	0
Peas + carrots—frzn, ckd	14	0.875	0.120	2.87	6.4	0.266	0.064	0.020	1.170	0
Green chili pepper—raw	11	0.557	0.057	2.68	5.0	0.340	0.026	0.026	0.504	0
Red chili peppers—raw/chopped	11	0.567	0.057	2.68	4.9	0.340	0.026	0.026	0.454	0
Jalapeno peppers—cnd/chopped	7	0.225	0.170	1.39	7.5	0.792	0.008	0.014	0.850	0
Baked potato with skin	31	0.653	0.028	7.16	2.8	0.386	0.030	0.009	0.660	0
Baked potato—flesh only	26	0.556	0.029	6.10	1.5	0.100	0.030	0.006	0.436	0
Potato skin—oven baked	56	1.220	0.029	13.20	9.8	1.080	0.035	0.034	1.130	0
Potato + peel—microwaved	30	0.692	0.028	6.83	3.1	0.350	0.034	0.009	0.660	0
Peeled potato—boiled	24	0.485	0.029	5.67	2.1	0.088	0.028	0.005	0.426	0
French fries—oven heated	63	0.980	2.480	9.64	2.3	0.380	0.035	0.009	0.567	0
French fries—frzn—veg oil	90	1.140	4.690	11.20	5.7	0.215	0.050	0.008	0.567	0
Cottage-fried potatoes	62	0.975	2.320	9.64	2.8	0.425	0.034	0.009	0.567	0
Hash-brown potatoes	30	0.343	1.980	3.02	1.1	0.115	0.010	0.003	0.567	0
Mashed potatoes prep/milk	22	0.548	0.166	4.98	7.4	0.077	0.025	0.011	0.405	0.5
Mashed potatoes—mlk & margarine	30	0.533	1.200	4.74	7.3	0.074	0.024	0.014	0.405	0.5

Vegetables (cont.)	kcal	Protein (g)	Fat (g)	CHO (g)	Ca (mg)	Fe (mg)	B_1 (mg)	B_2 (mg)	Fiber (g)	Cholesterol (mg)
Potato pancakes	88	1.730	4.700	9.85	7.8	0.451	0.039	0.035	0.563	34.7
Potatoes au gratin mix	26	0.653	1.170	3.65	23.5	0.090	0.006	0.023	0.487	1.4
Scalloped potatoes—recipe	24	0.813	1.040	3.05	16.2	0.163	0.020	0.026	0.289	3.4
Potato chips	148	1.590	10.000	14.70	7.0	0.339	0.040	0.006	1.360	0
Potato flour	100	2.260	0.226	22.60	9.3	4.880	0.119	0.040	0.317	0
Pumpkin—canned	10	0.311	0.080	2.28	7.4	0.394	0.007	0.015	0.519	0
Red radishes	4	0.170	0.151	1.01	5.7	0.082	0.001	0.013	0.624	0
Rutabaga—cooked cubes	10	0.314	0.053	2.19	12.0	0.133	0.020	0.010	0.434	0
Sauerkraut—canned w/ liqd	5	0.258	0.040	1.21	8.7	0.417	0.006	0.006	0.529	0
Soybeans—mature, raw	37	3.700	1.900	3.17	19.4	0.599	0.096	0.033	0.656	0
Spinach—cooked from fresh	7	0.843	0.074	1.06	38.4	1.010	0.027	0.067	0.702	0
Summer squash—raw slices	6	0.334	0.061	1.23	5.7	0.130	0.018	0.010	0.425	0
Zucchini squash—cooked	5	0.181	0.014	1.11	3.6	0.099	0.012	0.012	0.567	0
Acorn squash—boiled/ mashed	10	0.190	0.023	2.49	7.5	0.159	0.028	0.002	0.680	0
Butternut squash—bkd—cube	12	0.256	0.026	2.97	11.6	0.170	0.020	0.005	0.794	0
Spaghetti squash—baked/boiled	8	0.187	0.073	1.83	6.0	0.095	0.010	0.006	0.794	0
Winter squash—boiled	10	0.319	0.050	2.40	5.2	0.136	0.018	0.006	0.794	0
Sweet potato—bkd in skin	29	0.487	0.032	6.89	8.0	0.129	0.020	0.036	0.850	0
Candied sweet potatoes	39	0.246	0.920	7.91	7.3	0.324	0.005	0.012	0.545	0
Tofu (soybean curd)	22	2.290	1.360	0.53	29.7	1.520	0.023	0.015	0.343	0
Tomato—fresh whole	6	0.251	0.060	1.23	2.1	0.136	0.017	0.014	0.415	0
Tomatoes—whole canned	6	0.265	0.070	1.22	7.4	0.171	0.013	0.009	0.298	0
Tomato sauce—canned	9	0.376	0.047	2.04	3.9	0.218	0.019	0.016	0.425	0
Tomato paste—canned	24	1.070	0.249	5.33	9.9	0.848	0.044	0.054	1.210	0
Tomato juice—canned	5	0.215	0.017	1.20	2.6	0.164	0.013	0.009	0.220	0
Turnip cubes—raw	8	0.255	0.028	1.76	8.5	0.085	0.011	0.009	0.587	0
Mixed vegetables—frzn, cooked	17	0.812	0.043	3.70	7.2	0.232	0.020	0.034	1.120	0
Vegetable juice cocktail	6	0.178	0.026	1.29	3.1	0.119	0.012	0.008	0.178	0
Water chestnuts—raw	30	0.398	0.027	6.77	3.2	0.170	0.040	0.057	0.869	0
Watercress—fresh	3	0.650	0.033	0.37	33.4	0.050	0.025	0.033	0.719	0
White yams—raw	34	0.438	0.049	7.90	8.7	0.153	0.032	0.009	0.822	0

Salad Bar	kcal	Protein (g)	Fat (g)	CHO (g)	Ca (mg)	Fe (mg)	B_1 (mg)	B_2 (mg)	Fiber (g)	Cholesterol (mg)
Alfalfa sprouts	8.59	1.130	0.196	1.070	9.45	0.272	0.021	0.036	1.030	0
Artichoke hearts, marinatd	28.00	0.680	2.250	2.180	6.50	0.270	0.010	0.029	1.780	0
Asparagus	6.35	0.867	0.062	1.050	6.35	0.193	0.032	0.035	0.432	0
Avocado	45.70	0.563	4.340	2.100	3.07	0.284	0.030	0.035	2.720	0
Bacon, regular	163.00	8.640	14.000	0.164	2.98	0.482	0.195	0.080	0	23.9
Bean sprouts	8.50	0.861	0.050	1.680	3.82	0.258	0.024	0.035	0.736	0
Beets	8.67	0.300	0.013	1.900	3.00	0.176	0.009	0.004	0.567	0
Beets, canned, diced	9.00	0.260	0.040	2.040	4.34	0.517	0.003	0.012	0.590	0
Broccoli, raw	7.73	0.844	0.097	1.490	13.50	0.251	0.019	0.034	0.934	0
Cabbage	6.48	0.340	0.049	1.520	13.00	0.162	0.015	0.009	0.680	0
Cabbage, red	7.70	0.393	0.073	1.740	14.60	0.142	0.018	0.009	0.648	0
Carrots, grated	12.40	0.289	0.052	2.880	7.73	0.142	0.027	0.016	0.907	0
Cauliflower	6.80	0.561	0.051	1.390	7.94	0.164	0.022	0.016	0.720	0
Celery	4.54	0.189	0.033	1.030	10.40	0.137	0.009	0.009	0.472	0

Salad Bar (cont.)	kcal	Protein (g)	Fat (g)	CHO (g)	Ca (mg)	Fe (mg)	B_1 (mg)	B_2 (mg)	Fiber (g)	Cholesterol (mg)
Chicken salad	96.70	3.820	8.900	0.469	5.92	0.239	0.012	0.028	0.109	17.3
Crab, cooked	23.90	5.050	0.561	0.140	12.90	0.104	0.012	0.044	0	18.0
Croutons, dry bread cubes	105.00	3.690	1.040	20.500	35.00	1.020	0.099	0.099	0.085	0
Cucumber slices	3.69	0.153	0.037	0.824	3.99	0.079	0.009	0.006	0.329	0
Egg, chopped	40.40	3.520	2.790	0.338	13.80	0.475	0.014	0.133	0	113
Escarole/curly endive	4.82	0.354	0.057	0.953	14.70	0.235	0.023	0.022	0.369	0
Garbanzo/chickpeas, cooked	46.50	2.500	0.735	7.780	13.80	0.819	0.033	0.018	1.920	0
Green pepper, sweet	6.80	0.244	0.130	1.500	1.70	0.357	0.024	0.014	0.454	0
Ham salad	51.50	5.000	3.000	0.880	2.00	0.280	0.244	0.072	0	16
Ham, minced	74.20	4.620	5.860	0.526	2.70	0.216	0.203	0.054	0	20.2
Leeks	17.30	0.425	0.085	4.000	16.70	0.594	0.017	0.008	0.688	0
Lettuce, butterhead	3.69	0.366	0.062	0.658	9.47	0.085	0.017	0.017	0.370	0
Lettuce, iceberg	3.69	0.287	0.054	0.592	5.37	0.142	0.013	0.009	0.370	0
Lettuce, loose leaf	5.11	0.369	0.085	0.992	19.20	0.397	0.014	0.023	0.391	0
Lettuce, Romaine	4.54	0.459	0.057	0.673	10.20	0.312	0.028	0.028	0.482	0
Lobster meat	27.80	5.800	0.168	0.364	17.20	0.111	0.020	0.019	0	20.3
Mushrooms, raw	7.09	0.593	0.119	1.320	1.42	0.352	0.029	0.127	0.508	0
Onions	9.57	0.335	0.074	2.070	7.09	0.105	0.017	0.003	0.454	0
Parmesan cheese, grated	129.00	11.800	8.500	1.060	389.00	0.270	0.013	0.109	0	22.0
Peas, cooked	22.30	1.460	0.078	4.040	6.73	0.443	0.080	0.050	1.280	0
Sesame seed kernels, dried	167.00	7.480	15.500	2.660	37.20	2.210	0.204	0.024	1.950	0
Shrimp, boiled	28.00	5.930	0.306	0	11.00	0.876	0.009	0.009	0	55.3
Spinach, fresh	6.23	0.810	0.099	0.992	28.00	0.770	0.022	0.054	0.947	0
Sunflower seeds, dry	162.00	6.460	14.000	5.320	32.90	1.920	0.650	0.070	1.970	0
Tomatoes	5.51	0.252	0.061	1.230	1.89	0.135	0.017	0.014	0.416	0
Tuna salad	53.00	4.550	2.630	2.670	4.84	0.282	0.009	0.019	0.340	3.73
Turkey meat	41.30	5.270	2.030	0.149	11.40	0.358	0.025	0.064	0	11.9

Variety	kcal	Protein (g)	Fat (g)	CHO (g)	Ca (mg)	Fe (mg)	B_1 (mg)	B_2 (mg)	Fiber (g)	Cholesterol (mg)
Chips & crackers										
Doritos—nacho flavor	139	2.20	6.79	18.00	17.0	0.399	0.040	0.030	1.10	0
Doritos—taco flavor	140	2.60	6.59	17.60	44.9	0.699	0.080	0.090	1.10	0
Potato chips—sour crm onion	153	2.40	9.48	14.60	21.0	0.474	0.040	0.055	1.35	1.0
Wheat cracker—thin	124	3.19	4.96	17.70	10.6	1.060	0.142	0.106	1.84	0
Whole wheat crackers	124	3.19	5.32	17.70	10.6	1.850	0.070	0.106	2.94	0
Condiments										
Catsup	30	0.52	0.11	7.17	6.2	0.228	0.026	0.020	0.45	0
Mustard	21	1.34	1.25	1.81	23.8	0.567	0.024	0.057	0.11	0
Soy sauce	14	1.46	0.02	2.40	4.7	0.567	0.014	0.036	0	0
Deli meats										
Bologna—beef	89	3.32	8.04	0.56	3.7	0.394	0.016	0.036	0	16.0
Brotwurst	92	4.05	7.90	0.84	13.8	0.292	0.070	0.064	0	17.8
Keilbasa sausage	88	3.76	7.70	0.61	12.0	0.414	0.064	0.061	0	18.5
Knockwurst sausage	87	3.37	7.88	0.50	2.9	0.258	0.097	0.040	0	16.3
Liverwurst	93	4.00	8.10	0.63	7.9	1.810	0.077	0.291	0	44.1
Pepperoni sausage	140	5.94	12.50	0.80	2.8	0.397	0.09	0.07		9.79
Polish sausage	92	3.99	8.13	0.46	3.0	0.409	0.142	0.042	0	20.0
Salami—beef	72	4.17	5.69	0.70	2.47	0.567	0.036	0.073	0	17.3
Salami—pork & beef	72	3.94	5.70	0.64	3.68	0.755	0.068	0.106	0	18.5
Salami—turkey	55	4.62	3.89	0.15	5.47	0.463	0.029	0.075	0	22.9
Salami—dry—beef & pork	120	6.49	9.75	0.74	2.84	0.425	0.170	0.082	0	22.7
Turkey pastrami	37	5.22	1.75	0.43	2.49	0.403	0.022	0.075	0	14.9

Variety (cont.)	kcal	Protein (g)	Fat (g)	CHO (g)	Ca (mg)	Fe (mg)	B_1 (mg)	B_2 (mg)	Fiber (g)	Cholesterol (mg)
Mexican foods										
Beef taco	75.2	4.94	4.80	3.67	30.9	0.469	0.01	0.049	0.407	16.2
Beef enchilada	69.0	3.09	3.26	3.69	60.2	0.418	0.017	0.039	0.465	8.93
Cheese enchilada	78.0	3.12	4.2	3.78	108.0	0.324	0.015	0.050	0.465	10.2
Chicken enchilada	63.6	3.38	2.48	3.69	60.5	0.359	0.018	0.036	0.465	9.10
Corn tortilla, enr, reg	61.4	1.89	0.964	12.30	39.7	0.567	0.047	0.028	2.27	0
Corn tortilla, enr, thin	61.0	1.64	0.95	12.30	39.8	0.567	0.046	0.028	2.26	0
Corn tortilla, enr, fried	82.2	2.08	2.84	12.30	39.7	0.567	0.047	0.028	2.27	0
Enchirito	60.4	3.15	2.75	3.31	51.5	0.410	0.015	0.037	0.748	9.18
Flour tortilla	84	2.07	2.15	15.50	17.0	0.440	0.102	0.062	0.800	0
Refried beans, canned	30.3	1.77	0.303	5.24	13.2	0.500	0.014	0.016	2.47	0
Nuts & seeds										
Almonds—dried, chopped	167	5.65	14.80	5.78	75.5	1.040	0.060	0.220	3.36	0
Almonds—whole, toasted	167	5.77	14.40	6.48	80.0	1.400	0.037	0.170	3.99	0
Sunflower seeds—dry	162	6.46	14.00	5.32	32.9	1.920	0.650	0.070	1.97	0
Oils & shortening										
Cocoa butter oil	251	0	28.40	0	0	0			0	0
Corn oil	251	0	28.40	0	0	0.001	0	0	0	0
Cottonseed oil	251	0	28.40	0	0	0	0	0	0	0
Olive oil	251	0	28.40	0	0.1	0.109	0	0	0	0
Palm oil	251	0	28.40	0	0.1	0.003	0	0	0	0
Palm kernel oil	251	0	28.40	0	0	0	0	0	0	0
Peanut oil	251	0	28.40	0	0	0.008	0	0	0	0
Safflower oil	251	0	28.40	0	0	0	0	0	0	0
Sesame oil	250	0	28.40	0	0	0	0	0	0	0
Soybean oil	251	0	28.40	0	0	0.007	0	0	0	0
Sunflower oil	251	0	28.40	0	0	0.	0	0	0	0
Walnut oil	251	0	28.40	0	0	0.	0	0	0	0
Wheat germ oil	250	0	28.40	0	0	0.	0	0	0	0
Vegetable shortening	251	0	28.40	0	0	0.	0	0	0	0
Pasta & noodles										
Spaghetti, ckd firm, hot	41	1.42	0.142	8.53	3.1	0.454	0.051	0.028	0.482	0
Spaghetti, ckd tender, hot	31	1.01	0.111	6.48	3.0	0.405	0.04	0.022	0.425	0
Whole wheat spaghetti, ckd	35	1.53	0.113	7.49	4.3	0.244	0.048	0.020	1.040	0
Spaghetti + sce + cheese, cnd	22	0.68	0.227	4.42	4.5	0.318	0.040	0.032	0.284	0.3
Spaghetti + sce + cheese, home	30	1.02	1.02	4.20	9.07	0.260	0.028	0.020	0.284	0.9
Spaghetti + sce + meat, canned	30	1.36	1.13	4.42	6.01	0.374	0.017	0.020	0.312	2.6
Spaghetti + sce + meat, home	38	2.17	1.37	4.46	14.20	0.423	0.029	0.034	0.314	10.2
Spaghetti sauce, home-made	23	0.77	1.25	2.95	6.70	0.380	0.026	0.017	0.343	0
Spaghetti sauce, canned	31	0.52	1.35	4.52	7.97	0.184	0.016	0.017	0.343	0
Spaghetti meat sauce,	30	1.03	1.30	3.72	4.95	0.385	0.028	0.022	0.193	2.3
Spaghetti sauce, dry, pkt	79	1.70	0.28	18.20	48.20	0.765	NA	0.162	0.057	0
Spaghetti sce + mshrm, pkt	85	2.84	2.55	13.90	113.00	0.510	NA	0.136	0.085	0
Egg noodles, cooked	35	1.17	0.35	6.60	3.19	0.400	0.039	0.023	0.624	8.9
Chow mein noodles, dry	139	3.72	6.93	16.40	8.82	0.252	0.032	0.019	1.100	3.2
Spinach noodles, dry	108	3.97	1.08	20.20	11.60	1.290	0.278	0.133	1.930	0

Variety (cont.)	kcal	Protein (g)	Fat (g)	CHO (g)	Ca (mg)	Fe (mg)	B_1 (mg)	B_2 (mg)	Fiber (g)	Cholesterol (mg)
Pasta & noodles (cont.)										
Spinach noodles, cooked	32	1.13	0.36	5.97	3.37	0.429	0.043	0.027	0.569	0
Chicken + noodles, recipe	43	2.60	2.13	3.07	3.07	0.278	0.006	0.020	0.142	12.2
Chicken + noodles, frozen	32	2.17	1.30	2.49	15.70	0.393	0.009	0.018	0.022	8.0
Noodles-ramen-beef, cooked	28	0.76	0.94	4.17	NA	NA	NA	NA	0.500	NA
Noodles, ramen, chicken, ckd	25	0.76	0.85	3.63	NA	NA	NA	NA	0.512	NA
Noodles, ramen, oriental	26	0.74	1.07	3.83					0.512	
Lasagna, frozen entree	38	2.32	1.71	2.61	34.00	0.343	0.026	0.045	0.194	12.4
Pizza										
Pizza—cheese	69	3.54	2.13	9.21	52.00	0.378	0.080	0.069	0.510	13.2
Pizza—mozzarella	80	7.60	4.67	0.89	207.00	0.076	0.006	0.097	0	15.0
Pizza—Canadian bacon	52	6.82	2.36	0.38	3.00	0.229	0.231	0.055	0	16.3
Pizza—pepperoni	140	5.94	12.50	0.81	2.80	0.397	0.090	0.070	0	9.8
Pizza—onion	10	0.34	0.07	2.07	7.10	1.105	0.017	0.003	0.450	0
Popcorn										
Popcorn—plain, air popped	106	3.50	1.42	21.30	3.50	0.709	0.106	0.035	4.600	0
Popcorn—cooked in oil/salted	142	2.32	7.99	15.50	7.70	0.696	0.026	0.052	3.090	0
Popcorn—syrup-coated	109	1.60	0.81	24.30	1.60	0.405	0.106	0.016	0.810	0
Rice										
Brown—dry	102	2.13	0.54	21.90	9.04	0.510	0.096	0.014	0.965	0
Brown—cooked	34	0.709	0.17	7.23	3.40	0.170	0.026	0.006	0.483	0
White—regular, dry	103	1.90	0.11	22.80	6.74	0.828	0.125	0.009	0.340	0
White—regular, cooked	31	0.567	0.03	6.86	2.84	0.397	0.03	0.003	0.102	0
White—converted, dry	105	2.10	0.15	23.00	17.00	0.828	0.124	0.010	0.624	0
White—converted, ckd	30	0.599	0.02	6.60	5.35	0.227	0.03	0.003	0.180	0
White—instant, dry	106	2.13	0.06	23.40	1.42	1.300	0.125	0.008	0.737	0
White—instant, prepd	31	0.624	0.03	6.86	0.85	0.227	0.037	0.003	0.216	0
Wild—cooked	26	1.02	0.06	5.39	1.42	0.312	0.031	0.045	0.709	0
Rice bran	78	3.77	5.44	14.40	21.50	5.500	0.64	0.070	6.150	0
Rice polish	75	3.43	3.62	16.40	19.40	4.560	0.521	0.051	0.680	0
Salad dressings										
Blue cheese salad dressing	143	1.37	14.80	2.09	22.90	0.057	0.003	0.028	0.020	7.6
Ceasar's salad dressing	126	2.66	12.70	0.67	44.40	0.239	0.007	0.025	0.050	33.9
French dressing	150	0.16	16.00	1.81	3.55	0.113	0	0	0.220	0
Italian dressing—lo cal	15	0.02	1.18	1.37	0.59	0.059	0	0	0.080	1.7
Mayonnaise	203	0.31	22.60	0.77	5.67	0.168	0.005	0.012	0	16.8
Imitation mayonnaise	66	0	5.67	3.78	0	0	0	0	0	7.6
Ranch salad dressing	104	0.86	10.70	1.31	28.40	0.075	0.010	0.040	0	11.1
Russian salad dressing	140	0.45	14.50	3.00	5.44	0.174	0.014	0.014	0.080	18.4
1000 island dressing	107	0.26	10.10	4.30	3.52	0.170	0.006	0.009	0.060	7.3
1000 island dressing—lo cal	45	0.22	3.00	4.58	3.12	1.174	0.006	0.008	0.340	3.4
Vinegar & oil dressing	124	0	14.20	0		0	0	0	0	0
Salads, prepared										
Chicken salad w/celery	97	3.82	8.90	0.47	5.92	0.239	0.012	0.028	0.110	17.3
Cole slaw	20	0.36	0.74	3.52	12.80	0.166	0.019	0.017	0.570	2.3
Egg salad	68	2.91	6.01	0.45	14.50	0.525	0.019	0.070	0	97.4
Ham salad spread	62	2.46	4.39	3.01	2.24	0.168	0.123	0.034	0.030	10.4

Variety (cont.)	kcal	Protein (g)	Fat (g)	CHO (g)	Ca (mg)	Fe (mg)	B_1 (mg)	B_2 (mg)	Fiber (g)	Cholesterol (mg)
Salads, prepared (cont.)										
Macaroni salad—no cheese	75	0.54	6.66	3.52	5.50	0.229	0.020	0.014	0.270	4.9
Potato salad w/mayo + eggs	41	0.76	2.32	3.16	5.44	0.185	0.022	0.017	0.420	19.3
Tuna salad	53	4.55	2.53	2.67	4.84	0.282	0.009	0.019	0.340	3.7
Waldorf salad	85	0.72	8.33	2.62	8.82	0.196	0.020	0.013	0.720	4.3
Sandwiches										
Avocado cheese sand—white	64	2.02	4.00	5.39	43.1	0.418	0.057	0.059	0.98	4.4
Avocado cheese sand—whole wheat	62	2.14	3.97	5.24	37.8	0.477	0.047	0.05		4.3
BLT Sandwich—whole wheat	68	2.49	3.77	6.45	11.4	0.570	0.077	0.043	1.55	4.1
BLT sandwich—white	70	2.30	3.77	6.70	18.2	0.489	0.092	0.055	0.43	4.2
Grilled cheese sand/wheat	91	4.22	5.37	7.10	87.4	0.565	0.057	0.076	1.59	11.8
Grilled cheese sand/part WW	95	4.39	5.82	6.59	103.0	0.526	0.067	0.093	0.61	13.3
Grilled cheese sand—white	97	4.22	5.79	6.88	103.0	0.441	0.068	0.092	0.30	13.3
Chicken salad sand—wheat	80	3.00	4.25	8.13	14.7	0.679	0.066	0.046	1.88	6.2
Chicken salad sand—white	85	2.83	4.63	8.05	22.7	0.552	0.080	0.060	0.39	7.1
Corn dog	84	2.55	5.10	6.97	8.7	0.495	0.072	0.043	0.03	9.5
Corned beef & swiss on rye	83	5.26	4.59	4.90	63.8	0.768	0.044	0.078	0.97	16.4
Engl mfn (egg/cheese/bacon)	74	3.70	3.70	6.37	40.5	0.637	0.095	0.103	0.32	43.8
Egg salad sand—wheat	79	2.60	4.56	7.44	17.0	0.744	0.063	0.059	1.67	48.8
Egg salad sand/soft white	83	2.41	4.90	7.25	24.5	0.636	0.075	0.074	0.30	41.6
Ham sandwich—rye bread	59	3.84	2.09	6.10	12.0	0.474	0.182	0.073	1.24	7.1
Ham sandwich—whole wheat	59	3.79	2.04	6.84	12.4	0.617	0.164	0.060	1.54	6.1
Ham sandwich—soft white	61	3.74	2.08	6.60	18.6	0.504	0.186	0.073	0.29	6.7
Ham & swiss sand/on rye	68	4.65	3.23	5.08	63.5	0.389	0.147	0.079	0.99	10.8
Ham & cheese sand—wheat	67	4.20	3.23	5.72	40.5	0.527	0.136	0.066	1.27	9.7
Ham & cheese sand—soft white	69	4.20	3.36	5.43	48.0	0.428	0.152	0.078	0.23	10.6
Ham salad sand—wheat	75	2.45	4.02	7.83	11.5	0.569	0.104	0.045	1.52	5.6
Ham salad sand—white	78	2.25	4.26	7.71	17.5	0.454	0.119	0.057	0.28	6.2
Hotdog/frankfurter & bun	87	2.80	5.10	7.04	19.6	0.570	0.095	0.062	0.40	7.6
Patty melt—ground beef/rye	91	5.09	6.07	3.96	36.5	0.533	0.040	0.072	0.81	17.1
Peanut butter & jam—whole wheat	92	3.40	3.85	12.30	15.4	0.751	0.070	0.045	2.29	0
Peanut butter & jam—white	98	3.29	4.14	12.80	23.4	0.632	0.085	0.059	0.85	0
Reuben sandwich—grilled	58	3.43	3.38	3.53	43.6	0.633	0.030	0.052	0.80	10.4
Roast beef sand—whole wheat	64	4.00	2.52	6.71	12.3	0.760	0.061	0.054	1.53	6.2

Variety (cont.)	kcal	Protein (g)	Fat (g)	CHO (g)	Ca (mg)	Fe (mg)	B_1 (mg)	B_2 (mg)	Fiber (g)	Cholesterol (mg)
Sandwiches (cont.)										
Roast beef sand—white	67	3.97	2.63	6.46	18.5	0.665	0.072	0.066	0.27	6.9
Tuna salad sand—wheat	72	3.29	3.29	8.03	13.0	0.667	0.057	0.040	1.74	5.5
Tuna salad sand—white	76	3.18	3.47	7.92	19.6	0.555	0.068	0.052	0.44	6.2
Turkey sand—whole wheat	62	4.09	2.33	6.67	11.6	0.554	0.056	0.044	1.53	6.0
Turkey sand—white	64	4.07	2.42	6.41	17.8	0.435	0.066	0.055	0.27	6.7
Turkey & ham sandwich—rye	58	3.74	2.12	6.18	12.3	0.743	0.060	0.079	1.23	8.4
Turkey & ham sand—whole wheat	59	3.71	2.07	6.90	12.6	0.846	0.060	0.064	1.54	7.2
Turkey & ham sand—white	60	3.65	2.10	6.67	18.8	0.762	0.071	0.078	0.28	8.0
Turkey & ham & cheese on rye	68	4.22	3.46	5.04	44.2	0.616	0.050	0.083	0.99	12.1
Turkey & ham & cheese—wheat	67	4.14	3.25	5.77	40.5	0.716	0.051	0.070	1.27	10.6
Turkey & ham & cheese—white	69	4.13	3.38	5.48	48.3	0.636	0.059	0.082	0.23	11.6
Sauces										
Bordelaise sauce	24	0.33	1.46	1.10	3.80	0.179	0.008	0.010	0.01	3.8
Hot chili sauce, red pepper	5	0.25	0.17	1.10	2.51	0.137	0.003	0.026	2.29	0
Teriyaki sauce	24	1.69	0.09	4.52	6.30	0.488	0.008	0.020	0	0
Seafood										
Anchovy, raw	37	5.78	1.37	0	41.7	0.921	0.016	0.073	0	19.6
Frog legs, raw meat	21	4.65	0.085	0	5.1	0.539	0.040	0.070	0	14.2
Lobster meat—cooked	28	5.80	0.17	0.36	17.2	0.111	0.020	0.019	0	20.3
Scampi—fried in crumbs	69	6.07	3.49	3.26	19.0	0.357	0.037	0.039	0.04	50.2
Shrimp—boiled	28	5.93	0.31	0	11.0	0.876	0.009	0.009	0	55.3
Squid (calamari), fried in flour	50	5.10	2.12	2.20	11.0	0.287	0.016	0.130	0	73.7
Soup										
Cream of celery soup	20	0.38	1.27	2.00	9.04	0.141	0.007	0.011	0.09	3.2
Chicken soup, chunky	20	1.43	0.75	1.95	2.71	0.195	0.010	0.020	0.03	3.4
Chicken + dumpling soup	23	1.30	1.28	1.39	3.34	0.144	0.004	0.017	0.10	7.6
Chicken gumbo soup	13	0.60	0.32	1.89	5.53	0.201	0.006	0.009	0.05	0.9
Chick-noodl soup—chunky	14	1.50	0.70	0.24	2.84	0.170	0.009	0.020	0.09	2.1
Chili with beans	32	1.62	1.56	3.38	13.20	0.973	0.014	0.030	0.91	4.8
Clam chowder—New England	19	1.08	0.75	1.90	21.40	0.169	0.008	0.027	0.11	2.5
Minestrone soup—chunky	15	0.60	0.33	2.45	7.20	0.209	0.006	0.014	0.12	0.6
Cream of mushroom soup	29	0.46	2.15	2.10	7.23	0.119	0.007	0.019	0.06	0.4
Mushroom-barley soup	14	0.43	0.51	1.69	2.82	0.113	0.006	0.020	0.17	0
Onion soup—canned	13	0.87	0.40	1.89	6.10	0.156	0.008	0.006	0.11	0
Oyster stew	14	0.49	0.89	0.94	4.96	0.227	0.005	0.008	0	3.1
Pea soup—prepared w/milk	27	1.40	0.79	3.59	19.30	0.224	0.017	0.030	0.07	2.0
Cream of potato soup	17	0.39	0.53	2.59	4.52	0.107	0.008	0.008	0.10	1.5
Split pea + ham soup	22	1.31	0.47	3.17	3.90	0.253	0.014	0.011	0.19	0.8
Tomato soup—canned	19	0.47	0.43	3.75	3.05	0.396	0.020	0.011	0.11	0
Tomato-beef-noodle soup	32	1.00	0.97	4.78	3.95	0.252	0.019	0.020	0.03	0.9

Variety (cont.)	kcal	Protein (g)	Fat (g)	CHO (g)	Ca (mg)	Fe (mg)	B_1 (mg)	B_2 (mg)	Fiber (g)	Cholesterol (mg)
Tomato bisque prep w/milk	22	0.71	0.75	3.32	21.00	0.099	0.013	0.030	0.01	2.5
Turkey soup—chunky	16	1.23	0.53	1.69	6.00	0.229	0.010	0.029	0.12	1.1
Turkey noodle soup	16	0.88	0.45	1.95	2.60	0.212	0.017	0.014	0.03	1.1
Cream vegetable soup—dry mix	126	2.27	6.84	14.80	1.42	0.539	1.470	0.127	0.22	1.2
Vegetable soup	16	0.49	0.45	2.77	4.96	0.249	0.012	0.010	0.37	0
Miscellaneous										
Garlic cloves	42	1.80	0.14	9.38	51.30	0.482	0.057	0.030	0.47	0
Gelatin salad/desert	17	0.43	0	3.99	0.50	0.024	0.002	0.002	0.02	0
Quiche lorraine—⅛th	97	2.09	7.73	4.67	34.00	0.226	0.018	0.052	0.09	45.9
Spinach souffle	45	2.29	3.84	0.59	47.90	0.279	0.019	0.064	0.79	38.4

PART 2. NUTRITIVE VALUES FOR ALCOHOLIC AND NONALCOHOLIC BEVERAGES

The nutritive values for alcoholic and nonalcoholic beverages are expressed in 1-ounce (28.4 g) portions. We have also included the nutritive values for the minerals calcium, iron, magnesium, phosphorus, and potassium and the vitamins thiamine, riboflavin, niacin, and cobalamin. The alcoholic beverages contain no cholesterol or fat.

ALCOHOLIC BEVERAGES (1 OUNCE)

				Minerals					Vitamins			
Beverage	kcal	Protein (g)	CHO (g)	Ca (mg)	Fe (mg)	Mg (mg)	P (mg)	K (mg)	B_1 (mg)	B_2 (mg)	Niacin (mg)	B_{12} (mg)
Beer, regular	12	0.072	1.1	1.4	0.009	1.83	3.50	7.09	0.002	0.007	0.128	0.005
Beer, light	8	0.057	0.4	1.4	0.011	1.42	3.44	5.13	0.003	0.008	0.111	0.002
Brandy	69	0	10.6	2.5	0.012		1.01	1.01	0.002	0.002	0.004	0
Champagne	22	0.043	0.6	1.6	0.093	2.40	1.90	22.60	0	0.003	0.019	0
Dessert wine, dry	36	0.057	1.2	2.3	0.068	2.55	2.55	26.20	0.005	0.005	0.060	0
Dessert wine, sweet	44	0.057	3.3	2.3	0.057	2.55	2.64	26.20	0.005	0.005	0.060	0
Gin, rum, vodka, scotch, whiskey, 80 proof	64	0	0	0	0.010	0	0	1.01	0	0	0	0
Gin, rum, vodka, scotch, whiskey, 86 proof	71	0	0	0	0.012	0	1.16	0.55	0.002	0.002	0.004	0
Gin, rum, vodka, scotch, whiskey, 90 proof	74	0	0	0	0.010	0	0	0.86	0	0	0	0
Sherry, dry	28	0.024	0.3	2.1	0.052	1.96	2.60	17.80	0.002	0.002	0.024	0
Sherry, medium	40	0.066	2.3	2.3	0.071	2.27	1.89	23.60	0.002	0.008	0.035	0
Vermouth, dry	34	0.028	1.6	2.0	0.096	1.42	1.89	11.30	NA	NA	0.011	0
Vermouth, sweet	44	0.014	4.5	1.7	0.099	1.13	1.65	8.50	NA	NA	0.011	0
Wine, dry white	19	0.029	0.2	2.6	0.093	2.62	1.67	17.40	0	0.001	0.019	0
Wine, medium white	19	0.028	0.2	2.5	0.085	3.03	3.84	22.60	0.001	0.001	0.019	0

ALCOHOLIC BEVERAGES (1 OUNCE)

				Minerals					Vitamins			
Beverage	kcal	Protein (g)	CHO (g)	Ca (mg)	Fe (mg)	Mg (mg)	P (mg)	K (mg)	B_1 (mg)	B_2 (mg)	Niacin (mg)	B_{12} (mg)
Wine, red	20	0.055	0.5	2.2	0.122	3.60	3.84	31.50	0.001	0.008	0.023	0.004
Wine, rosé	20	0.055	0.4	2.4	0.108	2.74	4.08	28.10	0.001	0.004	0.020	0.002
Creme de menthe	105	0	11.8	0	0.023	0	0	0	0	0	0.001	0
Bloody mary	22	0.153	0.9	1.9	0.105	2.10	4.02	41.40	0.010	0.006	0.123	0
Bourbon and soda	26	0	0	1.0		0.24	0.48	0.48	0	0	0.005	0
Daiquiri	52	0	1.9	0.9	0.043	0.47	1.89	6.14	0.004	0	0.012	0
Manhattan	64	0	0.9	0.5	0.025	0.01	1.99	7.46	0.003	0.001	0.026	0
Martini	63	0	0.1	0.4	0.024	0.40	0.81	5.26	0	0	0.004	0
Pina colada	53	0.120	8.0	2.2	0.062		2.01	20.10	0.008	0.004	0.033	0
Screwdriver	23	0.160	2.5	2.1	0.023	2.26	3.86	43.30	0.018	0.004	0.046	0
Tequila	31	0.099	2.4	1.7	0.077	1.98	2.80	29.30	0.010	0.005	0.054	0
Tom collins	16	0.013	0.4	1.3	NA	0.38	0.12	2.30	0	0	0.004	0
Whiskey sour	42	0	3.7	0.3	0.021	0.26	1.60	5.08	0.003	0.002	0.006	0
Coffee + cream liqueur	93	0.784	5.9	4.2	0.036	0.60	13.90	9.05	0	0.016	0.022	0
Coffee liqueur	95	0	13.3	0.5	0.016	0.54	1.64	8.18	0.001	0.003	0.040	0

NONALCOHOLIC BEVERAGES (1 OUNCE)

				Minerals					Vitamins			
Beverage	kcal	Protein (g)	CHO (g)	Ca (mg)	Fe (mg)	Mg (mg)	P (mg)	K (mg)	B_1 (mg)	B_2 (mg)	Niacin (mg)	B_{12} (mg)
Hot cocoa with whole milk	25	1.030	2.9	33.8	0.088	6.350	30.60	54.400	0.012	0.049	0.041	0.099
Cocoa mix + water-diet	7	0.561	1.3	13.3	0.110	4.870	19.80	59.800	0.006	0.030	0.024	0
Coffee-brewed	0.2	0.016	0.1	0.5	0.113	1.590	0.32	15.400	0	0.002	0.063	0
Coffee-instant dry powder	1.4	0.016	0.3	0.8	0.019	1.100	2.05	67.70	0	0	0.061	0
Coffee, capuchino	9.2	0.059	1.6	1.0	0.022	1.330	3.84	17.600	0	0	0.048	0
Coffee, Swiss mocha	7.7	0.078	1.3	1.1	0.036	1.360	4.37	17.900	0	0	0.039	0
Coffee whitener, nondairy, liquid	38.5	0.284	3.2	2.6	0.009	0.060	18.20	54.1	0	0	0	0
powder	155	1.360	15.6	6.3	0.326	1.200	120.00	230.0	0	0.047	0	0
Cola beverage, regular	12	0	3.0	0.7	0.009	0.230	3.52	0.306	0	0	0	0
Diet cola-w/ aspartame	0	0	0	1.0	0.009	0.319	2.40	0	0.001	0.007	0	0
Club soda	0	0	0	1.4	0.012	0.319	0	0.479	0	0	0	0
Cream soda	15	0	3.8	1.5	0.015	0.229	0	0.306	0	0	0	0
Diet soda-avg assorted	0	0	0.0	1.1	0.011	0.200	3.03	0.559	0	0	0	0
Egg nog—commercial	38	1.080	3.8	36.8	0.057	5.250	31.00	46.900	0.010	0.054	0.030	0.127
Five Alive citrus	13	0.135	3.1	1.7	0.021	1.950	2.70	34.000	0.015	0.003	0.060	0
Fruit flavored soda pop	13	0	3.2	1.1	0.020	0.305	0.15	1.520	0	0	0.002	0
Fruit punch drink—canned	13	0.015	3.4	2.1	0.058	0.610	0.31	7.160	0.006	0.006	0.006	0
Gatorade	5	0	1.3	2.8	NA	NA	0	2.840	NA	NA	NA	0
Ginger ale	10	0.008	2.5	0.9	0.051	0.232	0.08	0.387	0	0	0	0

NONALCOHOLIC BEVERAGES (1 OUNCE)

Beverage	kcal	Protein (g)	CHO (g)	Minerals Ca (mg)	Fe (mg)	Mg (mg)	P (mg)	K (mg)	Vitamins B_1 (mg)	B_2 (mg)	Niacin (mg)	B_{12} (mg)
Grape soda, carbonated	12	0	3.2	0.9	0.024	0.305	0	0.229	0	0	0	0
Koolade w/ NutraSweet	0	0	0	0	0	0.028	0	0	0	0	0	0
Koolade w/sugar added	12	0	3.0	0	0	0	0	0	0	0	0	0
Lemon-lime soda	12	0	3.0	0.7	0.019	0.154	0.08	0.308	0	0	0.004	0
Lemonade drink from dry	11	0	2.9	7.6	0.016	0.322	3.65	3.540	0	0	0.004	0
Lemonade frozen conc	51	0.078	13.3	1.9	0.205	1.420	2.46	19.200	0.007	0.027	0.020	0
Limeade frozen conc	53	0.052	14.0	1.4	0.029	7.800	1.69	16.800	0.003	0.003	0.028	0
Chocolate milkshake	36	0.962	5.8	32.0	0.088	4.700	28.90	56.800	0.016	0.069	0.046	0.097
Strawberry milkshake	32	0.952	5.4	32.0	0.030	3.600	28.40	51.700	0.013	0.055	0.050	0.088
Vanilla milkshake	32	0.982	5.1	34.5	0.026	3.500	29.00	49.300	0.013	0.052	0.052	0.101
Orange drink/ carbonated	14	0	3.5	1.5	0.018	0.305	0.31	0.686	0	0	0	0
Pepper-type soda	12	0	2.9	0.9	0.010	0.077	3.16	0.154	0	0	0	0
Root beer	12	0.008	3.0	1.5	0.014	0.306	0.15	0.230	0	0	0	0
Pineapple grape-fruit drink	13	0.068	3.3	2.0	0.087	1.700	1.59	17.500	0.009	0.005	0.076	0
Pineapple orange drink	14	0.352	3.3	1.5	0.076	1.590	1.13	13.200	0.009	0.005	0.059	0
Tang orange juice crystals	13	0.170	0.06	3.1	4.57	0.002	0.02	0.008	0	0	0	0
Tonic water/Quinine water	10	0	2.5	0.4	0.019	0.077	0	0.077	0	0	0	0
Tea-brewed	0	0.001	0.1	0	0.006	0.796	0.16	10.500	0	0.004	0.012	0
Herbal tea, brewed	0	0	0	0.6	0.022	0.319	0	2.390	0.003	0.001	0	0
Perrier water	0	0	0	3.8	0	0.148	0	0	0	0	0	0
Poland Springs bottle water	0	0	0	0.4	0.001	0.239	0	0	0	0	0	0

Note: Alcoholic beverages contain no fat or cholesterol; light beer contains 0.5 g fiber and regular beer contains 1.2 g fiber. All of the other nonmixed alcoholic beverages have no fiber.

Note: Other nonalcoholic beverages are listed in the sections on fruits and vegetables.

PART 3. NUTRITIVE VALUES FOR SPECIALTY AND FAST-FOOD ITEMS

Nutrient information was kindly provided by the manufacturer or its representative. Unlike Parts 1 and 2, nutritive values are not given for 1-ounce portions but for the actual amounts of the foods as sold commercially. To make a direct comparison of the kcal values and the various nutrients, we recommend that the weight of the food and its nutrients be expressed relative to 1-ounce (28.4 g) portions.

SPECIALTY AND FAST FOOD ITEMS (DASHES INDICATE INFORMATION NOT PROVIDED BY SOURCES.)

ARBY'S

Food item	Serving size (g)	kcal	Protein (g)	Fat (g)	CHO (g)	Ca	Fe	Vit A	Vit C	Vit B_1	Vit B_2
Bac'n Cheddar Deluxe	225	561	28	34	78	—	—	—	—	—	—
Baked Potato											
Plain	312	290	8	1	0	—	—	—	—	—	—
Beef 'n Cheddar	190	490	24	21	51	—	—	—	—	—	—
Chicken Breast Sandwich	210	592	28	27	57	—	—	—	—	—	—
Chocolate Shake	300	384	9	11	32	—	—	—	—	—	—
French Fries	71	211	2	8	6	—	—	—	—	—	—
Hot Ham 'n Cheese Sandwich	161	353	26	13	50	—	—	—	—	—	—
Jamocha Shake	305	424	8	10	31	—	—	—	—	—	—
Junior Roast Beef	86	218	12	8	22	—	—	—	—	—	—
King Roast Beef	192	467	27	19	49	—	—	—	—	—	—
Potato Cakes	85	201	2	14	13	—	—	—	—	—	—
Regular Roast Beef	147	353	22	15	32	—	—	—	—	—	—
Super Roast Beef	234	501	25	22	40	—	—	—	—	—	—
Superstuffed Potato											
Broccoli and Cheddar	340	541	13	22	24	—	—	—	—	—	—
Superstuffed Potato											
Deluxe	312	648	18	38	72	—	—	—	—	—	—
Superstuffed Potato											
Mushroom and Cheese	300	506	16	22	21	—	—	—	—	—	—
Superstuffed Potato											
Taco	425	619	23	27	145	—	—	—	—	—	—
Turkey Deluxe	197	375	24	17	39	—	—	—	—	—	—
Vanilla Shake	250	295	8	10	30	—	—	—	—	—	—

Source: Arby's Inc. Nutritional information provided by Consumer Affairs, Arby's Inc., Atlanta, GA, 1986.

BURGER KING

Food item	Serving size (g)	kcal	Protein (g)	CHO (g)	Fat (g)	Cholesterol (mg)	Vit A (mg)	Vit C (mg)	Thia (mg)	Ribo (mg)	Nia (mg)	Ca (mg)	Fe (mg)
Burgers													
Whopper Sandwich	270	614	27	45	36	91	11	20	24	24	34	8	27
Whopper Sandwich with Cheese	294	706	32	47	44	116	19	20	24	28	34	22	27
Double Whopper Sandwich	351	844	46	45	53	170	11	20	25	33	52	0	40
Double Whopper Sandwich with Cheese	375	935	51	47	61	195	19	20	25	37	52	24	40
Cheeseburger	121	318	17	28	15	50	7	5	15	17	19	11	15
Cheeseburger Deluxe	151	390	18	29	23	56	10	9	15	17	19	11	15
Hamburger	108	272	15	28	11	37	3	5	15	15	19	4	15
Hamburger Deluxe	138	344	15	28	19	43	5	9	15	15	19	4	15
Bacon Double Cheeseburger	160	507	33	26	30	108	8	*	23	29	36	18	21
Bacon Double Cheeseburger Deluxe	195	584	33	28	38	114	12	5	23	29	37	18	22
Double Cheeseburger	172	483	30	29	27	100	11	5	16	24	29	18	21
Burger Buddies (pair)	129	349	18	31	17	52	9	8	32	24	23	11	19
Sandwich/side orders													
BK Broiler Chicken Sandwich	154	267	22	28	8	45	4	6	45	45	60	4	15
Chicken Sandwich	229	685	27	56	40	60	3	*	32	18	49	8	19

BURGER KING

Food item	Serving size (g)	kcal	Protein (g)	CHO (g)	Fat (g)	Cholesterol (mg)	Vit A (mg)	Vit C (mg)	Thia (mg)	Ribo (mg)	Nia (mg)	Ca (mg)	Fe (mg)
Sandwich/side orders (cont.)													
Ocean Catch Fish Filet Sandwich	165	479	16	31	33	45	*	*	48	25	48	5	13
Chicken Tenders (6 piece)	90	236	16	14	13	38	2	*	7	5	40	*	4
Chef Salad†	273	178	17	7	9	103	95	25	18	15	20	16	9
Chunky Chicken Salad†	258	142	20	8	4	49	92	34	10	10	47	4	7
Garden Salad†	223	95	6	8	5	15	100	58	5	6	4	15	6
Side Salad†	135	25	1	5	0	0	88	20	3	*	3	3	3
French Fries (medium, salted)	116	372	5	43	20	0	*	5	5	*	12	*	7
Onion Rings	97	339	5	38	19	0	15	*	10	6	12	11	3
Apple Pie	125	311	3	44	14	4	*	8	18	9	3	*	7
Cherry Pie	128	360	4	55	13	0	6	10	15	10	2	*	6
Lemon Pie	92	290	6	49	8	35	*	*	2	8	4	10	2
Snickers Ice Cream Bar	57	220	5	20	14	15	2	*	*	6	4	6	2
Drinks													
Vanilla Shake	284	334	9	51	10	33	*	*	7	35	*	31	*
Chocolate Shake	284	326	9	49	10	31	7	4	6	28	*	31	4
Chocolate Shake (syrup added)	312	409	10	68	11	33	*	*	7	35	*	31	*
Strawberry Shake (syrup added)	312	394	9	66	10	33	*	*	7	35	*	31	*
Coca-Cola Classic (medium)	22 (oz)	264	0	70	0	0	*	*	*	*	*	*	*
Diet Coke (medium)	22 (oz)	1	0	0	0	0	*	*	*	*	*	*	*
Sprite (medium)	22 (oz)	264	0	66	0	0	*	*	*	*	*	*	*
Orange Juice	183	82	1	20	0	0	3	119	10	*	*	*	*
Coffee	244	2	0	0	0	0	*	*	*	*	4	*	*
Milk-2% Low Fat	244	121	8	12	5	18	10	4	6	24	*	30	*
Breakfast													
Croissan'wich with Bacon, Egg and Cheese	118	353	16	19	23	230	10	*	23	27	15	14	10
Croissan'wich with Sausage, Egg and Cheese	159	534	21	22	40	258	10	*	24	25	22	15	16
Croissan'wich with Ham, Egg and Cheese	144	351	19	20	22	236	10	*	44	36	33	14	12
Breakfast Buddy with Sausage, Egg and Cheese	84	255	11	15	16	127	5	*	19	17	13	8	10
French Toast Sticks	141	538	10	53	32	52	*	*	16	16	18	8	16
Hash Browns	71	213	2	25	12	0	12	9	7	4	10	*	2
Mini Muffins—Blueberry	95	292	4	37	14	72	*	*	8	8	5	4	7
Sandwich Condiments/ Toppings													
Processed American Cheese	25	92	5	1	7	25	8	*	*	5	*	14	*
Lettuce	21	3	0	0	0	0	*	*	*	*	*	*	*
Tomato	28	6	0	1	0	0	4	9	*	*	*	*	*
Onion	14	5	0	1	0	0	*	*	*	*	*	*	*
Pickles	14	1	0	0	0	0	*	*	*	*	*	*	*
Ketchup	14	17	0	4	0	0	5	8	*	*	*	*	*
Mustard	3	2	0	0	0	0	*	*	*	*	*	*	*
Mayonnaise	28	194	0	2	21	17	*	*	*	*	*	*	*
Tartar Sauce	28	134	0	2	14	15	*	*	*	*	*	*	*
BK Broiler Sauce	11	37	0	1	4	5	*	*	*	3	*	*	*
Bull's Eye Barbecue Sauce	14	22	0	5	0	0	*	*	*	*	*	*	*
Bacon Bits	3	16	1	0	1	5	*	*	*	*	*	*	*
Croutons	7	31	1	5	1	—	*	*	*	*	*	*	*

BURGER KING

Food item	Serving size (g)	kcal	Protein (g)	CHO (g)	Fat (g)	Cholesterol (mg)	Vit A (mg)	Vit C (mg)	Thia (mg)	Ribo (mg)	Nia (mg)	Ca (mg)	Fe (mg)
Salad Dressings													
Thousand Island	63	290	1	15	26	36	64	*	*	*	*	*	*
French	64	290	0	23	22	0	31	*	*	*	*	*	*
Ranch	57	350	1	4	37	20	*	*	*	*	*	*	*
Bleu Cheese	59	300	3	2	32	58	*	*	*	*	*	*	*
Olive Oil and Vinegar	56	310	0	2	33	0	*	*	*	*	*	*	*
Reduced Calorie Light Italian	59	170	0	3	18	0	*	*	*	*	*	*	*
Dipping Sauces													
A.M. Express Dip	28	84	0	21	0	0	*	*	*	*	*	*	*
Honey	28	91	0	23	0	0	*	*	*	*	*	*	*
Ranch	28	171	0	2	18	0	*	*	*	*	*	*	*
Barbecue	28	36	0	9	0	0	3	4	*	*	*	*	*
Sweet & Sour	28	45	0	11	0	0	*	*	*	*	*	*	*

* Less than 2% of the U.S. RDA.
† Without salad dressing.
— = Negligible.
Source: From Burger King Corporation, Miami, FL, 1991. For additional information, call 1-800-937-1800.

DAIRY QUEEN

Food item	Serving size (g)	Description	kcal	Protein (g)	Fat (g)	CHO (g)	Ca (mg)	Fe (mg)	Vit A (IU)	Vit C (mg)	Vit B_1 (mg)	Vit B_2 (mg)
Banana Split	383		540	9	11	103	—	—	—	—	—	—
Big Brazier Deluxe	213		470	28	24	36	111	5.2	—	<2.5	0.34	0.37
Big Brazier Regular	184		184	27	23	37	113	5.2	—	<2.0	0.37	0.39
Big Brazier w/Cheese	213		553	32	30	38	268	5.2	495	<2.3	0.34	0.53
Blizzard Banana Split	—	regular	763	—	—	—	—	—	—	—	—	—
Blizzard Banana Split	—	large	1333	—	—	—	—	—	—	—	—	—
Blizzard Chocolate Sandwich Cookies	—	regular	600	—	—	—	—	—	—	—	—	—
Blizzard Chocolate Sandwich Cookies	—	large	1050	—	—	—	—	—	—	—	—	—
Blizzard German Chocolate	—	regular	794	—	—	—	—	—	—	—	—	—
Blizzard German Chocolate	—	large	1460	—	—	—	—	—	—	—	—	—
Blizzard, Heath	—	regular	824	—	—	—	—	—	—	—	—	—
Blizzard, Heath	—	large	1212	—	—	—	—	—	—	—	—	—
Blizzard, M&M	—	regular	766	—	—	—	—	—	—	—	—	—
Blizzard, M&M	—	large	1154	—	—	—	—	—	—	—	—	—
Brazier Cheese Dog	113		330	15	19	24	168	1.6	—	—	—	0.18
Brazier Chili Dog	128		330	13	20	25	86	2.0	—	11.0	0.15	0.23
Brazier Dog	99		273	11	15	23	75	1.5	—	11.0	0.12	0.15
Brazier French Fries	71		200	2	10	25	tr	0.4	tr	3.6	0.06	tr
Brazier French Fries	113		320	3	16	40	tr	0.4	tr	4.8	0.09	0.03
Brazier Onion Rings	85		300	6	17	33	20	0.4	tr	2.4	0.09	tr
Brazier Regular	106		260	13	9	28	70	3.5	—	<1.0	0.28	0.26
Brazier w/Cheese	121		318	18	14	30	163	3.5	—	<1.2	0.29	0.29
Buster Bar	149		460	10	29	41	—	—	—	—	—	—
Chicken Sandwich	220		670	29	41	46	—	—	—	—	—	—
Cone, large	213		340	9	10	57	—	—	—	—	—	—
Cone, regular	142		240	6	7	38	—	—	—	—	—	—
Cone, small	85		140	3	4	22	—	—	—	—	—	—
Dairy Queen Parfait	284		460	10	11	81	300	1.8	400	tr	0.12	0.43
Dilly Bar	85		240	4	15	22	100	0.4	100	tr	0.06	0.17

DAIRY QUEEN

Food item	Serving size (g)	Description	kcal	Protein (g)	Fat (g)	CHO (g)	Ca (mg)	Fe (mg)	Vit A (IU)	Vit C (mg)	Vit B_1 (mg)	Vit B_2 (mg)
Dilly Bar	85		210	3	13	21	—	—	—	—	—	—
Dipped Cone, large	234		510	9	24	64	—	—	—	—	—	—
Dipped Cone, regular	156		340	6	16	42	—	—	—	—	—	—
Dipped Cone, small	92		190	3	9	25	—	—	—	—	—	—
Double Delight	255		490	9	20	69	—	—	—	—	—	—
Double Hamburger	210		530	36	28	33	—	—	—	—	—	—
Double w/Cheese	239		650	43	37	34	—	—	—	—	—	—
Chocolate Dipped Cone	234	large	450	10	20	58	300	0.4	400	tr	0.12	0.51
Chocolate Dipped Cone	156	medium	300	7	13	40	200	0.4	300	tr	0.09	0.34
Chocolate Dipped Cone	78	small	150	3	7	20	100	tr	100	tr	0.03	0.17
Chocolate Malt	588	large	840	22	28	125	600	5.4	750	6.0	0.15	0.85
Chocolate Malt	418	medium	600	15	20	89	500	3.6	750	3.6	0.12	0.60
Chocolate Malt	241	small	340	10	11	51	300	1.8	400	2.4	0.06	0.34
Chocolate Sundae	248	large	400	9	9	71	300	1.8	400	tr	0.09	0.43
Chocolate Sundae	184	medium	300	6	7	53	200	1.1	300	tr	0.06	0.26
Chocolate Sundae	106	small	170	4	4	30	100	0.7	100	tr	0.03	0.17
Cone	213	large	340	10	10	52	300	tr	400	tr	0.15	0.43
Cone	142	medium	230	6	7	35	200	tr	300	tr	0.09	0.26
Cone	71	small	110	3	3	18	100	tr	100	tr	0.03	0.14
Float	397		330	6	8	59	200	tr	100	tr	0.12	0.17
Freeze	397		520	11	13	89	300	tr	200	tr	0.15	0.34
Sandwich	60		140	3	4	24	60	0.4	100	tr	0.03	0.14
Fiesta Sundae	269		570	9	22	84	200	tr	200	tr	0.23	0.26
Fish Sandwich	170		400	20	17	41	60	1.1	tr	tr	0.15	0.26
Fish Sandwich w/cheese	177		440	24	21	39	150	0.4	100	tr	0.15	0.26
Float	397		410	5	7	82	—	—	—	—	—	—
Freeze	397		500	9	12	89	—	—	—	—	—	—
French Fries	71		200	2	10	25	—	—	—	—	—	—
French Fries	113	large	320	3	16	40	—	—	—	—	—	—
Frozen Dessert	113		180	4	6	27	—	—	—	—	—	—
Hot Dog	100		280	11	16	21	—	—	—	—	—	—
Hot Dog w/Cheese	114		330	15	21	21	—	—	—	—	—	—
Hot Dog w/Chili	128		320	13	20	23	—	—	—	—	—	—
Hot Fudge Brownie Delight	266		600	9	25	85	—	—	—	—	—	—
Malt, large	588		1060	20	25	187	—	—	—	—	—	—
Malt, regular	418		760	14	18	134	—	—	—	—	—	—
Malt, small	291		520	10	13	91	—	—	—	—	—	—
Mr. Misty	439	large	340	0	0	84	—	—	—	—	—	—
Mr. Misty	330	regular	250	0	0	63	—	—	—	—	—	—
Mr. Misty	248	small	190	0	0	48	—	—	—	—	—	—
Mr. Misty Float	404		440	6	8	85	200	tr	120	tr	0.12	0.17
Mr. Misty Float	411		390	5	7	74	—	—	—	—	—	—
Mr. Misty Freeze	411		500	9	12	91	—	—	—	—	—	—
Mr. Misty Kiss	89		70	0	0	17	—	—	—	—	—	—
Onion Rings	85		280	4	16	31	—	—	—	—	—	—
Parfait	283		430	8	8	76	—	—	—	—	—	—
Peanut Buster Parfait	305		740	16	34	94	—	—	—	—	—	—
Shake, large	588		990	19	26	168	—	—	—	—	—	—
Shake, regular	418		710	14	19	120	—	—	—	—	—	—
Shake, small	291		490	10	13	82	—	—	—	—	—	—
Single Hamburger	148		360	21	16	33	—	—	—	—	—	—
Single w/Cheese	162		410	24	20	33	—	—	—	—	—	—
Strawberry Shortcake	312		540	10	11	100	—	—	—	—	—	—
Sundae, large	248		440	8	10	78	—	—	—	—	—	—
Sundae, regular	177		310	5	8	56	—	—	—	—	—	—
Sundae, small	106		190	3	4	33	—	—	—	—	—	—
Super Brazier	298		783	53	48	35	282	7.3	—	<3.2	0.39	0.69
Super Brazier Chili Dog	210		555	23	33	42	158	4.0	—	18.0	0.42	0.48

DAIRY QUEEN

Food item	Serving size (g)	Description	kcal	Protein (g)	Fat (g)	CHO (g)	Ca (mg)	Fe (mg)	Vit A (IU)	Vit C (mg)	Vit B_1 (mg)	Vit B_2 (mg)
Super Brazier Dog	182		518	20	30	41	158	4.3	tr	14.0	0.42	0.44
Super Brazier Dog w/Cheese	203		593	26	36	43	297	4.4	—	14.0	0.43	0.48
Super Hot Dog	175		520	17	27	44	—	—	—	—	—	—
Super Hot Dog w/Cheese	196		580	22	34	45	—	—	—	—	—	—
Super Hot Dog w/Chili	218		570	21	32	47	—	—	—	—	—	—
Triple Hamburger	272		710	51	45	33	—	—	—	—	—	—
Triple w/Cheese	301		820	58	50	34	—	—	—	—	—	—

Source: International Dairy Queen, Inc., Minneapolis, MN, 1982. Nutritional information reviewed and edited by Dr. David J. Aulik in cooperation with Raltech Scientific Services.

JACK IN THE BOX

Food item	Serving size (g)	Description	kcal	Protein (g)	Fat (g)	CHO (g)	Ca (mg)	Fe (mg)	Vit A (IU)	Vit C (mg)	Vit B_1 (mg)	Vit B_2 (mg)
1000 Island Dressing	—		250	0	24	9	—	—	—	—	—	—
Apple Turnover	—		410	4	24	45	—	—	—	—	—	—
Bacon	—	2 slices	70	3	6	0	—	—	—	—	—	—
Bacon Cheeseburger Supreme	—		724	34	46	44	—	—	—	—	—	—
Bleu Cheese Dressing	—		210	0	18	11	—	—	—	—	—	—
Breakfast Jack	—		307	18	13	30	—	—	—	—	—	—
Buttermilk House Dressing	—		290	0	29	6	—	—	—	—	—	—
Canadian Crescent	—		452	19	31	25	—	—	—	—	—	—
Cheese Nachos	—		571	15	35	49	—	—	—	—	—	—
Cheeseburger	—		323	16	15	32	—	—	—	—	—	—
Chicken Strips Dinner	—		689	40	30	65	—	—	—	—	—	—
Chicken Supreme	—		601	31	36	39	—	—	—	—	—	—
Chocolate Shake	—		330	11	7	55	—	—	—	—	—	—
Club Pita	—		284	22	8	30	—	—	—	—	—	—
Grape Jelly	—		38	0	0	9	—	—	—	—	—	—
Ham & Swiss Burger	—		638	36	39	37	—	—	—	—	—	—
Hamburger	—		276	13	12	30	—	—	—	—	—	—
Jumbo Jack	—		485	26	26	38	—	—	—	—	—	—
Jumbo Jack w/Cheese	—		630	32	35	45	—	—	—	—	—	—
Ketchup	—		10	0	2	0	—	—	—	—	—	—
Milk	—		137	10	5	14	—	—	—	—	—	—
Moby Jack	—		444	16	25	39	—	—	—	—	—	—
Mushroom Burger	—		477	28	27	30	—	—	—	—	—	—
Onion Rings	—		382	5	23	39	—	—	—	—	—	—
Orange Juice	—		80	1	0	20	—	—	—	—	—	—
Pancake Breakfast	—		630	16	27	79	—	—	—	—	—	—
Pasta Seafood Salad	—		394	15	22	32	—	—	—	—	—	—
Regular French Fries	—		221	2	12	27	—	—	—	—	—	—
Regular Taco	—		191	8	11	16	—	—	—	—	—	—
Sausage Crescent	—		584	22	43	28	—	—	—	—	—	—
Scrambled Eggs Breakfast	—		720	26	44	55	—	—	—	—	—	—
Shrimp Dinner	—		731	22	37	77	—	—	—	—	—	—
Sirloin Steak Dinner	—		699	38	27	75	—	—	—	—	—	—
Strawberry Shake	—		320	10	7	55	—	—	—	—	—	—
Super Taco	—		288	12	17	21	—	—	—	—	—	—
Supreme Crescent	—		547	20	40	27	—	—	—	—	—	—
Supreme Nachos	—		718	23	40	66	—	—	—	—	—	—
Swiss & Bacon Burger	—		643	33	43	31	—	—	—	—	—	—
Taco Salad	—		377	31	24	10	—	—	—	—	—	—
Vanilla Shake	—		320	10	6	57	—	—	—	—	—	—

Source: Jack In The Box; nutritional information provided by Foodmaker, Inc., San Diego, CA.

KENTUCKY FRIED CHICKEN

Food item	Serving Size (g)	kcal	Protein (g)	CHO (g)	Fat (g)	Cholesterol (mg)	Vit A (mg)	Vit C (mg)	Thia (mg)	Ribo (mg)	Nia (mg)	Ca (mg)	Fe (mg)
Original Recipe Chicken													
Wing	55	178	12.2	6.0	11.7	64	<100	<1.0	0.03	0.08	3.7	47.9	1.2
Side Breast	90	267	18.8	10.8	16.5	77	<100	<1.0	0.06	0.13	6.9	68.0	1.2
Center Breast	115	283	27.5	8.8	15.3	93	<100	<1.0	0.09	0.17	11.5	68.0	1.0
Drumstick	57	146	13.1	4.2	8.5	67	<100	<1.0	0.05	0.12	3.2	21.2	1.1
Thigh	104	294	17.9	11.1	19.7	123	104	<1.0	0.08	0.30	5.5	65.1	1.3
Extra Tasty Crispy Chicken													
Wing	65	254	12.4	9.3	18.6	67	<100	<1.0	0.04	0.06	3.3	17.8	0.6
Side Breast	110	343	21.7	14.0	22.3	81	<100	<1.0	0.09	0.10	8.5	30.4	0.8
Center Breast	135	342	33.0	11.7	19.7	114	<100	<1.0	0.11	0.13	13.1	33.3	0.8
Drumstick	69	204	13.6	6.1	13.9	71	<100	<1.0	0.06	0.12	3.7	12.9	0.7
Thigh	119	406	20.0	14.4	29.8	129	131	<1.0	0.10	0.21	6.5	49.0	1.2
Kentucky Nuggets	16	46	2.8	2.2	2.9	11.9	<100	<1.0	<0.01	0.03	1.00	2.4	0.1
Barbeque sauce	28.3	35	0.3	7.1	0.6	<1.0	<370	<1.0	<0.01	0.01	0.19	6.1	0.2
Sweet 'n Sour	28.3	58	0.1	13.0	0.6	<1.0	<100	<1.0	<.01	0.02	0.04	4.7	0.2
Honey	14.2	49	0.0	12.1	<0.01	<1.0	<100	<1.0	<0.01	0.00	0.04	0.6	0.1
Mustard	28.3	36	0.9	6.1	0.9	<1.0	<100	<1.0	<0.01	0.01	0.16	10.2	0.3
Chicken Littles	47	169	5.7	13.8	10.1	18	<100	<1.0	0.16	0.12	2.2	22.6	1.7
Buttermilk biscuits	65	235	4.5	28.0	11.7	1	<100	<1.0	0.24	0.19	2.6	95.0	1.6
Mashed potatoes w/gravy	98	71	2.4	11.7	1.6	<1	<100	<1.0	<0.01	0.04	1.2	21.8	0.04
French Fries	77	244	3.2	31.1	11.9	2	<100	15.7	0.15	0.05	2.0	12.5	0.06
Corn on the Cob	143	176	5.1	31.9	3.1	<1	272	2.3	0.14	0.11	1.8	7.2	0.08
Cole Slaw	91	119	1.5	13.2	6.6	5	310	21.5	0.03	0.03	0.2	32.8	0.02
Colonel's Chicken Sandwich	166	482	20.8	38.6	27.3	47	<100	<1.0	0.38	0.27	11.1	46.1	1.3

Source: Public Affairs Department, KFC Corporation, Louisville, KY.

LONG JOHN SILVER'S

Food item	Serving size (g)	Description	kcal	Protein (g)	Fat (g)	CHO (g)	Ca (mg)	Fe (mg)	Vit A (IU)	Vit C (mg)	Vit B_1 (mg)	Vit B_2 (mg)
3 Pc. Nugget Dinner		6 chicken nuggets, Fryes, slaw	699	23	45	54	—	—	—	—	—	—
Apple Pie	113		280	2	11	43	—	—	—	—	—	—
Barbecue Sauce	34		45	0	0	11	—	—	—	—	—	—
Battered Shrimp Dinner		6 battered shrimp, Fryes, slaw	711	17	45	60	—	—	—	—	—	—
Bleu Cheese Dressing	45		225	4	23	3	—	—	—	—	—	—
Breaded Clams			465	13	25	46	—	—	—	—	—	—
Breaded Fish Sandwich Platter		Fish sandwich, Fryes, slaw	835	30	42	84	—	—	—	—	—	—
Breaded Oysters		6 pc.	460	14	19	58	—	—	—	—	—	—
Breaded Shrimp Platter		Breaded shrimp, Fryes, slaw, 2 hush puppies	962	20	57	93	—	—	—	—	—	—
Cherry Pie	113		294	3	11	46	—	—	—	—	—	—
Chicken Planks		4 pc.	458	27	23	35	—	—	—	—	—	—

LONG JOHN SILVER'S

Food item	Serving size (g)	Description	kcal	Protein (g)	Fat (g)	CHO (g)	Ca (mg)	Fe (mg)	Vit A (IU)	Vit C (mg)	Vit B_1 (mg)	Vit B_2 (mg)
Clam Chowder	187		128	7	5	15	—	—	—	—	—	—
Clam Dinner		Clams, Fryes, slaw	955	22	58	100	—	—	—	—	—	—
Cole Slaw			138	1	8	16	—	—	—	—	—	—
Cole Slaw, drained on fork	98		182	1	15	11	—	—	—	—	—	—
Combo Salad		4.25 oz seafood salad, 2 oz salad shrimp, 6 oz lettuce, 2.4 oz tomato, 1 pkg crackers	397	27	29	21	—	—	—	—	—	—
Corn on the Cob	150	1 ear	176	5	4	29	—	—	—	—	—	—
Fish & Chicken		1 fish, 2 tender chicken planks, Fryes, slaw	935	36	55	73	—	—	—	—	—	—
Fish & Fryes		3 fish, Fryes	853	43	48	64	—	—	—	—	—	—
Fish & Fryes		2 pc fish, Fryes	651	30	36	53	—	—	—	—	—	—
Fish & More		2 fish, Fryes, slaw, 2 hush puppies	978	34	58	92	—	—	—	—	—	—
Fish w/Batter		2 pc	319	19	19	19	—	—	—	—	—	—
Fish w/Batter		3 pc	477	28	28	28	—	—	—	—	—	—
Four Nuggets and Fryes			427	16	24	39	—	—	—	—	—	—
Fryes	85		247	4	12	31	—	—	—	—	—	—
Fryes			275	4	15	32	—	—	—	—	—	—
Honey–Mustard Sauce	35		56	—	—	14	—	—	—	—	—	—
Hush Puppies	47	2 pieces	145	3	7	18	—	—	—	—	—	—
Hush Puppies		3 pc	158	1	7	20	—	—	—	—	—	—
Kitchen–Breaded Fish (Three Piece Dinner)		3 kitchen breaded fish, Fryes, slaw, 2 hush puppies	940	35	52	84	—	—	—	—	—	—
Kitchen–Breaded Fish (Two Piece Dinner)		2 kitchen–breaded fish, Fryes, slaw, 2 hush puppies	818	26	46	76	—	—	—	—	—	—
Lemon Meringue Pie	99		200	2	6	37	—	—	—	—	—	—
Ocean Chef Salad		6 oz. lettuce, 1.25 oz shrimp, 2 oz. seafood blend, 2 tomato wedges, 3/4 oz cheese	229	27	8	13	—	—	—	—	—	—
Ocean Scallops		6 pieces	257	10	12	27	—	—	—	—	—	—
One Fish and Fryes			449	16	24	42	—	—	—	—	—	—
One Fish, Two Nuggets, and Fryes			539	23	30	46	—	—	—	—	—	—
Oyster Dinner		6 oysters, Fryes, slaw	789	17	45	78	—	—	—	—	—	—
Pecan Pie	113		446	5	22	59	—	—	—	—	—	—
Peg Leg w/Batter		5 pieces	514	25	33	30	—	—	—	—	—	—

LONG JOHN SILVER'S

Food item	Serving size (g)	Description	kcal	Protein (g)	Fat (g)	CHO (g)	Ca (mg)	Fe (mg)	Vit A (IU)	Vit C (mg)	Vit B_1 (mg)	Vit B_2 (mg)
Pumpkin Pie	113		251	4	11	34	—	—	—	—	—	—
Reduced Calorie Italian Dressing	49		20	0	1	3	—	—	—	—	—	—
Scallop Dinner		6 scallops, Fryes, slaw	747	17	45	66	—	—	—	—	—	—
Sea Salad Dressing	45		220	4	21	5	—	—	—	—	—	—
Seafood Platter		1 fish, 2 battered shrimp, 2 scallops, Fryes, slaw	976	29	58	85	—	—	—	—	—	—
Seafood Salad		5.6 oz seafood salad, 6 oz lettuce, 2.4 oz tomato	426	19	30	22	—	—	—	—	—	—
Shrimp & Fish Dinner		1 fish, 3 battered shrimp, Fryes, slaw, 2 hush puppies	917	27	55	80	—	—	—	—	—	—
Shrimp Salad		4.5 oz salad shrimp, 6 oz lettuce, 2.4 oz tomato	203	28	3	16	—	—	—	—	—	—
Shrimp w/Batter		5 pieces	269	9	13	31	—	—	—	—	—	—
Sweet–n–Sour Sauce	30		—	—	—	—	—	—	—	—	—	—
Tartar Sauce	30		117	—	11	5	—	—	—	—	—	—
Tender Chicken Plank Dinner		3 chicken planks, Fryes, slaw	885	32	51	72	—	—	—	—	—	—
Tender Chicken Plank Dinner		4 chicken planks, Fryes, slaw	1037	41	59	82	—	—	—	—	—	—
Thousand Island Dressing	48		223	—	22	8	—	—	—	—	—	—
Three Piece Fish Dinner		3 fish, Fryes, slaw, 2 hush puppies	1180	47	70	93	—	—	—	—	—	—
Treasure Chest		2 pc fish, 2 Peg Legs	467	25	29	27	—	—	—	—	—	—
Two Planks and Fryes			551	22	28	51	—	—	—	—	—	—

Source: Long John Silver's Seafood Shoppes, sampling and nutrient analysis conducted independently by the Department of Nutrition and Food Science, University of Kentucky, April 10, 1986.

McDONALD'S

Food Item	Serving Size (g)/(oz)	kcal	Protein (g)	CHO (g)	Fat (g)	Cholesterol (mg)	Percentage of U.S. RDA: Vit A (mg)	Vit C (mg)	Thia (mg)	Ribo (mg)	Nia (mg)	Ca (mg)	Fe (mg)
Sandwiches													
Hamburger	102 g	255	12	30	9	37	4	4	20	10	20	10	15
Cheeseburger	116 g	305	15	30	13	50	8	4	20	15	20	20	15
Quarter Pounder	166 g	410	23	34	20	85	4	6	25	15	35	15	20
Quarter Pounder w/Cheese	194 g	510	28	34	28	115	15	6	25	20	35	30	20

McDONALD'S

Food Item	Serving Size (g)/(oz)	kcal	Protein (g)	CHO (g)	Fat (g)	Choles-terol (mg)	Percentage of U.S. RDA						
							Vit A (mg)	Vit C (mg)	Thia (mg)	Ribo (mg)	Nia (mg)	Ca (mg)	Fe (mg)
Sandwiches (cont.)													
McLean Deluxe	206 g	320	22	35	10	60	10	10	25	20	35	15	20
McLean Deluxe w/Cheese	219 g	370	24	35	14	75	15	10	25	20	35	20	20
Big Mac	215 g	500	25	42	26	100	6	2	30	25	35	25	20
Filet-O-Fish	141 g	370	14	38	18	50	2	*	20	8	45	15	10
McChicken	187 g	415	19	39	20	50	2	4	60	10	45	15	15
Chicken Fajitas	82 g	185	11	20	8	35	2	8	10	10	20	8	4
French fries													
Small	68 g	220	3	26	12	0	*	15	10	*	10	*	2
Medium	97 g	320	4	36	17	0	*	20	15	*	15	*	4
Large	122 g	400	6	46	22	0	*	25	15	*	15	*	6
Chicken McNuggets/ Sauces													
Chicken McNuggets	6 pce	270	20	17	15	55	*	*	8	8	40	*	6
Hot Mustard Sauce	1.05 oz	70	0	8	3.6	5	*	*	*	*	*	2	*
Barbeque Sauce	1.12 oz	50	0	12	0.5	0	4	4	*	*	*	*	2
Sweet 'N Sour Sauce	1.12 oz	60	0	14	0.2	0	6	*	*	*	*	*	*
Honey	0.50 oz	45	0	12	0	0	*	*	*	*	*	*	*
Salads													
Chef Salad	265 g	170	17	8	9	111	100	35	20	15	20	15	8
Garden Salad	189 g	50	4	6	2	65	90	35	6	6	2	4	8
Chunky Chicken Salad	255 g	150	25	7	4	78	170	45	15	10	45	4	6
Side Salad	106 g	30	2	4	1	33	80	20	4	4	*	2	4
Croutons	11 g	50	1	7	2	0	*	*	4	*	2	*	*
Bacon Bits	3 g	15	1	0	1	1	*	*	*	*	*	*	*
Salad dressings													
Bleu Cheese	1/2 oz†	50	0	1	4	7	*	*	*	*	*	*	*
Ranch	1/2 oz†	55	0	1	5	5	*	*	*	*	*	*	*
1000 Island	1/2 oz†	45	0	4	3	8	*	*	*	*	*	*	*
Lite Vinaigrette	1/2 oz†	12	0	2	0.5	0	*	*	*	*	*	*	*
Red French Reduced Calorie	1/2 oz†	40	0	5	2	0	*	*	*	*	*	*	*
Breakfast													
Egg McMuffin	135 g	280	18	28	11	235	10	*	30	20	20	25	15
Sausage McMuffin	135 g	345	15	27	20	57	4	*	35	15	25	20	15
Sausage McMuffin w/Egg	159 g	430	21	27	25	270	10	*	35	25	25	25	20
English Muffin w/Spread	58 g	170	5	26	4	0	2	*	20	8	10	15	8
Sausage Biscuit	118 g	420	12	32	28	44	*	*	30	10	20	8	10
Sausage Biscuit w/Egg	175 g	505	19	33	33	260	6	*	30	20	20	10	20
Bacon, Egg & Cheese Biscuit	153 g	440	15	33	26	240	10	*	25	20	10	20	15
Biscuit w/Biscuit Spread	75 g	260	5	32	13	1	*	*	15	6	8	8	8
Sausage	43 g	160	7	0	15	43	*	*	15	6	10	*	4
Scrambled Eggs (2)	100 g	140	12	1	10	425	10	*	4	15	*	6	10
Hash Brown Potatoes	53 g	130	1	15	7	0	*	2	4	*	4	*	*
Hotcakes w/Margarine & Syrup (2 pats)	174 g	440	8	74	12	8	4	*	20	20	15	10	10
Breakfast Burrito	105 g	280	12	21	17	135	10	10	20	15	10	10	8
Muffins/Danish													
Fat-Free Apple Bran Muffin	75 g	180	5	40	0	0	*	*	10	10	10	4	6
Apple Danish	115 g	390	6	51	17	25	*	25	20	10	10	*	8
Iced Cheese Danish	110 g	390	7	42	21	47	4	*	20	15	10	4	8
Cinnamon Raisin Danish	110 g	440	6	58	21	34	*	6	20	15	15	4	10
Raspberry Danish	117 g	410	6	62	16	26	*	6	20	10	10	*	8

McDONALD'S

Food Item	Serving Size (g)/(oz)	kcal	Protein (g)	CHO (g)	Fat (g)	Choles-terol (mg)	Percentage of U.S. RDA: Vit A (mg)	Vit C (mg)	Thia (mg)	Ribo (mg)	Nia (mg)	Ca (mg)	Fe (mg)
Desserts/Milk shakes													
Vanilla Lowfat Frozen Yogurt Cone	3 oz	105	4	22	1	3	2	*	2	10	2	10	*
Strawberry Lowfat Frozen Yogurt Sundae	6 oz	210	6	49	1	5	4	2	4	20	*	20	*
Hot Fudge Lowfat Frozen Yogurt Sundae	6 oz	240	7	50	3	6	4	*	6	20	*	25	*
Hot Caramel Lowfat Frozen Yogurt Sundae	6 oz	270	7	59	3	13	6	*	6	20	*	20	*
Apple Pie	3 oz	260	2	30	15	6	*	20	4	*	*	*	4
McDonaldland Cookies	2 oz	290	4	47	9	0	*	*	15	10	10	*	10
Chocolaty Chip Cookies	2 oz	330	4	42	15	4	*	*	10	10	10	2	10
Vanilla Lowfat Milk Shake	10.4 oz	290	11	60	1.3	10	6	*	8	30	*	35	*
Chocolate Lowfat Milk Shake	10.4 oz	320	11	66	1.7	10	6	*	8	30	*	35	*
Strawberry Lowfat Milk Shake	10.4 oz	320	11	67	1.3	10	6	*	8	30	*	35	*
Milk/Juices													
1% Lowfat Milk	8 fl oz	110	9	12	2	10	10	4	8	30	*	30	*
Orange Juice	6 fl oz	80	1	19	0	0	*	120	10	*	*	*	*
Grapefruit Juice	6 fl oz	80	1	19	0	0	*	100	4	2	2	*	*
Apple Juice	6 fl oz	90	0	23	0	0	*	2	2	*	*	*	4*

* = less than 2% of U.S. RDA.
Source: McDonald's Corporation. Nutritional analysis reported by Hazelton Labatories, Inc., 1993.

PIZZA HUT

Food Item (1 slice)	Serving Size (g)	kcal	Protein (g)	Fat (g)	CHO (g)	Ca (mg)	Fe (mg)	Vit A (IU)	Vit C (mg)	Vit B_1 (mg)	Vit B_2 (mg)
Thick 'N' Chewy, Beef		620	38	20	73	400	7.2	750	<1.2	0.68	0.60
Thick 'N' Chewy, Cheese		560	34	14	71	500	5.4	1000	<1.2	0.68	0.68
Thick 'N' Chewy, Pepperoni		560	31	18	68	400	5.4	1250	3.6	0.68	0.68
Thick 'N' Chewy, Pork		640	36	23	71	400	7.2	750	1.2	0.90	0.77
Thick 'N' Chewy, Supreme		640	36	22	74	400	7.2	1000	9.0	0.75	0.85
Thin 'N' Crispy, Beef		490	29	19	51	350	6.3	750	<1.2	0.30	0.60
Thin 'N' Crispy, Cheese		450	25	15	54	450	4.5	750	<1.2	0.30	0.51
Thin 'N' Crispy, Pepperoni		430	23	17	45	300	4.5	1000	<1.2	0.30	0.51
Thin 'N' Crispy, Pork		520	27	23	51	350	6.3	1000	<1.2	0.38	0.68
Thin 'N' Crispy, Supreme		510	27	21	51	350	7.2	1250	2.4	0.38	0.68

Source: Research 900 and Pizza Hut, Inc., Wichita, KS.

ROY ROGERS

Food Item	Serving Size (g)	Description	kcal	Protein (g)	Fat (g)	CHO (g)	Ca (mg)	Fe (mg)	Vit A (IU)	Vit C (mg)	Vit B_1 (mg)	Vit B_2 (mg)
Apple Danish	71		249	4.5	11.6	31.6	—	—	—	—	—	—
Bacon Cheeseburger	180		581	32.3	39.2	25.0	—	—	—	—	—	—
Biscuit	63		231	4.4	12.1	26.2	—	—	—	—	—	—
Breakfast Crescent Sandwich	127		401	13.3	27.3	25.3	—	—	—	—	—	—

ROY ROGERS

Food Item	Serving Size (g)	Description	kcal	Protein (g)	Fat (g)	CHO (g)	Ca (mg)	Fe (mg)	Vit A (IU)	Vit C (mg)	Vit B_1 (mg)	Vit B_2 (mg)
Breakfast Crescent Sandwich w/bacon	133		431	15.4	29.7	25.5	—	—	—	—	—	—
Breakfast Crescent Sandwich w/ham	165		557	19.8	41.7	25.3	—	—	—	—	—	—
Breakfast Crescent Sandwich w/sausage	162		449	19.9	29.4	25.9	—	—	—	—	—	—
Breast & Wing	196		604	43.5	36.5	25.4	—	—	—	—	—	—
Brownie	64		264	3.3	11.4	37.3	—	—	—	—	—	—
Caramel Sundae	145		293	7.0	8.5	51.5	—	—	—	—	—	—
Cheese Danish	71		254	4.9	12.2	31.4	—	—	—	—	—	—
Cheeseburger	173		563	29.5	37.3	27.4	—	—	—	—	—	—
Cherry Danish	71		271	4.4	14.4	31.7	—	—	—	—	—	—
Chicken Breast	144		412	33.0	23.7	16.9	—	—	—	—	—	—
Chocolate Shake	319		358	7.9	10.2	61.3	—	—	—	—	—	—
Cole Slaw	99		110	1.0	6.9	11.0	—	—	—	—	—	—
Crescent Roll	70		287	4.7	17.7	27.2	—	—	—	—	—	—
Egg and Biscuit Platter	165		394	16.9	26.5	21.9	—	—	—	—	—	—
Egg and Biscuit Platter w/bacon	173		435	19.7	29.6	22.1	—	—	—	—	—	—
Egg and Biscuit Platter w/ham	200		442	23.5	28.6	22.5	—	—	—	—	—	—
Egg and Biscuit Platter w/sausage	203		550	23.4	40.9	21.9	—	—	—	—	—	—
French Fries	85		268	3.9	13.5	32.0	—	—	—	—	—	—
Hamburger	143		456	23.8	28.3	65.6	—	—	—	—	—	—
Hot Chocolate	8 oz		123	3.0	2.0	22.0	—	—	—	—	—	—
Hot Fudge Sundae	151		337	6.5	12.5	53.3	—	—	—	—	—	—
Hot Topped Potato plain	227		211	5.9	0.2	47.9	—	—	—	—	—	—
Hot Topped Potato w/bacon 'n cheese	248		397	17.1	21.7	33.3	—	—	—	—	—	—
Hot Topped Potato w/broccoli 'n cheese	312		376	13.7	18.1	39.6	—	—	—	—	—	—
Hot Topped Potato w/oleo	236		274	5.9	7.3	47.9	—	—	—	—	—	—
Hot Topped Potato w/sour cream 'n chives	297		408	7.3	20.9	47.6	—	—	—	—	—	—
Hot Topped Potato w/taco beef 'n cheese	359		463	21.8	21.8	45.0	—	—	—	—	—	—
Large Fries	113		357	5.3	18.4	42.7	—	—	—	—	—	—
Large Roast Beef	182		360	33.9	11.9	29.6	—	—	—	—	—	—
Large Roast Beef w/Cheese	211		467	39.6	20.9	30.3	—	—	—	—	—	—
Leg	53		140	11.5	8.0	5.5	—	—	—	—	—	—
Macaroni	100		186	3.1	10.7	19.4	—	—	—	—	—	—
Milk	8 oz		150	8.0	8.2	11.4	—	—	—	—	—	—
Orange Juice	8 oz		99	1.5	0.2	22.8	—	—	—	—	—	—
Orange Juice	8 oz		136	2.0	0.3	31.3	—	—	—	—	—	—
Pancake Platter (w.syrup, butter)	165		452	7.7	15.2	71.8	—	—	—	—	—	—
Pancake Platter (w.syrup, butter) w/bacon	173		493	10.4	18.3	72.0	—	—	—	—	—	—
Pancake Platter (w.syrup, butter) w/ham	200		506	14.3	17.3	72.4	—	—	—	—	—	—
Pancake Platter (w.syrup, butter) w/sausage	203		608	14.2	29.6	71.8	—	—	—	—	—	—
Potato Salad	100		107	2.0	6.1	10.9	—	—	—	—	—	—
Roast Beef Sandwich	154		317	27.2	10.2	29.1	—	—	—	—	—	—
Roast Beef Sandwich w/Cheese	182		424	32.9	19.2	29.9	—	—	—	—	—	—
RR Bar Burger	208		611	36.1	39.4	28.0	—	—	—	—	—	—
Salad Bar 1,000 Island	—	2 T	160	NA	16.0	4.0	—	—	—	—	—	—
Salad Bar Bacon 'n Tomato	—	2 T	136	NA	12.0	6.0	—	—	—	—	—	—
Salad Bar Bacon Bits	—	1 T	24	4.0	1.0	38.0	—	—	—	—	—	—

ROY ROGERS

Food Item	Serving Size (g)	Description	kcal	Protein (g)	Fat (g)	CHO (g)	Ca (mg)	Fe (mg)	Vit A (IU)	Vit C (mg)	Vit B_1 (mg)	Vit B_2 (mg)
Salad Bar Blue Cheese Dressing	—	2 T	150	2.0	16.0	2.0	—	—	—	—	—	—
Salad Bar Cheddar Cheese	—	¼ cup	112	5.8	9.0	0.8	—	—	—	—	—	—
Salad Bar Chinese Noodles	—	¼ cup	55	1.5	2.8	6.5	—	—	—	—	—	—
Salad Bar Chopped Eggs	—	2 T	55	4.0	4.0	0.7	—	—	—	—	—	—
Salad Bar Croutons	—	2 T	132	5.5	0	31.0	—	—	—	—	—	—
Salad Bar Cucumbers	—	5–6 slices	4	NA	0	1.0	—	—	—	—	—	—
Salad Bar Green Peas	—	¼ cup	7	0.5	0	1.2	—	—	—	—	—	—
Salad Bar Green Peppers	—	2 T	4	0.3	0	1.0	—	—	—	—	—	—
Salad Bar Lettuce	—	1 cup	10	NA	0	4.0	—	—	—	—	—	—
Salad Bar Lo–cal Italian	—	2 T	70	NA	6.0	2.0	—	—	—	—	—	—
Salad Bar Macaroni Salad	—	2 T	60	1.0	3.6	6.2	—	—	—	—	—	—
Salad Bar Mushrooms	—	¼ cup	5	0.5	0	0.7	—	—	—	—	—	—
Salad Bar Potato Salad	—	2 T	50	1.0	3.0	5.5	—	—	—	—	—	—
Salad Bar Ranch	—	2 T	155	NA	14.0	4.0	—	—	—	—	—	—
Salad Bar Shredded Carrots	—	¼ cup	12	0.6	0	24.0	—	—	—	—	—	—
Salad Bar Sliced Beets	—	¼ cup	16	0.5	0	3.8	—	—	—	—	—	—
Salad Bar Sunflower Seeds	—	2 T	101	4.0	9.0	5.0	—	—	—	—	—	—
Salad Bar Tomatoes	—	3 slices	20	0.8	0	4.8	—	—	—	—	—	—
Strawberry Shake	312		315	7.6	10.2	49.4	—	—	—	—	—	—
Strawberry Shortcake	205		447	10.1	19.2	59.3	—	—	—	—	—	—
Strawberry Sundae	142		216	5.7	7.1	33.1	—	—	—	—	—	—
Thigh	98		296	18.4	19.5	11.7	—	—	—	—	—	—
Thigh & Leg	151		436	29.9	27.5	17.2	—	—	—	—	—	—
Vanilla Shake	306		306	8.0	10.7	45.0	—	—	—	—	—	—
Wing	52		192	10.5	12.8	8.5	—	—	—	—	—	—

Source: Roy Rogers Restaurants, Marriott Corporation, Washington, DC. Nutritional data furnished by Lancaster Laboratories, 1985.

TACO BELL

Food Item	Serving Size (g)	kcal	Protein (g)	CHO (g)	Fat (g)	Cholesterol (mg)	Vit A (IU)	Vit C (mg)	Thia (mg)	Ribo (mg)	Nia (mg)	Ca (mg)	Fe (mg)
Tacos and Tostadas													
Taco	78	183	10	11	11	32	350	1	0.1	0.1	1.2	84	1
Soft Taco	92	225	12	18	12	32	200	1	0.4	0.2	2.8	116	2
Soft Taco Supreme	124	272	13	19	16	32	450	3	0.4	0.3	2.8	142	2
Tostada	156	243	9	27	11	16	650	45	0.1	0.2	0.6	180	2
Chicken Soft Taco	107	213	14	19	10	52	200	2	0.2	0.2	3.4	80	6
Taco Supreme	92	230	11	12	15	32	550	3	0.1	0.2	1.2	110	1
Burritos													
Bean	206	385	15	63	14	9	350	53	0.4	2.0	2.8	190	4
Beef	206	431	25	48	21	57	500	2	0.4	2.1	4.2	150	4
Burrito Supreme	255	440	20	55	22	52	450	26	0.4	0.1	4.4	110	8
Combo burrito	198	407	18	46	16	33	900	27	0.4	2.1	3.6	119	4
Chicken burrito	171	334	17	38	12	33	450	11	0.2	0.3	3.2	150	3
Specialty items													
Nachos Bellgrande	287	649	22	61	35	36	1150	58	0.1	0.3	2.2	297	3
Nachos Supreme	145	367	12	41	27	18	700	30	0.1	0.2	0.2	260	tr
Nachos	106	346	7	37	18	9	550	2	tr	0.2	0.6	191	1
Beef Meximelt	106	266	13	19	15	38	800	2	0.4	0.2	2.4	250	2
Chicken Meximelt	107	257	14	19	15	48	500	2	0.2	0.2	1.4	220	4
Mexican Pizza	223	575	21	40	37	52	1000	31	0.3	0.3	3	257	4
Pintos 'N Cheese	128	190	9	19	9	16	450	52	0.1	0.2	0.4	156	1

TACO BELL

Food Item	Serving Size (g)	kcal	Protein (g)	CHO (g)	Fat (g)	Choles-terol (mg)	Vit A (IU)	Vit C (mg)	Thia (mg)	Ribo (mg)	Nia (mg)	Ca (mg)	Fe (mg)
Specialty items (cont.)													
Chilito	156	383	18	36	18	47	850	tr	0.2	0.2	2.8	270	3
Taco Salad	575	905	34	55	61	80	1650	75	0.5	0.6	4.8	320	6
Taco Salad without Shell	520	484	28	22	31	80	1650	74	0.2	0.4	3.2	290	4
Cinnamon Twists	35	171	2	24	8	0	tr	tr	tr	tr	tr	tr	tr
Side orders													
Taco Sauce	11	2	0	0	0	0	200	tr	tr	tr	tr	2	tr
Hot Taco Sauce	11	3	0	0	0	0	150	tr	tr	tr	tr	2	tr
Salsa	10	18	1	4	0	0	250	tr	tr	0.1	tr	36	1
Pico de Gallo	28	6	0	1	0	1	550	2	tr	tr	tr	10	tr
Sour Cream	21	46	1	1	4	0	150	tr	tr	tr	tr	20	tr
Guacamole	21	34	1	3	2	0	100	3	tr	tr	tr	10	tr
Ranch Dressing	74	236	2	1	25	35	250	tr	tr	0.1	tr	29	1
Jalapeño Peppers	100	20	1	4	0	0	250	2	tr	tr	tr	40	tr
Nacho Cheese Sauce	56	103	4	5	8	9	150	1	tr	0.1	tr	110	tr
Red Sauce	28	10	0	2	0	0	250	1	tr	tr	tr	11	tr
Green Sauce	28	4	0	1	0	0	100	tr	tr	tr	tr	tr	tr

tr = trace.
Source: From Taco Bell Corporation, Irvine, CA, 1992. For more information, call 714-863-2200.

WENDY'S

Food Item	Serving Size (g)	kcal	Protein (g)	CHO (g)	Fat (g)	Choles-terol (mg)	Percentage of U.S. RDA						
							Vit A (mg)	Vit C (mg)	Thia (mg)	Ribo (mg)	Nia (mg)	Ca (mg)	Fe (mg)
Sandwiches													
¼ lb. hamburger patty	74	180	19	—	12	65	—	—	4	—	20	—	20
Plain single	126	340	24	30	15	65	—	—	25	20	30	10	30
Single with everything	210	420	25	35	21	70	5	15	25	20	30	10	30
Wendy's Big Classic	260	570	27	47	33	90	10	20	30	25	35	15	35
Jr. Hamburger	111	260	15	33	9	34	2	4	25	20	20	10	20
Jr. Cheeseburger	125	310	18	33	13	34	2	4	25	50	20	10	20
Jr. bacon cheeseburger	155	430	22	32	25	50	2	15	30	50	25	10	20
Jr. Swiss deluxe	163	360	18	34	18	40	4	10	25	60	20	20	20
Kids' meal hamburger	104	260	15	32	9	35	2	2	25	20	20	10	20
Kids'meal cheeseburger	116	300	18	33	13	35	2	2	25	50	20	10	20
Grilled chicken fillet	70	100	18	—	3	55	—	—	4	4	35	—	6
Grilled chicken sandwich	175	340	24	36	13	60	2	8	30	25	50	10	20
Chicken breast fillet	99	220	21	11	10	55	—	—	8	8	60	—	70
Chicken sandwich	219	430	26	41	19	60	2	8	30	25	70	10	80
Chicken club sandwich	205	506	30	42	25	70	2	15	35	30	80	10	80
Fish fillet sandwich	170	460	18	42	25	55	2	2	40	35	20	10	15
Kaiser bun	65	200	6	37	3	10	—	—	25	20	10	10	10
White bun	56	160	5	30	3	tr	—	—	20	20	10	10	10
Sandwich Toppings													
American cheese slice	18	70	4	—	6	15	6	—	—	4	—	12	—
Bacon	6	30	2	—	3	5	—	4	4	—	2	—	—
Ketchup	14	17	—	4	—	N/A	4	4	—	—	—	—	—
Lettuce	10	1	—	—	—	0	—	—	—	—	—	—	—
Mayonnaise	13	90	—	—	10	10	—	—	—	—	—	—	—
Mustard	5	4	—	—	—	0	—	—	—	—	—	—	—
Onion	10	4	—	—	—	0	—	—	—	—	—	—	—
Pickles	14	2	—	—	—	0	—	—	—	—	—	—	—
Tomatoes	21	4	—	—	—	0	—	6	—	—	—	—	—

WENDY'S

Food Item	Serving Size (g)	kcal	Protein (g)	CHO (g)	Fat (g)	Cholesterol (mg)	Percentage of U.S. RDA						
							Vit A (mg)	Vit C (mg)	Thia (mg)	Ribo (mg)	Nia (mg)	Ca (mg)	Fe (mg)
Sandwich Toppings (cont.)													
Honey mustard	14	71	—	4	6	5	—	—	—	—	—	—	—
Tartar sauce	21	120	—	—	14	15	—	—	15	10	—	—	—
Superbar—Pasta													
Alfredo sauce	56	35	1	5	1	tr	—	—	—	—	—	6	—
Fettucini	56	190	4	27	3	10	—	—	10	6	6	—	6
Garlic toast	18.3	70	2	9	3	tr	4	—	6	2	2	2	2
Pasta medley	56	60	2	9	2	tr	6	15	6	4	4	—	4
Rotini	56	90	3	15	2	tr	—	—	6	4	6	—	4
Spaghetti sauce	56	28	—	7	0	tr	—	—	—	—	—	—	—
Spaghetti meat sauce	56	60	4	8	2	10	4	4	—	2	4	—	4
Garden Spot Salad Bar													
Alfalfa sprouts	28	8	1	1	0	0	—	4	—	2	—	—	—
Applesauce, chunky	28	22	—	6	—	0	—	—	—	—	—	—	—
Bacon bits	14	40	5	—	14	10	—	2	6	4	6	—	—
Bananas	28	26	—	7	—	0	—	4	—	2	—	—	—
Breadsticks	7.5	30	1	5	1	0	—	—	2	2	2	2	2
Broccoli	43	12	1	2	0	0	6	65	2	2	—	2	2
Cantaloupe	57	20	—	5	0	0	20	30	—	—	—	—	—
Carrots	27	12	—	2	0	0	80	4	2	—	—	—	—
Cauliflower	57	14	1	3	0	0	—	70	4	2	2	2	2
Cheddar chips	28	160	3	12	12	5	—	—	2	—	4	6	2
Cheese, shredded (imitation)	28	90	6	1	6	tr	4	—	—	15	—	20	—
Chicken salad	56	120	7	4	8	tr	—	4	—	4	6	—	2
Chives	28	71	6	18	1	0	195	313	15	25	8	25	30
Chow mein noodles	14	74	1	8	4	0	—	—	6	4	4	—	4
Cole slaw	57	70	—	8	5	5	4	25	—	—	—	2	—
Cottage cheese	105	108	13	3	4	15	6	—	—	10	—	6	—
Croutons	14	60	2	8	3	—	—	—	4	4	4	—	4
Cucumbers	14	2	—	—	0	0	—	—	—	—	—	—	—
Eggs (hard cooked)	20	30	3	—	2	90	4	—	—	6	—	—	—
Garbanzo beans	28	46	3	8	1	0	—	—	2	—	—	—	6
Green peas	28	21	1	4	0	0	4	8	6	2	—	—	2
Green peppers	37	10	—	2	0	0	2	60	2	—	—	—	—
Honeydew melon	57	20	—	5	0	0	—	25	2	—	2	—	—
Jalapeno peppers	14	2	—	—	0	0	—	—	—	—	—	—	—
Lettuce—iceberg	55	8	—	1	0	0	2	4	2	—	—	—	2
Lettuce—romaine	55	9	1	1	0	0	15	20	4	4	—	2	4
Mushrooms	17	4	—	—	0	0	—	—	—	4	4	—	—
Olives, black	28	35	—	2	3	0	—	—	—	—	—	2	4
Oranges	56	26	—	7	0	0	—	50	4	—	—	2	—
Parmesan cheese	28	130	12	1	9	20	6	—	—	6	—	40	—
Parmesan cheese (imitation)	28	80	9	4	3	tr	20	—	—	—	—	50	—
Pasta salad	57	35	2	6	—	0	—	—	—	2	2	—	2
Peaches	57	31	—	8	0	0	2	2	—	—	2	—	—
Pepperoni, sliced	28	140	5	2	12	35	—	—	160	4	10	—	2
Pineapple chunks	100	60	—	16	0	0	—	15	6	—	—	—	2
Potato salad	57	125	—	6	11	10	—	10	2	—	2	—	2
Pudding—butterscotch	57	90	1	11	4	tr	—	—	—	—	—	6	2
Pudding—chocolate	57	90	—	12	4	tr	—	—	2	2	—	15	2
Red onions	9	2	—	—	0	0	—	—	—	—	—	—	—
Red peppers, crushed	28	120	5	15	4	0	200	15	10	15	20	2	15
Seafood salad	56	110	4	7	7	tr	—	2	—	2	—	20	2
Strawberries	56	17	—	4	0	0	—	50	—	2	—	—	—

WENDY'S

Food Item	Serving Size (g)	kcal	Protein (g)	CHO (g)	Fat (g)	Choles-terol (mg)	Percentage of U.S. RDA Vit A (mg)	Vit C (mg)	Thia (mg)	Ribo (mg)	Nia (mg)	Ca (mg)	Fe (mg)
Garden Spot Salad Bar (cont.)													
Sour topping	28	58	—	2	5	0	—	—	—	—	—	—	—
Sunflower seeds & raisins	28	140	5	6	10	0	—	—	30	4	6	2	10
Three bean salad	57	60	1	13	—	—	4	—	—	—	—	—	2
Tomatoes	28	6	—	1	0	0	2	10	—	—	—	—	—
Tuna salad	56	100	8	4	6	tr	—	4	—	4	25	—	2
Turkey ham	28	35	5	—	1	15	—	—	—	4	6	—	4
Watermelon	57	18	—	4	0	0	2	10	4	—	—	—	—
Salad Dressings													
Blue cheese	15	9	—	—	10	10	—	—	—	—	—	—	—
Celery seed	15	70	—	3	6	5	—	—	—	—	—	—	—
French	15	60	—	4	6	0	—	—	—	—	—	—	—
French, sweet red	15	70	—	5	6	0	—	—	—	—	—	—	—
Hidden Valley ranch	15	50	—	—	6	5	—	—	—	—	—	—	—
Italian Caesar	15	80	—	—	9	5	—	—	—	—	—	—	—
Italian, golden	15	45	—	3	4	0	—	—	—	—	—	—	—
Salad oil	28	250	0	0	28	0	—	—	—	—	—	—	—
Thousand island	15	70	—	2	7	5	—	—	—	—	—	—	—
Wine vinegar	15	2	—	—	0	0	—	—	—	—	—	—	—
Red. Cal. bacon & tomato	15	45	—	3	4	—	—	—	—	—	—	—	—
Reduced calorie Italian	15	25	—	2	2	0	—	—	—	—	—	—	—
Prepared Salads													
Chef salad	331	180	15	10	9	120	110	110	15	25	6	25	15
Garden salad	277	102	7	9	5	0	110	110	10	20	6	20	10
Taco salad	791	660	40	46	37	35	80	80	30	45	25	80	35
Superbar—Mexican Fiesta (where available)													
Cheese sauce	56	39	1	5	2	tr	—	—	—	—	—	6	—
Picante sauce	56	18	—	4	—	N/A	10	30	2	—	2	—	2
Refried beans	56	70	4	10	3	tr	—	—	4	2	—	2	6
Rice, Spanish	56	70	2	13	1	tr	6	—	45	—	8	4	10
Taco chips	40	260	4	40	10	0	—	—	2	4	—	8	4
Taco meat	56	110	10	4	7	25	—	—	8	6	10	4	10
Taco sauce	28	16	—	3	—	tr	4	2	—	—	—	—	—
Taco shells	11	45	—	6	3	0	—	—	—	—	—	—	—
Tortilla, flour	37	110	3	19	3	N/A	—	—	4	2	2	8	2
French fries (small) 3.2 oz**	91	240	3	33	12	0	—	10	10	2	10	—	4
Chili (regular) 9 oz	255	220	21	23	7	45	15	15	8	10	10	8	35
Cheddar cheese, shredded	28	110	7	1	10	30	10	—	—	6	—	20	—
Sour cream	28	60	1	1	6	10	6	—	—	2	—	4	—
Crispy chicken nuggets (6)	93	280	14	12	20	50	—	—	6	6	30	4	4
Nugget sauces													
Barbeque	28	50	—	11	—	0	6	—	—	—	—	—	4
Honey	14	45	—	12	—	0	—	—	—	—	—	—	—
Sweet & sour	28	45	—	11	—	0	—	—	—	—	—	—	2
Sweet mustard	28	50	—	9	1	0	—	—	—	—	—	—	—
Hot Stuffed Baked Potatoes													
Plain	250	270	6	63	—	0	—	50	20	6	20	2	20
Bacon & cheese	362	520	20	70	18	20	10	60	35	15	35	8	24
Broccoli & cheese	350	400	8	58	16	tr	14	60	20	10	20	10	15
Cheese	318	420	8	66	15	10	10	50	20	100	20	6	20
Chili & cheese	403	500	15	71	18	25	15	60	20	100	25	8	28
Sour cream & chives	323	500	8	67	23	25	50	75	20	10	20	10	20

WENDY'S

Food Item	Serving Size (g)	kcal	Protein (g)	CHO (g)	Fat (g)	Choles-terol (mg)	Percentage of U.S. RDA Vit A (mg)	Vit C (mg)	Thia (mg)	Ribo (mg)	Nia (mg)	Ca (mg)	Fe (mg)
Beverages													
Frosty, small***	243	400	8	59	14	50	10	—	8	30	2	30	6
Cola, sm	8*	100	0	25	0	0	—	—	—	—	—	—	—
Lemon-lime soft drink, sm	8*	100	0	24	0	0	—	—	—	—	—	—	—
Diet cola	8*	1	0	—	0	0	—	—	—	—	—	—	—
Coffee	6*	2	0	—	0	0	—	—	—	—	—	—	—
Decaf coffee	6*	2	0	—	0	0	—	—	—	—	—	—	—
Hot chocolate	6*	110	2	22	1	tr	—	—	—	8	—	6	2
Lemonade	8*	90	0	24	0	0	—	15	—	4	—	—	2
Choc milk	8*	160	7	24	5	15	15	4	6	20	—	25	4
Milk, 2%	8*	110	8	11	4	20	10	4	6	20	—	30	—
Tea (hot or ice)	6*	1	0	0	0	0	—	—	—	—	—	—	—
Chocolate chip cookie	64	275	3	40	13	15	2	—	8	8	6	2	8

* Fluid ounces.

** To determine nutritional information for a large order of Fries, multiply figures by 1.3; Biggie Fries, multiply by 1.87; large Chilli, multiply by 1.5; 9-piece Nuggets, multiply by 1.5; 20-piece Nuggests, multiply by 3.3

*** To determine nutritional information for a medium Frosty, multiply figures by 1.3; large Frosty, multiply by 1.7. For medium soft drink, multiply by 1.5; large soft drink, multiply by 2. For Biggie soft drink, multiply by 3.5.

Source: Consumer Relations, Wendy's International, Dublin, OH.

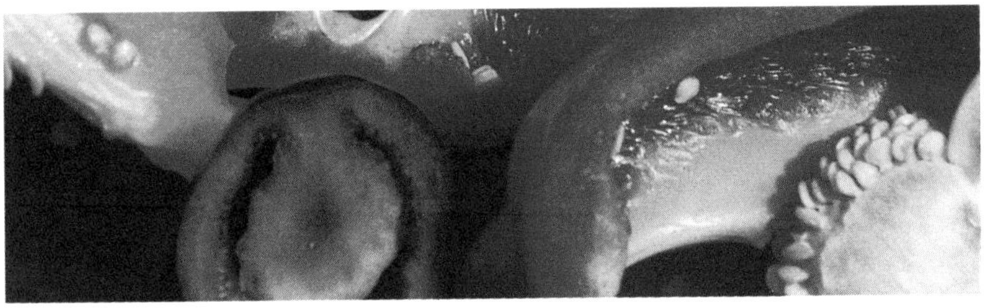

C

EVALUATION OF BODY COMPOSITION

This appendix contains the age- and gender-specific equations to predict body fat percentage based on three girth measurements. There are four charts, one each for young and older men and women. A cloth tape is preferred over a metal one because there is little skin compression when applying a cloth tape to the skin's surface at a relatively constant tension. Take each measurement at least twice, and use an average to represent the girth score. Refer to Figure 14–6 in Chapter 14 for the precise anatomical sites for taking the girth measurements.

To use the Appendix C charts, measure the three girths for your age and gender as follows:

AGE, YEARS	GENDER	SITE A	SITE B	SITE C
17–26	M	Right upper arm	Abdomen	Right forearm
	F	Abdomen	Right thigh	Right forearm
27–50	M	Buttocks	Abdomen	Right forearm
	F	Abdomen	Right thigh	Right calf

A step-by-step explanation of how to compute the relative and absolute values for body fat, lean body mass, and desirable body mass from the Appendix C charts is presented on pages 241 to 245 in Chapter 14. The specific equation to predict percent body fat with its corresponding constant is presented at the bottom of each of the Appendix C charts.

CHART C–1. CONVERSION CONSTANTS TO PREDICT PERCENT BODY FAT FOR YOUNG MEN*

UPPER ARM			ABDOMEN			FOREARM		
in	cm	Constant A	in	cm	Constant B	in	cm	Constant C
7.00	17.78	25.91	21.00	53.34	27.56	7.00	17.78	38.01
7.25	18.41	26.83	21.25	53.97	27.88	7.25	18.41	39.37
7.50	19.05	27.76	21.50	54.61	28.21	7.50	19.05	40.72
7.75	19.68	28.68	21.75	55.24	28.54	7.75	19.68	42.08
8.00	20.32	29.61	22.00	55.88	28.87	8.00	20.32	43.44
8.25	20.95	30.53	22.25	56.51	29.20	8.25	20.95	44.80
8.50	21.59	31.46	22.50	57.15	29.52	8.50	21.59	46.15
8.75	22.22	32.38	22.75	57.78	29.85	8.75	22.22	47.51
9.00	22.86	33.31	23.00	58.42	30.18	9.00	22.86	48.87

CHART C–1. *continued*

UPPER ARM			ABDOMEN			FOREARM		
in	cm	Constant A	in	cm	Constant B	in	cm	Constant C
9.25	23.49	34.24	23.25	59.05	30.51	9.25	23.49	50.23
9.50	24.13	35.16	23.50	59.69	30.84	9.50	24.13	51.58
9.75	24.76	36.09	23.75	60.32	31.16	9.75	24.76	52.94
10.00	25.40	37.01	24.00	60.96	31.49	10.00	25.40	54.30
10.25	26.03	37.94	24.25	61.59	31.82	10.25	26.03	55.65
10.50	26.67	38.86	24.50	62.23	32.15	10.50	26.67	57.01
10.75	27.30	39.79	24.75	62.86	32.48	10.75	27.30	58.37
11.00	27.94	40.71	25.00	63.50	32.80	11.00	27.94	59.73
11.25	28.57	41.64	25.25	64.13	33.13	11.25	28.57	61.08
11.50	29.21	42.56	25.50	64.77	33.46	11.50	29.21	62.44
11.75	29.84	43.49	25.75	65.40	33.79	11.75	29.84	63.80
12.00	30.48	44.41	26.00	66.04	34.12	12.00	30.48	65.16
12.25	31.11	45.34	26.25	66.67	34.44	12.25	31.11	66.51
12.50	31.75	46.26	26.50	67.31	34.77	12.50	31.75	67.87
12.75	32.38	47.19	26.75	67.94	35.10	12.75	32.38	69.23
13.00	33.02	48.11	27.00	68.58	35.43	13.00	33.02	70.59
13.25	33.65	49.04	27.25	69.21	35.76	13.25	33.65	71.94
13.50	34.29	49.96	27.50	69.85	36.09	13.50	34.29	73.30
13.75	34.92	50.89	27.75	70.48	36.41	13.75	34.92	74.66
14.00	35.56	51.82	28.00	71.12	36.74	14.00	35.56	76.02
14.25	36.19	52.74	28.25	71.75	37.07	14.25	36.19	77.37
14.50	36.83	53.67	28.50	72.39	37.40	14.50	36.83	78.73
14.75	37.46	54.59	28.75	73.02	37.73	14.75	37.46	80.09
15.00	38.10	55.52	29.00	73.66	38.05	15.00	38.10	81.45
15.25	38.73	56.44	29.25	74.29	38.38	15.25	38.73	82.80
15.50	39.37	57.37	29.50	74.93	38.71	15.50	39.37	84.16
15.75	40.00	58.29	29.75	75.56	39.04	15.75	40.00	85.52
16.00	40.64	59.22	30.00	76.20	39.37	16.00	40.64	86.88
16.25	41.27	60.14	30.25	76.83	39.69	16.25	41.27	88.23
16.50	41.91	61.07	30.50	77.47	40.02	16.50	41.91	89.59
16.75	42.54	61.99	30.75	78.10	40.35	16.75	42.54	90.95
17.00	43.18	62.92	31.00	78.74	40.68	17.00	43.18	92.31
17.25	43.81	63.84	31.25	79.37	41.01	17.25	43.81	93.66
17.50	44.45	64.77	31.50	80.01	41.33	17.50	44.45	95.02
17.75	45.08	65.69	31.75	80.64	41.66	17.75	45.08	96.38
18.00	45.72	66.62	32.00	81.28	41.99	18.00	45.72	97.74
18.25	46.35	67.54	32.25	81.91	42.32	18.25	46.35	99.09
18.50	46.99	68.47	32.50	82.55	42.65	18.50	46.99	100.45
18.75	47.62	69.40	32.75	83.18	42.97	18.75	47.62	101.81
19.00	48.26	70.32	33.00	83.82	43.30	19.00	48.26	103.17
19.25	48.89	71.25	33.25	84.45	43.63	19.25	48.89	104.52
19.50	49.53	72.17	33.50	85.09	43.96	19.50	49.53	105.88
19.75	50.16	73.10	33.75	85.72	44.29	19.75	50.16	107.24
20.00	50.80	74.02	34.00	86.36	44.61	20.00	50.80	108.60
20.25	51.43	74.95	34.25	86.99	44.94	20.25	51.43	109.95
20.50	52.07	75.87	34.50	87.63	45.27	20.50	52.07	111.31
20.75	52.70	76.80	34.75	88.26	45.60	20.75	52.70	112.67
21.00	53.34	77.72	35.00	88.90	45.93	21.00	53.34	114.02
21.25	53.97	78.65	35.25	89.53	46.25	21.25	53.97	115.38
21.50	54.61	79.57	35.50	90.17	46.58	21.50	54.61	116.74
21.75	55.24	80.50	35.75	90.80	46.91	21.75	55.24	118.10
22.00	55.88	81.42	36.00	91.44	47.24	22.00	55.88	119.45
			36.25	92.07	47.57			
			36.50	92.71	47.89			
			36.75	93.34	48.22			
			37.00	93.98	48.55			
			37.25	94.61	48.88			
			37.50	95.25	49.21			

CHART C–1. *continued*

UPPER ARM			ABDOMEN			FOREARM		
in	cm	Constant A	in	cm	Constant B	in	cm	Constant C
			37.75	95.88	49.54			
			38.00	96.52	49.86			
			38.25	97.15	50.19			
			38.50	97.79	50.52			
			38.75	98.42	50.85			
			39.00	99.06	51.18			
			39.25	99.69	51.50			
			39.50	100.33	51.83			
			39.75	100.96	52.16			
			40.00	101.60	52.49			
			40.25	102.23	52.82			
			40.50	102.87	53.14			
			40.75	103.50	53.47			
			41.00	104.14	53.80			
			41.25	104.77	54.13			
			41.50	105.41	54.46			
			41.75	106.04	54.78			
			42.00	106.68	55.11			

Note: Percent fat = Constant A + Constant B − Constant C − 10.2

CHART C–2. CONVERSION CONSTANTS TO PREDICT PERCENT BODY FAT FOR OLDER MEN*

BUTTOCKS			ABDOMEN			FOREARM		
in	cm	Constant A	in	cm	Constant B	in	cm	Constant C
28.00	71.12	29.34	25.50	64.77	22.84	7.00	17.78	21.01
28.25	71.75	29.60	25.75	65.40	23.06	7.25	18.41	21.76
28.50	72.39	29.87	26.00	66.04	23.29	7.50	19.05	22.52
28.75	73.02	30.13	26.25	66.67	23.51	7.75	19.68	23.26
29.00	73.66	30.39	26.50	67.31	23.73	8.00	20.32	24.02
29.25	74.29	30.65	26.75	67.94	23.96	8.25	20.95	24.76
29.50	74.93	30.92	27.00	68.58	24.18	8.50	21.59	25.52
29.75	75.56	31.18	27.25	69.21	24.40	8.75	22.22	26.26
30.00	76.20	31.44	27.50	69.85	24.63	9.00	22.86	27.02
30.25	76.83	31.70	27.75	70.48	24.85	9.25	23.49	27.76
30.50	77.47	31.96	28.00	71.12	25.08	9.50	24.13	28.52
30.75	78.10	32.22	28.25	71.75	25.29	9.75	24.76	29.26
31.00	78.74	32.49	28.50	72.39	25.52	10.00	25.40	30.02
31.25	79.37	32.75	28.75	73.02	25.75	10.25	26.03	30.76
31.50	80.01	33.01	29.00	73.66	25.97	10.50	26.67	31.52
31.75	80.64	33.27	29.25	74.29	26.19	10.75	27.30	32.27
32.00	81.28	33.54	29.50	74.93	26.42	11.00	27.94	33.02
32.25	81.91	33.80	29.75	75.56	26.64	11.25	28.57	33.77
32.50	82.55	34.06	30.00	76.20	26.87	11.50	29.21	34.52
32.75	83.18	34.32	30.25	76.83	27.09	11.75	29.84	35.27
33.00	83.82	34.58	30.50	77.47	27.32	12.00	30.48	36.02
33.25	84.45	34.84	30.75	78.10	27.54	12.25	31.11	36.77
33.50	85.09	35.11	31.00	78.74	27.76	12.50	31.75	37.53
33.75	85.72	35.37	31.25	79.37	27.98	12.75	32.38	38.27
34.00	86.36	35.63	31.50	80.01	28.21	13.00	33.02	39.03
34.25	86.99	35.89	31.75	80.64	28.43	13.25	33.65	39.77
34.50	87.63	36.16	32.00	81.28	28.66	13.50	34.29	40.53
34.75	88.26	36.42	32.25	81.91	28.88	13.75	34.92	41.27
35.00	88.90	36.68	32.50	82.55	29.11	14.00	35.56	42.03
35.25	89.53	36.94	32.75	83.18	29.33	14.25	36.19	42.77

CHART C–2. *continued*

BUTTOCKS		
in	cm	Constant A
35.50	90.17	37.20
35.75	90.80	37.46
36.00	91.44	37.73
36.25	92.07	37.99
36.50	92.71	38.25
36.75	93.34	38.51
37.00	93.98	38.78
37.25	94.61	39.04
37.50	95.25	39.30
37.75	95.88	39.56
38.00	96.52	39.82
38.25	97.15	40.08
38.50	97.79	40.35
38.75	98.42	40.61
39.00	99.06	40.87
39.25	99.69	41.13
39.50	100.33	41.39
39.75	100.96	41.66
40.00	101.60	41.92
40.25	102.23	42.18
40.50	102.87	42.44
40.75	103.50	42.70
41.00	104.14	42.97
42.25	104.77	43.23
41.50	105.41	43.49
41.75	106.04	43.75
42.00	106.68	44.02
42.25	107.31	44.28
42.50	107.95	44.54
42.75	108.58	44.80
43.00	109.22	45.06
43.25	109.85	45.32
43.50	110.49	45.59
43.75	111.12	45.85
44.00	111.76	46.12
44.25	112.39	46.37
44.50	113.03	46.64
44.75	113.66	46.89
45.00	114.30	47.16
42.25	114.93	47.42
45.50	115.57	47.68
45.75	116.20	47.94
46.00	116.84	48.21
46.25	117.47	48.47
46.50	118.11	48.73
46.75	118.74	48.99
47.00	119.38	49.26
47.25	120.01	49.52
47.50	120.65	49.78
47.75	121.28	50.04
48.00	121.92	50.30
48.25	122.55	50.56
48.50	123.19	50.83
48.75	123.82	51.09
49.00	124.46	51.35

ABDOMEN		
in	cm	Constant B
33.00	83.82	29.55
33.25	84.45	29.78
33.50	85.09	30.00
33.75	85.72	30.22
34.00	86.36	30.45
34.25	86.99	30.67
34.50	87.63	30.89
34.75	88.26	31.12
35.00	88.90	31.35
35.25	89.53	31.57
35.50	90.17	31.79
35.75	90.80	32.02
36.00	91.44	32.24
36.25	92.07	32.46
36.50	92.71	32.69
36.75	93.34	32.91
37.00	93.98	33.14
37.25	94.61	33.36
37.50	95.25	33.58
37.75	95.88	33.81
38.00	96.52	34.03
38.25	97.15	34.26
38.50	97.79	34.48
38.75	98.42	34.70
39.00	99.06	34.93
39.25	99.69	35.15
39.50	100.33	35.38
39.75	100.96	35.59
40.00	101.60	35.82
40.25	102.23	36.05
40.50	102.87	36.27
40.75	103.50	36.49
41.00	104.14	36.72
41.25	104.77	36.94
41.50	105.41	37.17
41.75	106.04	37.39
42.00	106.68	37.62
42.25	107.31	37.87
42.50	107.95	38.06
42.75	108.58	38.28
43.00	109.22	38.51
43.25	109.85	38.73
43.50	110.49	38.96
43.75	111.12	39.18
44.00	111.76	39.41
44.25	112.39	39.63
44.50	113.03	39.85
44.75	113.66	40.08
45.00	114.30	40.30

FOREARM		
in	cm	Constant C
14.50	36.83	43.53
14.75	37.46	44.27
15.00	38.10	45.03
15.25	38.73	45.77
15.50	39.37	46.53
15.75	40.00	47.28
16.00	40.64	48.03
16.25	41.27	48.78
16.50	41.91	49.53
16.75	42.54	50.28
17.00	43.18	51.03
17.25	43.81	51.78
17.50	44.45	52.54
17.75	45.08	53.28
18.00	45.72	54.04
18.25	46.35	54.78

Note: Percent fat = Constant A + Constant B − Constant C − 15.0

CHART C–3. CONVERSION CONSTANTS TO PREDICT PERCENT BODY FAT FOR YOUNG WOMEN*

ABDOMEN			THIGH			FOREARM		
in	cm	Constant A	in	cm	Constant B	in	cm	Constant C
20.00	50.80	26.74	14.00	35.56	29.13	6.00	15.24	25.86
20.25	51.43	27.07	14.25	36.19	29.65	6.25	15.87	26.94
20.50	52.07	27.41	14.50	36.83	30.17	6.50	16.51	28.02
20.75	52.70	27.74	14.75	37.46	30.69	6.75	17.14	29.10
21.00	53.34	28.07	15.00	38.10	31.21	7.00	17.78	30.17
21.25	53.97	28.41	15.25	38.73	31.73	7.25	18.41	31.25
21.50	54.61	28.74	15.50	39.37	32.25	7.50	19.05	32.33
21.75	55.24	29.08	15.75	40.00	32.77	7.75	19.68	33.41
22.00	55.88	29.41	16.00	40.64	33.29	8.00	20.32	34.48
22.25	56.51	29.74	16.25	41.27	33.81	8.25	20.95	35.56
22.50	57.15	30.08	16.50	41.91	34.33	8.50	21.59	36.64
22.75	57.78	30.41	16.75	42.54	34.85	8.75	22.22	37.72
23.00	58.42	30.75	17.00	43.18	35.37	9.00	22.86	38.79
23.25	59.05	31.08	17.25	43.81	35.89	9.25	23.49	39.87
23.50	59.69	31.42	17.50	44.45	36.41	9.50	24.13	40.95
23.75	60.32	31.75	17.75	45.08	36.93	9.75	24.76	42.03
24.00	60.96	32.08	18.00	45.72	37.45	10.00	25.40	43.10
24.25	61.59	32.42	18.25	46.35	37.97	10.25	26.03	44.18
24.50	62.23	32.75	18.50	46.99	38.49	10.50	26.67	45.26
24.75	62.86	33.09	18.75	47.62	39.01	10.75	27.30	46.34
25.00	63.50	33.42	19.00	48.26	39.53	11.00	27.94	47.41
25.25	64.13	33.76	19.25	48.89	40.05	11.25	28.57	48.49
25.50	64.77	34.09	19.50	49.53	40.57	11.50	29.21	49.57
25.75	65.40	34.42	19.75	50.16	41.09	11.75	29.84	50.65
26.00	66.04	34.76	20.00	50.80	41.61	12.00	30.48	51.73
26.25	66.67	35.09	20.25	51.43	42.13	12.25	31.11	52.80
26.50	67.31	35.43	20.50	52.07	42.65	12.50	31.75	53.88
26.75	67.94	35.76	20.75	52.70	43.17	12.75	32.38	54.96
27.00	68.58	36.10	21.00	53.34	43.69	13.00	33.02	56.04
27.25	69.21	36.43	21.25	53.97	44.21	13.25	33.65	57.11
27.50	69.85	36.76	21.50	54.61	44.73	13.50	34.29	58.19
27.75	70.48	37.10	21.75	55.24	45.25	13.75	34.92	59.27
28.00	71.12	37.43	22.00	55.88	45.77	14.00	35.56	60.35
28.25	71.75	37.77	22.25	56.51	46.29	14.25	36.19	61.42
28.50	72.39	38.10	22.50	57.15	46.81	14.50	36.83	62.50
28.75	73.02	38.43	22.75	57.78	47.33	14.75	37.46	63.58
29.00	73.66	38.77	23.00	58.42	47.85	15.00	38.10	64.66
29.25	74.29	39.10	23.25	59.05	48.37	15.25	38.73	65.73
29.50	74.93	39.44	23.50	59.69	48.89	15.50	39.37	66.81
29.75	75.56	39.77	23.75	60.32	49.41	15.75	40.00	67.89
30.00	76.20	40.11	24.00	60.96	49.93	16.00	40.64	68.97
30.25	76.83	40.44	24.25	61.59	50.45	16.25	41.27	70.04
30.50	77.47	40.77	24.50	62.23	50.97	16.50	41.91	71.12
30.75	78.10	41.11	24.75	62.86	51.49	16.75	42.54	72.20
31.00	78.74	41.44	25.00	63.50	52.01	17.00	43.18	73.28
31.25	79.37	41.78	25.25	64.13	52.53	17.25	43.81	74.36
31.50	80.01	42.11	25.50	64.77	53.05	17.50	44.45	75.43
31.75	80.64	42.45	25.75	65.40	53.57	17.75	45.08	76.51
32.00	81.28	42.78	26.00	66.04	54.09	18.00	45.72	77.59
32.25	81.91	43.11	26.25	66.67	54.61	18.25	46.35	78.67
32.50	82.55	43.45	26.50	67.31	55.13	18.50	46.99	79.74
32.75	83.18	43.78	26.75	67.94	55.65	18.75	47.62	80.82
33.00	83.82	44.12	27.00	68.58	56.17	19.00	48.26	81.90
33.25	84.45	44.45	27.25	69.21	56.69	19.25	48.89	82.98
33.50	85.09	44.78	27.50	69.85	57.21	19.50	49.53	84.05
33.75	85.72	45.12	27.75	70.48	57.73	19.75	50.16	85.13
34.00	86.36	45.45	28.00	71.12	58.26	20.00	50.80	86.21

CHART C–3. continued

ABDOMEN			THIGH			FOREARM		
in	cm	Constant A	in	cm	Constant B	in	cm	Constant C
34.25	86.99	45.79	28.25	71.75	58.78			
34.50	87.63	46.12	28.50	72.39	59.30			
34.75	88.26	46.46	38.75	73.02	59.82			
35.00	88.90	46.79	29.00	73.66	60.34			
35.25	89.53	47.12	29.25	74.29	60.86			
35.50	90.17	47.46	29.50	74.93	61.38			
35.75	90.80	47.79	29.75	75.56	61.90			
36.00	91.44	48.13	30.00	76.20	62.42			
36.25	92.07	48.46	30.25	76.83	62.94			
36.50	92.71	48.80	30.50	77.47	63.46			
36.75	93.34	49.13	30.75	78.10	63.98			
37.00	93.98	49.46	31.00	78.74	64.50			
37.25	94.61	49.80	31.25	79.37	65.02			
37.50	95.25	50.13	31.50	80.01	65.54			
37.75	95.88	50.47	31.75	80.64	66.06			
38.00	96.52	50.80	32.00	81.28	66.58			
38.25	97.15	51.13	32.25	81.91	67.10			
38.50	97.79	51.47	32.50	82.55	67.62			
38.75	98.42	51.80	32.75	83.18	68.14			
39.00	99.06	52.14	33.00	83.82	68.66			
39.25	99.69	52.47	33.25	84.45	69.18			
39.50	100.33	52.81	33.50	85.09	69.70			
39.75	100.96	53.14	33.75	85.72	70.22			
40.00	101.60	53.47	34.00	86.36	70.74			

Note: Percent fat = Constant A + Constant B − Constant C − 19.6

CHART C–4F–5. CONVERSION CONSTANTS TO PREDICT PERCENT BODY FAT FOR OLDER WOMEN*

ABDOMEN			THIGH			CALF		
in	cm	Constant A	in	cm	Constant B	in	cm	Constant C
25.00	63.50	29.69	14.00	35.56	17.31	10.00	25.40	14.46
25.25	64.13	29.98	14.25	36.19	17.62	10.25	26.03	14.82
25.50	64.77	30.28	14.50	36.83	17.93	10.50	26.67	15.18
25.75	65.40	30.58	14.75	37.46	18.24	10.75	27.30	15.54
26.00	66.04	30.87	15.00	38.10	18.55	11.00	27.94	15.91
26.25	66.67	31.17	15.25	38.73	18.86	11.25	28.57	16.27
26.50	67.31	31.47	15.50	39.37	19.17	11.50	29.21	16.63
26.75	67.94	31.76	15.75	40.00	19.47	11.75	29.84	16.99
27.00	68.58	32.06	16.00	40.64	19.78	12.00	30.48	17.35
27.25	69.21	32.36	16.25	41.27	20.09	12.25	31.11	17.71
27.50	69.85	32.65	16.50	41.91	20.40	12.50	31.75	18.08
27.75	70.48	32.95	16.75	42.54	20.71	12.75	32.38	18.44
28.00	71.12	33.25	17.00	43.18	21.02	13.00	33.02	18.80
28.25	71.75	33.55	17.25	43.81	21.33	13.25	33.65	19.16
28.50	72.39	33.84	17.50	44.45	21.64	13.50	34.29	19.52
28.75	73.02	34.14	17.75	45.08	21.95	13.75	34.92	19.88
29.00	73.66	34.44	18.00	45.72	22.26	14.00	35.56	20.24
29.25	74.29	34.73	18.25	46.35	22.57	14.25	36.19	20.61
29.50	74.93	35.03	18.50	46.99	22.87	14.50	36.83	20.97
29.75	75.56	35.33	18.75	47.62	23.18	14.75	37.46	21.33
30.00	76.20	35.62	19.00	48.26	23.49	15.00	38.10	21.69

CHART C–4F–5. *continued*

ABDOMEN			THIGH			CALF		
in	cm	Constant A	in	cm	Constant B	in	cm	Constant C
30.25	76.83	35.92	19.25	48.89	23.80	15.25	38.73	22.05
30.50	77.47	36.22	19.50	49.53	24.11	15.50	39.37	22.41
30.75	78.10	36.51	19.75	50.16	24.42	15.75	40.00	22.77
31.00	78.74	36.81	20.00	50.80	24.73	16.00	40.64	23.14
31.25	79.37	37.11	20.25	51.43	25.04	16.25	41.27	23.50
31.50	80.01	37.40	20.50	52.07	25.35	16.50	41.91	23.86
31.75	80.64	37.70	20.75	52.70	25.66	16.75	42.54	24.22
32.00	81.28	38.00	21.00	53.34	25.97	17.00	43.18	24.58
32.25	81.91	38.30	21.25	53.97	26.28	17.25	43.81	24.94
32.50	82.55	38.59	21.50	54.61	26.58	17.50	44.45	25.31
32.75	83.18	38.89	21.75	55.24	26.89	17.75	45.08	25.67
33.00	83.82	39.19	22.00	55.88	27.20	18.00	45.72	26.03
33.25	84.45	39.48	22.25	56.51	27.51	18.25	46.35	26.39
33.50	85.09	39.78	22.50	57.15	27.82	18.50	46.99	26.75
33.75	85.72	40.08	22.75	57.78	28.13	18.75	47.62	27.11
34.00	86.36	40.37	23.00	58.42	28.44	19.00	48.26	27.47
34.25	86.99	40.67	23.25	59.05	28.75	19.25	48.89	27.84
34.50	87.63	40.97	23.50	59.69	29.06	19.50	49.53	28.20
34.75	88.26	41.26	23.75	60.32	29.37	19.75	50.16	28.56
35.00	88.90	41.56	24.00	60.96	29.68	20.00	50.80	28.92
35.25	89.53	41.86	24.25	61.59	29.98	20.25	51.43	29.28
35.50	90.17	42.15	24.50	62.23	30.29	20.50	52.07	29.64
35.75	90.80	42.45	24.75	62.86	30.60	20.75	52.70	30.00
36.00	91.44	42.75	25.00	63.50	30.91	21.00	53.34	30.37
36.25	92.07	43.05	25.25	64.13	31.22	21.25	53.97	30.73
36.50	92.71	43.34	25.50	64.77	31.53	21.50	54.61	31.09
36.75	93.35	43.64	25.75	65.40	31.84	21.75	55.24	31.45
37.00	93.98	43.94	26.00	66.04	32.15	22.00	55.88	31.81
37.25	94.62	44.23	26.25	66.67	32.46	22.25	56.51	32.17
37.50	95.25	44.53	26.50	67.31	32.77	22.50	57.15	32.54
37.75	95.89	44.83	26.75	67.94	33.08	22.75	57.78	32.90
38.00	96.52	45.12	27.00	68.58	33.38	23.00	58.42	33.26
38.25	97.16	45.42	27.25	69.21	33.69	23.25	59.05	33.62
38.50	97.79	45.72	27.50	69.85	34.00	23.50	59.69	33.98
38.75	98.43	46.01	27.75	70.48	34.31	23.75	60.32	34.34
39.00	99.06	46.31	28.00	71.12	34.62	24.00	60.96	34.70
39.25	99.70	46.61	28.25	71.75	34.93	24.25	61.59	35.07
39.50	100.33	46.90	28.50	72.39	35.24	24.50	62.23	35.43
39.75	100.97	47.20	28.75	73.02	35.55	24.75	62.86	35.79
40.00	101.60	47.50	29.00	73.66	35.86	25.00	63.50	36.15
40.25	101.24	47.79	29.25	74.29	36.17			
40.50	102.87	48.09	29.50	74.93	36.48			
40.75	103.51	48.39	29.75	75.56	36.79			
41.00	104.14	48.69	30.00	76.20	37.09			
41.25	104.78	48.98	30.25	76.83	37.40			
41.50	105.41	49.28	30.50	77.47	37.71			
41.75	106.05	49.58	30.75	78.10	38.02			
42.00	106.68	49.87	31.00	78.74	38.33			
42.25	107.32	50.17	31.25	79.37	38.64			
42.50	107.95	50.47	31.50	80.01	38.95			
42.75	108.59	50.76	31.75	80.64	39.26			
43.00	109.22	51.06	32.00	81.28	39.57			
43.25	109.86	51.36	32.25	81.91	39.88			
43.50	110.49	51.65	32.50	82.55	40.19			
43.75	111.13	51.95	32.75	83.18	40.49			
44.00	111.76	52.25	33.00	83.82	40.80			
44.25	112.40	52.54	33.25	84.45	41.11			

CHART C–4F–5. *continued*

ABDOMEN			THIGH			CALF		
in	cm	Constant A	in	cm	Constant B	in	cm	Constant C
44.50	113.03	52.84	33.50	85.09	41.42			
44.75	113.67	53.14	33.75	85.72	41.73			
45.00	114.30	53.44	34.00	86.36	42.04			

Note: Percent fat = Constant A + Constant B − Constant C − 18.4

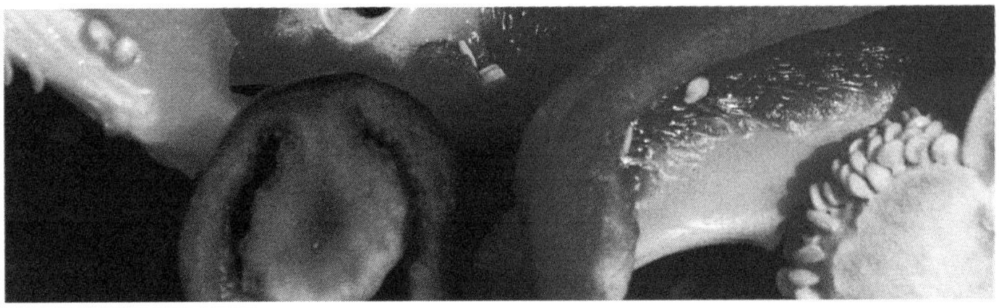

D

COMPUTERIZED MEAL AND EXERCISE PLAN*

Your FITCOMP nutrition program (on the "a" diet plan) is designed so you will lose about 1.8 pounds a week and achieve your goal weight of 138.0 pounds in 110 days. Your personalized meal plan provides an optimal blend of carbohydrates (sugars), fats, proteins, vitamins, and minerals. Your total food intake each day will equal 1576 Calories. If you faithfully follow your nutrition and exercise program, your weight should decrease according to the pattern shown in the graph below.

Notice that you should weigh 151 pounds on or about Monday, Sept. 16, 1993, and achieve your goal weight of 138.0 pounds during the week of Nov 3, 1993. GOOD LUCK.

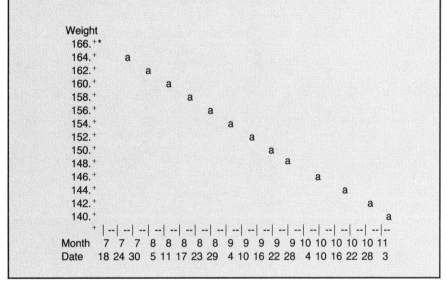

```
Weight
 166.+*
 164.+   a
 162.+      a
 160.+         a
 158.+            a
 156.+               a
 154.+                  a
 152.+                     a
 150.+                        a
 148.+                          a
 146.+                               a
 144.+                                   a
 142.+                                       a
 140.+                                          a
     + |--| --| --| --| --| --| --| --| --| --| --| --| --| --| --| --| --| --|--
Month  7  7  7  8  8  8  8  8  9  9  9  9  9 10 10 10 10 10 11
Date  18 24 30  5 11 17 23 29  4 10 16 22 28  4 10 16 22 28  3
```

Example of weight loss curve. For this individual who initially weighed 165 lb, the desired weight loss was 27 lb.

Examples of food items selected from the questionnaire.

Meat (amount for 70 calories)	
Canadian bacon	1 ounce
Farmer's cheese	1 ounce
Ricotta cheese	1 ounce
Mozzarella cheese	1 ounce
Egg	1
Peanut butter	2 tbsp
Cottage cheese	¼ cup
Tuna	¼ cup
Salmon—canned	¼ cup
Turkey	1 ounce
Chicken	1 ounce
Lamb shoulder	1 ounce
Lamb roast	1 ounce
Lamb chops	1 ounce
Lamb leg	1 ounce
Sirloin	1 ounce
Rump steak	1 ounce
Round steak	1 ounce
Tenderloin	1 ounce
Flank steak	1 ounce
Chuck steak	1 ounce
Veal—chops	1 ounce
Veal—cutlets	1 ounce
Pork roast	1 ounce
Pork chops	1 ounce
Pork—ham	1 ounce
Pork—leg	1 ounce
Ground round	1 ounce
Ground beef	1 ounce
Scallops	1 ounce
Shrimp	1 ounce
Fish—fresh/frzn	1 ounce
Cornish hen	1 ounce

Treats (amount for 80 calories)	
Popcorn (popped)	3 cup
Oatmeal cookies	1½ 2″ dia
Choc chip cookies	1½ 2″ dia
Chocolate fudge	1 sml pc
Candy bar, choc	1 small
Cupcake-icing	1 small

Alcohol (amount for 80 calories)	
Cognac	1½ ounce
Wine red/white	3½ ounce
Sherry	1½ ounce
Port	1½ ounce
Liquor	1½ ounce
Beer	6 ounce
Ale	6 ounce

Fruit (amount for 40 calories)	
Papaya	¾ cup
Apricot juice	½ cup
Prune juice	¼ cup
Prunes	2
Pineapple juice	⅓ cup
Orange juice	½ cup
Banana	½ small
Apple juice	⅓ cup
Raisins	2 tbsp
Oranges	1 small
Dates	2
Cider—any kind	⅓ cup
Raspberries	½ cup
Apple	1 small
Tangerines	1 medium
Pineapple	½ cup
Nectarines	1 small
Watermelon	1 cup
Honeydew	⅙ small
Cantaloupe	¼ small
Apple sauce	½ cup

The vegetable, bread and fat selections are not shown. The caloric values are a close approximation to actual values.

****

1576 Calorie Food Plan

Nutrient Composition

Carbohydrate...	261 grams or	64% of your total calories
Protein........	71 grams or	17% of your total calories
Fat...........	35 grams or	19% of your total calories

	Breakfast	Lunch	Dinner
Day	Cooked grits	Bread-any kind	Candy bar, choc
1	1½ cup	3 slice	1 small
	Milk, skim	Milk, skim	Mashed potato
	1 cup	1 cup	1 cup
	Cream-light	Pork—ham	Milk, skim
	4 tbsp	1 ounce	1 cup
	Apricot juice	Cauliflower	Veal—cutlets
	1 cup	½ cup	2 ounce
		Raisins	Rhubarb
		6 tbsp	1½ cup
			Radishes
			no limit
			Diet margarine
			4 tsp
			Tangerines
			2 medium

	Breakfast	Lunch	Dinner
Day	Toast	Bread—any kind	Beer
2	3 slice	3 slice	6 ounce
	Milk, skim	Milk, skim	Baked potato
	1 cup	1 cup	1 small
	Bacon—crisp	Peanut butter	Milk, skim
	2 strip	2 tbsp	1 cup
	Prune juice	Celery	Pork roast
	½ cup	½ cup	2 ounce
		Oranges	Artichokes
		3 small	1½ cup
			Lettuce
			no limit
			Diet margarine
			4 tsp
			Pineapple
			1 cup

This is an example of the first two days of a 1,576 calorie food plan. The usual procedure is to generate a 14-day plan; because foods are arranged as exchanges within a given food category, each exchange is assigned a specific calorie value. Therefore, one can exchange any one food within a food category with any other food in that category. In addition, any one complete breakfast, lunch, or dinner can be interchanged for any other breakfast, lunch, or dinner. This makes the number of food combinations for a given day equal to 14 factorial.

STEP 9 Walk for 2½ miles in 47 minutes 24 seconds (18 min 58 sec/mile)
This exercise burns 280 calories.

Cycle 3½ miles in 19 minutes 26 seconds (10.80 miles/hour)
Repeat this 2 times. This exercise burns 229 calories.

Swim 275 yards in 9 minutes 50 seconds (28 yards/min)
Repeat this 5 times. This exercise burns 290 calories.

The following alternative activities will expend approximately the same number of calories as the aerobic activities above:

Racquetball	for	51 minutes
Circuit Training	for	22 minutes
Squash	for	38 minutes
Badminton	for	92 minutes
Basketball	for	34 minutes
Downhill Skiing	for	40 minutes
Tennis	for	82 minutes
Golf	for	47 minutes
Aerobic Dancing	for	28 minutes

Example for Step 9 of the beginner aerobic exercise plan to accompany the daily meal plans. With this program, individuals proceed to the next week's exercise after they complete their choice of exercise at least 3 times in the same week. Caloric expenditure represents average values for a particular body weight.

This kind of computer-generated output gives the person freedom to exchange activities for any given workout; it offers flexibility and variety in planning workouts to meet individual preferences. The major advantage, however, is the maintenance of caloric equivalency between the different activities that is linked with caloric input from the menus. If inclement weather prohibits jogging or cycling, then swimming or racquetball, for example, can be substituted without altering either the required calorie output (activity) or the required calorie input (food) side of the energy balance equation. In this way, the individual stays in phase with his or her tailor-made weight loss curve. The exercise prescription is sensitive to individual differences because it considers age, gender, and current level of physical activity (relative fitness status).

HOW TO ORDER THE COMPUTERIZED MEAL AND EXERCISE PLAN

1. Send $17 (check, money order, or business, school, or university purchase order only) to the following address:

Computer Meal and Exercise Plan
PO Box 431
Amherst, MA 01004

2. Make payable to: FITCOMP.
3. Outside continental USA add $2 for postage and bank handling (total $19).

Please note: Questionnaires are processed within 48 hours; you should receive the printout, under normal mail conditions, within 10 days. The $17 cost for the program applies until Dec 31, 1995. Thereafter, price subject to change and availability. For updated information after this date, write to: Computer Plan/Katch, McArdle, Lea & Febiger, 200 Chester Field Parkway, Malvern, PA 19355-9725. The computer meal and exercise plan is an exclusive product of Fitcomp, ® Fitness Technologies, Inc, PO Box 431, Amherst, MA 01004.

More detailed information about the FITCOMP computerized meal and exercise plan can be found in the following articles:

Katch FI, Katch VL. Computer technology to evaluate body composition, nutrition, and exercise. *Preventive Medicine 12*:619, 1983

Katch, FI: Nutrition for the athlete. In: Welsh RP and Shephard RJ (eds). *Current Therapy in Sports Medicine.* Toronto, BC Decker, 1985

Katch, FI: *FITCOMP* computerized assessment system to evaluate body composition, nutrition, and exercise. In: Katch FI (ed): *Sport, Health, and Nutrition,* The 1984 Olympic Scientific Congress Proceedings, Vol 2. Champaign, IL, Human Kinetics Publishers, 1986.

COMPUTERIZED MEAL PLAN AND EXERCISE QUESTIONNAIRE

Please print with a pen.

1. Name ____
   (First) (Last)
2. Address ____
   (Street Number and Name) (Apt. #)

   ______________ ______________ ______________
   City State Zip
3. Age __________
   (years)
4. a. ______Female b. ______Male
5. Current body weight __________
   (nearest pound)
6. Height (nearest ¼ in.) ____ ______ ________
   feet inches fraction
7. How much you would like to weigh ______________
   (nearest pound)
8. Place an X next to the exercises you would like for your program. Select at least one from Group 1. Group 2 are optional.
9. Place an X next to the *one* section which best describes your current level of daily physical activity:
   - a. ______ **Inactive:** You have a sit-down job and no regular physical activity.
   - b. ______ **Relatively Inactive:** Three to four hours of walking or standing per day are usual. You have *no* regular organized physical activity during leisure time.
   - c. ______ **Light Physical Activity:** You are sporadically involved in recreational activities such as weekend golf or tennis, occasional jogging, swimming, or cycling.
   - d. ______ **Moderate Physical Activity:** Usual job activities might include lifting or stair climbing, or you participate regularly in recreational/fitness activities such as jogging, swimming, or cycling at least three times per week for 30 to 60 minutes each time.
   - e. ______ **Very Vigorous Physical Activity:** You participate in *extensive* physical activity for 60 minutes or more at least four days per week.

Group 1. a. ____ Walking, Jogging, Running; b. ____Swimming; c. ____ Cycling.

Group 2. d. ____ Racquetball; e. ____ Circuit Weight Training; f. ____ Squash; g. ____ Badminton; h. ____ Basketball; i. ____ Downhill Skiing; j. ____ Tennis; k. ____ Golf; l. ____ Aerobic Dancing.

FOOD PREFERENCE LIST

Select the foods you want as part of your daily diet from the Food Groups below. Mark an X in the box next to the food items you wish within each Group. You *must* select at least *one* item from Groups 1 through 18. To ensure menu variety, be sure to select all the foods you would like to eat. If you omit a choice from one of the required groups, the computer will make a selection for you. *Please note:* The computer *cannot* make vegetarian menus. You may select none, or as many choices as you wish from Groups 19, 20, and 21—these are optional.

Group 1	**A** ☐ milk, skim	**B** ☐ milk, non-fat	**C** ☐ milk, 2%	
Group 2	**A** ☐ yogurt, skim milk **B** ☐ yogurt, 2% milk	**C** ☐ yogurt, regular milk **D** ☐ yogurt, fruit	**E** ☐ whole milk **F** ☐ choc. milk, non-fat	**G** ☐ buttermilk **H** ☐ ice milk
Group 3	**A** ☐ egg **B** ☐ mozzarella cheese	**C** ☐ ricotta cheese **D** ☐ farmer's cheese	**E** ☐ cheddar cheese **F** ☐ American cheese	**G** ☐ Swiss cheese **H** ☐ Canadian bacon
Group 4	**A** ☐ chicken **B** ☐ turkey **C** ☐ hot dog	**D** ☐ corned beef **E** ☐ salmon, canned **F** ☐ tuna	**G** ☐ crab, canned **H** ☐ oysters	**I** ☐ cottage cheese **J** ☐ peanut butter
Group 5	**A** ☐ chuck steak **B** ☐ flank steak **C** ☐ tenderloin	**D** ☐ round steak **E** ☐ rump steak **F** ☐ sirloin	**G** ☐ lamb leg **H** ☐ lamb chops	**I** ☐ lamb roast **J** ☐ lamb shoulder
Group 6	**A** ☐ Cornish hen **B** ☐ fish, fresh and frzn. **C** ☐ shrimp **D** ☐ scallops	**E** ☐ ground beef **F** ☐ ground round **G** ☐ pork leg **H** ☐ pork/ham	**I** ☐ pork chops **J** ☐ pork roast **K** ☐ pork shoulder **L** ☐ veal shoulder	**M** ☐ veal cutlets **N** ☐ veal chops **O** ☐ veal roast
Group 7	**A** ☐ avocado **B** ☐ olives	**C** ☐ almonds **D** ☐ pecans	**E** ☐ peanuts, dry roast **F** ☐ walnuts	**G** ☐ cream cheese **H** ☐ bacon, crisp
Group 8	**A** ☐ diet margarine			
Group 9	**A** ☐ cream, light **B** ☐ French dressing	**C** ☐ 1000 island dressing **D** ☐ Italian dressing	**E** ☐ mayonnaise **F** ☐ sour cream	**G** ☐ blue cheese dressing **H** ☐ Tartar sauce
Group 10	**A** ☐ raisin bread **B** ☐ bagel **C** ☐ English muffin	**D** ☐ toast **E** ☐ bran flakes **F** ☐ cereal, dry	**G** ☐ puffed cereal **H** ☐ cooked cereal	**I** ☐ cooked grits **J** ☐ donut, plain
Group 11	**A** ☐ bread, any kind **B** ☐ cooked barley	**C** ☐ arrowroot crackers **D** ☐ graham crackers	**E** ☐ matzo **F** ☐ soda crackers	**G** ☐ plain muffin **H** ☐ cooked rice
Group 12	**A** ☐ cooked spaghetti **B** ☐ cooked noodles **C** ☐ cooked macaroni **D** ☐ beans, cooked **E** ☐ lentils, cooked	**F** ☐ corn, off cob **G** ☐ corn, on cob **H** ☐ lima beans **I** ☐ parsnips	**J** ☐ peas **K** ☐ baked potato **L** ☐ mashed potato **M** ☐ squash	**N** ☐ biscuit **O** ☐ corn bread **P** ☐ corn muffins **Q** ☐ yam
Group 13	**A** ☐ apple juice **B** ☐ banana **C** ☐ grapefruit juice	**D** ☐ grapefruit **E** ☐ grape juice **F** ☐ orange juice	**G** ☐ pineapple juice **H** ☐ prunes **I** ☐ prune juice	**J** ☐ apricot juice **K** ☐ papaya
Group 14	**A** ☐ apple **B** ☐ apricot **C** ☐ apricot, dried **D** ☐ blackberries	**E** ☐ blueberries **F** ☐ raspberries **G** ☐ strawberries **H** ☐ cider, any kind	**I** ☐ dates **J** ☐ mango **K** ☐ orange **L** ☐ peach	**M** ☐ pear **N** ☐ plum **O** ☐ raisins
Group 15	**A** ☐ apple sauce **B** ☐ cherries **C** ☐ grapes	**D** ☐ cantaloupe **E** ☐ honeydew	**F** ☐ watermelon **G** ☐ nectarine	**H** ☐ pineapple **I** ☐ tangerine
Group 16	**A** ☐ cucumber **B** ☐ vegetable juice	**C** ☐ tomato **D** ☐ tomato juice	**E** ☐ carrots **F** ☐ green pepper	**G** ☐ celery **H** ☐ cauliflower
Group 17	**A** ☐ asparagus **B** ☐ bean sprouts	**C** ☐ beets **D** ☐ broccoli	**E** ☐ brussels sprouts **F** ☐ cabbage	**G** ☐ eggplant
Group 18	**A** ☐ collards **B** ☐ kale **C** ☐ mustard greens **D** ☐ spinach	**E** ☐ turnip greens **F** ☐ mushrooms **G** ☐ okra	**H** ☐ string beans **I** ☐ artichokes **J** ☐ rutabaga	**K** ☐ sauerkraut **L** ☐ turnips **M** ☐ zucchini
		Optional Choices		
Group 19	**A** ☐ lettuce **B** ☐ radishes	**C** ☐ chicory **D** ☐ endive	**E** ☐ escarole **F** ☐ parsley	**G** ☐ watercress
Group 20	**A** ☐ ale **B** ☐ beer	**C** ☐ liquor **D** ☐ port	**E** ☐ sherry **F** ☐ wine, red/white	**G** ☐ cognac
Group 21	**A** ☐ cake, angel food **B** ☐ cake, fruit **C** ☐ cake, pound	**D** ☐ cupcake, with icing **E** ☐ candy bar, choc **F** ☐ chocolate fudge	**G** ☐ marshmallows, reg **H** ☐ choc chip cookies **I** ☐ oatmeal cookies	**J** ☐ sugar cookies **K** ☐ pudding **L** ☐ popcorn, popped

E

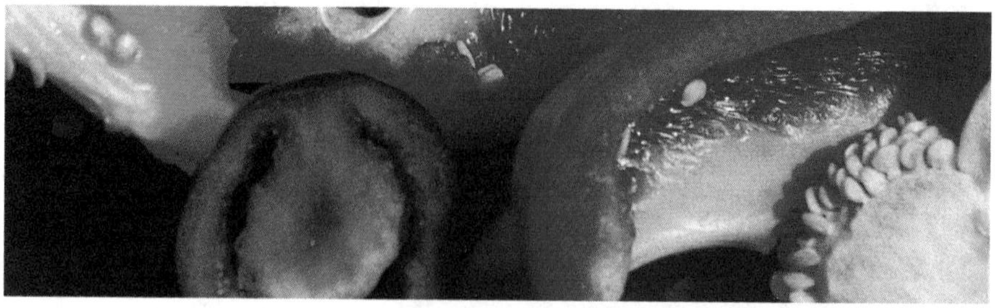

JOURNALS AND NEWSLETTERS RELATED TO NUTRITION, EXERCISE, AND HEALTH

Nutrition, exercise, and health encompasses numerous but interrelated scientific areas of inquiry. The following scientific journals (with their common abbreviations) and specialized newsletters (with subscription information) have been useful in our own library searches on a variety of topic areas. For convenience, the scientific journals are grouped into the broad categories of nutrition, exercise, and health.

JOURNALS

JOURNAL	ABBREVIATION
Nutrition	
American Journal of Clinical Nutrition	Am J Clin Nutr
Annual Reviews of Nutrition	Annu Rev Nutr
Appetite	Appetite
British Journal of Nutrition	Br J Nutr
Ecology of Food and Nutrition	Ecol Food Nutr
FDA Consumer	FDA Consumer
Food Engineering	Food Engin
Human Nutrition: Applied Nutrition	Hum Nutr: Appl Nutr
Human Nutrition: Clinical Nutrition	Hum Nutr: Clin Nutr
International Journal of Obesity	Int J Obes
International Journal of Vitamin Research	Int J Vitamin Res
Journal of Food Science	J Food Sci
Journal of Food Technology	J Food Technol
Journal of Human Nutrition and Dietetics	J Hum Nutr Diet
Journal of Lipid Research	J Lipid Res
Journal of Nutrition Education	J Nutr Educ
Journal of Nutrition for the Elderly	J Nutr Elderly
Journal of Parenteral and Enteral Nutrition	JPEN
Nutrition (cont.)	
Journal of the American Dietetic Association	J Am Diet Assoc
Journal of the Canadian Dietetic Association	J Can Diet Assoc
Nutrition Abstracts and Reviews	Nutr Abstr Rev
Nutrition and Metabolism	Nutr Metab
Nutrition Reviews	Nutr Rev
Nutrition Today	Nutr Today
Proceedings of the Nutrition Society	Proc Nutr Soc
The Journal of Nutrition	J Nutr
Exercise	
American Journal of Sports Medicine	Am J Sports Med
British Journal of Sports Medicine	Br J Sports Med
Canadian Journal of Applied Sports Sciences	Can J Appl Sport Sci
Human Movement Science	Hum Move Sci
International Journal of Sports Medicine	Int J Sports Med
Journal of Applied Sport Science Research	J Appl Sport Sci Res

JOURNAL	ABBREVIATION	JOURNAL	ABBREVIATION
Exercise and Health (cont.)		**Health (cont.)**	
Journal of Human Movement Studies	J Hum Move Studies	Atherosclerosis	Atherosclerosis
Journal of Sports Medicine	J Sports Med	Aviation and Environmental Medicine	Aviat Environ Med
Journal of Sports Medicine and Physical Fitness	J Sports Med Phys Fitness	Clinical Science	Clin Sci
Journal of Sports Psychology	J Sport Psychol	Diabetes	Diabetes
Medicine and Science in Sports and Exercise	Med Sci Sports Exerc	Endocrinology	Endocrinology
Pediatric Exercise Science	Ped Exerc Sci	Ergonomics	Ergonomics
Physician and Sports Medicine	Phys Sportsmed	European Journal of Applied Physiology	Eur J Appl Physiol
Research Quarterly for Exercise and Sports	Res Q Exerc Sport	Federal Proceedings	Fed Proc
Scandinavian Journal of Sports Science	Scand J Sprot Sci	Geriatrics	Geriatrics
Sports Medicine	Sports Med	Growth	Growth
		Human Biology (now American Journal of Human Biology)	Hum Biol (Am J Hum Biol)
Health		Journal of Applied Physiology	J Appl Physiol
Acta Physiologica Scandinavica	Acta Physiol Scand	Journal of Clinical Investigation	J Clin Invest
American Heart Journal	Am Heart J	Journal of Gerontology	J Gerontol
American Journal of Epidemiology	Am J Epidemiol	Journal of Pediatrics	J Pediatr
American Journal of Human Biology (formerly Human Biology)	Am J Hum Biol (Hum Biol)	Journal of Physical and Medical Rehabilitation	J Phys Med Rehabil
American Journal of Nursing	Am J Nurs	Journal of Physiology	J Physiol
American Journal of Physical Anthropology	Am J Phys Anthropol	Journal of the American Medical Association	JAMA
American Journal of Physiology	Am J Physiol	Lancet [British]	Lancet
American Journal of Public Health	Am J Publ Health	Nature [British]	Nature
American Scientist	Am Sci	New England Journal of Medicine	N Engl J Med
Annals of Human Biology	Ann Hum Biol	Pediatrics	Pediatrics
Annals of the New York Academy of Sciences	Ann NY Acad Sci	Physical Therapy Reviews	Phys Ther Rev
Annual Reviews of Medicine	Ann Rev Med	Physiological Reviews	Physiol Rev
Archives of Environmental Health	Arch Environ Health	Postgraduate Medicine	Postgrad Med
		Preventive Medicine	Prev Med
		Psychosomatic Medicine	Psychosom Med
		Public Health Reports	Publ Health Rep
		Science	Science
		Science News	Sci News
		Scientific American	Sci Am

NEWSLETTERS

There are numerous newsletters that cover topic areas related to nutrition, exercise, and health. In our experience, reliable information about the interrelated aspects of nutrition, exercise, and health can be obtained from the following sampling of newsletters.

Contemporary Nutrition
Contemporary Nutrition
General Mills, Inc
PO Box 1112, Dept 65
Minneapolis, MN 55440

Diary Council Digest
National Dairy Council
6300 North River Road
Rosemont, IL 60018-4233

Food and Nutrition News
National Livestock and Meat Board
444 North Michigan Avenue
Chicago, IL 60611

Harvard Medical School Health Letter
Harvard Medical School Health Letter
Department of Continuing Education
25 Shattuck Street
Boston, MA 02115

Dietetic Currents
Director of Professional Services
Ross Laboratories
625 Cleveland Avenue
Columbus, OH 43216

FDA Consumer
Superintendent of Documents
Government Printing Office
Washington, DC 20402

International Obesity Newsletter
Subscription Department
Healthy Living Institute
Route 1, Box 6A
Hettinger, ND 58639

National Council Against Health Fraud
National Council Against Health Fraud
PO Box 1276
Loma Linda, CA 92354

Sports Science Exchange
Gatorade Sports Science Institute
PO Box 049005
Chicago, IL 60604

Tufts University Diet and Nutrition Letter
Tufts University Diet and Nutrition Letter
PO Box 10948
Des Moines, IA 50940

University of California at Berkeley Wellness Letter
Wellness Letter Subscription Department
PO Box 420148
Palm Coast, FL 32142

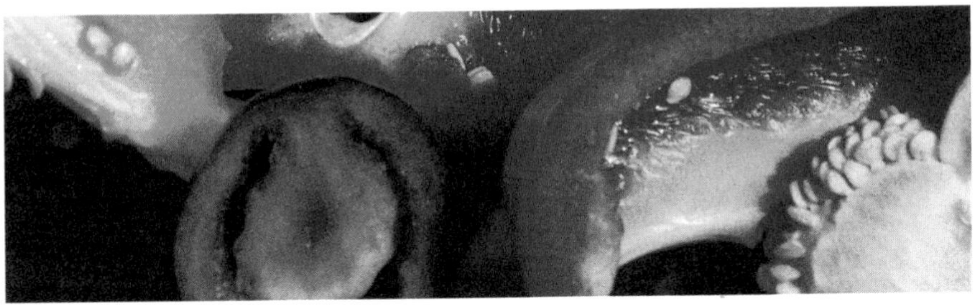

F

RELIABLE SOURCES OF INFORMATION ABOUT NUTRITION, EXERCISE, AND HEALTH

We are grateful to the following organizations for responding to a request for information about their consumer efforts in relation to nutrition, exercise, and health.

American Dietetic Association
216 West Jackson Boulevard, Suite 800
Chicago, IL 60606-6995
(312) 899-0040

The American Dietetic Association is a professional organization whose main goal is to promote optimal health and nutritional status of the population by providing leadership for quality dietetic practice, education, and research. *The Journal of the American Dietetic Association* contains research articles in the fields of nutrition and dietetics. A variety of resource materials are available at a nominal cost (with discounts for professional members). These include clinical publications (e.g., *Sports Nutrition; Diet, Exercise, and Coronary Heart Disease*), publications that deal with management (e.g., *Quantity Food Preparation: Standardizing Recipes and Controlling Ingredients*), and publications for private practice (e.g., *Becoming an Entrepreneur in Your Own Setting*), community practice (e.g., *Nutrition at the Worksite*), and basic client nutrition information (e.g., *Exchange Lists for Meal Planning, Healthy Food Choices, Lowfat Living: A Guide to Enjoying a Healthy Diet, Recommendations of Food Choices for Women, Feeding Your Baby: The First Year, The New Cholesterol Countdown*). The National Center for Nutrition and Dietetics, a public education initiative of the American Dietetic Association, sponsors National Nutrition Month and the Eat Right America program.

American Council on Science and Health
1995 Broadway, 16th Floor
New York, NY 10023-5860
(212) 362-7044
(212) 362-4919 (fax)

The American Council on Science and Health (ACSH) is a public education group directed and advised mostly by scientists and physicians. The goal of ACSH is to provide consumers with up-to-date, scientifically sound information on the relationship between chemicals, foods, nutrition, lifestyle, and the environment and human health. The ACSH produces a wide range of publications on topics such as baby foods, microwave ovens, food allergies, hypertension, premenstrual syndrome, sugars and health, and diet and coronary heart disease. The ACSH also publishes peer-reviewed reports in health and environmental issues and *Priorities,* a quarterly magazine. Examples of recent articles are: Dietary Supplement Frauds Deserve Greater FDA Priority, The Lowdown on Food Labeling, Overseas Tobacco Sales, The Biochemistry of Migraine Headaches, Electromagnetic Fields, and Smokers' Rights: The Tobacco Companies' Latest Gasp for Survival.

Anorexia Nervosa and Related Eating Disorders, Inc
PO Box 5102
Eugene, OR 97405

Anorexia Nervosa and Related Eating Disorders (ANRED) has provided information and services since 1979. The services include a monthly newsletter (The ANRED Alert); an information telephone line (503) 344-1144; referral information about how to find physicians, psychotherapists, and counselors in different areas of the United States; and support groups and workshops.

American Anorexia and Bulimia Association, Inc
418 East 76th Street
New York, NY 10021

The American Anorexia and Bulimia Association (AABA) is a nonprofit organization for the prevention, treatment, and cure of eating disorders. Its mission is to help sufferers, families, and friends through support groups in several states (Florida, New Jersey, New York, Pennsylvania, and Virginia), a referral network, recovery panels, public information, education programs and materials (quarterly newsletter that reviews books, videos, articles by specialists, and research developments), and professional training. The AABA offers the following reading materials: *Anorexia & Bulimia: The Potential Devastation of Dieting, Nutrition and Eating Disorders: Guidelines for the Patient with Anorexia Nervosa and Bulimia Nervosa,* and *When Will We Laugh Again? Living and Dealing with Anorexia Nervosa and Bulimia.*

American College of Sports Medicine
PO Box 1440
Indianapolis, IN 46206-1440
(317) 637-9200
(317) 634-7817 (fax)

The American College of Sports Medicine (ACSM) is a multidisciplinary professional and scientific society dedicated to the generation and dissemination of knowledge concerning the motivation, responses, adaptation, and health aspects of persons engaged in sports and exercise. Specifically, the ACSM is concerned with the following areas of inquiry:

- Basic physiologic, biomechanical, biomedical, structural, and behavioral mechanisms
- Improvement and maintenance of functional capacities for daily living
- Prevention and rehabilitation of chronic and degenerative diseases
- Evaluation and conditioning of athletes
- Prevention and treatment of injuries related to sport and exercise

Since its founding in 1954 by 11 physicians, physiologists, and educators, the ACSM currently represents over 50 different professions and has a worldwide membership of nearly 13,000. There are 3,000 undergraduate and graduate student members and 900 foreign members from 57 countries. Approximately 7% of the membership are Fellows of the College, recognized for their professional achievement and competence via published works, professional practice, and a demonstrated commitment to sports medicine.

Within the ACSM, there are 12 regional chapters that act as authorized components of the College. The regional chapters conduct or assist with various public and professional programs, provide a member forum, and publish various educational and news materials for both public and professional use. Membership in the ACSM includes the following:

- Professional and student members receive the College's scientific journal, *Medicine and Science in Sports and Exercise*
- Those members also receive the annual hardcover series *Exercise and Sport Sciences Reviews*
- All members receive the quarterly newsmagazine *Sports Medicine Bulletin*
- All members receive the annual *Membership Directory*
- Members have access to a comprehensive selection of other ACSM publications, including *Guidelines for Exercise Testing and Prescription*, *Resource Manual for Guidelines for Exercise Testing and Prescription*, and official ACSM position papers
- Members receive a discount on subscriptions to *Career Services Bulletin*
- Registration discounts are available for ACSM's conferences, including the Annual Meeting and the Team Physician Course
- Discounts are available for ACSM's Certification Programs, which include Health/Fitness Instructor, Health/Fitness Director, Exercise Leader, Exercise Specialist, Exercise Test Technologist, and Preventive and Rehabilitative Program Director
- The American College of Sports Medicine endorses Continuing Education programs including regional workshops, conferences, seminars, and lecture tours. Continuing Medical Education credits (CMEs) and Continuing Education Credits (CECs) are offered

American Heart Association
Inquiries Coordinator
7272 Greenville Avenue
Dallas, TX 75231-4596
(214) 373-6300
(214) 706-1341 (fax)

The mission of the American Heart Association (AHA), established in 1924, is to reduce disability and death from cardiovascular diseases and stroke. The AHA has about 3.5 million volunteers who are involved either nationally or with the association's nearly 2000 state and metropolitan affiliates, divisions, and branches. The AHA has three priority enterprises: (1) cardiovascular research (in addition to funding basic and applied research, the AHA develops and disseminates current scientific information through statements, publications, and conferences), (2) cardiovascular education and community programs, and (3) revenue generation.

Examples of consumer education booklets include *Facts About Stroke, Cigarette Smoking and Cardiovascular Disease, How to Make Your Heart Last a Lifetime, About High Blood Pressure, "E" is for Exercise,* and *The American Heart Association Diet: An Eating Plan for Healthy Americans.* The AHA also publishes *Research Facts, Research Facts Update,* and *Heart and Stroke Facts.* These excellent publications provide a wealth of factual information. For example, in the publication *1992 Heart and Stroke Facts,* topics include major types of heart and blood vessel disorders, how many Americans are affected, how victims are diagnosed and treated, and what can be done to reduce risk.

The consumer education booklets and research publications provide up-to-date information. The materials can be easily incorporated as handouts in most educational programs that deal with nutrition, exercise, and health. The national office provides samples of publications. Contact the state affiliate of the AHA for requests that require prepayment, quantities of materials, price quotations, catalog listings, or other special handling.

Consumer Information Center
U.S. General Services Administration
18th and F Streets NW
Washington, DC 20405
(202) 501-1794
(202) 501-4281 (fax)

The Consumer Information Center (CIC) was established in 1970 to help Federal agencies and departments develop, promote, and distribute consumer information to the public. The most useful information for an individual is the *Consumer Information Catalog,* published four times yearly. Each issue has descriptive listings of more than 200 free or low-cost booklets available from a variety of Federal agencies. The *Consumer Information Catalog* is free; to order, write to Catalog, Pueblo, CO 81009, or call (719) 948-4000. Other responsibilities of the CIC are to assist agencies in planning, revising, and evaluating their publications; to help produce consumer information booklets in cooperation with government and private agencies; to cooperate in media advertising efforts; and to maintain a media hotline (202) 501-1794 that assists reporters in researching consumer storires.

Egg Nutrition Center
2301 M Street, NW, Suite 410
Washington, DC 20037
(202) 833-8850

The Egg Nutrition Center provides useful nutrition education materials for the health and media communities about eggs and the importance of a healthful diet and exericse. The handouts are free upon request; these include camera-ready copy and one-page fold-out pamphlets (*The Egg Lov-*

er's Heart Healthy Cookbook, The Egg Lover's Heart Healthy Recipes, The Diet Balancing Act, Eggs: Choices and Changes for Heart Healthy Diets, Questions and Answers about Cholesterol and Heart Disease, and *Nutrient Density and the Egg*).

Food and Nutrition Information Center
National Agriculture Library
Room 304
10301 Baltimore Blvd
Beltsville, MD 20705
(301) 504-5719
(301) 504-5472 (fax)

The Food and Nutrition Information Center serves persons seeking information or educational materials in the area of food and human nutrition. Its many outstanding services include:

- Provides answers to specific food and nutrition questions
- Lends books and audiovisuals
- Provides computerized literature searches; these include brief reading lists designed to help locate information or resources on a given topic. The lists include the Quick Bibliography Series and the Special Reference Briefs Series, both making use of the National Agriculture Library database (AGRICOLA) and other databases. The list can be tailored for the consumer, educator, or health professional. An example would be: *Childhood Obesity and Cardiovascular Disease,* January 1985 to May 1990, 212 citations (update available winter 1992).
- Maintains a food- and nutrition-related microcomputer software collection for on-site use
- Prepares publications that list reference materials on various food and nutrition topics
- Publishes an annotated bibliography of educational materials
  Publishes adult patient educational materials. Examples in the Nutri-Topics/Pathfinders series include Sports Nutrition, Vegetarian Nutrition, Nutrition and the Elderly, Anorexia Nervosa and Bulimia, and Sensible Nutrition. Single copies are free.

Food Service Inspection Service
U.S. Department of Agriculture
14th Street & Independence Avenue, SW
Room 1165, South Building
Washington, DC 20250
Meat and Poultry Hotline (800) 535-4555

The Food Service Inspection Service (FSIS) of the U.S. Department of Agriculture is responsible for ensuring that meat and poultry products are safe, wholesome, and accurately labeled. The FSIS performs mandatory inspection in meat and poultry slaughtering and processing plants. It also issues publications and other informational materials for consumers about its programs and the safe handling of meat and poultry.

Examples of free publications include *Preventing Foodborne Illness, A Quick Consumer Guide to Safe Food Handling, Talking About Turkey, Food News for Consumers,* and *Meat and Poultry Products: A Guide to Content and Labeling Requirements.* The FSIS publishes *Food News,* a quarterly magazine that reports how FSIS acts to protect public safety, covering research findings and regulatory efforts important in understanding how the agency works and how consumers can protect themselves against foodborne illness. Fact sheets are available on salmonella and food safety, inspection of meat and poultry imports, and bacteria that cause foodborne illness. A teaching kit for use by high school science and health educators, "The Danger Zone," includes a videotape, teaching materials, and a poster.

The Meat and Poultry Hotline (800-535-4555) should be called with questions about proper handling of meat and poultry, how to tell if they are safe to eat, how to better understand meat and poultry labels, how to report problems with meat and poultry products in your home or market, how to cope when the refrigerator or freezer fails, safe cooking and storage times and temperatures, and how to care for special foods such as ham, marinades, mayonnaise, canned goods, hamburger, turkey, chicken and duck with stuffing, hot dogs and luncheon meats, and eggs and egg-rich foods.

Contact the following agencies to obtain further information about foods issues:

- U.S. Food and Drug Administration: safety, labeling, and ingredients of food products *not* containing meat or poultry
- U.S. Environmental Protection Agency: pesticides
- U.S. Federal Trade Commission: suspected false advertising
- Cooperative Extension Service (listed in local telephone books under county government or state university): questions about food handling, nutrition, and storage
- City, county, or state health agencies: sanitation of restaurants and food stores

Gerber Products Company
Consumer Relations
445 State Street
Fremont, MI 49413
(616) 924-2000
(800) 443-7237

Consumers can obtain answers to questions on feeding and caring for babies by calling the toll-free number at any time throughout the year. Gerber's provides a deatiled 53-page booklet on their baby and toddler food products that gives the average nutrient values per 100 grams and the average nutrient values as a percent of U.S. Recommended Daily Allowances for infants.

Grand Metropolitan
Consumer Relations
PO Box 550
Minneapolis, MN 55440-9843
(800) 767-4466

The Pillsbury Company provides a toll-free number on all product packages. The 800 number is staffed with representatives who provide product information, including nutrition compilations and printed material, on calories, fiber, complex carbohydrates, sodium, fat, and cholesterol. To obtain detailed information, write or call the Consumer Relations Department.

Heinz USA
Consumer Relations
PO Box 57
Pittsburgh, PA 15230

For information about Heinz baby foods, consumers can call (800) 872-2229. Write to Heinz to receive the pamphlet *Guide to Good Nutrition* and additional product information. Nutrition information about Weight Watchers products can be obtained by writing to Weight Watchers Food Company, Consumer Affairs, PO Box 41, Boise, ID 83707.

National Dairy Council
Dairy Center
6300 North River Road
Rosemont, IL 60018-4233
(800) 426-8271
(708) 696-1033 (fax)

The National Dairy Council is a division of the United Dairy Industry Association. The National Dairy Council and its affiliated Diary Council units provide a wide variety of nutrition education materials for the professional market, educators, and consumers. An excellent catalog is available concerning a wide variety of nutrition education materials (e.g., school curriculum packages for grades 1 through high school, colorful brochures and posters, videotapes, and the LifeSteps Weight Management Program). Of particular interest is *Food Power: A Coach's Guide to Improving Performance.* This well-researched information packet has 7 chapters and 12 handouts on topics related to nutrition and specific sports such as baseball/softball, basketball, bicycling, bowling, boxing, figure skating, field hockey, football, golf, ice hockey, jogging and running, rowing/crew, soccer, skiing, racquet sports, swimming, tennis, track and field, volleyball, weight lifting, and wrestling.

National Heart, Lung, and Blood Institute
Information Center
PO Box 30105
Bethesda, MD 20824-0105
(301) 951-3260

The Information Center is a service of the National Heart, Lung, and Blood Institute (NHLBI). It is a resource that can help the public and health profession find the most current and accurate information about cardiopulmonary and related disease. Its services include dissemination of public education materials and scientific information for the health professions. The Information Center database contains programmatic information on high blood pressure, cholesterol, smoking, asthma, blood resources, obesity, and heart attack. The Information Center is part of the Combined Health Information Database (CHID), which is available through BRS Information Technologies. Serial publications include "Infomemo," which provides program updates about cholesterol, high blood pressure, asthma, smoking, and heart attack, as well as "InfoLine," which describes the activities of the national Blood Resources Education Program.

National Council Against Health Fraud, Inc
PO Box 1276
Loma Linda, CA 92354-9983
(714) 824-4690

The National Council Against Health Fraud (NCAF) is a nonprofit organization comprising health professionals, educators, researchers, attorneys, and concerned citizens who wish to actively oppose misinformation, fraud, and quackery in the health marketplace. The purposes of the Council are as follows:

- Conduct studies and investigations to evaluate claims made for health products and services
- Educate consumers, professionals, business people, legislators, law enforcement personnel, organizations, and agencies about health fraud, misinformation, and quackery
- Provide a center for communication between individuals and organizations concerned about health misinformation, fraud, and quackery
- Support sound consumer health laws and oppose legislation that undermines consumer rights
- Encourage and aid in legal actions against those who violate consumer health protection law

Members receive a newsletter as well as discounts on publications, buttons, and T-shirts, and they have ready access to experts on health fraud and quackery.

An extensive list is available of resource materials in the area of nutrition and health, including the "NCAF Newsletter," a hard-hitting, pull-no-punches resource that deals with various aspects of fraud and quackery in the health industry.

National Potato Board
1385 South Carolina Boulevard, Suite 512
Denver, CO 80222
(303) 758-7783
(303) 756-9256 (fax)

The National Potato Board provides consumer information about various facets of the potato industry including nutrition information about the potato, suggestions for recipes, storage and handling, and classroom educational materials.

Nestlé Information Service
2020 Pennsylvania Avenue, NW, Suite 167
Washington, DC 20006

Nestlé Information Service publishes "Worldview," a newsletter that covers a variety of topics related to nutrition and health. For example, these topics were covered in a recent issue: AIDS and Nutrition: Fighting the Wasting Disease, Vitamins: Building Blocks of Better Health, When Nutrition Loses Its Appeal: Nutrition and the Elderly, Food Safety, The Chilled Food Challenge, Antioxidants, Mother Knew Best. A poster-size chart, Vitamin Facts, is available upon request from the above address.

NutraSweet Company
Supervisor, Consumer Affairs
Box 830
1751 Lake Cook Road
Deerfield, IL 60015-5239
(800) 323-5316

The mission of the NutraSweet Consumer Affairs department is to promote trust, consumer intent to purchase, and brand loyalty by disseminating information about the safety, benefits, and use of its products. Information is provided by specially trained staff and registered dietitians on such topics as cooking and baking, product safety, and use by persons with diabetes.

Office on Smoking and Health
National Center for Chronic Disease Prevention and Health Promotion
Mail Stop K-50
Centers for Disease Control
1600 Clifton Road, NE
Atlanta, GA 30333
(404) 488-5705

The Office on Smoking and Health (OSH), an agency of the U.S. Public Health Service, collects and distributes information on the health risks associated with smoking and tobacco products as well as materials on smoking prevention and cessation methods. OSH provides the following services:

- OSH designs and conducts periodic national surveys on smoking behavior in the United States and on the attitudes, knowledge, and beliefs of adults and teenagers regarding the health consequences of smoking.
- The Technical Information Center can assist with comprehensive research on topics of current interest in smoking and health.
- Free publications are available in small quantities to health professionals and the general public. Materials emphasize the relationship between smoking and the development of cardiovascular disease, lung disease, cancer, and complications during pregnancy. Emphasis is also placed on the health benefits of smoking cessation. Annual reports from OSH include the Smoking and Health Bibliography and Health Consequences of Smoking: A Report of the Surgeon General. A listing of materials is available upon request.

Produce Marketing Association
1500 Casho Mill Road
PO Box 6036
Newark, DE 19714-6036
(302) 738-7100
(302) 731-2409 (fax)

The Produce Marketing Association provides a Fresh Facts Education Kit. This informative kit contains pamphlets and brochures about a variety of vegetables (Belgian endive, broccoli, iceberg lettuce, onions, peppers, potatoes, tofu), nuts (pistachios), and fruits (apples, bananas, citrus fruits, dates, figs, grapes, kiwifruit, melons, nectarines, peaches, pears, plums, prunes, strawberries, tomatoes, tropical fruits, and watermelons).

Sunkist Growers, Inc
Consumer Affairs
PO Box 7888
Van Nuys, CA 91409-7888

Sunkist Growers provides a variety of helpful consumer-oriented educational materials about oranges, tangerines, grapefruits, and lemons. Materials include the *Fresh Citrus Handbook,* booklets with recipes, nutrition research papers, posters, and educational materials for students.

United Fresh Fruit and Vegetable Association
727 North Washington Street
Alexandria, VA 22314
(800) 336-7745
(703) 836-7745 (fax)

The United Fresh Fruit and Vegetable Association is the national trade organization that represents all sectors of the fresh fruit and vegetable industry. One of its services, the United Information Center, provides data on all aspects of the fresh produce industry. This includes consumption trends, industry practices, and marketing statistics. The service is available free to members and on a fee basis for nonmembers. Pamphlets, fact sheets, videotapes, posters and charts, and a newsletter are available. Examples of materials include *Fresh Ideas for Schools,* an 80-slide training program with audiocassette and script for school food service operators; *Facts and Pointers on Fruits and Vegetables,* a 1200-page report on over 80 fresh fruits and vegetables; and *Excite Your Senses: Discover Fresh Fruits and Vegetables,* a complete multimedia kit for teaching high school students (included are two 80-frame film strips, activity sheets, teacher's guide, and camera-ready masters on selection and care of fresh fruit and vegetables. Contact the association for a catalog and price list.

University of Alabama at Birmingham
Nutrition Information Service
Webb Building, Room 447
UAB Station
Birmingham, AL 35294
(800) 231-DIET

The Nutrition Information Service (NIS), staffed by UAB faculty, registered dietitians, and a dietetic technician in the Department of Nutrition Sciences, distributes and translates research findings into practical information for the public and professional practitioner. Last year, 25,000 individuals received information from NIS. Examples include a series of fact sheets on various nutrition topics, access to a computer database, providing materials and speakers for continuing education of allied health practitioners and practicing physicians, and a toll-free telephone service to fulfill rquests for educational materials, make referrals, and assist in program planning.

FEDERAL AGENCIES AND COMMITTEES

In addition to various public and private agencies that deal with nutrition, exercise, and health, the three divisions of the Federal government—the House of Representatives, the Senate, and the Executive Branch—also have various committees and agencies that oversee activities dealing with nutrition, exercise, and health. The following table lists some of the congressional committees and the agency in the Executive branch that deal with oversight of the various programs. For more information about a particular program, contact your state Senator or member of the House of Representatives.

GOVERNMENTAL AGENCIES AND LEGISLATIVE COMMITTEES INVOLVED WITH VARIOUS PROGRAMS RELATED TO NUTRITION AND HEALTH

PROGRAM AREA	EXECUTIVE BRANCH	SENATE COMMITTEE	HOUSE COMMITTEE
Health claims	FDA; FTC; DHHS	LHR; Commerce, Science, and Transportation	Energy and Commerce
Labeling of meat and poultry	Marketing and Inspection Service of USDA	Agriculture, Nutrition, and Forestry	Agriculture
General nutrition labeling	FDA; DHHS	LHR	Energy and Commerce
National cholesterol education project	National Heart, Lung, and Blood Institute; DHHS	Appropriations; LHR	Appropriations; Energy and Commerce
Cancer	National Cancer Institute; DHHS	Appropriations; LHR	Appropriations; Energy and Commerce
Dietary guidelines	Human Nutrition Information Service, Office of Disease Prevention and Health Promotion; DHHS	Agriculture, Nutrition, and Forestry; Appropriations; LHR	Appropriations; Agriculture
Nutrition education resources	Food and Nutrition Information Center, National Agriculture Library; USDA	Agriculture, Nutrition, and Forestry; Appropriations	Appropriations; Agriculture

FDA = Food and Drug Administration; FTC = Federal Trade Commission; DHHS = Department of Health and Human Services; LHR = Labor and Human Resources; USDA = US Department of Agriculture. The listings in this table represent a small sample of many excellent programs sponsored by the Federal government.

G

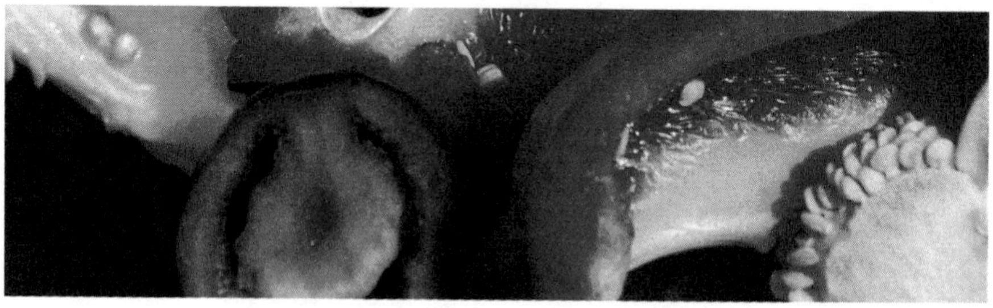

THE METRIC SYSTEM AND CONVERSION CONSTANTS IN NUTRITION, EXERCISE, AND HEALTH

Appendix G has two parts. Part 1 deals with the metric system, and Part 2 discusses le Système International d'Unités (SI units). We have also included common household conversions in Table G-1. These should be helpful in meal preparation, shopping, and planning dietary programs.

PART 1

THE METRIC SYSTEM

Most measurements in science are expressed in terms of the metric system. This system uses units that are related to one another by some power of 10. The prefix "centi" means one hundredth, "milli" means one thousandth, whereas the prefix "kilo" is derived from a word that means one thousand. In the following sections, we show the relationship between metric units and English units of measurement that are relevant to the material presented in this book.

UNITS OF LENGTH

METRIC UNIT	EQUIVALENT METRIC UNIT	EQUIVALENT ENGLISH UNIT
meter (m)	100 cm 1000 mm	39.37 in. (3.28 ft; 1.09 yd)
centimeter (cm)	0.01 m 10 mm	0.3937 in.
millimeter (mm)	0.001 m 0.1 cm	0.03937 in.

Use the following conversions for common units of weight and volume. For example, 1 ounce = 0.06 pound. Two ounces would therefore equal 2 × 0.06 = 0.12 pound, and 16 ounces = 0.96 pound (16 × 0.06).

UNITS OF WEIGHT

METRIC UNIT	EQUIVALENT METRIC UNIT	EQUIVALENT ENGLISH UNIT
kilogram (kg)	1000 g 1,000,000 mg	35.3 oz (2.2046 lb)
gram (g)	0.001 kg 1000 mg	0.0353 oz
milligram (mg)	0.000001 kg 0.001 g	0.0000353 oz

UNITS OF VOLUME

METRIC UNIT	EQUIVALENT METRIC UNIT	EQUIVALENT ENGLISH UNIT
liter (L)	1000 mL	1.057 qt
milliliter (mL) or cubic centimeter (cc)	0.001 L	0.001057 qt

TEMPERATURE

To convert a Fahrenheit temperature to Celsius:
°C = (°F − 32) ÷ 1..8

To convert a Celsius temperature to Fahrenheit:
°F = (1.8 × °C) + 32

With the Fahrenheit scale, the freezing point of water is 32°F and the boiling point 212°F. On the Celsius scale, the freezing point of water is 0°C and the boiling point is 100°C.

UNITS OF SPEED

MPH	$Km \cdot Hr^{-1}$	$M \cdot S^{-1}$	MPH	$Km \cdot Hr^{-1}$	$M \cdot S^{-1}$
1	1.6	0.47	11	17.7	5.17
2	3.2	0.94	12	19.3	5.64
3	4.8	1.41	13	20.9	6.11
4	6.4	1.88	14	22.5	6.58
5	8.0	2.35	15	24.1	7.05
6	9.6	2.82	16	25.8	7.52
7	11.2	3.29	17	27.4	7.99
8	12.8	3.76	18	29.0	8.46
9	14.4	4.23	19	30.6	8.93
10	16.0	4.70	20	32.2	9.40

COMMON EXPRESSIONS OF WORK, ENERGY, AND POWER

WATTS	KILOCALORIES (kcal)	FOOT-POUNDS (ft-lb)
1 watt = 0.73756 ft-lb $\cdot s^{-1}$	1 kcal = 3086 ft-lb	1 ft-lb = 3.2389×10^{-3} kcal
1 watt = 0.01433 kcal $\cdot min^{-1}$	1 kcal = 426.8 kg-m	1 ft-lb = 0.13825 kg-m
1 watt = 1.341×10^{-3} hp or 0.0013 hp	1 kcal = 3087.4 ft-lb	1 ft-lb = 5.050×10^{-3} hp $\cdot h^{-1}$
1 watt = 6.12 kg-m $\cdot min^{-1}$	1 kcal = 1.5593 $\times 10^{-3}$ hp $\cdot h^{-1}$	

COMMON HOUSEHOLD CONVERSIONS

Often, it is convenient to use common household conversions for purposes of meal preparation, shopping, and planning dietary programs that make use of the food exchange plan. Instead of relying on the SI system, the American system often uses measurements such as cups, pints, quarts, glasses, and teaspoons and tablespoons. The following conversions are helpful in converting from the American to metric system. While 1 ounce is equivalent to 28.4 grams, for ease in computation we have let 1 ounce equal 30 grams. In addition, 1 gram (g) = 1 milliliter (ml) = 1 cubic centimeter (cc). Thus, 1 ounce of cottage cheese would be approximately equivalent to 30 g or 30 cc.

TABLE G–1 COMMON HOUSEHOLD CONVERSIONS

AMERICAN MEASURE (WEIGHT)	METRIC EQUIVALENT (APPROXIMATE)
1 teaspoon	5 g
1 tablespoon	15 g
4 ounces	120 g
8 ounces	240 g
½ cup	120 g
1 cup	240 g
1 pint	480 g
1 quart	960 g

The following conversions for level measures and weights are especially helpful during cooking and shopping.

AMERICAN MEASURE (VOLUME)	APPROXIMATE EQUIVALENT
1 teaspoon	5cc; 5g
3 teaspoons	1 tablespoon; 15 g; 15 cc
2 tablespoons	1 fluid ounce; 30 g; 30 cc
4 tablespoons	¼ cup; 60 g; 60 cc
8 tablespoons	½ cup; 120 g; 120 cc
16 tablespoons	1 cup; 240 g; 8 fluid ounces; ½ pound
2 cups	1 pound; 16 fluid ounces; 480 mL; 480 g
4 cups	1 kilogram (2.2 pounds); 960 g; 960 cc
4 quarts	1 gallon

UNITS OF WEIGHT	OUNCE	POUND	GRAM	KILOGRAM
1 ounce	1.0	0.06	28.4	0.028
1 pound	16.0	1.0	454	0.454
1 gram	0.035	0.002	1.0	0.001
1 kilogram	35.3	2.2	1000	1.0

UNITS OF VOLUME	OUNCE	PINT	QUART	MILLILITER	LITER
1 ounce	1.0	0.062	0.031	29.57	0.029
1 pint	16.0	1.0	0.5	437	0.473
1 quart	32.0	2.0	1.0	946	0.946
1 milliliter	0.034	0.002	0.001	1.0	0.001
1 liter	33.8	2.112	1.056	1000	1.0

TABLE G–2. CONVERSION FACTORS FOR USE IN THE NUTRITION, HEALTH, AND EXERCISE SCIENCES

TO CONVERT	INTO	MULTIPLY BY
A		
angstrom units	inches	3.937×10^{-9}
angstrom units	meters	1×10^{-10}
angstrom units	microns	1×10^{-4}
B		
Btu	ergs	1.0550×10^{10}
Btu	foot-lb	778.3
Btu	gram-calories	252.0
Btu	joules	1,054.8
Btu	kilogram-calories	0.2520
Btu	kilogram-meters	107.5
Btu/min	foot-lb/second	12.96
Btu/min	kilowatts	0.01757
Btu/min	watts	17.57
C		
centigrade	Fahrenheit	$(C° \times 9/5) + 32$
centigrams	grams	0.01
centimeters	feet	3.281×10^{-2}
centimeters	inches	0.3937
centimeters	kilometers	1×10^{-5}
centimeters	meters	0.01
centimeters	miles	6.214×10^{-6}
centimeters	millimeters	10.0
centimeters	yards	1.094×10^{-2}
cubic centimeters	cu feet	3.531×10^{-5}
cubic centimeters	cu inches	0.06102
cubic centimeters	cu meters	1×10^{-6}
cubic centimeters	cu yards	1.308×10^{-6}
cubic centimeters	gallons (U.S. liq.)	2.642×10^{-4}
cubic centimeters	liters	0.001
cubic centimeters	pints (U.S. liq.)	2.113×10^{-3}
cubic centimeters	quarts (U.S. liq.)	1.057×10^{-3}
D		
decigrams	grams	0.1
deciliters	liters	0.1
decimeters	meters	0.1
dynes	grams	1.020×10^{-3}
E		
ergs	Btu	9.480×10^{-11}
ergs	dyne-centimeters	1.0
ergs	foot-pounds	7.3670×10^{-8}
ergs	gram-calories	0.2389×10^{-7}
ergs	grams-cm	1.020×10^{-3}
ergs	horsepower hours	3.7250×10^{-14}
ergs	joules	1×10^{-7}
ergs	kg-calories	2.389×10^{-11}
ergs	kg-meters	1.020×10^{-8}
ergs	kilowatt-hours	0.2778×10^{-13}
ergs	watt-hours	0.2778×10^{-10}

TABLE G–2. *continued*

TO CONVERT	INTO	MULTIPLY BY
F		
feet	centimeters	30.48
feet	kilometers	3.048×10^{-4}
feet	meters	0.3048
feet	miles (naut.)	1.645×10^{-4}
feet	miles (stat.)	1.894×10^{-4}
feet	millimeters	304.8
foot-pounds	Btu	1.286×10^{-3}
foot-pounds	ergs	1.356×10^{7}
foot-pounds	gram-calories	0.3238
foot-pounds	joules	1.356
foot-pounds	kg-calories	3.24×10^{-4}
foot-pounds	kg-meters	0.1383
foot-pounds	kilowatt-hours	3.766×10^{-7}
foot-pounds/min	Btu/min	1.286×10^{-3}
foot-pounds/min	foot-pounds/sec	0.01667
foot-pounds/min	horsepower	3.030×10^{-5}
foot-pounds/min	kg-calories/min	3.24×10^{-4}
foot-pounds/min	kilowatts	2.260×10^{-5}
foot-pounds/second	Btu/hour	4.6263
foot-pounds/second	Btu/min	0.07717
foot-pounds/second	horsepower	0.818×10^{-3}
foot-pounds/second	kg-calories/min	1.01945
foot-pounds/second	kilowatts	1.356×10^{-3}
G		
gallons	cu cm	3,785.0
gallons	cu feet	0.1337
gallons	cu inches	231.0
gallons	cu meters	3.785×10^{-3}
gallons	cu yards	4.951×10^{-3}
gallons	liters	3.785
gallons (liq. British imp.)	gallons (U.S. liq.)	1.20095
gallons (U.S.)	gallons (imp.)	0.83267
gallons of water	pounds of water	8.3453
gallons/min	cu ft/sec	2.228×10^{-3}
gallons/min	liters/sec	0.06308
gallons/min	cu ft/hour	8.0208
grams	dynes	980.7
grams	grains	15.43
grams	joules/cm	9.807×10^{-5}
grams	joules/meter (newtons)	9.807×10^{-3}
grams	kilograms	0.001
grams	milligrams	1,000.0
grams	ounces (avoirdupois)	0.03527
grams	ounces (troy)	0.03215
grams	pounds	2.205×10^{-3}
gram-calories	Btu	3.9683×10^{-3}
gram-calories	ergs	4.1868×10^{7}
gram-calories	foot-pounds	3.0880
gram-calories	horsepower-hours	1.5596×10^{-6}
gram-calories	kilowatt-hours	1.1630×10^{-6}
gram-calories	watt-hours	1.1630×10^{-3}
gram-centimeters	Btu	9.297×10^{-8}
gram-centimeters	ergs	980.7
gram-centimeters	joules	9.807×10^{-5}
gram-centimeters	kg-cal	2.343×10^{-8}
gram-centimeters	kg-meters	1×10^{-5}

TABLE G–2. *continued*

TO CONVERT	INTO	MULTIPLY BY
H		
horsepower	Btu/min	42.44
horsepower	foot-lb/min	33,000.0
horsepower	foot-lb/sec	550.0
(542.5 ft lb/second)	(550 ft lb/sec)	
(550 ft lb/second)	(542.5 ft lb/sec)	
horsepower	kg-calories/min	10.68
horsepower	kilowatts	0.7457
horsepower	watts	745.7
I		
inches	centimeters	2.540
inches	meters	2.540×10^{-2}
inches	millimeters	25.40
inches	yards	2.778×10^{-2}
inches of mercury	atmospheres	0.03342
inches of mercury	feet of water	1.133
inches of water (at 4°C)	atmospheres	2.458×10^{-3}
inches of water (at 4°C)	inches of mercury	0.07355
J		
joules	Btu	9.480×10^{-4}
joules	ergs	1×10^{7}
joules	foot-pounds	0.7376
joules	kg-calories	2.389×10^{-4}
joules	kg-meters	0.1020
joules	watt-hours	2.778×10^{-4}
K		
kilograms	dynes	980,665.0
kilograms	grams	1,000.0
kilograms	joules/cm	0.09807
kilograms	joules/meter (newtons)	9.807
kilograms	pounds	2.205
kilogram-calories	Btu	3.968
kilogram-calories	foot-pounds	3,088.0
kilogram-calories	joules	4,186.0
kilogram-calories	kg-meters	426.9
kilogram-calories	kilojoules	4.186
kilogram-calories	kilowatt-hours	1.163×10^{-3}
kilogram-meters	Btu	9.294×10^{-3}
kilogram-meters	ergs	9.804×10^{7}
kilogram-meters	foot-pounds	7.233
kilogram-meters	joules	9.804
kilogram-meters	kg-caloies	2.342×10^{-3}
kilogram-meters	kilowatt-hours	2.723×10^{-6}
kilometers	centimeters	1×10^{5}
kilometers	feet	3,281.0
kilometers	inches	3.937×10^{4}
kilometers	meters	1,000.0
kilometers	miles	0.6214
kilometers	millimeters	1×10^{6}
kilometers	yards	1,094.0
kilowatts	Btu/min	56.92
kilowatts	foot-lb/min	4.426×10^{4}
kilowatts	foot-lb/second	737.6
kilowatts	kg-calories/min	14.34
kilowatts	watts	1,000.0
kilowatt-hr	Btu	3,413.0
kilowatt-hr	ergs	3.600×10^{13}

TABLE G–2. *continued*

TO CONVERT	INTO	MULTIPLY BY
K		
kilowatt-hr	foot-lb	2.655×10^{6}
kilowatt-hr	gram-calories	859,850.0
kilowatt-hr	horsepower-hours	1.341
kilowatt-hr	joules	3.6×10^{6}
kilowatt-hr	kg-calories	860.5
kilowatt-hr	kg-meters	3.671×10^{5}
L		
liters	bushels (U.S. dry)	0.02838
liters	cu cm	1,000.0
liters	cu feet	0.03531
liters	cu inches	61.02
liters	cu meters	0.001
liters	cu yards	1.308×10^{-3}
liters	gallons (U.S. liq.)	0.2642
liters	pints (U.S. liq.)	2.113
liters	quarts (U.S. liq.)	1.057
liters/min	cu ft/second	5.886×10^{-4}
liters/min	gals/second	4.403×10^{-3}
M		
meters	centimeters	100.0
meters	feet	3.281
meters	inches	39.37
meters	kilometers	0.001
meters	miles (nautical)	5.396×10^{-4}
meters	miles (statute)	6.214×10^{-4}
meters	millimeters	1,000.0
meters	yards	1.094
meters/min	cms/second	1.667
miles (statute)	centimeters	1.609×10^{5}
miles (statute)	feet	5,280.0
miles (statute)	inches	6.336×10^{4}
miles (statute)	kilometers	1.609
miles (statute)	meters	1,609.0
miles (statute)	miles (nautical)	0.8684
miles (statute)	yards	1,760.0
miles/hour	cm/second	44.70
miles/hour	feet/min	88.0
miles/hour	feet/second	1.467
miles/hour	km/hour	1.609
miles/hour	km/min	0.02682
miles/hour	knots	0.8684
miles/hour	meters/min	26.82
miles/hour	miles/min	0.1667
millimicrons	meters	1×10^{-9}
milligrams	grains	0.01543236
milligrams	grams	0.001
milliliters	liters	0.001
millimeters	centimeters	0.1
millimeters	feet	3.281×10^{-3}
millimeters	inches	0.03937
millimeters	kilometers	1×10^{-6}
millimeters	meters	0.001
millimeters	miles	6.214×10^{-7}
millimeters	yards	1.094×10^{-3}
N		
newtons	dynes	1×10^{5}

TABLE G–2. *continued*

TO CONVERT	INTO	MULTIPLY BY
O		
ounces	drams	16.0
ounces	grains	437.5
ounces	grams	28.349527
ounces	pounds	0.0625
ounces	ounces (troy)	0.9115
ounces	tons (long)	2.790×10^{-5}
ounces	tons (metric)	2.835×10^{-5}
ounces (fluid)	cu inches	1.805
ounces (fluid)	liters	0.02957
ounces (troy)	grains	480.0
ounces (troy)	grams	31.103481
ounces (troy)	ounces (avoirdupois)	1.09714
ounces (troy)	pennyweights (troy)	20.0
ounces (troy)	pounds (troy)	0.08333
P		
pints (liquid)	cu cm	473.2
pints (liquid)	cu feet	0.01671
pints (liquid)	cu inches	28.87
pints (liquid)	cu meters	4.732×10^{-4}
pints (liquid)	cu yards	6.189×10^{-4}
pints (liquid)	gallons	0.125
pints (liquid)	liters	0.4732
pints (liquid)	quarts (liquid)	0.5
pounds (avoirdupois)	ounces (troy)	14.5833
pounds	drams	256.0
pounds	dynes	44.4823×10^{4}
pounds	grains	7,000.0
pounds	grams	453.5924
pounds	joules/cm	0.04448
pounds	joules/meter (newtons)	4.448
pounds	kilograms	0.4536
pounds	ounces	16.0
pounds	ounces (troy)	14.5833
pounds	pounds (troy)	1.21528
pounds	tons (short)	0.0005
pounds of water	gallons	0.1198
Q		
quarts (dry)	cu inches	67.20
quarts (liquid)	cu cm	946.4
quarts (liquid)	cu feet	0.03342
quarts (liquid)	cu inches	57.75
quarts (liquid)	cu meters	9.464×10^{-4}
quarts (liquid)	cu yards	1.238×10^{-3}
quarts (liquid)	gallons	0.25
quarts (liquid)	liters	0.9463
R		
revolutions	degrees	360.0
revolutions	radians	6.283
revolutions/min	degrees/second	6.0
revolutions/min	radians/second	0.1047
revolutions/min	revolutions/second	0.01667
revolutions/second	degrees/second	360.0
revolutions/second	rev/min	60.0

TABLE G–2. continued

TO CONVERT	INTO	MULTIPLY BY
S		
square centimeters	square feet	1.076×10^{-3}
square centimeters	square inches	0.1550
square centimeters	square meters	0.0001
square centimeters	sq miles	3.861×10^{-11}
square centimeters	sq millimeters	100.0
square centimeters	sq yards	1.196×10^{-4}
square feet	sq cm	929.0
square feet	sq inches	144.0
square feet	sq meters	0.09290
square feet	sq miles	3.587×10^{-8}
square feet	sq millimeters	9.290×10^{4}
square feet	sq yards	0.1111
square inches	sq cm	6.452
square inches	sq feet	6.944×10^{-3}
square inches	sq millimeters	645.2
square meters	sq cm	1×10^{4}
square meters	sq feet	10.76
square meters	sq inches	1,550.0
square meters	sq miles	3.861×10^{-7}
square meters	sq millimeters	1×10^{6}
square meters	sq yards	1.196
T		
temperature (°F) + 460	absolute temperature (°F)	1.0
temperature (°F) − 32	temperature (°C)	5/9
temperature (°F) + 460	absolute temperature (°F)	1.0
temperature (°F) − 32	temperature (°C)	5.9
tons (metric)	kilograms	1,000.0
tons (metric)	pounds	2,205.0
W		
watts	Btu/hour	3.4129
watts	Btu/min	0.05688
watts	ergs/second	107.0
watts	foot-lb/min	44.27
watts	foot-lb/second	0.7378
watts	horsepower	1.341×10^{-3}
watts	horsepower (metric)	1.360×10^{-3}
watts	kg-calories/min	0.01433
watts	kilowatts	0.001
Y		
yards	centimeters	91.44
yards	kilometers	9.144×10^{-4}
yards	meters	0.9144
yards	miles (nautical)	4.934×10^{-4}
yards	miles (statute)	5.682×10^{-4}
yards	millimeters	914.4

TERMINOLOGY AND UNITS OF MEASUREMENT

The American College of Sports Medicine suggests that the following terminology and units of measurement be used in scientific endeavors to promote consistency and clarity of communication, and to avoid ambiguity. The terms defined below utilize the units of measurement of the Système International d'Unités (SI).

Exercise: Any and all activity involving generation of force by the activated muscle(s) which results in disruption of a homeostatic state. In dynamic exercise, the muscle may perform shortening (concentric) contractions or be overcome by external resistance and perform lengthening (eccentric) contractions. When muscle force results in no movement, the contraction should be termed static or isometric.

Exercise intensity: A specific level of maintenance of muscular activity that can be quantified in terms of power (energy expenditure or work performed per unit of time), isometric force sustained, or velocity of progression.

Endurance: The time limit of a person's ability to maintain either a specific isometric force or a specific power level involving combinations of concentric or eccentric muscular contractions.

Mass: A quantity of matter of an object, a direct measure of the object's inertia (note: mass = weight ÷ acceleration due to gravity; units: gram or kilogram).

Weight: The force with which a quantity of matter is attracted toward Earth by normal acceleration of gravity (traditional unit: kilogram of weight).

Energy: The capability of producing force, performing work, or generating heat (unit: joule or kilojoule).

Force: That which changes or tends to change the state of rest or motion in matter (unit: newton).

Speed: Total distance travelled per unit of time (units: meter per second).

Velocity: Displacement per unit of time. A vector quantity requiring that direction be stated or strongly implied (units: meter per second or kilometer per hour).

Work: Force expressed through a distance but with no limitation on time (unit: joule or kilojoule). Quantities of energy and heat expressed independently of time should also be presented in joules. The term "work" should *not* be employed synonymously with muscular exercise.

Power: The rate of performing work; the derivative of work with respect to time; the product of force and velocity (unit: watt). Other related processes such as energy release and heat transfer should, when expressed per unit of time, be quantified and presented in watts.

Torque: The effectiveness of a force to produce rotation about an axis (unit: newton-meter).

Volume: A space occupied, for example, by a quantity of fluid gas (unit: liter or milliliter). Gas volumes should be indicated as ATPS, BTPS, or STPD.

Amount of a substance: The amount of a substance is frequently expressed in moles. A mole is the quantity of a chemical substance that has a weight in mass units (e.g., grams) numerically equal to the molecular weight, or that in the case of a gas has a volume occupied by such a weight under specified conditions. One mole of a respiratory gas is equal to 22.4 liters at STPD.

PART 2

SI UNITS

The uniform system of reporting numerical values is known as le Système International d'Unités, or its abbreviation, SI. The SI was developed through international cooperation to create a universally acceptable system for units of measurement. The SI ensures that units of measurement are uniform in concept and style. The SI system permits quantities in common use to be more easily compared. Many scientific organizations endorse the concept of the SI, and leading journals in nutrition, health, and exercise science now require that laboratory data be presented in SI units. The information in this appendix has been summarized from a detailed description about the SI published in the following article:

Young DS: Implementation of SI units for clinical laboratory data. Style specifications and conversion tables. *Ann Intern Med,* 106:114, 1987

DEFINITIONS OF COMMON SI UNITS

Degree Celsius (°C)	The degree Celsius is equivalent to K − 273.15.
Radian (rad)	The radian is the plane angle between two radii of a circle which subtend on the circumference an arc equal in length to the radius.
Joule (J)	The joule is the work done when the point of application of a force of one newton is displaced through a distance of one meter in the direction of the force. 1 J = 1 Nm.
Kelvin (K)	The kelvin is the fraction 1/273.16 of the thermodynamic temperature of the triple point of water.
Kilogram (kg)	The kilogram is a unit of mass equal to the mass of the international prototype of the kilogram.
Meter (m)	The meter is the length equal to 1,650,763.73 wavelengths in vacuum of the radiation that corresponds to the transition between the levels $2p_{10}$ and $5d_5$ of the krypton 86 atom.
Newton (N)	The newton is that force which, when applied to a mass of one kilogram, gives it an acceleration of one meter per second squared. 1 N = 1 kg · m/s^2.
Pascal (pa)	The pascal is the pressure produced by a force of one newton applied, with uniform distribution, over an area of one square meter. 1 Pa = 1 N/m^2.
Second (s)	The second is the duration of 9,192,631,770 periods of the radiation that corresponds to the transition between the two hyperfine levels of the ground state of the cesium 133 atom.
Watt (W)	The watt is the power that in one second gives rise to the energy of one joule. 1 W = 1 J/s.

TABLE G–3. BASE UNITS OF SI NOMENCLATURE

PHYSICAL QUANTITY	BASE UNIT	SI SYMBOL
Length	meter	m
Mass	kilogram	kg
Time	second	s
Amount of substance	mole	mol
Thermodynamic temperature	kelvin	K
Electric current	ampere	A
Luminous intensity	candela	cd

TABLE G–4. GENERAL SI STYLE GUIDELINES

GUIDELINES	EXAMPLE	INCORRECT STYLE	CORRECT STYLE
Use lowercase for symbols or abbreviations	kilogram	Kg	kg
Exceptions:			
	kelvin	k	K
	ampere	a	A
	liter	l	L
Symbols are not followed by period	meter	m.	m
	mole	mol.	mol
Exception: end of sentence			
Do not pluralize symbols	kilograms	kgs	kg
	meters	ms	m
Names and symbols are not to be combined	force	kilogram · meter · s^{-2}	kg · m · s^{-2}
			kg · m/s^2
When numbers are printed, symbols are preferred		100 meters	100 m
		2 moles	2 mol
Space between number and symbol		50ml	50 mL
The product of units is indicated by a dot above the line		kg × m/s^2	kg · m · s^{-2}
			kg · m/s^2
Use only one solidus (/) per expression		mmol/L/s	mmol/(L · s)
Place zero before decimal		.01	0.01
Decimal numbers are preferable to fractions		¾	0.75
		75%	0.75
Spaces are used to separate long numbers		1,500,000	1 500 000
Exception: optional with four-digit number		1,000	1000 or 1 000

For SI units in nutrition, exercise, and health, the term *body weight* is properly referred to as mass (kg), height should be referred to as stature (m), second is s, minute is min, hour is h, week is wk, month is mo, year is y, day is d, gram is g, liter is L, hertz is Hz, joule is J, kilocalorie is kcal, ohm is Ω, pascal is Pa, revolutions per minute is rpm, volt is V, and watt is W. These abbreviations or symbols are used for the singular or plural form.

Table G-5 lists common values in clinical hematology/clinical chemistry and nutrition. The table lists the present reference intervals, the present unit, the conversion factor, the SI reference intervals, the SI unit symbol, the significant digits, and the suggested minimum increment.

TABLE G–5. SI CONVERSION TABLE FOR COMMON VALUES IN CLINICAL HEMATOLOGY/CLINICAL CHEMISTRY AND NUTRITION

COMPONENT	PRESENT REFERENCE INTERVALS (EXAMPLES)	PRESENT UNIT	CONVERSION FACTOR	SI REFERENCE INTERVALS	SI UNIT SYMBOL	SIGNIFICANT DIGITS	SUGGESTED MINIMUM INCREMENT
Hemoglobin (B)							
Mass concentration							
—female	12.0–15.0	g/dL	10	120–150	g/L	XXX	1 g/L
—male	13.6–17.2	g/dL	10	136–172	g/L	XXX	1 g/L
Substance conc. Hb [Fe]							
—female	12.0–15.0	g/dL	0.6206	7.45–9.30	mmol/L	XX.XX	0.05 mmol/L
—male	13.6–17.2	g/dL	0.6206	8.45–10.65	mmol/L	XX.XX	0.05 mmol/L
Alkaline phosphatase (S)	30–120	U/L	0.01667	0.5–2.0	μkat/L	X.X	0.1 μkat/L
Amino acid nitrogen (P)	4.0–6.0	mg/dL	0.7139	2.9–4.3	mmol/L	X.X	0.1 mmol/L
Amino acid nitrogen (U)	50–200	mg/24 h	0.07139	3.6–14.3	mmol/d	X.X	0.1 mmol/d
Androstenedione (S)							
—male >18 years	0.2–3.0	μg/L	3.492	0.5–10.5	mmol/L	XX.X	0.5 nmol/L
—female >18 years	0.8–3.0	μg/L	3.492	3.0–10.5	nmol/L	XX.X	0.5 nmol/L
Bilirubin, total (S)	0.1–1.0	mg/dL	17.10	2–18	μmol/L	XX	2 μmol/L
Calcium (S)							
—male	8.8–10.3	mg/dL	0.2495	2.20–2.58	mmol/L	X.XX	0.02 mmol/L
—female <50 years	8.8–10.0	mg/dL	0.2495	2.20–2.50	mmol/L	X.XX	0.02 mmol/L
—female >50 years	8.8–10.2	mg/dL	0.2495	2.20–2.56	mmol/L	X.XX	0.02 mmol/L
Calcium (U), normal diet	<250	mg/24 h	0.02495	<6.2	mmol/d	X.X	0.1 mmol/d
Cholesterol (P)							
—<29 years	<200	mg/dL	0.02586	<5.20	mmol/L	X.XX	0.05 mmol/L
—30–39 years	<225	mg/dL	0.02586	<5.85	mmol/L	X.XX	0.05 mmol/L
—40–49 years	<245	mg/dL	0.02586	<6.35	mmol/L	X.XX	0.05 mmol/L
—>50 years	<265	mg/dL	0.02586	<6.85	mmol/L	X.XX	0.05 mmol/L
Ferritin (S)	18–300	ng/mL	1.00	18–300	μg/L	XX0	10 μg/L
Glucose (P)—fasting	70–110	mg/dL	0.05551	3.9–6.1	mmol/L	XX.X	0.1 mmol/L
Hemoglobin (B)							
—male	14.0–18.0	g/dL	10.0	140–180	g/L	XXX	1 g/L
—female	11.5–15.5	g/dL	10.0	115–155	g/L	XXX	1 g/L
Insulin (P,S)	5–20	μU/mL	7.175	35–145	pmol/L	XXX	5 pmol/L
	5–20	mU/L	7.175	35–145	pmol/L	XXX	5 pmol/L
	0.20–0.84	μg/mL	172.2	35–145	pmol/L	XXX	5 pmol/L
Iron (S)							
—male	80–180	μg/dL	0.1791	14–32	μmol/L	XX	1 μmol/L
—female	60–160	μg/dL	0.1791	11–29	μmol/L	XX	1 μmol/L
Lipoproteins (P)							
Low density [LDL]—as cholesterol	50–190	mg/dL	0.02586	1.30–4.90	mmol/L	X.XX	0.05 mmol/L
High density [HDL]—as cholesterol							
Male	30–70	mg/dL	0.02586	0.80–1.80	mmol/L	X.XX	0.05 mmol/L
Female	30–90	mg/dL	0.02586	0.80–2.35	mmol/L	X.XX	0.05 mmol/L
Testosterone (P)							
—female	0.6	ng/mL	3.467	2.0	nmol/L	XX.X	0.5 nmol/L
—male	4.6–8.0	ng/mL	3.467	14.0–28.0	nmol/L	XX.X	0.5 nmol/L
Thyroid tests:							
Thyroid stimulating hormone [TSH] (S)	2–11	μU/mL	1.00	2–11	mU/L	XX	1 mU/L
Thyroxine [T_4] (S)	4.0–11.0	μg/dL	12.87	51–142	nmol/L	XXX	1 nmol/L
Thyroxine binding globulin [TBG] (S)—[as thyroxine]	12.0–28.0	μg/dL	12.87	150–360	nmol/L	XX0	1 nmol/L
Thyroxine, free (S)	0.8–2.8	ng/dL	12.87	10–36	pmol/L	XX	1 pmol/L

TABLE G–5. *continued*

COMPONENT	PRESENT REFERENCE INTERVALS (EXAMPLES)	PRESENT UNIT	CONVERSION FACTOR	SI REFERENCE INTERVALS	SI UNIT SYMBOL	SIGNIFICANT DIGITS	SUGGESTED MINIMUM INCREMENT
Hemoglobin (B) (cont.)							
Thyroid tests: (cont.)							
Triiodothyronine $[T_3]$ (S)	75–220	ng/dL	0.01536	1.2–3.4	nmol/L	X.X	0.1 nmol/L
T_3 uptake (S)	25–35	%	0.01	0.25–0.35	1	0.XX	0.01
Tolbutamide (P)—therapeutic	50–120	mg/L	3.699	180–450	μmol/L	XX0	10 μmol/L
Transferrin (S)	170–370	mg/dL	0.01	1.70–3.70	g/L	X.XX	0.01 g/L
Triglycerides (P) [as triolein]	<160	mg/dL	0.01129	<1.80	mmol/L	X.XX	0.02 mmol/L
Vitamin A [retinol] (P,S)	10–50	μg/dL	0.03491	0.35–1.75	μmol/L	X.XX	0.05 μmol/L
Vitamin B_1 [thiamine hydrochloride] (U)	60–500	μg/24 h	0.002965	0.18–1.48	μmol/d	X.XX	0.01 μmol/d
Vitamin B_2 [riboflavin] (S)	2.6–3.7	μg/dL	26.57	70–100	nmol/L	XXX	5 nmol/L
Vitamin B_6 [pyridoxinel] (B)	20–90	ng/mL	5.982	120–540	nmol/L	XXX	5 nmol/L
Vitamin B_{12} [cyanocobalamin] (P,S)	200–1000	pg/mL	0.7378	150–750	pmol/L	XX0	10 pmol/L
		ng/dL	7.378		pmol/L		
Vitamin C (ascorbic acid)	0.6–2.00	mg/dL	56.78	30–110	μmol/L	X0	10 μmol/L
Vitamin D_3 [cholecalciferol] (P)	24–40	μg/mL	2.599	60–105	nmol/L	XXX	5 nmol/L
25 OH-cholecalciferol	18–36	ng/mL	2.496	45–90	nmol/L	XXX	5 mmol/L
Vitamin E [alpha-tocopherol] (P,S)	0.78–1.25	mg/dL	23.22	18–29	μmol/L	XX	1 μmol/L

B = blood, S = serum, P = plasma, U = urine.

INDEX

Page numbers in *italics* indicate figures; t indicates tables.